CRITICAL CARE *procedures and protocols*

A NURSING PROCESS APPROACH

CAROL BATTEN PERSONS, R.N., M.S.N., Ed.D.

Quality Assurance/Utilization Review Coordinator, Veterans Administration Medical Center, Amarillo, Texas;

Assistant Professor, Graduate Program, School of Nursing, West Texas State University, Canyon, Texas

WITH 16 CONTRIBUTORS

J. B. LIPPINCOTT COMPANY PHILADELPHIA

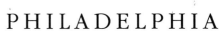

| LONDON | MEXICO CITY | NEW YORK | ST. LOUIS | SAO PĀULO | SYDNEY |

CRITICAL CARE

procedures and protocols

A NURSING PROCESS APPROACH

Sponsoring Editor: Diana Intenzo
Developmental Editor: Eleanor Faven
Manuscript Editor: Margaret E. Maxwell
Indexer: Alberta Morrison
Design Director: Tracy Baldwin
Design Coordinator: Earl Gerhart
Designer: Arlene Putterman
Production Supervisor: J. Corey Gray
Production Coordinator: Kathleen R. Diamond
Compositor: Progressive Typographers
Printer/Binder: The Murray Printing Company
Cover Printer: Philips Offset

6 5 4 3 2

Library of Congress Cataloging-in-Publication Data
Main entry under title:

Critical care procedures and protocols.

Includes index.
1. Intensive care nursing—Handbooks, manuals, etc.
I. Persons, Carol Batten. [DNLM: 1. Critical Care—
methods—nurses' instruction. 2. Nursing Process—
methods. WY 154 C9335]
RT120.I5C77 1987   616'.028   85-23959
ISBN 0-397-54565-7

The authors and publisher have exerted every effort to ensure that drug selection and dosage set forth in this text are in accord with current recommendations and practice at the time of publication. However, in view of ongoing research, changes in government regulations, and the constant flow of information relating to drug therapy and drug reactions, the reader is urged to check the package insert for each drug for any change in indications and dosage and for added warnings and precautions. This is particularly important when the recommended agent is a new or infrequently employed drug.

To my parents, Gordon and Millie Batten, with love

CONTRIBUTORS

NEIL R. ALLEN, R.R.T., B.A.
Clinical Coordinator, Respiratory Therapy Program, Amarillo College, Amarillo, Texas
Chapter 19, Airway Management; Chapter 20, Ventilatory Support; Chapter 22, Sections on Postural Drainage, and Chest Percussion and Vibration

ALICIA WHITE BAILEY, R.N., B.S.N., C.C.R.N.
Formerly Coordinator of Nursing Education, Critical Care, High Plains Baptist Hospital, Amarillo, Texas
Chapter 7, Artificial Pacemakers

THERESA BECKETT, R.N., M.S.N.
Director of Continuing Education Program, School of Nursing, West Texas State University, Canyon, Texas
Chapter 9, Pericardiocentesis; Chapter 13, Gastrointestinal Intubation; Chapter 14, Upper Gastrointestinal Bleeding; Chapter 15, Abdominal Paracentesis; Chapter 22, Section on Thoracentesis

DOROTHY BRITTING, R.N., B.S.N.
Formerly Enterostomal Therapist, Don and Sibyl Harrington Cancer Center, Amarillo, Texas
Chapter 30, Stoma and Draining Wound Techniques; Chapter 32, Positioning/Immobility Techniques

JEANETTE K. CHAMBERS, R.N., M.S., C.S.
Renal Clinical Nurse Specialist, Riverside Methodist Hospital, Columbus, Ohio
Chapter 27, Hemodialysis Techniques

DEBORAH O'GORMAN DAVENPORT, R.N., M.S.N., C.C.R.N.
Instructor, School of Nursing, West Texas State University, Canyon, Texas; C. E. Faculty, School of Nursing, West Texas State University; Staff Nurse, Northwest Texas Hospital, Amarillo, Texas
Chapter 31, Thermal Trauma Techniques; Chapter 35, Organ Harvesting

MARY E. LOUGH, R.N., M.S., C.C.R.N.
Nursing Education Coordinator, Cardiovascular Intensive Care Unit, Stanford University Hospital, Stanford, California
Chapter 12, Heart Transplantation

SUSAN MECKSTROTH, R.N., B.S.N.
Infection Control Coordinator, Formerly Assistant Head Nurse, Education and Training, Dialysis Unit, Riverside Methodist Hospital, Columbus, Ohio
Chapter 27, Hemodialysis Techniques

BARBARA PARKER, R.N., M.S.N., C.C.R.N.
Instructor, Division of Nursing, Amarillo College, Amarillo, Texas
Chapter 28, Peritoneal Dialysis; Chapter 29, Continuous Bladder Irrigation
(Murphy Drip)

ANTONIA VIRGINIA REYES, R.N., M.S.N., C.C.R.N.
Instructor, Critical Care, Veterans Administration Medical Center, Albuquerque,
New Mexico
Chapter 3, Mega Code (Advanced Cardiac Life Support)

DEBORAH WRIGHT SHPRITZ, R.N., M.S., C.C.R.N.
Instructor, Undergraduate Studies, School of Nursing, University of Maryland,
Baltimore, Maryland; Doctoral Candidate, College of Education, University of
Maryland, College Park, Maryland
Chapter 23, Neurologic Assessment; Chapter 24, Fixed Skeletal Traction; Chapter
25, Neurologic Diagnostic Techniques; Chapter 26, Controlling Body Temperature:
Hypothermia and Hyperthermia

MARY E. SLAVIK, R.N., M.S.N.
Associate Chief of Nursing Service/Education, Veterans Administration Medical
Center, Reno, Nevada
Chapter 5, Section on Noninvasive Techniques; Chapter 6, Section on Noninvasive
Techniques

ROXIE TABOR, R.N., B.S.N., C.I.C.
Certified in Infection Control, Infection Control Nurse, Veterans Administration
Medical Center, Amarillo, Texas; Formerly Infection Control Nurse, Veterans
Administration Medical Center, Biloxie, Mississippi
Chapter 4, Sections on Infection Control Protocol for Invasive Vascular Devices
and Infection Control Protocol for Blood/Body Fluid Precautions; Chapter 16,
Infection Control for Gastrointestinal Techniques (Enteric Precautions); Chapter
21, Infection Control for Respiratory Techniques; Chapter 33, Section on
Miscellaneous Infection Control Techniques

CAROL TORCZON, R.N., B.S.N., C.C.R.N.
Critical Care Education Coordinator, High Plains Baptist Hospital, Amarillo, Texas
Chapter 22, Section on Chest Tube and Water-Seal Drainage; Chapter 33, Section
on Electric Safety Protocol

JAN VANDERLAAN, R.N., B.S.N.
Team Leader, Coronary Care Unit, High Plains Baptist Hospital, Amarillo, Texas
Chapter 10, Blood/Blood Component Administration

WILLIAM A. YOUNG, R.R.T., M.S.
Director, Respiratory Therapy Department, Amarillo College, Amarillo, Texas
Chapter 19, Airway Management; Chapter 20, Ventilatory Support; Chapter 22,
Sections on Postural Drainage, and Chest Percussion and Vibration

PREFACE

Unlike other current texts on critical care nursing, *Critical Care Procedures and Protocols: A Nursing Process Approach* is designed to be a generic technique manual. The essence of procedures routinely performed in the critical care arena has been condensed to provide a rapid reference and step-by-step guidelines for the skills required by critical care nurses. The text is not designed to stand alone, but rather to augment available texts in critical care and subspecialties. Selected references provided at the conclusion of each section direct the reader to current literature and books in which in-depth information on each technique is readily available.

Critical Care Procedures and Protocols has been written using the nursing process as a framework, that is, assessment, planning, implementation, and evaluation. The implementation section of each technique description is written using a two-column format to provide rationale side by side with nursing actions. The evaluation section is presented as expected outcomes for the technique. Precautions are included with each technique and are highlighted in boldface to draw attention to them. Product availability is presented at the end of each section. The text is liberally illustrated with photographs and line drawings to clarify proposed nursing actions. The following headings are used to present the techniques and protocols:

BACKGROUND
  Objectives
ASSESSMENT PHASE
  PRECAUTIONS
PLANNING PHASE
  Equipment
  Client/Family Teaching
IMPLEMENTATION PHASE
  Nursing Actions   Rationale/Amplification
EVALUATION PHASE
  Anticipated Outcomes   Nursing Actions
PRODUCT AVAILABILITY
SELECTED REFERENCES

The focus of the text is on adult clients. Caring for neonates or children in the critical care setting is a subspecialty in itself, and an attempt to cover this area would be too vast an undertaking. The resultant text is manageable, and its usefulness in the clinical setting, where quick reference and clarification are essential, is enhanced.

Principles of infection control as recommended by the Centers for Disease Control (CDC) have been incorporated within the technique descriptions. Additionally, infection control protocols have been presented for each system. Although it is recognized that good handwashing is one of the most effective ways of preventing nosocomial infections, this is not repeated over and over throughout the technique descriptions.

The reader should consult institutional policies on matters regarding informed consent, the qualifications and licensure of personnel who can perform specific techniques, and procedures requiring a physician's order. Institutional policies will be guided by existing laws and regulations, and these may vary from state to state. It is also critical that personnel consult instruction manuals provided by the manufacturers of biomedical equipment before employing such equipment in caring for clients. The overwhelming array of available instrumentation makes a generic text desirable because the material presented is applicable regardless of which manufacturer supplies the equipment.

Throughout the book the generic names for medications are used. In most cases dosages are not specified because these often require individual adjustments. Nurses who are administering medications should consult package-insert information or other appropriate literature before administering medications. Measurements are presented in metric terms with appropriate equivalents in parentheses.

In the interest of space, descriptions of the techniques of basic life support have been purposely omitted. These techniques are available in basic medical–surgical texts and are presently taught to the public. This book focuses instead on advanced cardiac life support (ACLS) techniques, many of which are specific to the role of the critical care nurse.

Although there is an emphasis on procedures in this book, the psychosocial aspects of giving nursing care should not be overlooked. Nursing care must be provided within the concept of holism, with genuine concern for the person's physical, biological, psychosocial, and cultural needs. As presented in this book, the family includes those persons important to the client rather than only those persons who are related through traditional family ties.

Current regulations in health care have created a trend toward early discharge from the hospital. The client's family members or significant others are now performing care in the home that would usually have been considered within the realm of the health professional. With this trend in mind, discharge planning and teaching must begin much earlier in the hospital stay, and they are receiving much more emphasis in the critical care areas. Client and family teaching is emphasized in each technique description. Adequate preparation and explanation before performing a procedure serves to allay the anxiety of the client and family members as well as to prepare the person for home care.

It should be kept in mind that any nursing technique will have to be adapted to meet the needs of the individual client. Because the fastest growing segment of the population in the United States is people over the age of 65, elderly clients will be seen in the critical care unit in greater numbers. Nurses must be aware of the special needs of the elderly who are admitted to the critical care unit and must be able to adapt nursing techniques to accommodate these needs.

Contributions of clinical experts in critical care have added dimension to *Critical Care Procedures and Protocols*. The information offered in this book is basic to critical care, and both beginning and advanced practitioners as well as educators should profit from its use.

Carol Batten Persons, R.N., M.S.N., Ed.D.

ACKNOWLEDGMENTS

I would like to thank Robert Bradshaw, R.N., Radiology Special Procedures Nurse, High Plains Baptist Hospital, Amarillo, Texas, and Ernie Farino, formerly Chief of Medical Media, Amarillo Veterans Administration Medical Center, for photography in many of the chapters of *Critical Care Procedures and Protocols: A Nursing Process Approach.* Steve Ackeroyd has been very willing to process film for photographs that appear in the text. Photographs for Chapter 31, Thermal Trauma Techniques, were provided by Dr. Charles R. Baxter, Professor of Surgery, University of Texas Health Sciences Center, Dallas, Texas. Carol Torczon, R.N., B.S.N., critically reviewed Chapter 28, Peritoneal Dialysis.

The publishing team at J. B. Lippincott has been most helpful in guiding me through the steps involved in producing a finished product. I would like to thank in particular those individuals with whom I have worked closely: Diana Intenzo, Eleanor Faven, and Peggy Maxwell.

CONTENTS

I *Cardiovascular techniques*

1 *Cardiac monitoring*

The standard 12-lead electrocardiogram (ECG) records the electric events of the heart from 12 different angles. The standard leads include six limb leads (leads I, II, III, aV_R, aV_L, and aV_F) and six precordial leads (leads V_1 through V_6) (Figs. 1–1 and 1–2).

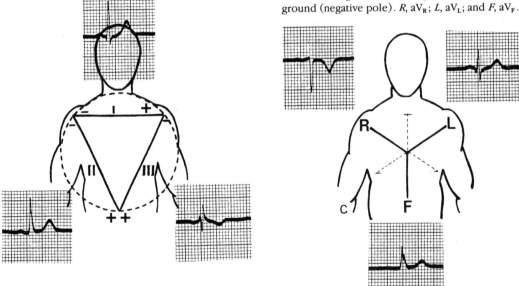

Fig. 1–1 Leads I, II, and III form Einthoven's triangle when superimposed on chest in frontal plane. Note positive and negative poles for each lead.

Fig. 1–2 Leads aV_R, aV_L, and aV_F record electrical activity in frontal plane. The right arm is positive pole for aV_R, the left arm is positive pole for aV_L, and left leg is positive pole for aV_F. For each lead the remaining electrodes represent a common ground (negative pole). *R*, aV_R; *L*, aV_L; and *F*, aV_F.

Leads II, III, and aV_F (augmented voltage of the left leg) record electric activity from the inferior surface of the left ventricle. Leads I and aV_L (augmented voltage of the left arm) reflect activity from the lateral wall of the left ventricle, and lead aV_R (augmented voltage of the right arm) reflects electric activity within the left ventricular muscle.

Leads V_1 and V_2 (right precordial leads) are positioned over the right side of the heart. Leads V_5 and V_6 (left precordial leads) are placed over the left side of the heart. Leads V_3 and V_4 (midprecordial leads) are placed over the interventricular septum. A reciprocal picture of the posterior surface of the heart, which may be required to identify posterior wall myocardial infarction (MI), is obtained through lead V_1 (Fig. 1–3).

The 12-lead ECG has a number of uses for the critical care nurse, including the differentiation of arrhythmias, left versus right ventricular complexes, bundle branch

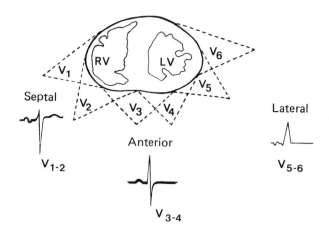

Fig. 1–3 Electrode positions for recording precordial leads. V_1 and V_2 are recorded from fourth intercostal space at right and left sternal borders respectively. V_4 is recorded at fifth intercostal space in midclavicular line. V_3 is recorded halfway between V_2 and V_4. V_6 is placed lateral to V_4 in midaxillary line, with V_5 midway between V_4 and V_6. The positive electrode is placed on anterior chest; the negative end of each chest lead is positioned toward client's back. (After Sharp L, Rabin B: Nursing in the Coronary Care Unit. Philadelphia, JB Lippincott, 1970)

block, hypertrophy, and injury, necrosis, and ischemia associated with MI. The calculation of the ventricular axis helps to determine pacemaker electrode position and reveals left anterior or left posterior hemiblock. Computer analysis of the 12-lead ECG by telephone is available in some facilities.

INSTRUMENTATION

An ECG is recorded using either a single-channel or a multichannel recorder. The single-channel recorder writes one lead at a time, and the lead-selector switch is manually operated. The precordial leads may be recorded by manually moving the suction-cup electrode to a standard position to write each lead. Newer models have six chest electrodes, which permit recording of the chest leads without moving the chest electrode each time. The multichannel recorder records three leads simultaneously, and once the ECG is initiated, no further operator input is necessary to switch leads.

CONTINUOUS ECG MONITORING

Two kinds of systems are presently used for continuous ECG monitoring. The first consists of hard-wire systems in which the client is connected directly to the cardiac monitor by a cable; the second consists of telemetry systems in which the client is connected to a compact, portable, battery-operated transmitter that sends the ECG to a central decoding station by an antenna system. The ECG is displayed on an oscilloscope at a central monitoring station for both hard-wire and telemetry systems. Hard-wire systems also provide a bedside oscilloscope that displays the ECG.

Components of a hard-wire bedside console include a rate indicator, an alarm-limit setting, sweep control (50 mm/second or 25 mm/second), control of adjustment of the height of the QRS complex (beginning of Q wave to end of S wave), control of the position of the ECG on the oscilloscope, a lead selector, remote control to document rhythm on demand at the central monitoring station, and a defibrillator jack for synchronized cardioversion (Fig. 1–4).

Features that are available with a central monitoring station include a slave oscilloscope, which displays the rhythms of several clients continuously; a recorder for documenting rhythms; storage capability, which permits retrieval of dysrhythmias 8 seconds to 60 seconds after their occurrence through tape loops or electronic memory; a time and date marker; a lead-failure indicator; alarm system; and a rate-change indicator, which is triggered by differences in the R–R (R wave to R wave) interval. These features are available for both hard-wire and telemetry systems monitored at a central monitoring station.

COMPUTERIZED ECG MONITORING

Computerized monitoring and dysrhythmia detection systems are used in many critical care units. These systems provide continuous monitoring of the client's rhythm while alerting the nurse to potential problem rhythms. However, a computerized system cannot replace the nurse's expertise in differentiating a false alarm and an emergency situation. Options available with computer monitoring include 24-hour monitoring with periodic updates of cardiac rhythm (Fig. 1–5), automatic detection of

Fig. 1–4 Hard-wire bedside console.

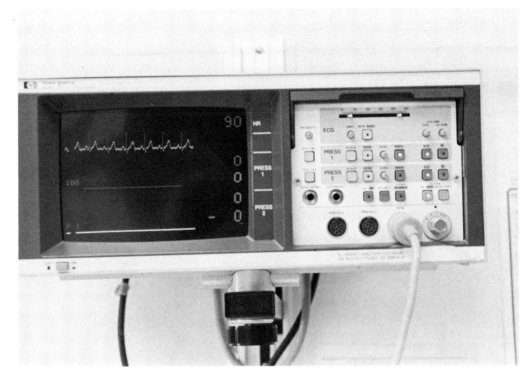

Fig. 1–5 Computer update of cardiac rhythm.

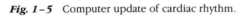

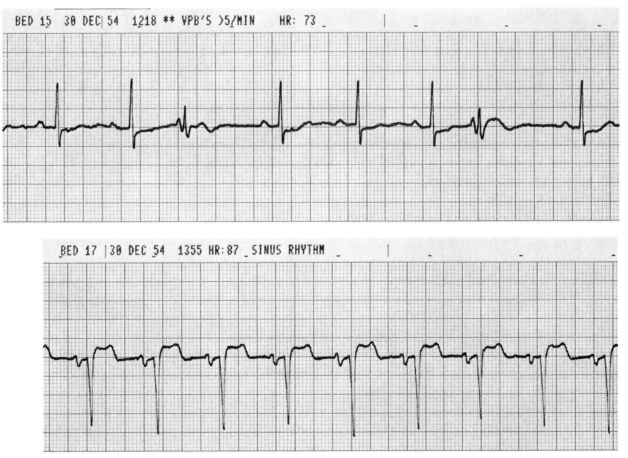

Fig. 1-6 Trend plot.

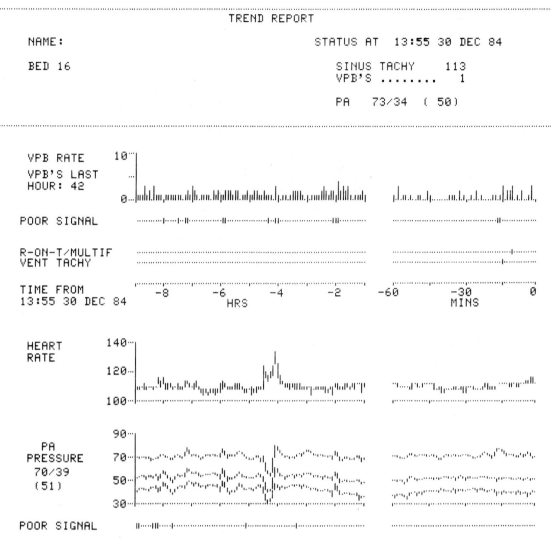

specific dysrhythmias, a priority alarm system with automatic documentation, detection of paced rhythms with a display of the total of paced and nonpaced complexes, and plotted trend displays of cardiac rate and significant events (Fig. 1–6). Specific instructions provided by the manufacturer should be consulted before operating the computer.

Electrocardiogram (ECG)

Objectives
To record cardiac electric events for diagnostic or documentary purposes
To record serial changes in cardiac activity (*e.g.,* those that occur in MI)

ASSESSMENT PHASE

- Has the client previously had an ECG?
- Will a portable (bedside) ECG be required, or can the client safely be transported to the electrocardiography department?
- Is the client receiving any medication (*e.g.,* digoxin, quinidine, thyroid medication) that can affect the ECG? Record this information on the ECG tracing or on the ECG request.
- What are the client's height and weight? Record this information on the ECG request and on the ECG report.

PRECAUTION   • **Ground the ECG recorder and all electric equipment to prevent electric shock.**

PLANNING PHASE   Single-channel or multichannel ECG recorder
EQUIPMENT   Four limb electrode plates and straps or suction cups
                          Electrode cable
                          Precordial suction-cup electrodes
                          Electrode paste
                          Alcohol sponges
                          Fine abrasive (optional)
                          Tissues
                          Washcloth, towel, and soap and water

CLIENT/FAMILY TEACHING   • Explain the procedure to the client and elicit cooperation.
                          • Explain that the ECG records the heartbeat.
                          • Reassure the client that an ECG causes no discomfort and that there is no danger of electrocution.
                          • Encourage the client to ask questions before beginning the ECG, because talking or movement during the ECG will produce artifacts on the tracing.
                          • Tell the client whether transportation to another department will be required.

**IMPLEMENTATION
PHASE**

NURSING ACTIONS	RATIONALE/AMPLIFICATION
1. Connect grounded ECG recorder (single-channel or multichannel) to power supply.	
2. Turn on power to ECG recorder.	
3. Place client supine.	Check that the client's feet do not touch the footboard of the bed. Make sure that the client is comfortable before beginning the recording. Muscle tremors will cause artifacts on the ECG tracing.
4. Drape client with sheet and expose limbs and precordium.	
5. Prepare electrode sites with alcohol sponge and allow to dry.	Alcohol cleans the skin and improves electrode contact.
a. Select inner aspect of each forearm and medial aspect of each leg.	Shave excessively hairy sites to decrease resistance to the current flow recorded by the electrodes.
b. Select standard precordial electrode positions.	
6. Abrade skin lightly with fine sandpaper pad (optional).	Abrading decreases resistance by removing surface cells and debris from electrode sites.
7. Apply electrode paste to electrode sites.	Paste decreases resistance caused by the skin barrier and reduces the occurrence of artifacts on the tracing.
8. Apply electrode plates to selected sites on extremities and secure with straps.	Suction-cup electrodes may be used. If the client is an amputee, connect extremity electrode to stump.
9. Connect electrode cable to plate or suction cup on appropriate extremity (Fig. 1–7).	Cable connectors are color coded and marked with abbreviations for each extremity (*e.g.*, LL for left leg, or V for precordial leads). The standard color code is RA, white; LA, black; RL, green; LL, red; and chest leads, brown. Make sure that the cable is secured without undue tension, which will produce artifacts. Draping the cable across the chest may cause a respiratory artifact to be recorded.

Fig. 1–7 Electrodes connected to ECG cable.

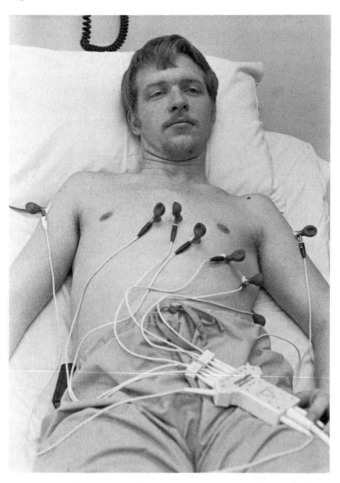

10. Connect cable to suction cups and apply leads to standard sites.

If a cable with only one extension for chest leads (single-channel recorder) is used, apply the electrode in the V_1 position. Turn off the recorder while rotating the chest leads and move the suction cup to the next position.

11. For a multichannel recorder position all leads before recording begins.

For a single-channel recorder, see step 17.

12. Press calibration button to check for standardization of tracing (Fig. 1–8).

Increase or decrease the gain to standardize the signal. The ECG is standardized to ensure that at 1 mV the deflection will be 10 mm. One-half standardization is occasionally required when ECG complexes are unusually tall (*e.g.*, as in ventricular hypertrophy). Write "½ standard" on the appropriate ECG lead to draw this to the attention of other care-givers.

13. Set paper speed at 25 mm/second.

14. Press button for automatic marking of leads.

15. Depress "Auto-run" button.

The 12 standard leads will be recorded automatically. If the ECG is interrupted for any reason, reset "Auto-run" and record ECG. Note clinical symptoms experienced by the client during the recording, for example, chest pain or palpitations.

16. If additional rhythm strips of selected leads are required, depress "Man-run" control and appropriate lead button.

Additional studies may help to identify dysrhythmias.

Fig. 1-8 Controls for multichannel ECG recorder.

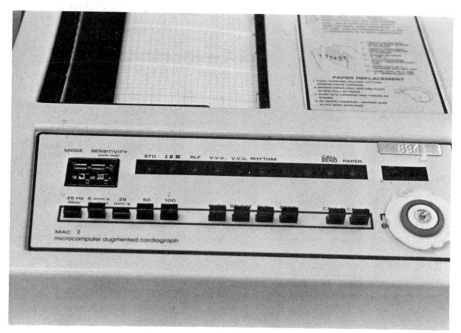

17. Technique adjustments for single-channel recorder induce the following:

   a. Turn selector switch to "Run."

   b. Turn lead selector to "STD" (standard).

   c. Adjust paper speed to 25 mm/second.

   d. Adjust stylus on ECG paper, if necessary, using position control.

   e. Press standardization button. Adjust standardization deflection to 1 mV if necessary.

   f. Turn power switch to "On."

    Paper flow will stop.

   g. Select lead I with lead selector.

   h. Turn power switch to "Run" and record for at least 6 seconds.

    Identify the lead in the margin of the ECG tracing using the marker button and standardized code. The standardized code is as follows:
Lead I __
Lead II __ __
Lead III __ __ __
aV_R _____
aV_L _____ _____
aV_F _____ _____ _____
Lead V_1 _____ _
Lead V_2 _____ _ _
Lead V_3 _____ _ _ _
Lead V_4 _____ _ _ _ _
Lead V_5 _____ _ _ _ _ _
Lead V_6 _____ _ _ _ _ _ _

   i. Turn power switch to "On" while selecting lead II.

    Repeat for all frontal plane leads.

   j. Select "V" leads with lead selector.

   k. Record chest leads V_1 through V_6, moving suction-cup electrode between recordings.

    Identify the leads using standardized code.

18. Turn off recorder.

19. Remove electrodes from client's chest and cleanse the site with tissues or soap and water.	If the ECG paste is gritty, the client may develop a skin irritation. Remove the paste with soap and water.

EVALUATION PHASE

ANTICIPATED OUTCOME	NURSING ACTIONS
Completion of a 12-lead ECG of diagnostic quality	Evaluate the electrodes for correct placement and for transposition of limb electrodes. Ground all electric equipment in the room. Evaluate for 60-cycle interference.

Hard-wire monitoring

Objectives
To continuously monitor changes in cardiac rhythm
To document cardiac dysrhythmias or changes in cardiac axis
To select an appropriate ECG lead to enhance diagnosis of cardiac abnormalities
To provide a clean ECG tracing that is free of extraneous artifacts

ASSESSMENT PHASE

- Has the client had previous experience with cardiac monitoring?
- Which lead system will be appropriate for continuous monitoring of this client? Using a five-lead system, modified versions of the twelve-lead ECG can be recorded. If a lead selector is available, rapid switching of leads can help document dysrhythmias and assist in interpretation. Select the appropriate three-lead system depending on individual requirements.
- Is the client diaphoretic, as, for example, during acute MI? If the client is diaphoretic, electrode contact will be impaired. Use diaphoretic electrodes (commercially available) or tincture of benzoin to enhance contact.

PRECAUTION

- **Ground all electric equipment to prevent accidental electric shock and to enhance the quality of the ECG tracing.**

PLANNING PHASE

EQUIPMENT

Bedside hard-wire monitor
Five-lead or three-lead ECG cable
Computerized ECG monitoring system (optional)
Pregelled disposable electrodes
Razor
Alcohol sponge
Fine abrasive pad or dry 4 × 4

CLIENT/FAMILY TEACHING

- Discuss the reasons for cardiac monitoring with the client and family.
- Answer questions about cardiac monitoring.
- Reassure the client that the cardiac rhythm is monitored continuously at the central monitoring station and that immediate assistance for rhythm problems is available.
- Instruct the client to report symptoms of chest pain or palpitations immediately. Document these symptoms with a rhythm strip or a 12-lead ECG as appropriate.

IMPLEMENTATION PHASE

NURSING ACTIONS	RATIONALE/AMPLIFICATION
1. Turn on bedside monitor and central monitoring station. Calibrate monitor according to manufacturer's instructions.	Check the manufacturer's instruction manual. Adjust the gain (size) control to provide a standardized tracing.
2. Select either three-lead or five-lead monitoring system (Figs. 1–9 and 1–10).	

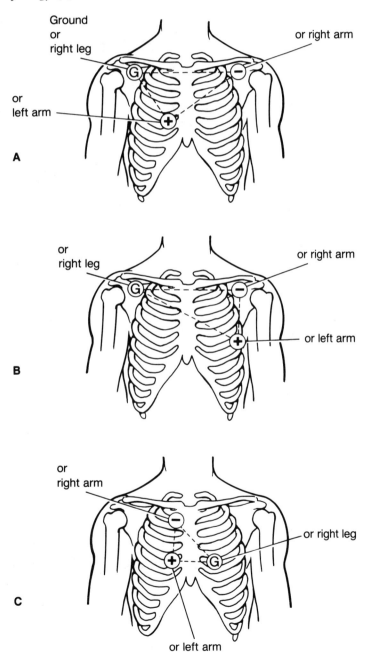

Fig. 1–9 (*A*) Marriott's MCL₁ allows differentiation of QRS morphology and bundle branch block. (*B*) MCL₆ enables differentiation of QRS morphology. (*C*) Lewis lead allows location of P waves.

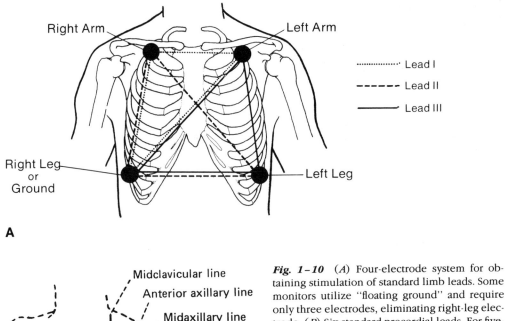

Fig. 1-10 (*A*) Four-electrode system for obtaining stimulation of standard limb leads. Some monitors utilize "floating ground" and require only three electrodes, eliminating right-leg electrode. (*B*) Six standard precordial leads. For five-lead system, apply "V" electrode to selected precordial site: V_1, V_2, V_3, V_4, V_5, or V_6. (After Bernreiter M: Electrocardiography. Philadelphia, JB Lippincott, 1963)

3. Prepare skin sites for electrode application.

   a. Shave if necessary.

   b. Avoid placement over muscle mass.

   Muscle movement causes artifacts on tracing.

   c. Swab skin with alcohol sponge and allow to dry.

   d. Abrade skin site with abrasive pad (optional).

   Prepackaged electrodes may come with abrasive pads. Skin sites may be abraded with dry gauze pads also. This decreases skin resistance to transmission of electric signals from the heart.

4. Connect electrodes to lead wires.

5. Peel protective backing from electrodes.

   Make sure that the electrode gel has not dried.

6. Place electrodes at preselected sites.

   Ensure good skin contact. Press the electrodes in place by pressing firmly in a circular pattern.

7. Observe monitor for clear ECG tracing and adequate R wave.

   An adequate R wave allows the monitor to count the client's heart rate accurately.

8. Set rate alarms.

   Follow the manufacturer's instructions.

9. Enter client data into computerized arrhythmia system if applicable.

RELATED NURSING CARE

NURSING ACTIONS	RATIONALE/AMPLIFICATION
1. Ensure that central monitoring station is constantly monitored by personnel and that alarms are activated at all times.	
2. Document arrhythmias as they occur.	
3. Document clinical symptoms such as chest pain with rhythm strip.	Clinical symptoms such as ischemia may be reflected in ECG changes.
4. Document rhythm regularly every 4 hours.	Regular documentation provides a serial record of the client's cardiac rhythm.
5. Check for tension on lead wires.	Tension on lead wires may cause fracture of the wires, which results in artifacts on the ECG tracing.
6. Replace electrodes every 24 to 48 hours as directed by manufacturer and check skin integrity.	Dried electrode gel causes poor signals. Rotate the electrode sites.

EVALUATION PHASE

ANTICIPATED OUTCOMES	NURSING ACTIONS
1. Completion of continuous clean ECG tracing with low incidence of false alarms.	Evaluate the tracing for artifacts and potential sources of false alarms.
	a. Artifacts may be caused by loose leads, movement, muscle tremors, damaged lead wires or cable, dry electrodes, or electric interference (Fig. 1–11).

Fig. 1–11 (*A*) Artifact caused by loose leads. (*B*) Sixty-cycle electrical interference.

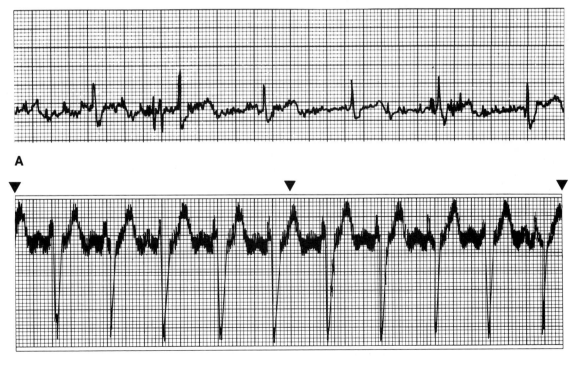

A

B

b. Incorrect sensing of R waves may be caused by an insufficient gain setting.

c. A wandering baseline may be caused by respiratory effort, which results in incorrect sensing of R waves.

d. Double sensing may be caused by excessive gain. Correct 60-cycle (electric) interference.

   (1) Check for electrode contact with skin or dried electrode gel.

   (2) Check for fractured lead wires or cable by exchanging one at a time for new equipment.

   (3) Eliminate one piece of electric equipment at a time while checking for the source of the problem.

e. Correct a wandering baseline by repositioning the electrodes.

f. Correct muscle artifacts by positioning the electrodes away from muscle mass.

2. Rapid detection of life-threatening dysrhythmias

Monitor the central monitoring station continuously.

3. Early detection of conduction disturbances or electric instability

---

PRODUCT AVAILABILITY   COMPLETE RANGE OF MONITORING EQUIPMENT

Hewlett-Packard
Marquette
Mennen

DIAPHORETIC ELECTRODES

NDM Corporation

Telemetry monitoring

Objectives
To continuously monitor changes in the cardiac rhythm in the ambulatory client
To provide freedom for the client from hard-wire attachment to the monitor
To document cardiac dysrhythmias

ASSESSMENT PHASE
- Why does the client require telemetry monitoring (*e.g.*, post-MI)?
- Does the client have clinical symptoms (*e.g.*, blackouts) that can be documented by telemetry?
- Is the client receiving medication (*e.g.*, digoxin) that can affect the ECG?
- Does the client have an artificial pacemaker?

PRECAUTION
- **Instruct the client to remain within the range of the telemetry system.**

PLANNING PHASE

EQUIPMENT

Transmitter
Battery
Battery tester
Lead wires—2 or 3
Electrodes—2 or 3
Telemetry bag and ties (or gown with telemetry pocket)

CLIENT/FAMILY TEACHING
- Describe telemetry monitoring to the client and answer any questions.
- Reassure the client and family that cardiac rhythm is monitored continuously at a central monitoring station.
- Instruct the client to notify personnel of clinical symptoms such as chest pain or dizziness. Some transmitters have a button that will activate a recording at the central monitoring station. Inform the client of this if applicable.
- Inform the client of the range of the telemetry transmitter and instruct him to stay within range.
- Tell the client not to shower while the transmitter is attached. If the physician permits the transmitter to be removed for showering, the central station monitor should be notified.

IMPLEMENTATION PHASE

NURSING ACTIONS	RATIONALE/AMPLIFICATION
1. Turn on telemetry channel at central monitoring station.	Follow the manufacturer's instructions.
2. Check battery with tester to ensure adequate charge.	
3. Place battery in transmitter.	Make sure that the positive (+) and negative (−) poles of the battery are placed as indicated on the transmitter.
4. Select three-lead monitoring system (see previous section on Hard-Wire Monitoring).	If the telemetry system requires only two electrodes, omit the ground electrode.
5. Connect lead wires to transmitter (Fig. 1 – 12).	Lead wires may be color coded to indicate negative and positive poles. Insert the appropriate lead wire as indicated on the transmitter.

Fig. 1–12 Telemetry transmitter.

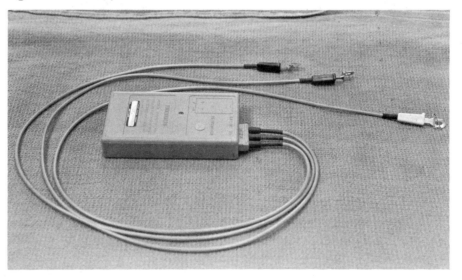

6. Prepare skin sites for electrode application.	See previous section on Hard-Wire Monitoring.
7. Peel backing from electrodes and apply to skin sites.	
8. Place transmitter in telemetry bag or telemetry pocket of client's gown (Fig. 1 – 13).	The telemetry bag and pocket protect the transmitter from damage and allow for ambulation.

Fig. 1–13   Transmitter secured in telemetry bag to permit ambulation.

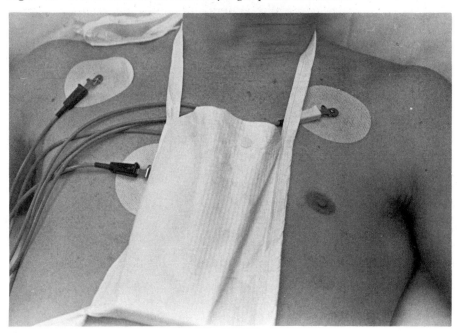

9.   Check for clear ECG tracing at central monitoring station.

10.   Enter client data into computerized monitoring system if applicable.

RELATED NURSING CARE   See previous section on Hard-Wire Monitoring.

EVALUATION PHASE   See previous section on Hard-Wire Monitoring.

PRODUCT AVAILABILITY   Hewlett-Packard
Mennen
Marquette

SELECTED REFERENCES

Dubin D: Rapid Interpretation of EKG's. Tampa, COVER Publishing Company, 1974
Guzzetta CE, Dossey BM: Cardiovascular Nursing Bodymind Tapestry, pp 222–223. St. Louis, CV Mosby, 1984

Hudak CM, Lohr T, Gallo BM: Critical Care Nursing, 3rd ed, pp 77–80 Philadelphia, JB Lippincott, 1982

2 *Cardioversion*

Defibrillation and elective cardioversion are used to terminate specific cardiac dys-rhythmias. In emergency situations these procedures are initiated by the critical care nurse. Disturbances of rhythm in which cardioversion may be effective include life-threatening cardiac dysrhythmias, tachyarrhythmias that result in low cardiac output and hemodynamic deterioration, and dysrhythmias that cannot be converted by phar-macologic intervention.

During defibrillation an electric current passes across the chest wall, causing simultaneous depolarization of myocardial muscle fibers. This disrupts all chaotic electric circuits, which are responsible for the dysrhythmia. Repolarization of each muscle fiber occurs, theoretically allowing the sinoatrial (SA) node or other potential pacemaker to regain control of cardiac rhythm.

Emergency countershock (defibrillation) is the treatment of choice for ventricu-lar fibrillation. During ventricular fibrillation myocardial muscle fibers depolarize independently, causing the myocardium to quiver (Fig. 2–1). As a result, the cardiac

Fig. 2–1 Ventricular fibrillation.

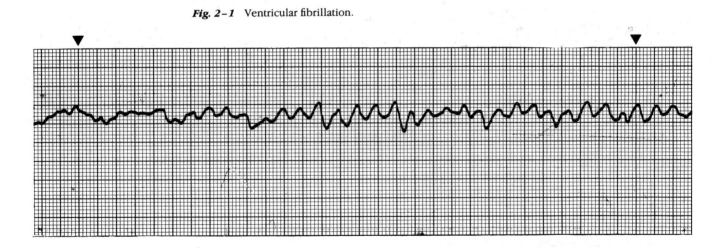

muscle is unable to maintain cardiac output. As the length of time that the client has been in ventricular fibrillation increases, defibrillation is progressively less likely to be successful. The presence of hypoxemia acidosis, electrolyte imbalance, hypother-mia, and drug toxicity makes countershock less effective. Hypoxemia, acidosis, and electrolyte levels are routinely evaluated and corrected during advanced life-support procedures.

During open-heart surgery sterile internal paddles are applied directly to the myocardium to fibrillate and defibrillate the heart. A significantly lower power setting (15 to 30 watt-seconds) is used during open-heart surgery than during normal defi-brillation.

Emergency synchronized cardioversion is used to convert dysrhythmias such as rapid ventricular rhythms or supraventricular rhythms, which result in hemodynamic deterioration (Fig. 2–2). The difference between synchronized cardioversion and defibrillation is that the defibrillator is synchronized to deliver an electric charge to the heart approximately 10 msec after the peak of the R wave. This avoids accidental delivery of the charge during the vulnerable portion of the T wave, which may induce ventricular fibrillation. From 50 to 200 watt-seconds of delivered energy is usually used during synchronized cardioversion. If repeated shocks are necessary, power levels recommended for defibrillation are usually used (200 to 300 watt-seconds).

Elective cardioversion is used to convert supraventricular dysrhythmias (rapid atrial fibrillation or atrial flutter) that do not respond to drug therapy (Fig. 2–3). The principles are similar to those of emergency synchronized cardioversion, but the procedure can be scheduled and carried out in a controlled environment.

Fig. 2–2 (*A, B*) Ventricular tachycardia. (*C*) Supraventricular tachycardia.

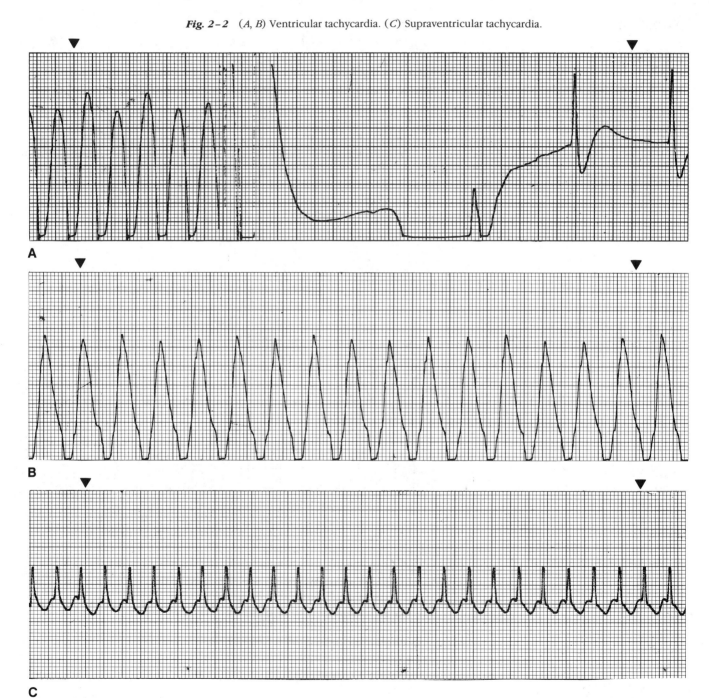

Fig. 2–3 (*A*) Atrial fibrillation. (*B*) Atrial flutter.

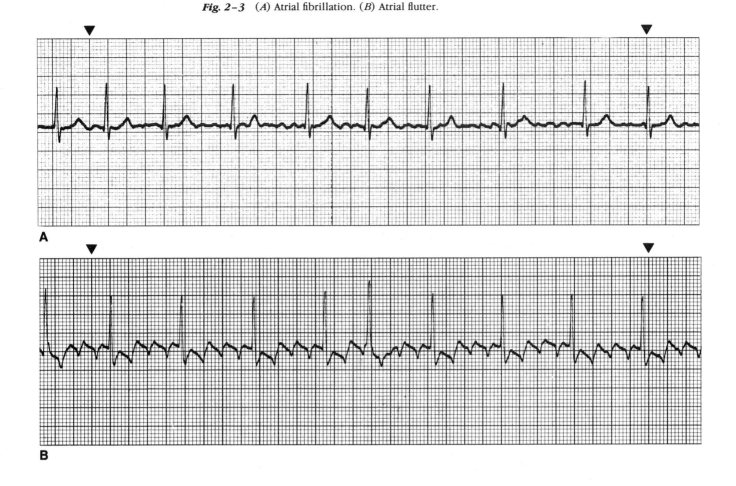

A

B

INSTRUMENTATION	The direct-current (DC) defibrillator consists of a power supply, an electric storage system (capacitor), and an appropriate electric discharge circuit (paddles). The defibrillator delivers several thousand volts of electricity to the paddles in 4 msec to 12 msec. The maximum amount of delivered energy (as opposed to stored energy) in most new defibrillators is 360 watt-seconds. Current research yields conflicting reports about the relationship between electric energy requirements for defibrillation and body weight and heart size. As a result, available defibrillators may not deliver enough energy to defibrillate some clients.

Light, effective, portable defibrillators that can be battery powered are available for emergency use outside the critical care unit. Many defibrillators now feature "quick look" paddles. Placing these paddles on the chest and turning on an oscilloscope provides a cardiac rhythm. They are helpful in assessing the client who is not attached to a cardiac monitor.

Defibrillation

Objective

To terminate ventricular fibrillation using electric countershock

ASSESSMENT PHASE

- Does the ECG rhythm strip indicate that the client is in ventricular fibrillation?
- Is the client unresponsive and pulseless? In a monitored adult client, administer a single precordial thump (Fig. 2–4). Start basic life support (BLS) and continue until a defibrillator is available.

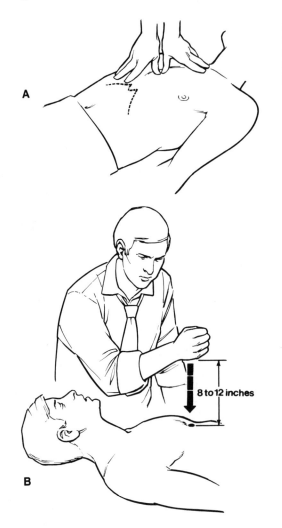

Fig. 2-4 (*A*) To determine position for precordial thump, estimate point halfway between suprasternal notch and xiphoid process. (*B*) Deliver sharp thump with closed fist from approximately 30 cm (12 inches) above chest.

8 to 12 inches

- Does the client have an intravenous (IV) infusion line? Start an IV infusion when personnel are available.
- Does the client have respiratory support? Provide immediate AMBU bag support when personnel are available.
- Is advanced cardiac life support (ACLS) available? (See ACLS Technique in Chap. 3.)
- Is cardiac medication (*e.g.*, sodium bicarbonate, epinephrine, lidocaine, procainamide, bretylium) available?

PRECAUTIONS
- **Personnel should not touch the client, equipment, or bed during defibrillation to avoid accidental electric shock.**
- **The defibrillator will not discharge during ventricular fibrillation if it is in the synchronized mode.**
- **Disconnect the temporary pacemaker or other electric equipment to prevent possible damage from defibrillation.**

PLANNING PHASE

EQUIPMENT

Defibrillator
External paddles
Conductive gel or saline pads
Emergency cart (with cardiac medications)
Airway-support equipment (see Intubation in Chap. 19)
Emergency pacing equipment

CLIENT/FAMILY TEACHING
- When personnel are available, a staff member should remain with family members to provide support.

IMPLEMENTATION PHASE

NURSING ACTIONS	RATIONALE/AMPLIFICATION
1. Initiate and continue BLS until defibrillator is available.	Cardiopulmonary resuscitation (CPR) maintains cardiac output.
2. Plug grounded defibrillator into electric outlet (unless equipped with battery pack).	
3. Turn on defibrillator.	
4. Check monitor again for ventricular fibrillation or use "quick look" paddles by placing them on client's chest and turning on oscilloscope.	
5. Apply conductive gel generously to metal portion of paddles. *Alternative:* Place prepared saline-soaked gauze pads in desired position on chest.	Skin provides resistance between heart and paddles. Conductive gel or saline pads increase current flow to myocardium and prevent skin burns. Prevent burns and arcing of current by avoiding excess gel or dripping saline.
6. Set defibrillator to deliver 200 to 300 watt-seconds.	Use the minimum setting required to convert rhythm, because defibrillation causes myocardial damage.
7. Charge defibrillator by activating charge button.	A digital display registers the electric charge selected.
8. Place paddles firmly on chest using approximately 25 pounds of pressure (Fig. 2–5).	One paddle is placed below the right clavicle at the sternoclavicular joint, and the second is placed to the left of the cardiac apex. Use an alternative placement if the client has a permanent pacemaker to prevent damage to the pacemaker generator (Fig. 2–6).

Fig. 2–5 Anterior placement of paddles.

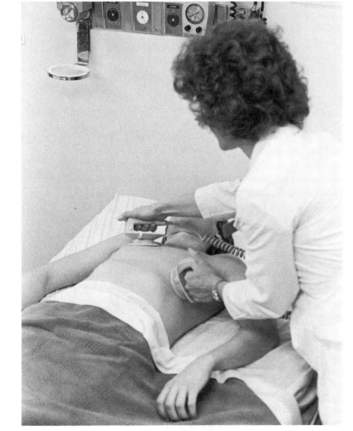

Fig. 2–6 Alternative paddle placement for client with implanted permanent pacemaker.

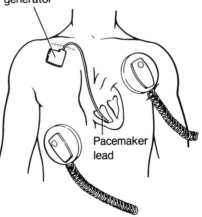

9. Reconfirm ventricular fibrillation on monitor. Record continuous ECG strip at central monitoring station if available.

10. Give command for personnel to stand clear of client, bed, and equipment.

Determine that all personnel are clear of the client, bed, and equipment. The operator should not be in contact with the client or bed.

11. Press buttons on both paddles simultaneously. Recharge paddles.

Hold the paddles firmly on the client's chest until the charge is delivered. Observe for skeletal muscle contractions.

12. Observe monitor for return of normal rhythm.

13. If first attempt is unsuccessful, repeat defibrillation attempt using 200 to 300 watt-seconds.

14. If normal rhythm does not return after second attempt, continue to administer BLS.

15. Intubate and ventilate client.

Hypoxemia may prevent successful defibrillation.

16. Administer epinephrine and sodium bicarbonate as appropriate.

Acidosis may prevent successful defibrillation.

17. Reapply conductive gel and defibrillate using 360 watt-seconds (delivered energy).

18. Observe monitor for return of normal rhythm and document with rhythm strip.

For an unsuccessful conversion, the physician may order lidocaine, procainamide, or bretylium.

19. Administer lidocaine bolus and start lidocaine drip as ordered after successful conversion.

20. Obtain 12-lead ECG.

This provides baseline data after defibrillation.

RELATED NURSING CARE

NURSING ACTIONS	RATIONALE/AMPLIFICATION
1. Monitor vital signs every 15 minutes until they are stable.	
2. Assess cardiovascular and respiratory functions hourly until they are stable.	
3. Monitor ECG rhythm continuously.	Continuous monitoring alerts personnel to recurrence of life-threatening arrhythmias.
4. Assess skin integrity for presence of burns.	

EVALUATION PHASE

ANTICIPATED OUTCOMES	NURSING ACTIONS
1. Correct functioning of defibrillator	If the defibrillator will not discharge or the rhythm fails to convert, evaluate the defibrillator for the following: **a.** Is the defibrillator in synchronized rather than unsynchronized mode? **b.** Is the battery power low or is the defibrillator unplugged? **c.** Is the equipment faulty? **d.** Is debris present on the paddles? (Debris impairs conductivity.)

e. Are low-amplitude fibrillatory waves, which are associated with longstanding ventricular fibrillation, present? Correct acidosis and hypoxia.

2. Restoration of sinus rhythm or acceptable cardiac rhythm

Evaluate a continuous rhythm strip. Monitor the client's vital signs and hemodynamic status. Evaluate the therapeutic effect of the lidocaine drip.

Synchronized cardioversion

Objective
To convert selected dysrhythmias using electric countershock

ASSESSMENT PHASE

- Why is the client a candidate for synchronized cardioversion? Selected supraventricular dysrhythmias or rapid ventricular dysrhythmias that cause hemodynamic deterioration, such as ventricular tachycardia, often require synchronized cardioversion.
- Has an informed consent been obtained?
- Is an IV line available? Start a keep-open IV of 5% dextrose in water (D_5W) or a medication ordered by the physician.
- Is respiratory support available? A respiratory therapist (if available) should be on standby to assist with ventilation.
- Are ACLS techniques available?
- Is the client NPO (*non per os;* nothing by mouth)? Keep NPO 6 hours before cardioversion unless an emergency intervenes.
- Is all equipment properly grounded to prevent possible current leakage and electric shock?
- What is the client's serum potassium level? Hypokalemia potentiates electric instability after cardioversion. Correct low potassium levels before beginning the procedure.
- Does time permit a digitalis-level determination? In the presence of digitalis toxicity, there is an increased incidence of lethal dysrhythmias after cardioversion. If an initial low-energy setting of 5 watt-seconds produces ventricular instability, the physician may decide to defer cardioversion.
- Is the client on continuous hard-wire monitoring?
- Has a 12-lead ECG been obtained to document precardioversion rhythm?
- Has a baseline assessment of vital signs, peripheral pulses, and neurologic status been completed?

PRECAUTIONS

- **See previous section on Defibrillation.**
- **Cardioversion should be done with the defibrillator in the synchronized mode to avoid countershock during the vulnerable portion of the T wave, which can cause ventricular fibrillation.**
- **If ventricular fibrillation occurs, switch the defibrillator to the unsynchronized mode before defibrillation.**

PLANNING PHASE

EQUIPMENT

See previous section on Defibrillation.

CLIENT/FAMILY TEACHING

- Reinforce the physician's explanation of cardioversion and answer questions for the client and family.
- Reassure the client that medication will be provided before the procedure to minimize discomfort.

IMPLEMENTATION PHASE

NURSING ACTIONS	RATIONALE/AMPLIFICATION
1. Place client supine.	
2. Remove dentures, if applicable.	Removal of dentures prevents airway obstruction.
3. Select monitoring lead with tall, positive R wave and minimal T wave.	The defibrillator will be synchronized to fire on the RS segment of the ventricular complex. New defibrillators may not require a positive R wave.
4. Plug defibrillator into electric outlet.	
5. Turn on defibrillator.	If a defibrillator tester is available, charge and test the defibrillator.
6. Set defibrillator on synchronized mode.	Observe the monitor for a flag (blip) on the downslope of the QRS complex. This indicates correct synchronization of the charge to the cardiac cycle.
7. Administer premedication as ordered.	Observe the client for drowsiness. Provide supplemental oxygen or an AMBU bag as required. Disconnect the oxygen before the cardioversion procedure begins.
8. Prepare paddles with conductive gel or place saline-soaked gauze pads on skin in appropriate position.	Avoid excessive gel or saline, which may cause arcing and burns.
9. Charge defibrillator to voltage ordered by physician.	A charge of 50 to 200 watt-seconds is usually prescribed for cardioversion. If this is not successful, power levels for defibrillation should be used in subsequent attempts.
10. Place paddles firmly on torso using approximately 10.9 kg (25 pounds) of pressure.	Paddles may be placed in the anterior position (see previous section on Defibrillation). For cardioversion the anteroposterior position is an alternative.
11. Give command for personnel to stand clear of client, bed, and equipment.	Make sure that personnel are clear of the client, bed, and equipment. Activate continuous ECG strip recording at the central monitoring station.
12. Discharge defibrillator by simultaneously pressing buttons on both paddles.	Wait until the charge is delivered before removing the paddles. This may take several seconds. Observe the client for skeletal muscle contraction.
13. Observe monitor for successful cardioversion.	If the client converts to ventricular fibrillation, switch the defibrillator to the desynchronized mode and defibrillate.
14. If cardioversion attempt is unsuccessful, ventilate client while preparing for another attempt.	
15. When client's rhythm has converted, document cardioversion with 12-lead ECG.	

RELATED NURSING CARE

NURSING ACTIONS	RATIONALE/AMPLIFICATION
1. After cardioversion provide respiratory support until client responds.	
2. Assess client's vital signs and rhythm every 15 minutes until stable. Then frequency may be decreased.	

3. Assess client's neurologic status every 15 minutes until stable. Reorient client as necessary.	Emboli may occur after conversion of longstanding atrial arrhythmias.
4. Continue to monitor client's ECG rhythm continuously.	The client may remain on the hard-wire monitor or may be placed on a telemetry transmitter.
5. Assess client's torso for burns.	
6. Maintain NPO for 6 hours to 12 hours after cardioversion.	Cardioversion may have to be repeated if the client reverts to precardioversion rhythm.

EVALUATION PHASE

ANTICIPATED OUTCOME	NURSING ACTION
Prevention of complications of cardioversion	Observe for symptoms of pulmonary, systemic, or cerebral emboli; lethal dysrhythmias; respiratory problems; or hypotension.

SELECTED REFERENCES

American Heart Association: Standards and Guidelines for Cardiopulmonary Resuscitation (CPR) and Emergency Cardiac Care (ECC). JAMA 244:453, 1980

Guzzetta CE, Dossey BM: Cardiovascular Nursing, Bodymind Tapestry. St. Louis, CV Mosby, 1984

McIntyre K, Lewis AJ (eds): Textbook of Advanced Cardiac Life Support. Dallas, American Heart Association, 1981

3

Mega code (advanced cardiac life support)

BACKGROUND

SUDDEN CARDIAC DEATH

An estimated one million people experience acute myocardial infarction (MI) each year in the United States. Of this number, 640,000 victims die of ischemic heart disease. Despite increased efforts directed toward public education, 60% to 70% of these persons die before hospitalization. The greatest risk of death for the heart attack victim is within the first 2 hours after the onset of symptoms. It is during this time that most life-threatening dysrhythmias occur. The cardiac emergencies that occur most commonly are ventricular fibrillation, ventricular tachycardia, and asystole. Death that occurs within the first 24 hours of acute MI is called *sudden cardiac death*.

BASIC AND ADVANCED LIFE SUPPORT

The number of deaths caused by acute MI may be decreased by preventive actions, early recognition of symptoms, and prompt seeking of medical treatment. Priority must be given to early therapy that is aimed at preventing life-threatening dysrhythmias, but once cardiac arrest has occurred, skilled, knowledgeable resuscitation of the client can decrease mortality.

The primary goal of any life-support skill is to restore spontaneous respirations and circulation with little or no neurologic impairment. This requires that basic life support (BLS) measures be implemented within 4 minutes to 6 minutes, followed promptly (within 8 minutes) by advanced cardiac life-support (ACLS) measures. The amount of time within which life-support measures are initiated is important; but the success of resuscitation is influenced by many other factors that must be assessed throughout the cardiac arrest.

Primarily, skillful management of the client's airway and circulation have a major impact on the success of resuscitative efforts. BLS is vitally important to the success of ACLS; it is virtually a holding status for ACLS measures. If quality BLS measures are not initiated early and maintained throughout resuscitation, the most skillful, knowledgeable ACLS measures will be of no avail. Oxygenation of the client is essential to prevent permanent neurologic impairment, but it is also necessary to ensure the responsiveness of the cardiac muscle to emergency cardiac drugs and to electric defibrillation. Without effective cardiac compressions, emergency cardiac drugs and oxygenated blood will not be circulated to the vital organs, specifically, to the brain and heart.

LEGAL ASPECTS OF ACLS

The degree to which nurses are permitted to perform ACLS measures is based on hospital policy and on regulations implemented by the state nursing-licensure body. In hospitals in which physicians are not readily available, it is expected that a physician will be notified immediately of a pending or occurring cardiac emergency. Upon arrival, the physician is identified as the care-giver in charge of the cardiac arrest team. Hospitals that do not have a physician in 24-hour residence must have an identified group of medical personnel qualified to manage a cardiopulmonary arrest. This team assumes responsibility for treating the cardiac arrest victim until a physician is available.

Objective

To provide emergency life-support measures to the client experiencing cardiopulmonary arrest

ASSESSMENT PHASE

- Has the client lost consciousness? Is the client unresponsive to stimulation?
- Are spontaneous respirations or pulse absent? Is the airway free of obstruction?
- Is the client connected to a cardiac monitoring system? What rhythm is displayed on the screen?
- Are personnel familiar with the correct use of the defibrillator, emergency-cart organization, and emergency drugs (*i.e.*, indications, dosage, route of administration, precautions, complications, and the sequence of their use)?

PRECAUTIONS

- **Avoid mixing or giving any drug in conjunction with sodium bicarbonate ($NaHCO_3$). The high pH of sodium bicarbonate will inactivate epinephrine. Ideally, two intravenous (IV) lines should be used for drug administration.**
- **Observe safety precautions when using the defibrillator (see Defibrillation in Chap. 2).**
- **Select the correct defibrillator paddle size for the client. The average adult-sized paddles are 10 cm to 13 cm in diameter.**
- **Apply a conductive medium to the paddles or to the client's chest to prevent burns and to decrease transthoracic skin resistance.**

PLANNING PHASE

EQUIPMENT

Cart supplied with standard equipment for treatment of cardiac arrest (Table 3–1)
Emergency cardiac arrest drugs (Table 3–2)
Defibrillator
Cardiac monitor

Table 3–1
Standard equipment for cardiac arrest cart*

Airway/breathing	Central:
Intubation tray	Subclavian catheter insertion tray
AMBU Bag	2-0 or 3-0 silk with cutting needle
Nasal airway	Xylocaine 1% injection
Oral airway	4×4s
McGill forceps	Povidone–iodine
Tongue blade	Infusion equipment:
Nasal prongs for O_2	Solusets (Buretrol sets)
O_2 mask	Macrodrip IV tubing
O_2 connecting tubing	IV extension tubing
Suctioning equipment:	Three-way stopcock connectors
Sterile gloves	D_5W—500 ml
Suction catheters	Ringer's lactate, 1000 ml
Yankover suction	Medication additive labels
Normal saline (for irrigation machine)	*Miscellaneous equipment*
Blood gas kits	Syringes and injection needles
	Nasogastric tube with 50-ml catheter-tip syringe
Circulation	Blood pressure cuff with stethoscope
Peripheral:	Sterile gloves
IV catheters (Nos. 16, 18, 20)	Spinal needles
Tourniquets	Defibrillator pads
Tape	ECG monitoring pads
Alcohol sponges	Chest board
Antibacterial ointment	Blood tubes for laboratory samples (optional)
2×2s	ECG paste, ECG paper (optional)

* Organization of the cart should be based on priority and accessibility of the equipment. Stock levels will be based on unit needs. Carts should not be cluttered with unnecessary equipment.

Table 3–2
Drugs used in cardiac arrest: how supplied, usual dose (average adult)

Drug	Concentration and volume of prefilled syringe	Dose	Infusion rate	Remarks
Atropine sulfate	0.1 mg/ml in 10-ml syringe	0.5 mg to 1 mg = 5 ml to 10 ml		Repeat at 5-min intervals to achieve desired rate. Generally, do not exceed 2 mg.
Bretylium tosylate	50 mg/ml in 10-ml ampule	5 mg/kg 350 mg to 500 mg as initial dose	500 mg in D$_5$W (in 250 ml = 2 mg/ml; in 500 ml = 1 mg/ml) Infusion: 2 mg to 3 mg/min	Infusion started after loading dose to control recurrent ventricular tachycardia or ventricular fibrillation.
Dopamine	200 mg in 5-ml syringe		200 mg in 250 ml D$_5$W 800 g/ml infusion = 2 to 10 g/kg/min	
Epinephrine (1:10,000)	0.1 mg/ml in 10-ml syringe	0.5 mg to 1 mg = 5 ml to ml IV or intratracheal	1 mg in 5% D$_5$W (in 250 ml = 4 g/ml; in 500 ml = 2 g/ml) Infusion: 1 g/min to maintain blood pressure	Avoid intracardiac injection. Repeat dose every 5 min as needed in cardiac arrest.
Isoproterenol	0.2 mg/ml in 5-ml ampule		1 mg in 5% D$_5$W (in 250 ml = 4 g/ml; in 500 ml = 2 g/ml) Infusion: 2 g to 20 g/min titrated	Watch for PVCs.
Lidocaine	For IV bolus: 1% (10 mg/ml) in 10 ml = 100 mg 2% (20 mg/ml) in 5 ml = 100 mg For infusion after bolus: 4% (40 mg/ml) in 25 ml = 1 g	1% in 75 mg = 7.70 ml 2% in 75 mg = 3.75 ml	2 g in 500 ml D$_5$W (or 1 g in 250 ml) = 4 mg/ml Infusion: 1 mg to 4 mg/min	For breakthrough ventricular ectopy, administer additional 50-mg bolus every 5 min (total of 225 mg) to suppress. Increase drip to 4 mg/min.
Procainamide	For IV bolus: 100 mg/ml in 10-ml ampule For infusion after bolus: 500 mg/ml in 2-ml ampules	20 mg/minute until: Dysrhythmia is suppressed, hypotension results, QRS widens by 50%, total dose of 1 g is administered.	1 g in 250 ml D$_5$W (4 mg/ml) Infusion: 1 mg to 4 mg/min	Monitor ECG and blood pressure. Administer cautiously in patients with acute MI.
Sodium bicarbonate	1 mEq/ml in 50 ml = 50 mEq	1 mEq/kg or 75 ml initial dose (average-size adult) or preferably according to pH		Repeat according to pH.

(From McIntyre K, Lewis AJ (eds): Textbook of Advanced Cardiac Life Support, p. 302. Dallas, American Heart Association, 1983. Used with permission.)

CLIENT/FAMILY TEACHING
- Provide for family support during the arrest situation. Use other family members, clergy, and staff.
- Explain to the client and family the purpose of the life-support devices that are used during the postresuscitation period.
- Keep the family informed of the client's condition and progress.

IMPLEMENTATION PHASE

NURSING ACTIONS	RATIONALE/AMPLIFICATION

CARDIAC ARREST: UNMONITORED SITUATION

1. Establish responsiveness by gently shaking client and shouting "Are you okay?"

The physical and verbal stimuli will be sufficient to arouse the client who is not in a coma or experiencing cardiac arrest.

2. If there is no response, initiate hospital's cardiac arrest notification procedure.

Obtaining qualified help as early as possible will increase the chances for successful resuscitation.

3. Place client supine.

The client must be supine and lying on a firm surface to provide adequate ventilation and cardiac compressions. Place a cardiac arrest board (if available) under the client's chest.

4. Open airway. Look, listen, and feel for breathing. If client is not breathing, give four full, quick breaths.

The airway is opened by hyperextending the head. Alternatively, the airway is opened using the jaw-tilt method in clients with cervical spine dysfunction (Fig. 3–1). Opening the airway is necessary to accurately assess ventilation. (The tongue is the primary cause of airway obstruction in the unconscious adult.)

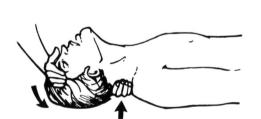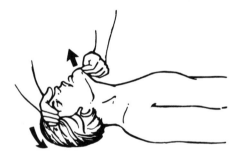

Fig. 3–1 Opening the airway *(Left)* Method of hyperextending head. *(Right)* Jaw-tilt method. (Brunner LS, Suddarth DS: The Lippincott Manual of Nursing Practice, 4th ed. Philadelphia, JB Lippincott, 1986)

5. Check for a carotid pulse.

Allow 5 seconds when checking for the carotid pulse. This is especially important because of the potential presence of bradycardia.

6. If no palpable pulse is present, initiate cardiopulmonary resuscitation (CPR). Begin ECG monitoring as soon as possible to confirm dysrhythmia (*i.e.*, ventricular fibrillation, ventricular tachycardia, or asystole).

Use the defibrillator paddles if they have the "quick look" feature. Otherwise, position the ECG electrodes and attach the client to a cardiac monitor.

7. Implement appropriate treatment.

MANAGEMENT OF VENTRICULAR FIBRILLATION

1. Verify ventricular fibrillation with "quick look" paddles or cardiac monitor if client is being monitored (see Fig. 2–1). Verify lack of pulse in large artery (*e.g.*, carotid or femoral).

2. Attach client to cardiac monitor or single-channel ECG machine for continuous monitoring throughout arrest procedure.

3. Confirm presence of ventricular fibrillation.

4. Prepare to defibrillate at earliest opportunity, before initiating CPR if defibrillator is readily available.

5. Apply conductive gel to appropriate sites on anterior chest.

See Defibrillation in Chapter 2.

6. Charge defibrillator to between 200 watt-seconds and 300 watt-seconds. Order personnel to stand clear of bed. Fire defibrillator.

The electric discharge from the defibrillator will take the path of least resistance to ground. Therefore personnel must not be in contact with the bed or the client.

7. After each defibrillation attempt, assess for the following results:

    a. Has change in rhythm occurred?

    b. Is pulse present in large artery (*e.g.*, femoral)?

8. If there has been no change in rhythm, immediately recharge defibrillator and deliver second charge.

9. Assess for change in rhythm and pulse; if there is no change, continue CPR.

10. Initiate IV therapy (if none is being administered) and initiate drug therapy.

Until the second unsuccessful attempt, emphasis is placed on defibrillation. Defibrillate early in the episode of ventricular fibrillation and in rapid sequence.

If the first two attempts at defibrillation are unsuccessful, the following two drugs should be administered.

    a. Epinephrine 0.5 mg to 1.0 mg intravenous push (IVP)

Epinephrine is administered for its effect on contractility and vasoconstriction. Epinephrine increases the amplitude of the fibrillatory waves and converts a fine ventricular fibrillation to a coarse fibrillation.

    b. Sodium bicarbonate 1 mEq/kg IVP (if indicated by arterial blood gas [ABG] determinations)

Sodium bicarbonate is given to alleviate metabolic acidosis. This is especially important in an unmonitored situation in which acidosis (both respiratory and metabolic) is likely to be present. Do not mix epinephrine and sodium bicarbonate because sodium bicarbonate will inactivate epinephrine. Use two IV infusion sites if available.

Continuing CPR will circulate drugs throughout cardiovascular system.

11. Reassess rhythm. If ventricular fibrillation continues, defibrillate a third time.

Use maximum energy output (approximately 360 watt-seconds).

12. If client remains in ventricular fibrillation, administration of an antiarrhythmic agent should be considered.

    a. Lidocaine 1 mg/kg IV bolus

Lidocaine is an antiarrhythmic drug that has been used extensively in managing cardiac dysrhythmias, particularly those of ventricular origin that occur after MI.

    b. Bretylium tosylate 5 mg/kg

The antiarrhythmic action of bretylium tosylate is not clearly understood. It is known to increase the fibrillation threshold and to increase both the action potential and the refractory period.

    c. Procainamide 100 mg IV (20 mg/minute)

Procainamide should be considered when lidocaine has been ineffective.

13. Attempt defibrillation at maximum output. Continue to assess for change in pulse rate or rhythm.

14. If no change occurs, continue CPR.

15. Determine whether repeat doses of epinephrine and sodium bicarbonate will be beneficial.

Epinephrine may be repeated at 5-minute intervals and sodium bicarbonate at 10- to 15-minute intervals as indicated by ABG analysis.

16. Repeat antiarrhythmic therapy.

    a. Lidocaine 0.5 mg/kg IV at 5- to 10-minute intervals

Alternative method: Start an IV infusion of lidocaine 2 g/500 ml dextrose 5% in water (D_5W) at a rate of 2 mg to 4 mg/minute. (Lidocaine boluses may be given until a maximum total dosage of 225 mg is reached.)

    b. Bretylium tosylate 10 mg/kg IV

Alternative method: Start an IV infusion of bretylium tosylate 2 g/500 ml D_5W at a rate of 1 mg to 4 mg/minute.

    c. Procainamide infusion of 2 g/500 ml D_5W at a rate of 1 mg to 4 mg/minute.

17. Reassess airway management. Draw blood for ABG analysis to assess ventilation and acid–base status.

18. Defibrillate at maximum output. Reassess rhythm. If no change occurs, repeat doses of epinephrine and sodium bicarbonate (if indicated by ABG determinations) and resume antiarrhythmic therapy.

Increase the dosage of the IV bolus of lidocaine to a maximum of 225 mg.

19. Continually assess ventilation and acid–base status.

MANAGEMENT OF MONITORED VENTRICULAR FIBRILLATION

1. Precede treatment described above with a precordial thump (see Defibrillation in Chap. 2).

The precordial thump is used only when the client attached to a cardiac monitor experiences ventricular fibrillation or ventricular tachycardia. It is performed when the myocardium is still sufficiently oxygenated to allow the jolt from the thump to convert the rhythm.

MANAGEMENT OF VENTRICULAR TACHYCARDIA

1. Confirm presence of ventricular tachycardia (Fig. 3–2).

Ventricular tachycardia occurs when three or more ventricular beats follow in rapid succession. The rate is generally greater than 100 beats per minute but does not exceed 220 beats per minute. At slower rates this dysrhythmia may be well tolerated and the client may remain conscious. Ventricular tachycardia becomes a life-threatening situation when loss of consciousness and pulselessness occur.

2. In conscious client with palpable pulse management of ventricular tachycardia is as follows:

    a. Administer precordial thump. Assess for change in pulse rate or rhythm.

    b. Notify physician.

    c. Initiate antiarrhythmic therapy with lidocaine 1 mg/kg IV bolus.

Lidocaine is a first-line antiarrhythmic drug that can be given rapidly without immediate detrimental side-effects.

    d. Assess for change in rhythm and notify physician.

Fig. 3-2 (*A*) Accelerated ventricular rhythm at a rate of 94 beats per minute. If cardiac output is adequate, client will remain conscious. (*B*) Ventricular tachycardia at a rate of 150 beats per minute.

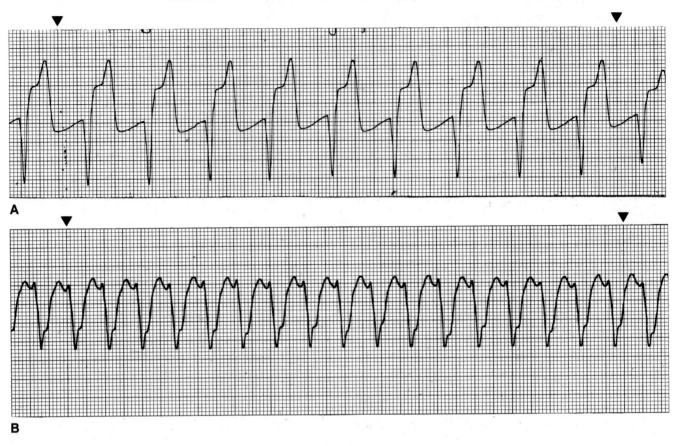

A

B

e. If there is no change in rhythm, prepare for cardioversion with 20 watt-seconds to 100 watt-seconds.

If time permits, the client may be mildly sedated before cardioversion. Set the defibrillator to the synchronized mode for cardioversion of ventricular tachycardia. This may reduce the energy requirements and alleviate secondary complicating dysrhythmias.

f. Deliver charge. Reassess pulse rate and rhythm.

g. Administer second dose of lidocaine 0.5 mg/kg IV bolus and follow with infusion of lidocaine 2 g/500 ml D₅W at rate of 2 mg to 4 mg/minute.

Give the second dose of lidocaine within 5 minutes to 10 minutes of the initial dose. Lidocaine 0.5 mg/kg may be given every 5 minutes to 10 minutes to a maximum dose of 225 mg.

3. In unconscious client management of ventricular tachycardia is as follows:

a. If client is connected to cardiac monitor, administer precordial thump. Assess for pulse rate or rhythm changes.

A precordial thump is administered *only* when ventricular tachycardia is documented by the cardiac monitor.

b. Attempt cardioversion at 200 watt-seconds.

c. Reassess rhythm and pulse rate for effectiveness of cardioversion. If no change occurs, prepare for immediate repeat of cardioversion at 200 watt-seconds.

d. If no change in rhythm occurs, insert IV line for administration of medications. Initiate CPR.

e. Administer lidocaine 1 mg/kg IV bolus.

The lidocaine bolus of 0.5 mg/kg should be repeated at 5- to 10-minute intervals to a maximum of 225 mg.

f. Circulate with CPR. Prepare to deliver third cardioversion at 200 watt-seconds.

g. Begin lidocaine infusion of 2 g/500 ml D₅W at rate of 2 mg to 4 mg/minute.

Alternative method: Administer bretylium tosylate 5 mg/kg IV bolus. Circulate with CPR. Attempt cardioversion. If attempt is unsuccessful, increase dose to 10 mg/kg IV bolus. Consider bretylium tosylate infusion 2 g/500 ml D₅W at 2 mg to 4 mg/minute.

h. Assess acid–base and ventilatory status.

i. Repeat cardioversion with 200 watt-seconds.

j. If ineffective, repeat dose of bretylium tosylate 10 mg/kg. Repeat cardioversion.

MANAGEMENT OF ASYSTOLE

1. Determine that client is unresponsive and pulseless.

Asystole is the third most frequently occurring dysrhythmia in cardiac emergency situations. Asystole indicates a lack of ventricular activity; no pulse will be felt in large arteries (Fig. 3–3).

2. Initiate CPR and ventilatory support, and prepare IV access site.

Establishing an IV line may be difficult because of vascular collapse.

3. Administer the following drugs:

a. Epinephrine 1 mg IV bolus

Occasionally, asystole is mistaken for fine ventricular fibrillation (Fig. 3–3). Administering epinephrine should convert the dysrhythmia to a coarse ventricular

Fig. 3–3 (*A*) Asystole. (*B*) Fine ventricular fibrillation.

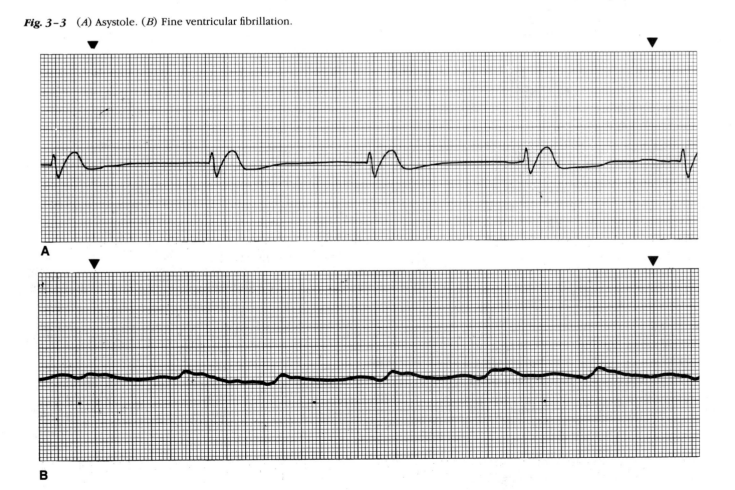

A

B

b. Sodium bicarbonate 1 mEq/kg IVP

4. Continue CPR. Continually assess for presence of pulse rate and change in rhythm.

5. If there is no response to drug therapy, administer 5 ml of calcium chloride 10% IV. Continue CPR.

6. If there is no response, repeat the following drugs as needed:

    a. Epinephrine every 5 minutes

    b. Sodium bicarbonate every 10 minutes to 15 minutes

    c. Atropine every 5 minutes

7. Draw ABG sample to assess ventilation and acid–base status.

8. If there is no response after second sequence of these drugs, consider infusion of isoproterenol 2 mg/500 ml D$_5$W at rate of 2 mcg to 20 mcg/minute.

9. If there is no response, repeat doses of epinephrine, sodium bicarbonate, and calcium chloride.

10. Continue to assess adequacy of ventilation and acid–base status frequently throughout arrest.

11. Normalize core body temperature if client is hypothermic.

12. Notify cardiologist if pacemaker insertion is necessary. (See Temporary Transvenous Pacemaker in Chap. 7.)

13. Continue resuscitative measures until resuscitation procedure is terminated by physician.

---

fibrillation. If the administration of epinephrine causes no change in the amplitude of the rhythm, treat the rhythm as asystole.

Give sodium bicarbonate if indicated by ABG determinations.

CPR circulates the drugs through the cardiovascular system.

The administration of sodium bicarbonate should be guided by ABG determinations.

Atropine is repeated only to a total dose of 2 mg.

Isoproterenol is primarily a β-adrenergic stimulator that produces positive inotropic (contractile) and chronotropic (heart-rate) effects. Once a rhythm has been established, these effects may not be desirable because they then affect myocardial oxygen requirements.

Hypothermia may affect the myocardial response to treatment.

Alternative method: Implement transcutaneous pacing. (See Temporary Transcutaneous Pacing in Chap. 7.)

The unresponsiveness of the cardiovascular system to BLS and ACLS must be taken into consideration when determining when to stop resuscitative efforts.

RELATED NURSING CARE

NURSING ACTIONS	RATIONALE/AMPLIFICATION
1. Document sequence of events and time that resuscitation was initiated and terminated.	The hospital cardiac-emergency protocol should designate one member of the arrest team as the "recorder."
2. Document therapies and outcomes.	Include drugs, dosage, and route and time of administration. Record the number of defibrillation attempts made, the amount of watt-seconds used, and the types of rhythms that resulted. Document airway management, ABG determinations, and vital signs.
3. During arrest, periodically call out amount of time that has elapsed since drug administration (*e.g.,* "It's been 5 minutes since the last epinephrine.").	This serves as a prompt for the person in charge of the arrest.
4. Anticipate need for hemodynamic monitoring (*e.g.,* prepare pulmonary artery catheter or arterial line).	Intravascular pressure monitoring will be required for accurate assessment and hemodynamic management.

5. Anticipate supportive therapy.	After successful resuscitation, supportive therapy will be required. A ventilator may be needed for ongoing pulmonary management. The cardiovascular system may require the support of vasopressors, vasodilators, or antiarrhythmic therapy. Ventricular failure may require an intra-aortic balloon pump.
6. Anticipate and prepare for subsequent cardiac emergency.	Myocardial damage, ventricular irritability, fluid and electrolyte imbalance, and acid–base imbalance may lead to another cardiac emergency.

EVALUATION PHASE

ANTICIPATED OUTCOMES	NURSING ACTIONS
1. Implementation of effective BLS and ACLS techniques	During the arrest, frequently assess the effectiveness of artificial circulation by checking for a pulse rate in a large artery (*e.g.*, femoral or carotid). Frequently assess the effectiveness of artificial ventilatory support. Observe for a rise in the client's chest with each ventilation. If the client is intubated, check for bilateral breath sounds. Monitor ABGs for oxygenation, ventilation, and acid–base status. Assess oxygenation by checking pupillary response.
2. Restoration of cardiopulmonary function	Evaluate the client's condition and follow the appropriate procedure. Evaluate all body systems. **a.** To evaluate the cardiovascular system, monitor vital signs, cardiac rate and rhythm, serum enzymes, and pulmonary artery pressures. **b.** To evaluate the pulmonary system, auscultate lung fields, and assess ventilatory perfusion and acid–base balance. **c.** The renal system can be evaluated by monitoring urinary output hourly. Decreased cardiac output during cardiac arrest may potentiate prerenal problems. Monitor urine electrolyte levels, blood urea nitrogen (BUN), and creatinine levels. **d.** The central nervous system can be evaluated by assessing pupillary response, movement, muscle strength, memory, and level of consciousness. **e.** To evaluate the gastrointestinal system, assess for the presence of bowel sounds.
3. Preservation of neurologic function	Compare neurologic function with prearrest baseline data.

SELECTED REFERENCES McIntyre K, Lewis AJ (eds): Textbook of Advanced Cardiac Life Support. Dallas, American heart Association, 1983

Standards and Guidelines for Cardiopulmonary Resuscitation (CPR) and Emergency Cardiac Care (ECC). JAMA 255(21):2905, 2992, June 1986

4

Invasive vascular techniques

BACKGROUND

Venipuncture is the invasive vascular technique performed most commonly by the critical care nurse. An intravenous (IV) line is a priority in caring for the critically ill client who is at risk for dysrhythmias, who requires fluid replacement, or who is receiving medications intravenously.

SELECTION OF INTRAVENOUS DEVICES

Selection of IV devices is based on the location of the vein to be used, the type and viscosity of fluid to be infused, and the medication to be injected. A flexible catheter is used if the IV line will be inserted in the antecubital area because of the movement of the joint, and an armboard will be needed to restrict mobility. High-viscosity fluids such as total parenteral nutrition (TPN) or blood require a larger bore catheter than a keep-open IV for emergency use does. Phlebitis due to antibiotic infusion or other sclerosing medication occurs less often if large deep veins are used.

INSTRUMENTATION

Several types of IV devices are available (Fig. 4–1). The catheter-over-the-needle device is a stainless steel needle within a catheter. The vein is punctured with the

Fig. 4–1 Types of infusion devices.

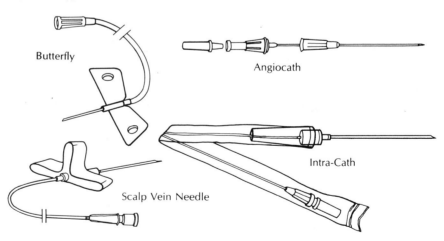

needle, which serves as a stylet for the catheter, and the catheter is threaded into the vein over the needle. The needle is then removed, and the IV tubing is connected to the catheter hub.

The catheter-through-the-needle device consists of a stainless steel needle through which the catheter is threaded into the vein. The catheter is protected by a plastic sleeve. Once the catheter is in place, the needle is withdrawn from the vein, and the hub is connected to the hub of the catheter. The plastic sleeve is removed, and the IV tubing is connected to the catheter hub. A protective clip is placed over the bevel of the needle to prevent damage to the catheter.

A butterfly device is not usually used in the critical care area because it is ineffective for long-term use and for infusion of large amounts of fluid. The device consists of a short stainless steel needle connected to plastic tubing. The IV tubing is connected directly to the hub of the plastic tubing.

An intermittent infusion set (IIS) is useful because it allows client mobility while maintaining vascular access. An IIS is similar to the butterfly device in design, but the hub is capped with a resealable injection cap. A catheter-over-the-needle device may be converted to an intermittent infusion device by disconnecting the IV tubing and attaching a resealable injection cap to the hub of the catheter. Intermittent infusion devices are kept patent by periodic flushing with a heparin solution. Before injecting medication into an IIS, check for backflow of blood into the tubing by applying pressure to the syringe. Once the medication is injected, clear the tubing with a heparin flush to prevent clotting in the device. An infusion can be administered using an IIS by connecting the IV tubing to a needle that is inserted into the resealable cap. Flush the device with a heparin solution when the infusion is complete.

IN-LINE FILTERS
IV fluids may be administered through an in-line filter that removes particulate matter and bacteria, depending on the type of filter. Both membrane and depth filters are available. Membrane filters will block the passage of air when wet. They are available in sizes that vary according to the pore size of the membrane — .45 micron and .22 micron filters. A .22 micron filter will remove most bacteria, but it may require a pump to maintain the IV infusion rate. Depth filters are assigned a rating according to the size of the particles that will be blocked 98% of the time.

Venipuncture

Objective
To administer parenteral fluids, medication, blood, or nutritional supplements

ASSESSMENT PHASE
- Why does the client require IV therapy? A client who is NPO (*non per os,* nothing by mouth) for surgery, who has dysrhythmias requiring IV medication, or who is dehydrated will require IV therapy.
- What gauge of IV device will be required? Blood administration and fluid and electrolyte replacement require an 18-gauge catheter. A 20-gauge device is appropriate for keep-open IVs and for drip rates of 75 ml/hour or less.
- What type of IV device will meet the client's needs? If the IV line will be inserted in the antecubital area, an intra-cath is the best choice because of increased movement over the joint.
- Is the client allergic to iodine? If so, use alcohol to prepare the skin.
- Does the client have impaired renal function as results, for example, post surgery, with renal disease, and post trauma (particularly head injury)? Monitor fluid balance with a Foley catheter and hourly urine measurements.
- Does the client have impaired cardiac function (*e.g.,* MI, congestive heart failure)? Use a microdrip and volume-control device to prevent accidental overload.

PLANNING PHASE

EQUIPMENT
IV solution
IV tubing (with volume-control device if required)
Infusion device
Heparin flush in syringe (if using intermittent infusion device)
Tourniquet
Razor or depilatory (if required)
Iodophor preparation sponges
Alcohol sponges
Sterile 4 × 4
Iodophor ointment (optional)
Tape

Padded armboard (if required)
Linen protector
IV pump/controller (if applicable)

CLIENT/FAMILY TEACHING
- Describe the procedure to the client.
- Answer questions about the reasons for administering IV therapy.
- Reassure the client that the IV infusion will cause discomfort but should not be excessively painful.
- Instruct the client to report pain and swelling at the infusion site.

IMPLEMENTATION PHASE

NURSING ACTIONS	RATIONALE/AMPLIFICATION
1. Prepare IV infusion apparatus and flush tubing. Suspend IV container on IV pole.	The drip chamber should be hung approximately 60 cm (24 inches) above the infusion site. Vein damage can result from higher pressures if the drip chamber is hung higher than 60 cm. Label the IV tubing with the date and time. Use the appropriate tubing, which is supplied by the manufacturer if a pump/controller is used.
2. Wash your hands. Determine appropriate venipuncture site (Fig. 4–2).	

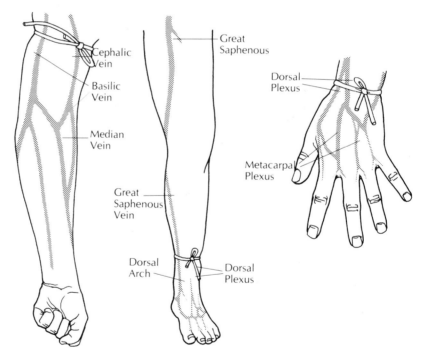

Fig. 4–2 Anatomic sites for venipuncture.

3. Apply tourniquet above planned infusion site.	The tourniquet should impede venous flow but should not affect arterial flow.
4. Select venipuncture site.	Prolonged application of the tourniquet may cause the vein to become tortuous. Sclerosed veins may be easier to puncture without a tourniquet.
5. Release tourniquet.	
6. Remove excess hair from site using razor or depilatory.	Shaving is optional. Microabrasions caused by shaving are potential sites of infection. Protect bed linen with linen protector.

7. Wash your hands. Prepare skin with iodophor sponge and allow to dry.

Remove iodophor with an alcohol sponge if the vein cannot be visualized.

8. Reapply tourniquet.

9. Hold needle bevel at 45-degree angle and puncture skin lateral to vein (Fig. 4–3).

Using your opposite hand support the extremity and anchor the vein.

Fig. 4–3   Venipuncture using catheter-through-the-needle device.

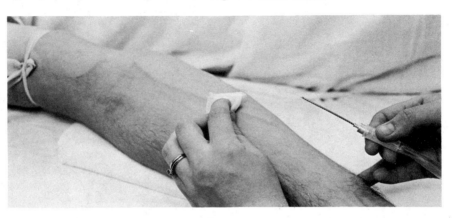

10. Reduce angle of needle and insert needle $\frac{1}{2}$ cm ($\frac{1}{4}$ inch) into vein.

11. Observe for retrograde flow into IV device.

Retrograde flow indicates successful venipuncture.

12. Advance IV device using appropriate technique.

13. For a catheter-through-the-needle device, proceed as follows:

    a. Stabilize needle with one hand.

    b. With opposite hand, advance catheter through needle and into vein until full length has been inserted.

A plastic sleeve protects the sterility of the catheter during advancement.

    c. Engage needle and catheter hub.

If the catheter cannot be inserted the full length, withdraw the needle over the catheter to engage the catheter hub.

    d. Withdraw needle and catheter from vein until 4 cm ($1\frac{1}{2}$ inches) of catheter is exposed.

    e. Remove plastic sleeve.

    f. Withdraw stylet.

    g. Attach primed IV tubing to catheter hub and start infusion.

    h. Apply needle guard over needle bevel (Fig. 4–4).

The needle guard protects the catheter from damage caused by the bevel. The catheter will be occluded if the needle and the catheter do not lie in the groove of the needle guard.

14. For a catheter-over-the-needle device, proceed as follows:

    a. Stabilize needle hub with one hand.

Stabilizing the needle prevents accidental removal of the device.

    b. With other hand, advance catheter over needle and into vein (Fig. 4–5).

Fig. 4-4 Intra-cath (Deseret) system with needle guard in place.

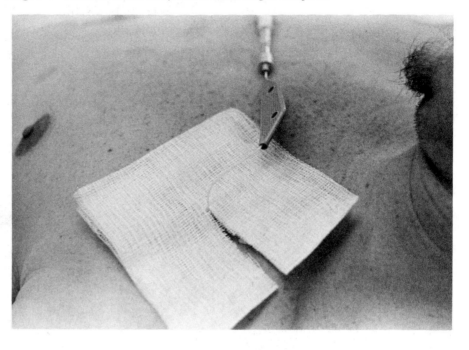

Fig. 4-5 Stabilizing needle hub with one hand while sliding catheter over needle and into vein.

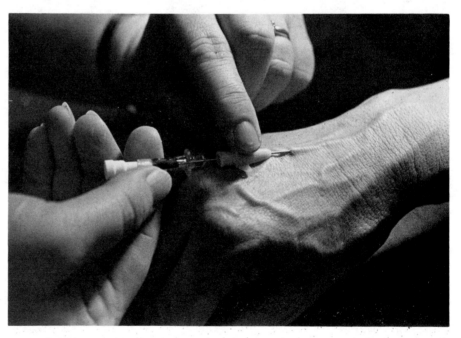

    c. Withdraw needle from catheter and connect primed IV tubing.

    d. Start infusion.

15. For a scalp vein (butterfly) device or an IIS, proceed as follows:

    a. Gently advance needle into vein until full length has been inserted.

Care must be taken not to puncture the vein.

Fig. 4-6 Flushing intermittent infusion device with heparin.

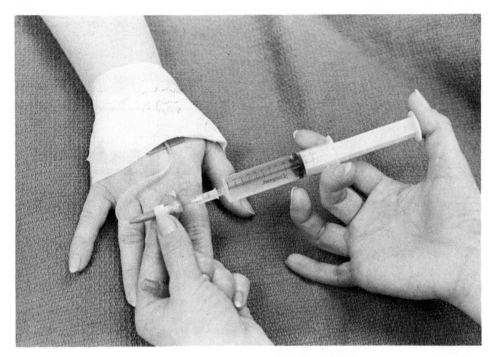

b. For scalp vein set, remove protective cap, connect primed IV tubing, and start infusion.

c. For IIS, flush tubing with heparin by piercing resealable cap (Fig. 4-6).

A heparin flush prevents clotting in the device. Use a premixed, commercially available heparin flush, or mix 1 ml normal saline and 1 unit heparin.

16. Secure infusion device with tape.

17. Apply iodophor ointment to insertion site (if used) and dress with sterile dressing.

18. Label tape with date, time, type of device, and name of care-giver starting IV infusion.

19. Adjust infusion rate.

RELATED NURSING CARE

NURSING ACTIONS	RATIONALE/AMPLIFICATION
1. Apply armboard to immobilize IV site, if applicable.	
2. Change IV tubing every 48 hours and IV fluid container every 24 hours.	Changing of tubing and container is an infection-control precaution.
3. Palpate IV site through dressing for tenderness and observe for signs of phlebitis every 8 hours.	
4. Change dressing every 48 to 72 hours.	
5. Monitor amount of time IV device is in place.	The maximum recommended time is 72 hours. The rate of infection increases significantly if the device is left in place longer.

EVALUATION PHASE

ANTICIPATED OUTCOMES	NURSING ACTIONS
1. Prevention of complications of IV therapy	
a. Fluid overload	Evaluate urinary output hourly if the client has renal, respiratory, or cardiac impairment.
	Evaluate insensible fluid loss.
	Use an IV pump/controller or a volume-control device if the client is at risk of fluid overload.
	Evaluate for signs of fluid overload (*e.g.*, increased pulse rate, increased fluid output, rales, congestive heart failure, or pulmonary edema).
b. Phlebitis, thrombus, or systemic infection	Change the IV apparatus and rotate the infusion site as recommended.
	Evaluate for signs of phlebitis (*e.g.*, redness, edema, pain, increased warmth).
	Monitor the client's temperature every 4 hours.
c. Air embolus	Clear the IV tubing of air before beginning infusion.
	Keep the drip chamber at least one-half full of fluid.
d. Hematoma	Evaluate the infusion site for bleeding after the infusion is discontinued.
e. Tissue sloughing due to fluid infiltration	Evaluate the IV infusion every 4 hours for patency.
	Use a pump/controller when one is available.
	Infuse medication that can cause tissue damage into a large vein (*e.g.*, Levophed, dopamine, antibiotics).

PRODUCT AVAILABILITY

IV DEVICES

Becton-Dickinson
Deseret
Bard
Jelco
Cutter Laboratories

IV FLUIDS

Abbott Laboratories
McGaw Laboratories
Travenol Laboratories, Inc.
Cutter Laboratories

IV PUMP/CONTROLLERS

Abbott Laboratories
IVAC Corporation
Biosearch

SELECTED REFERENCES

Metheny NM, Snively WD: Nurses' Handbook of Fluid Balance, 4th ed. Philadelphia, JB Lippincott, 1983

Infection control protocol for invasive vascular devices

BACKGROUND

Critical care clients are at significant risk of nosocomial (hospital-acquired) bacteremia. Multiple invasive vascular devices provide microorganisms with direct access to the client's bloodstream. These microorganisms are capable of causing serious illness and death. The Centers for Disease Control (CDC) have developed guidelines for infection control in intravascular therapy and hemodynamic pressure monitoring.

Objective

To prevent the development of nosocomial bacteremia related to invasive vascular devices

ASSESSMENT PHASE

- What are the mechanisms through which microorganisms potentially enter the client's bloodstream (*e.g.*, transvenous pacemaker, pulmonary artery catheter, IV infusion)?
- What precautions will be required to limit access of microorganisms to the client's bloodstream (*e.g.*, tubing changes, use of sterile transducers, handwashing)?
- Are signs of bacteremia/sepsis associated with the use of intravascular devices present (*e.g.*, redness, swelling, and pain at insertion site; discharge from insertion site; elevated temperature)?

PLANNING PHASE

EQUIPMENT

Iodophor solution*
Replacement tubing
IV fluids
Intravascular catheters/devices
Dressing
Tape
Iodophor ointment (optional)

CLIENT/FAMILY TEACHING

- Briefly explain to the client the various procedures necessary to protect against infection.
- Caution the client and family against the manipulation of tubing or insertion sites.
- Listen attentively to complaints of pain or irritation at the insertion sites because these may be a sign of infiltration, phlebitis, or infection.

IMPLEMENTATION PHASE

NURSING ACTIONS	RATIONALE/AMPLIFICATION
1. Wash your hands before inserting any vascular device or before manipulating tubing or sites.	Handwashing is the most important infection-control procedure.
2. Prepare insertion site.	
a. Scrub vigorously with antiseptic for at least 30 seconds before inserting device.	Tincture of iodine (3%) is the antiseptic of choice. Iodophors, chlorhexidine, or alcohol may also be used.
b. Allow site to dry at least 30 seconds before inserting device.	
3. Apply antiseptic ointment to site immediately after insertion.	This step is optional.
4. Secure cannula or needle adequately.	Unnecessary movement at the insertion site causes irritation, which predisposes the tissue to infection.
5. Dress insertion site with sterile dressing.	Either sterile gauze or a sterile transparent dressing is acceptable.
6. Record date of insertion and type and length of vascular device on tape.	This information alerts personnel to the date the site should be changed and allows the care-giver removing the device to determine if the device has been removed completely.

* Alcohol may be used if the client is allergic to iodine.

7. Label tubing and solution container with date and time.

8. Maintain closed system as much as possible.

9. Avoid flushing or irrigating systems to improve flow.

Disinfect the insertion ports before entering the system.

This can be damaging to the vein or artery and can cause clots to enter the vascular system. Pressure-monitoring lines require continuous flushing to maintain patency.

10. Do not withdraw blood specimens from lines being used for IV therapy.

There is a risk of contaminating the line, and the specimen may be diluted with IV fluid.

11. Evaluate insertion site at least daily by palpating over dressing for pain and observing area around dressing for redness or swelling.

Remove the dressing and visually inspect the area if there is unexplained fever or pain or tenderness at the site.

12. Change peripheral IV sites every 72 hours or earlier if signs of infiltration, phlebitis, or infection appear.

The potential for infection increases after 72 hours. If the site cannot be changed because no other site is available, notify the physician and document the reason.

13. Change intravascular devices that are inserted in unsterile emergency conditions at earliest opportunity.

14. Change dressing every 48 to 72 hours. Palpate site through dressing to check for inflammation.

The only exception is total parenteral nutrition (TPN), which should be changed every 24 to 48 hours.

15. Change tubing every 48 hours and after administration of blood, blood products, or lipid emulsions.

Adhesion of cells inside the tubing is a potential source of infection.

16. Change entire system including cannula, tubings, and fluid containers immediately if purulent thrombophlebitis, cellulitis or bacteremia related to use of intravascular device is suspected.

17. Culture cannula tip if system is changed because of suspected infection (Fig. 4–7).

Send the cannula tip to the laboratory for culture and sensitivity testing.

18. Prepare admixtures only in emergency situations if pharmacy has admixture program.

The pharmacy usually has a laminar hood to ensure sterility control as well as a quiet environment with limited access.

19. Refrigerate all admixed fluids or start infusion within 6 hours.

Admixed fluids may be stored in the refrigerator for a week before use if refrigeration is continuous and is

Fig. 4–7 To culture cannula tip when bacteremia is suspected, use sterile scissors to clip off 2 cm (¼ inch) of cannula tip and allow it to drop into sterile container.

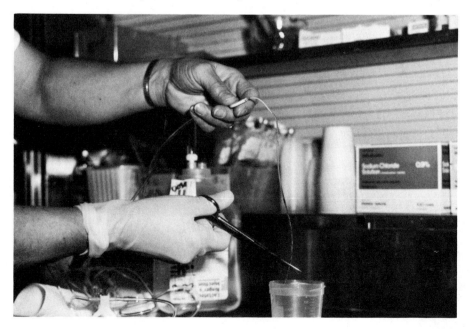

20. Remove and discard any solution that has been hanging for 24 hours.

21. Complete infusions of lipid emulsions within 12 hours.

22. Special precautions for intravascular pressure monitoring include the following:

    a. Use disposable components that are preassembled and sterile-packaged by manufacturer if possible.

    b. Use sterile transducer.

    c. Set up pressure-monitoring device just before use.

    d. Leave space between transducer head and dome dry unless priming is specified by the manufacturer.

    e. Use closed, continuous flush solution of fluid other than glucose.

    f. Maintain sterility of fluid column within cannula and tubing during calibration.

    g. Keep entire system closed as much as possible.

    h. If it is necessary to obtain blood specimen for analysis other than blood gas analysis, draw both samples at same time to minimize entry into system (Fig. 4–8).

begun immediately after preparation. Other factors such as the stability of the ingredients may dictate a shorter storage time.

IV solutions as well as flush solutions for pressure monitoring should be discarded after 24 hours.

Although the transducer head is not in direct contact with the fluid column, this precaution prevents cross-contamination from previous use of the transducer with another client.

Preparing the device hours or days in advance allows microorganisms to multiply during storage.

If priming is required, use bacteriostatic water. Glucose solutions support the growth of contaminating microorganisms. Saline causes the transducer head to rust.

Systems that require the use of a stopcock and syringe to flush need more frequent opening of the system than systems that do not.

Fig. 4–8 Obtaining blood sample from intravascular catheter.

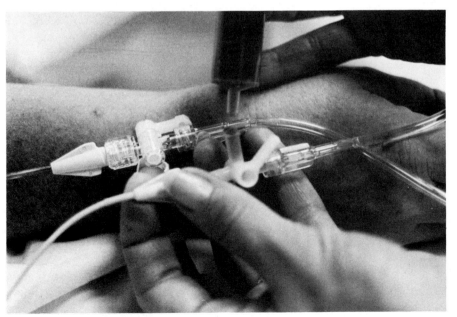

i. Replace tubing and dome if reflux of blood occurs during or after countershock.

j. Change or help physician to change devices used for pressure monitoring.

k. Carefully follow manufacturer's recommendations for appropriate disinfection or sterilization of reusable transducers.

23. Consult with physician about removal of any system that is no longer medically indicated.

Defibrillation or cardioversion may damage the protective membranes of some disposable domes.

Peripheral artery cannulas inserted through peripheral lines should be changed every 48 hours to 72 hours. Any cannula that is associated with infection should be changed immediately.

EVALUATION PHASE

ANTICIPATED OUTCOME	NURSING ACTIONS
Avoidance of infectious complications associated with intravascular devices	Evaluate vital signs every 4 hours to detect signs of infection. Suspect the intravascular system if the client develops fever or other signs of sepsis without known cause.

SELECTED REFERENCES   Guidelines for Prevention of Intravascular Infections. Atlanta, US Department of Health and Human Services (HHS Publication No. (CDC) 83-8314, 1983)

Roderick MA (ed): Infection Control in Critical Care. Rockville, MD, Aspen Publications, 1983

Infection control protocol for blood/body fluid precautions

BACKGROUND

Critical care clients and care-givers are at risk of exposure to disease that is transmitted by blood and body fluids. These infections include hepatitis B, hepatitis non-A and non-B, Creutzfeldt–Jakob disease, and Acquired Immune Deficiency Syndrome (AIDS).

The Centers for Disease Control (CDC) have issued guidelines for isolation that include blood/body fluid precautions as a specific category. The use of these protocols affords appropriate protection for both clients and staff. It is prudent professional practice to use these precautions during every exposure to blood or body fluids. It is the unknown carrier or asymptomatic client who is a serious infectious risk.

Objective

To prevent hospital cross-infection of diseases that may be transmitted by direct or indirect contact with infectious blood or body fluids

ASSESSMENT PHASE

- Does the client have an infectious disease that has been transmitted through blood or body fluids? (See list of diseases requiring precautions.)
- Is the client's hygiene poor? If so, a private room may be required.

PLANNING PHASE

EQUIPMENT

Gloves
Gowns
Puncture-resistant container for needle disposal (Fig. 4–9)
5.25% solution of sodium hypochlorite (household bleach)
CDC blood/body fluid precautions sign

CLIENT/FAMILY TEACHING

- Inform the client and family of the precautions and the rationale behind them.
- Assure them that the precautions will not alter the quality of the client's care. Stress

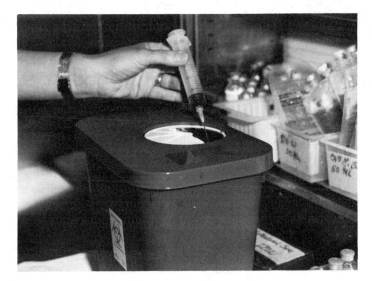

Fig. 4-9 Place intact needles and syringes in puncture-resistant container after use.

that it is the infectious agent—not the client—that will be isolated. Be nonjudgmental about the source of the client's infection (*e.g.,* AIDS).

Diseases requiring blood/body fluid precautions*

Acquired immune deficiency syndrome (AIDS)
Arthropodborne viral fevers (for example, dengue, yellow fever, and Colorado tick fever)
Babesiosis
Creutzfeldt-Jakob disease
Hepatitis B (including HBsAg antigen carrier)

Hepatitis, non-A, non-B
Leptospirosis
Malaria
Rat-bite fever
Relapsing fever
Syphilis, primary and secondary with skin and mucous membrane lesions

* A private room is indicated for blood/body fluid precautions if patient hygiene is poor. A patient with poor hygiene does not wash hands after touching infective material, contaminates the environment with infective material, or shares contaminated articles with other patients. In general, patients infected with the same organism may share a room. See Guideline for Isolation Precautions in Hospitals for details and for how long to apply precautions. (CDC Guidelines: Nosocomial Infections)

IMPLEMENTATION PHASE

NURSING ACTIONS	RATIONALE/AMPLIFICATION
1. Place "Blood/Body Fluid Precautions" sign on door or bed.	The sign is a guide for the client, family, and personnel.
2. Label outside of client's record with blood/body fluid precautions sticker.	
3. Label all interdepartmental communications (*e.g.,* laboratory or x-ray film requests) "Blood/Body Fluid Precautions."	Labeling alerts other departments to precautions.
4. Follow specifications on front of CDC card (see list of blood/body fluid precautions).	

EVALUATION PHASE

ANTICIPATED OUTCOMES	NURSING ACTIONS
1. Prevention of nosocomial transmission of blood/body fluid diseases	
2. Prevention of transmission of blood/body fluid diseases to hospital personnel	Monitor the infection-control techniques of hospital personnel as necessary.

SELECTED REFERENCES

Batten (Persons) C, Tabor R: Nursing the patient with AIDS. Canadian Nurses Journal 79:19–22, 1983

CDC Guidelines for Isolation Precautions in Hospitals. Atlanta, US Department of Health and Human Services (HHS Publication No. (CDC) 83-8314, 1983.

Blood/body fluid precautions

VISITORS—REPORT TO NURSES' STATION BEFORE ENTERING ROOM

1. Masks are not indicated.
2. Gowns are indicated if soiling with blood or body fluids is likely.
3. Gloves are indicated for touching blood or body fluids.
4. HANDS SHOULD BE WASHED IMMEDIATELY IF THEY ARE POTENTIALLY CONTAMINATED WITH BLOOD OR BODY FLUIDS AND BEFORE TAKING CARE OF ANOTHER PATIENT.
5. Articles contaminated with blood or body fluids should be discarded or bagged and labeled before being sent for decontamination and reprocessing.
6. Care should be taken to avoid needle-stick injuries. Used needles should not be recapped or bent; they should be placed in a prominently labeled, puncture-resistant container designated specifically for such disposal.
7. Blood spills should be cleaned up promptly with a solution of 5.25% sodium hypochlorite diluted 1:10 with water.

Hemodynamic pressure monitoring

INVASIVE TECHNIQUES

BACKGROUND

Invasive pressure-monitoring systems are widely used for bedside monitoring of hemodynamic changes in critically ill clients. One component of an intravascular monitoring system is a fluid-filled catheter, one end of which is placed within the vascular system. The catheter is connected to a transducer, which is an electronic device that converts physiological events (alterations in pressure) to electronic signals that can be displayed on an oscilloscope (Fig. 5–1).

Fig. 5–1 Transducer with disposable dome. (Courtesy Gould Inc., Oxnard, CA)

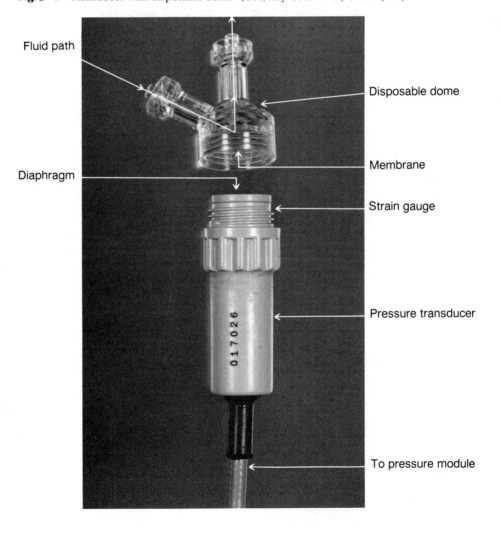

Fluid path

Disposable dome

Diaphragm

Membrane

Strain gauge

Pressure transducer

017026

To pressure module

To ensure accuracy and to allow for changes in atmospheric pressure, the transducer is periodically balanced and recalibrated. When measuring pressures, the transducer should be positioned at the level of the cardiac chamber in which the catheter tip is positioned. If the transducer is positioned too high, hydrostatic pressure and gravity will cause an erroneously low reading. A false high reading will result if the transducer is positioned too low, because of hydrostatic pressure on the transducer. The transducer should be positioned at the *phlebostatic axis,* which is measured from the fourth intercostal space in the midaxillary line, for accurate monitoring. This is the level of the right atrium. Mark this point with a magic marker to establish a consistent reference point (Fig. 5–2). Use a carpenter's level to check the position of the transducer in relation to the mark on the chest. Readings can be taken in any position, although the supine position is preferred. Take serial readings in the same position.

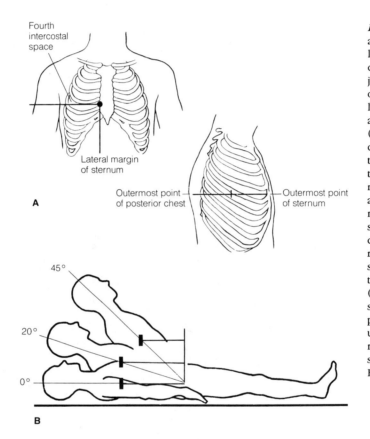

Fig. 5–2 (*A*) The phlebostatic axis is crossing of two reference lines: a line from fourth intercostal space at point where it joins sternum, drawn out to side of body beneath axilla; and a line midway between anterior and posterior surfaces of chest. (*B*) The phlebostatic level is indicated by a horizontal line through phlebostatic axis. The transducer or zero mark on manometer must be level with this axis to record accurate measurements. As client moves from supine to erect position, the chest moves and therefore the reference level. The phlebostatic level remains horizontal through same reference point. (After Shinn JA, Woods SL, Huseby JS: Effect of intermittent positive pressure ventilation upon pulmonary artery and pulmonary capillary wedge pressures in acutely ill patients. Heart Lung 8(2):324, 1979)

A variety of equipment is available for pressure monitoring, and much of this equipment is disposable. A continuous low-pressure flush system is used to prevent clot formation within arterial catheters. Clot formation inhibits free transmission of pressure waves and increases the risk of embolization. To minimize the risk of contamination or air leaks and to increase accuracy, use high-pressure tubing with as few connections and stopcocks as possible.

HEMODYNAMIC PARAMETERS

Hemodynamic parameters that are commonly used to assess critically ill clients include the peripheral arterial pressure, central venous pressure, pulmonary artery pressure, pulmonary capillary wedge pressure, left atrial pressure, cardiac output, cardiac index, and mixed venous oxygen saturation.

ARTERIAL PRESSURE

Continuous arterial pressure is monitored by cannulating an artery using an intravenous (IV) cannula. The device is sutured or taped in place and connected to a continuous flush device to maintain patency. An arterial waveform is displayed on the oscilloscope if the system is free of air bubbles, clots, and tubing kinks (Fig. 5–3). The

Fig. 5-3 Arterial pressure tracing.

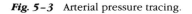

Systolic peak

Dicrotic notch

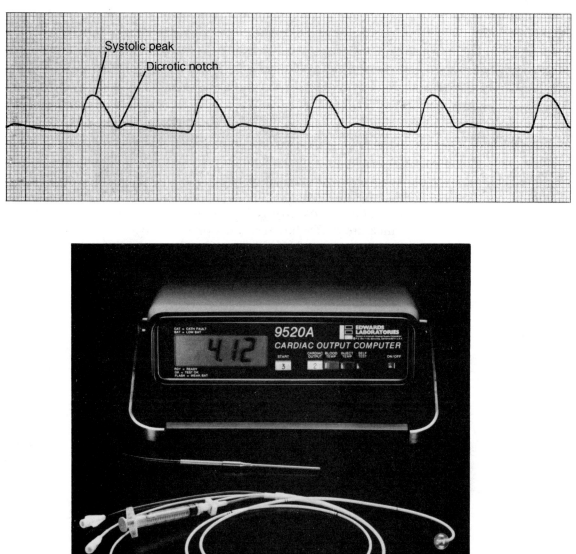

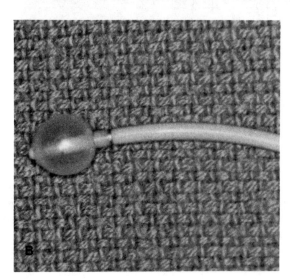

Fig. 5-4 (*A*) Swan–Ganz thermodilution catheter and cardiac output computer. (*B*) Enlargement of tip of Swan–Ganz pulmonary artery catheter. (*A*, courtesy American Edwards Laboratories, Santa Ana, CA; *B*, photograph taken by Keith Mitchell, Amarillo VA Medical Center)

normal range for arterial pressure is 100 mm Hg to 140 mm Hg systolic, 60 mm Hg to 80 mm Hg diastolic, and 70 mm Hg to 90 mm Hg mean.

PULMONARY ARTERY AND CENTRAL VENOUS PRESSURES

Pulmonary artery (PA) pressure is monitored continuously using a balloon-tipped, flow-directed pulmonary artery catheter (Fig. 5–4). The PA catheter is inserted into the PA under fluoroscopy through an intrathoracic vein. Inflation of the balloon helps to position the catheter in the PA. With the balloon deflated, the PA pressure is continuously displayed on the oscilloscope using the distal port on the catheter. Momentary inflation of the balloon wedges the catheter in the PA and provides a typical pulmonary capillary wedge (PCW) pressure tracing on the monitor (PCW pressure may also be referred to as pulmonary artery wedge [PAW] pressure.) (Fig. 5–5). The catheter that opens beyond the inflated balloon indirectly reflects pressures distal to the PA, that is, the left atrial filling pressure. The PCW pressure therefore measures left ventricular function indirectly; mean PCW pressure and left atrial pressure (LAP) closely approximate left ventricular end-diastolic pressure (LVEDP) in clients who have normal left ventricular and mitral valve function.

Fig. 5–5   Flow-directed catheter positions with corresponding pressure tracings. *RA*, right atrium; *RV*, right ventricle; *PA*, pulmonary artery; *PAW*, pulmonary artery wedge.

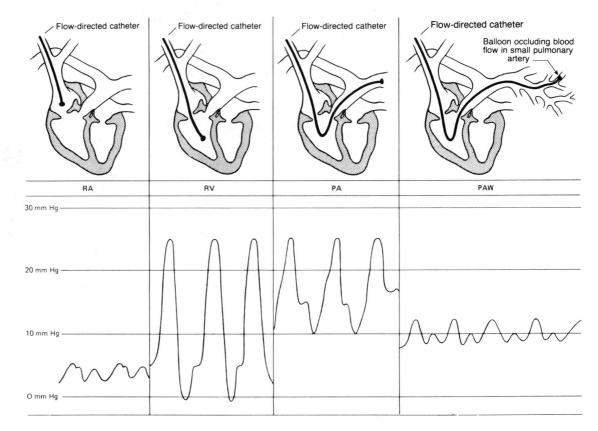

The normal range for PA pressure is 20 mm Hg to 30 mm Hg systolic and 8 mm Hg to 12 mm Hg diastolic. The range for PCW pressure is 4 mm Hg to 12 mm Hg, with a gradient of less than 5 mm Hg between PA diastolic and PCW pressures. PA catheters are available with a thermistor tip for cardiac output (CO) measurements and with a pacing electrode if pacing is required.

Central venous pressure (CVP) is determined using the proximal port that terminates in the right atrium. CVP can also be monitored using a fluid-filled manometer connected to a subclavian catheter and can be kept patent by a continuous IV infusion. The normal range for CVP is 2 mm Hg to 6 mm Hg (3 cm to 8 cm water pressure). To convert mm Hg to cm water pressure, multiply mm Hg by 1.34.

LEFT ATRIAL PRESSURE

Left atrial pressure (LAP) is monitored by a catheter that is inserted into the left atrium (LA) during open-heart surgery. Monitoring LAP is more hazardous than monitoring other hemodynamic pressures because the potential for an embolus to be released into the systemic circulation exists. Particular attention should be given to preventing air bubbles in the lines. The normal range for LAP is 4 mm Hg to 12 mm Hg (mean). LA catheters are also connected to continuous flush devices to prevent clotting.

CARDIAC OUTPUT AND CARDIAC INDEX

The cardiac output (CO) is a measure of the amount of blood pumped by the heart and is expressed as liters per minute. The normal resting CO is 4 liters to 8 liters/minute. The output of the left ventricle (LV) and right ventricle (RV) is essentially the same, unless an intracardiac shunt is present. Methods for measuring CO include the Fick method, the thermodilution method, and the indicator-dilution method. With the advent of flow-directed PA catheters, it is practical to use the indicator-dilution method in the critical care area. When divided by body surface area (BSA), which is obtained using a nomogram, CO becomes the cardiac index (CI). A normal CI is more than 2.8 liters/minute/square meter.

A range of hemodynamic parameters can be used to calculate other parameters. Calculators that can be programmed to compute hemodynamic parameters are available. The systemic vascular resistance (SVR), an indicator of vasoconstriction or vasodilation, can be hand calculated using the following formula:

$$\frac{(\text{Mean arterial pressure} - \text{PCW pressure}) \times 80}{\text{CO}}$$

The normal range is 900 dynes to 1440 dynes/sec/cm^{-5}. If the SVR is high, warming a cold vasoconstricted client may help to reduce impedance against ventricular functioning. A vasodilator such as sodium nitroprusside may be required, or, in extreme cases, the afterload may be reduced by using an intra-aortic balloon pump (IABP). Vasopressors may be required if the SVR is low.

PRELOAD AND AFTERLOAD

Preload is defined as the initial stretch of the fibers of the LV before ventricular contraction, which is called the *Frank–Starling mechanism*. Measures of PCW pressure, left ventricular filling pressure, and end-diastolic volume are indicators of preload. *Afterload* is the resistance (aortic pressure) against which the LV must pump in order to eject blood. An increase in the afterload causes a corresponding reduction in CO.

Both mechanical (IABP) and pharmacologic means are used to increase CO by increasing preload and decreasing afterload. Increasing preload increases myocardial fiber stretch, which improves myocardial contractility. In an effort to support the pumping action of the failing heart, dopamine may be administered to increase contractility (preload), while sodium nitroprusside is administered concurrently to decrease afterload. The net effect is an increase in stroke volume and CO.

Unfortunately, left ventricular pressures cannot be measured at the bedside because of the danger of embolism. Left ventricular performance may be evaluated clinically by administering a fluid challenge. In uncomplicated hypovolemia, fluids may be administered until both PCW pressure and CVP are adequate. The client who is experiencing heart failure will remain hypotensive in the presence of rising CVP and PCW pressure.

CONTINUOUS MEASUREMENT OF MIXED VENOUS OXYGEN SATURATION

Mixed venous oxygen saturation can be measured continuously using a five-lumen, 7.5F, balloon-tipped, thermodilution, fiberoptic PA catheter. The ability to measure the oxygen saturation *in vivo* is important in the early detection of hemodynamic changes. Changes in the mixed venous oxygen saturation ($S\bar{v}O_2$) occur up to 30 minutes before clinical symptoms appear. Hard copy is available so that trends can be recorded.

Transducer setup: up to two pressures

Objective
To continuously monitor a single intravascular pressure, or two pressures alternately

ASSESSMENT PHASE
- Why does the client require intravascular pressure monitoring (*e.g.*, heart failure, open-heart surgery, shock)?
- How many pressures will be monitored? Will a single transducer be adequate, or will a multiple transducer setup be required?

PRECAUTIONS
- **Be sure that all air bubbles are eliminated from the lines. This could be a source of air embolus or inaccurate pressure readings.**
- **Maintain the sterility of the fluid path of the pressure-monitoring setup.**

PLANNING PHASE

EQUIPMENT
Pressure transducer (sterile)*
Transducer holder mounted on IV stand
Disposable dome*
Intraflow (or similar constant flush device)*
IV administration set (microdrip)*
Heparinized normal saline (250 ml normal saline/250 units heparin)
Three-way stopcocks — 2*
Protective stopcock caps*
Pressure tubing (approximately 60 cm [24 inches])*
Bacteriostatic water in syringe
Pressure-administration cuff
Pressure-monitoring module
For a transducer with direct client mounting, substitute the following:
    Direct-mounting transducer (sterile)
    Transducer mounting clip
    Pressure tubing (approximately 15 cm [6 inches])

CLIENT/FAMILY TEACHING
- Answer the client's questions about the reasons for pressure monitoring.
- Explain the pressure monitoring setup using diagrams and intravascular devices as appropriate. If the client's condition does not allow participation, discuss the procedure with family members.
- Reassure the client and family about the complex equipment and extra alarms that may be used to monitor pressure.
- Reassure the client that the monitoring devices should not cause discomfort.

IMPLEMENTATION PHASE

NURSING ACTIONS	RATIONALE/AMPLIFICATION
1. Prepare transducer.	
a. Remove protective cap from transducer.	
b. Place a few drops of sterile water on transducer diaphragm (Fig. 5–6).	Normal saline may cause rust. Use alcohol if directed by manufacturer's instructions.
c. Screw on transducer dome firmly (Fig. 5–7).	
2. Place prepared transducer in transducer holder on IV stand.	For a transducer with direct client mounting, connect the transducer to the mounting clip.

* Double quantity is needed if two pressures will be monitored from the same transducer.

Fig. 5-6 (*A*) Priming transducer dome with sterile water. (*B*) Priming client-mounting transducer dome.

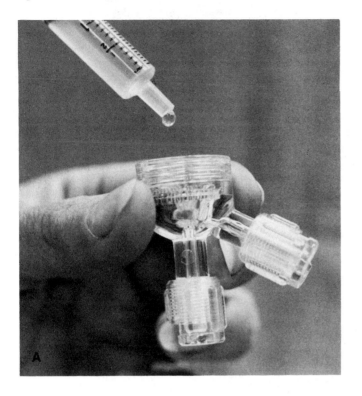

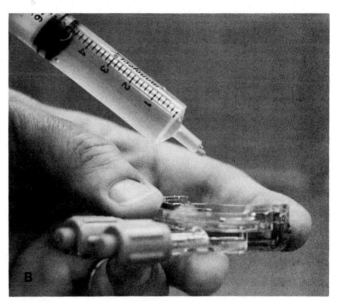

Fig. 5-7 (*A*) Connecting disposable dome to transducer. (*B*) Connecting disposable dome to client-mounting transducer.

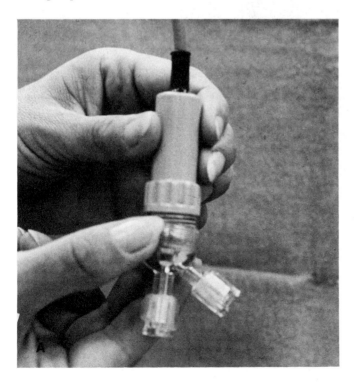

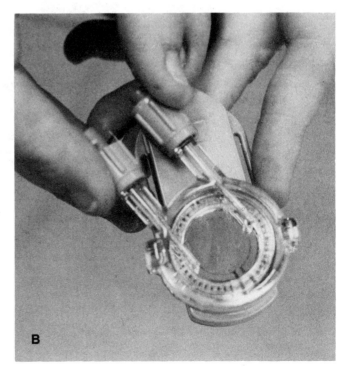

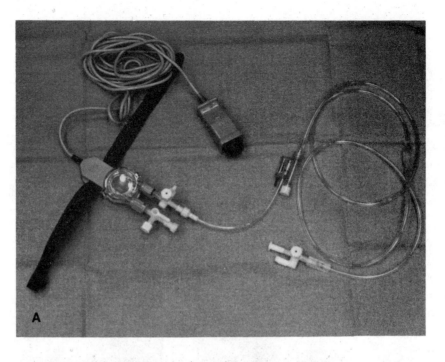

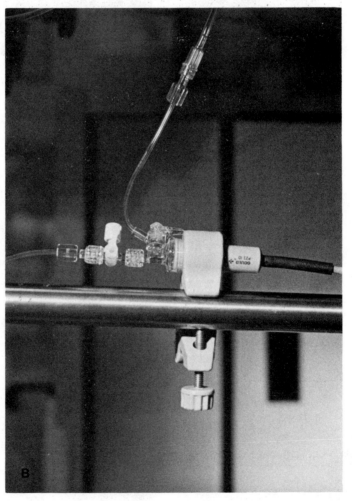

Fig. 5-8 (*A*) Assembled transducer. (*B*) Disposable dome.

3. Connect transducer cable to pressure module. Turn on pressure module.

4. Assemble transducer, sterile stopcocks, continuous infusion device, and pressure tubing as shown in Figure 5–8.

5. Connect IV tubing to normal saline solution and invert bag. Squeeze bag to displace air into IV tubing.

6. Hang normal saline solution on IV stand. Prime tubing and close clamp.

7. Connect IV tubing to continuous infusion device (Fig. 5–8). Open IV clamp.

8. Fast flush system to remove air from stopcock ports and lines using gravity pressure only (Fig. 5–9).

Allow at least 5 minutes for transducer to warm up.

Maintain the sterility of the fluid path at all times. Be sure that the connections are secure to prevent air from entering the system.

If an air-free solution source is not used, air may be forced into the monitoring line when the solution is exhausted, causing an air embolus.

Do not use a solution containing glucose because of the potential for microbial growth.

For a transducer with client mounting, proceed with the following steps:

a. Attach continuous infusion device to the flush solution.

b. Attach the stopcock to the male adapter or to continuous infusion device.

c. Flush air from continuous infusion device with the fast-flush valve.

d. Wet the transducer dome with the flush solution.

e. Attach the transducer to the female adapter of continuous infusion device.

Fig. 5–9 Flushing air from stopcock port.

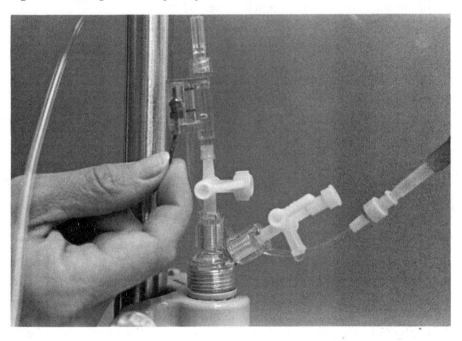

9. Alternately open and close stopcocks and remove protective cap from pressure tubing while flushing.

10. Cap client connection of pressure tubing again.

11. Pressurize solution source by pumping pressure administration cuff to 300 mm Hg.

Using a piece of pressure tubing longer than 120 cm (48 inches) adversely affects the system's response.

Make sure that the drip chamber does not fill completely during pressurization.

12. Balance transducer.

   a. Place transducer level with right atrium.

   b. Turn transducer venting stopcock so that transducer is open to air. Close remaining stopcock to continuous infusion device.

   c. Balance transducer at zero according to manufacturer's instructions.

   Observe the oscilloscope and adjust it to zero on the scale.

13. Calibrate transducer (if required).

   Some transducers are precalibrated.

   a. Set pressure range on control module.

   PA/venous pressures should be set at 0 to 75 mm Hg. Arterial pressures should be set at 0 to 300 mm Hg.

   b. Calibrate transducer according to manufacturer's instructions, adjusting appropriate control on pressure module.

   During calibration the transducer output is compared with a pressure of known value. Use a carpenter's level to align the air–fluid interface with the right atrium (RA). This is the level of the phlebostatic axis.

   c. Close transducer venting stopcock to air.

   d. Cover all stopcock ports with sterile caps.

   This reduces the chance of contamination.

14. Join client connector on pressure tubing with invasive pressure device.

   Be sure that the transducer is positioned level with the RA.

15. Open remaining stopcock to transducer and client.

   Observe the monitor for the appropriate waveform.

16. Rebalance and recalibrate transducer 30 minutes after monitoring begins.

17. If client will not be connected to transducer at this time, leave transducer venting stopcock open to air after balancing/calibration. Leave other stopcock closed to continuous infusion device and pressure tubing.

   Venting the transducer to air prevents pressure buildup and potential damage to the transducer.

18. When ready to connect client to transducer, rebalance and recalibrate transducer.

19. To monitor two pressures using one transducer, proceed as follows:

   a. Assemble a second flush system (steps 4 through 10).

   Connect additional IV tubing to the medication port of the IV bag.

   b. Connect continuous infusion device assembly to transducer venting stopcock (Fig. 5–10).

RELATED NURSING CARE

NURSING ACTIONS	RATIONALE/AMPLIFICATION
1. Periodically check system visually for proper fluid source pressure, flow rate, and leaks.	A small leak can result in a misrepresentation of the actual continuous flow through the catheter.
2. Periodically test system for dynamic response by observing pressure waveform on oscilloscope while alternately activating fast-flush valve.	Observe for a high-quality square waveform. If the fast flush shows an overdampened system, check the system for air in the line, leaks, or electronic equipment malfunction.
3. Change tubing and continuous flush device every 48 hours, when changing dressing on insertion site.	Changing of tubing and continuous flush device is an infection-control precaution.
4. Change flush solution and dressing every 48 to 72 hours.	Changing of the flush solution prevents microbial growth.
5. Label tubing and flush solution with date and time of change.	

Fig. 5–10   Setup for monitoring two pressures using one transducer.

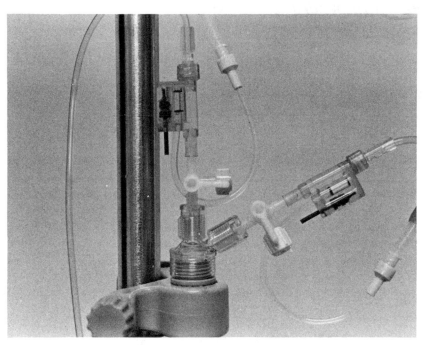

EVALUATION PHASE

ANTICIPATED OUTCOMES	NURSING ACTIONS
1. Prevention of complications of invasive pressure monitoring	Monitor for potential complications including sepsis, hemorrhage/tubing separation, thrombus formation, air embolism, vascular damage, and electromicroshock. Evaluate the arterial/venous insertion site for infection during each shift. Palpate through the dressing for excessive tenderness. Culture the intravascular device if it is removed for suspected infection.
2. Titration of fluid and medications according to serial pressure readings	Ensure the accuracy of readings. Record serial pressures and discuss changes requiring alterations in therapy with the physician.

PRODUCT AVAILABILITY

INTRAFLOW CONTINUOUS FLUSH SYSTEM

Sorenson Research Company

PRESSURE TUBING

North American Instrument Corporation, Medical Products Division
Cobe Laboratories

DISPOSABLE PRESSURE MONITORING SET

Gould Inc., Medical Products Division

PRESSURE MONITORING EQUIPMENT

Hewlett-Packard, Medical Products Group

MICROCOMPUTER PROGRAMS

American Edwards Laboratories
CV Mosby Co

Transducer setup: multiple pressures

Objective
To continuously monitor multiple intravascular pressures

ASSESSMENT PHASE
- Why does the client require intravascular pressure monitoring (*e.g.*, open-heart surgery, left ventricular failure with IABP)?
- How many pressures will be monitored? Will a single transducer setup be preferable to a manifold/multiple pressure setup?

PRECAUTIONS
- **Be certain that air is flushed from the lines. Air that remains in the lines can cause an air embolism.**
- **Maintain the sterility of the fluid path to prevent sepsis.**

PLANNING PHASE

EQUIPMENT
Multiple-channel pressure module
Sterile manifold mounted on IV stand
Heparinized normal saline (250 ml normal saline/250 units heparin) Two lines can be flushed from each bag of normal saline (see Fig. 5–10).
Pressure-administration cuff—1 cuff for each IV bag
Bacteriostatic water in syringe
Transducer (sterile)*
Intraflow continuous flush system (or similar constant infusion device)*
IV administration set, microdrip*
High-pressure tubing (60 cm, or 24 inches, in length)
Stopcocks—2*
Protective stopcock caps—2*
10-ml syringe

CLIENT/FAMILY TEACHING
See previous section on Transducer Setup: Up to Two Pressures.

IMPLEMENTATION PHASE

NURSING ACTIONS	RATIONALE/AMPLIFICATION
1. Prepare transducers.	
a. Remove protective cap from transducer.	
b. Place few drops of sterile water on transducer diaphragm.	Normal saline may cause rust. Use alcohol if directed by manufacturer's instructions.
c. Screw on transducer dome firmly.	Excessive force will crack the dome.
2. Secure prepared transducers to manifold.	
3. Connect transducer cables to pressure module. Turn on module.	Allow at least 5 minutes for the transducers to warm up so that they may be accurately calibrated.
4. Assemble transducer, sterile stopcocks, continuous infusion device, pressure tubing, manifold, and 10-ml syringe as shown in Figure 5–11.	Assemble a separate setup for each pressure to be monitored.
5. Connect IV tubing to normal saline solution. Invert bag. Squeeze bag to displace air into IV tubing.	If an air-free solution source is not used, air may be forced into the monitoring line when the solution is exhausted, causing an embolus.
6. Prime IV tubing and close clamp. Insert normal saline in pressure cuff and hang on IV stand.	Pressurize the normal saline solution to 300 mm Hg.

* Double quantity is required for each pressure to be monitored.

Fig. 5-11 Assembled transducer connected to manifold. (*A*) Manifold. (*B*) Air–fluid interface. (*C*) Transducer dome stopcock. (*D*) Disposable dome. (*E*) Air-venting stopcock. (*F*) Transducer. (*G*) Ten-milliliter syringe. (*H*) Tubing to intravascular device. (*I*) Tubing to IV flush solution. (*J*) High-pressure tubing. (*K*) Ten-milliliter syringe. (*L*) Cable to monitor. (*M*) Continuous infusion device. (*N*) Manifold stopcock. (Drawing by Ann Kime)

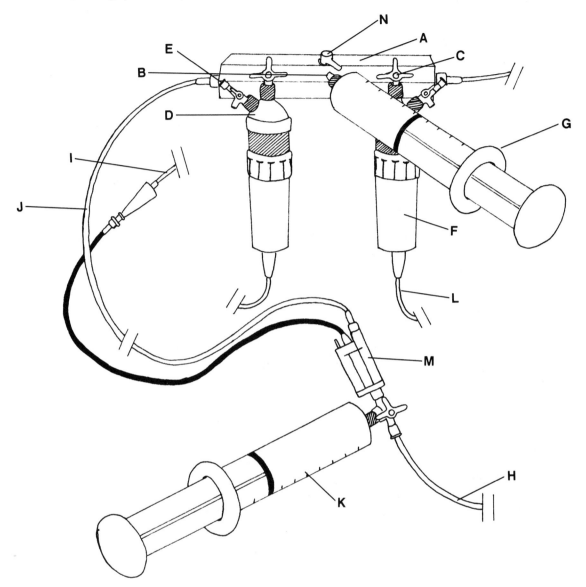

7. Connect IV tubing to continuous infusion device.

8. Open manifold stopcocks to syringe and one preassembled pressure monitoring setup.

9. Open IV clamp. Flush air from system with a fast-flush valve.

Alternately open and close the stopcocks. Observe and control the filling of the syringe.

10. Close manifold stopcock to primed system.

11. Open manifold stopcock to prefilled syringe and transducer. Open transducer stopcock to air.

12. Flush transducer dome and stopcock using syringe.

13. Close transducer stopcock to air, and close manifold stopcock to transducer.

Repeat steps 6 to 13 for each pressure system.

14. Balance each transducer.

   a. Place air–fluid interface stopcock of transducer level with RA.

The RA is at the level of the phlebostatic axis.

   b. Close manifold stopcocks to syringe and client system.

   c. Open transducer stopcock to air.

   d. Balance system according to manufacturer's instructions.

Adjust the tracing to zero on the monitor. The system should be balanced at room temperature to ensure accuracy. Changes in barometric pressure affect the pressure-monitoring system.

15. If client will not be connected at this time, leave system open to air. Cap stopcocks.

This step prevents pressure buildup in transducer.

16. Calibrate each transducer (if necessary).

Some transducers are calibrated automatically, and this step is not required.

   a. Set pressure range on control module.

PA/venous pressures should be set at 0 to 75 mm Hg. Arterial pressures should be set at 0 to 300 mm Hg.

   b. Calibrate according to manufacturer's instructions.

Adjust the pressure tracing on the module to preassigned values.

   c. Close transducer stopcock to air.

During calibration the transducer output is compared with a pressure of known value.

   d. Open manifold stopcocks to transducer and client.

17. Remove client connector cap and attach pressure monitoring system to intravascular device while flushing with fast-flush valve.

This prevents air from entering the system. Observe for an appropriate tracing on the monitor.

18. Cap all stopcock ports.

Repeat steps 14 to 18 for each pressure to be monitored.

19. Rebalance and recalibrate transducer 30 minutes after monitoring begins.

Be sure that the transducer is at the level of the phlebostatic axis.

RELATED NURSING CARE   See previous section on Transducer Setup: Up to Two Pressures.

EVALUATION PHASE   See previous section on Transducer Setup: Up to Two Pressures.

Disposable transducer setup

Objective
To continuously monitor a single intravascular pressure using a disposable transducer

ASSESSMENT PHASE
- Why does the client require intravascular pressure monitoring (*e.g.*, heart failure, open-heart surgery, shock)?
- How many pressures will be monitored continuously? Will a single- or a multiple-pressure setup be required?

PRECAUTION
- **Inspect all fluid-filled portions of the system, including the tubing and stopcock ports, to verify that bubbles have been eliminated. This could be a source of air embolism.**

PLANNING PHASE

EQUIPMENT

Pressure-monitoring module
IV flush solution (250 ml normal saline/250 units aqueous heparin)
Pressure infusion cuff

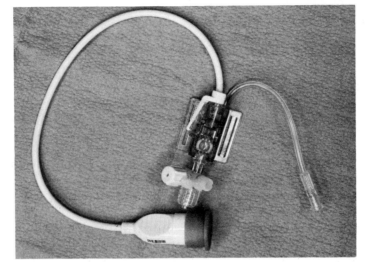

Fig. 5–12 Disposable transducer.

IV tubing (microdrip)
Pressure tubing
Stopcocks
Disposable transducer (Fig. 5–12)
Transducer mount (for IV pole or individual client mounting)
IV stand

CLIENT/FAMILY TEACHING   See previous section on Transducer Setup: Up to Two Pressures.

**IMPLEMENTATION
PHASE**

NURSING ACTIONS	RATIONALE/AMPLIFICATION
1. Connect IV tubing to normal saline solution and invert bag. Squeeze bag to displace air into IV tubing.	If an air-free solution source is not used, air may be forced into the monitoring line when the solution is exhausted, causing an air embolus.
2. Prime tubing and close clamp.	
3. Insert solution bag into pressure infusion cuff and hang on IV stand. Pressurize solution to 300 mm Hg.	Note that the drip chamber does not fill completely during pressurization because this will prevent verification of the flow rate.
4. Attach IV tubing to short length of IV tubing attached to transducer. Attach pressure tubing to client connector of transducer.	
5. Hold transducer vertically with stopcock at top. Open IV clamp and flush system using fast-flush valve.	Gently tap the system to help eliminate bubbles.
6. Replace all vented caps on side ports of stopcocks and distal end of pressure tubing with nonvented caps.	
7. Mount transducer on IV pole with stopcock level with phlebostatic axis.	*Alternative method:* Mount the transducer directly on client.
8. Attach electrical connector of transducer to monitor cable. Turn on monitor.	
9. Balance and calibrate system according to manufacturer's instructions.	Use the transducer three-way stopcock as the air–fluid interface. Open the unused port to air and remove the nonvented cap before balancing.
10. Close transducer to air and calibrate transducer.	The transducer will be calibrated to a known value.

11. Connect distal end of pressure tubing to intravascular device while flushing with fast-flush valve.

This prevents an air embolus.

12. Change disposable transducer every 48 hours, when tubing and dressing are changed.

This prevents potential bacterial growth.

RELATED NURSING CARE   See previous section on Transducer Setup: Up to Two Pressures.

EVALUATION PHASE   See previous section on Transducer Setup: Up to Two Pressures.

PRODUCT AVAILABILITY   DISPOSABLE TRANSDUCER SYSTEM
Gould Inc.

Arterial line

Objectives
To obtain continuous data that reflect the hemodynamic status of the critically ill client
To assess therapeutic interventions through continuous arterial pressure monitoring
To obtain repeated arterial blood samples with minimal discomfort to the client

ASSESSMENT PHASE
- Does an Allen's test demonstrate that arterial circulation will not be compromised by insertion of a catheter into the radial or brachial artery?
- Will circulation to the lower extremity be compromised by the insertion of an arterial line into the femoral artery?
- What is the arterial pressure as measured by a sphygmomanometer? Direct arterial pressure should be approximately 10 mm Hg higher than this reading because direct arterial pressure can be measured more accurately.

PRECAUTIONS
- **Be sure that all air bubbles are flushed from the system. Air bubbles can cause air embolus or inaccurate readings.**
- **Check the system for tight connections to avoid severe blood loss.**

PLANNING PHASE
EQUIPMENT
IV cannula (18-gauge, catheter-over-needle type)
Razor and soap
Iodophor solution
Xylocaine 1%
Skin suture on small curved cutting needle
Sterile gloves
Minor-procedure tray
    Syringes and needles
    Sterile towels
    Suture instruments
    4 × 4s
Calibrated and balanced transducer (See previous section on Transducer Setup: Up to Two Pressures.)
Sterile stopcocks — 2
Pressure monitor and recorder
Hypoallergenic tape or transparent dressing

CLIENT/FAMILY TEACHING
- Answer questions about arterial pressure monitoring.
- Reassure the client and family regarding the complex equipment required for monitoring, as well as additional alarms.
- Reassure the client that the procedure should cause only minor discomfort and that a local anesthetic will be administered.

IMPLEMENTATION PHASE

NURSING ACTIONS	RATIONALE/AMPLIFICATION
1. Shave insertion site and prepare with iodophor solution.	
2. Open minor-procedure tray on bedside table to provide a sterile field.	
3. Assist physician with sterile gloves and help to draw up Xylocaine 1%.	
4. Provide support to client during procedure.	The physician will inject a local anesthetic. The IV cannula is inserted into the chosen artery after palpating the pulse. When backflow is observed, the catheter is threaded into the artery over the needle, and the needle is removed. Backflow is prevented by occluding the catheter with a gloved finger.
5. Remove protective cap from pressure tubing that is connected to transducer setup. Attach two stopcocks and flush ports by pulling fast-flush valve while alternately opening and closing stopcock ports. Open stopcocks to client.	Observe the drip chamber and the client connector for a continuous flush of approximately 3 ml/hour.
6. Allow catheter to backflow and pull fast-flush valve while attaching connector to catheter.	This prevents the introduction of air into the system. The physician should support the catheter during this procedure to prevent accidental removal.
7. Observe for arterial tracing on monitor.	
8. After physician has sutured catheter in place, dress insertion site with iodophor ointment (if used), 4 × 4, and occlusive dressing.	*Alternate method:* Apply a transparent dressing directly to the insertion site.
9. Rebalance and recalibrate transducer to ensure accuracy.	Place the transducer at the phlebostatic axis (see Fig. 5–2).
10. Monitor arterial pressure.	Select systolic, diastolic, or mean on the pressure monitor and set the alarm limits 20 mm Hg above and below client's range. The normal range for arterial pressure is 100 mm Hg to 140 mm Hg systolic, and 70 mm Hg to 90 mm Hg diastolic.
11. Check appearance of arterial waveform.	The dicrotic notch should be at least one third the height of the systolic peak. Low CO is indicated by a dicrotic notch that is less than one third the height of the systolic peak. Decreased myocardial contractility, aortic stenosis, and a dampened tracing are indicated by a delay in the rising of the anacrotic notch. Physiological effects include variations in arterial waves caused by respiration, hypotension, and arrhythmias.

RELATED NURSING CARE

NURSING ACTIONS	RATIONALE/AMPLIFICATION
1. Flush with fast flush each time line is manipulated, or every hour.	Flushing maintains the patency of the line.

2. Control infusion rate at 3 ml to 4 ml/hour.

Check pressurization of system periodically. Do not record the amount of flush solution used on input and output form because it is not a significant amount.

3. If clotting of catheter is suspected, attach syringe and attempt to withdraw clot.

Caution: Flushing the arterial line with a syringe may introduce an embolism.

4. If air bubbles are observed in line, remove by flushing with fast flush through open stopcock port.

Air bubbles may cause an embolism.

5. Integrate arterial pressure readings with other hemodynamic parameters.

Report significant changes in the client's condition or response to therapy to the physician.

6. Recalibrate transducer each time client is moved with respect to transducer, and recalibrate once during each shift.

7. Rebalance once during each shift.

8. Check arterial-line pressure against cuff pressure every 4 hours.

Arterial-line pressure should be approximately 10 mm Hg higher than cuff pressure because arterial-line pressure can be measured more accurately than cuff pressure. Evaluate the possible reasons for this difference (*e.g.*, catheter position, dampened tracing, inaccurately balanced and calibrated transducer, transducer unaligned with phlebostatic axis).

9. Change dressing and pressure monitoring setup, including tubing, disposable dome, stopcocks, and continuous infusion device, every 48 hours.

This controls infection. Label setup with time and date of change.

10. Change flush solution every 24 hours. Label bag with date and time of change.

This prevents bacterial growth.

11. Discontinue arterial line.

a. Remove dressing.

Frequently assess arterial circulation and check the pressure dressing following discontinuation of the arterial line.

b. Close transducer stopcock that is nearest to client.

c. Remove sutures with sterile suture set.

d. Withdraw arterial cannula and hold pressure on site for 5 minutes or until bleeding stops.

e. Apply sterile pressure dressing.

EVALUATION PHASE

ANTICIPATED OUTCOMES	NURSING ACTIONS
1. Prevention of complications of arterial monitoring	Evaluate for signs and symptoms of complications (*e.g.*, sepsis, bleeding/tubing separation, embolus, electromicroshock, and vascular damage).
2. Titration of fluids and medication according to serial pressure readings	Record serial pressure readings. Report significant readings to the physician.

Obtaining blood sample from arterial line

Objective
To obtain an arterial blood sample aseptically and without discomfort to the client

ASSESSMENT PHASE	• Is an arterial pressure line in place? • If a specimen is needed for arterial blood gas (ABG) analysis, has the laboratory or respiratory therapy been notified so that a blood gas analyzer can be prepared? • Is an arterial sample suitable for the required laboratory test?
PRECAUTIONS	• **Use sterile technique.** • **Avoid introduction of air into the lines.**
PLANNING PHASE EQUIPMENT	10-ml syringe 6-ml syringe Needle Blood tube (if required) Emesis basin with ice
CLIENT/FAMILY TEACHING	• Tell the client that the sample will be drawn through an arterial catheter and explain the technique. • Answer questions regarding the proposed laboratory tests.

IMPLEMENTATION PHASE

NURSING ACTIONS	RATIONALE/AMPLIFICATION
1. If double stopcock setup is not in place, insert two stopcocks into line nearest to arterial catheter.	The double stopcock setup allows blood to be obtained using a closed system.
2. Remove stopcock caps and keep sterile.	Turn off the arterial pressure alarms.
3. Insert 10-ml syringe into proximal stopcock port to clear line.	
4. Insert 6-ml syringe into distal stopcock port to obtain blood sample.	
5. Close stopcocks to transducer so that blood and flush solution can be drawn into 10-ml syringe (Fig. 5–13).	This clears the line of saline solution, which would cause inaccurate laboratory results.
6. Close distal stopcock to 10-ml syringe and open it to 6-ml syringe. Allow arterial pressure to fill sample syringe (Fig. 5–14).	
7. Readjust stopcocks and flush line with fast-flush valve.	
8. Remove specimen syringe.	
9. Attach needle to specimen syringe and fill blood tube. If specimen is to be used for ABG analysis, remove air bubbles from syringe and cap immediately.	Place the ABG blood sample on ice during transportation.
10. Adjust stopcock to allow flushing of stopcock to 10-ml syringe.	
11. Close stopcock to 10-ml syringe. Remove syringe and attach it to specimen stopcock (Fig. 5–15).	
12. Flush specimen stopcock, close stopcock to syringe and remove syringe.	
13. Return stopcocks to monitoring position. Flush line with fast-flush valve. Cap stopcock ports.	
14. Reset arterial pressure alarms.	Observe the monitor for the return of an arterial pressure tracing.

Fig. 5-13 Close stopcocks to transducer and aspirate 10-ml syringe to clear line of flush solution.

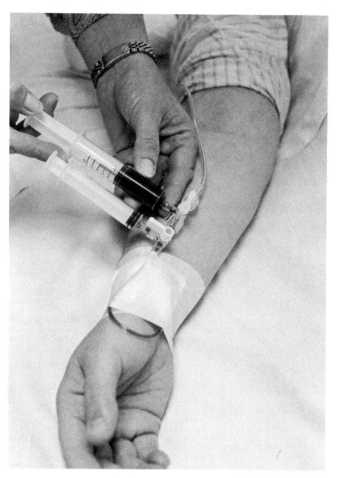

Fig. 5-14 Open stopcocks to catheter and 6-ml sample syringe. Arterial pressure will fill sample syringe.

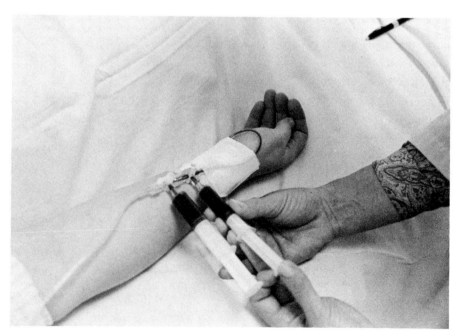

Fig. 5-15 Remove flush syringe and attach to specimen stopcock.

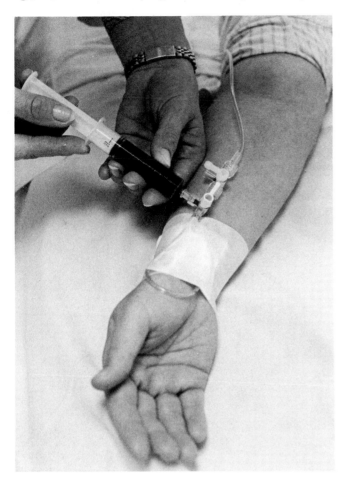

EVALUATION PHASE

ANTICIPATED OUTCOMES	NURSING ACTIONS
1. Prevention of client discomfort caused by frequent venipunctures	Evaluate which blood samples can be obtained from an arterial line.
2. Prevention of infection caused by break in system	Monitor for breaks in technique and evaluate for signs of infection.

Pulmonary artery catheter

Objectives

To assess LVEDP indirectly (when mitral valve function is normal) using a balloon-tipped, flow-directed catheter inserted by a cutdown into the PA

To assess hemodynamic changes in response to therapeutic intervention

To assess CO

To obtain mixed venous blood samples

ASSESSMENT PHASE
- Why does the client require PA pressure monitoring (*e.g.,* heart failure, shock, open-heart surgery)?
- How many parameters will be monitored? Set up transducers using a single system or a multiple-pressure system.
- Will a PA catheter with pacing electrodes or thermistor tip for CO be required?

- Will continuous S$\bar{v}$O$_2$ be measured? Use the appropriate five-lumen fiberoptic PA catheter.
- Which vein will be used for insertion: brachial, subclavian, jugular, or femoral? The brachial vein is the site used most commonly.

PRECAUTIONS

- **Do not inflate the balloon with fluid.**
- **If the balloon is inflated for an extended period, necrosis of the PA can occur.**

PLANNING PHASE

EQUIPMENT*

Pressure module
Prepared transducer/pressure-monitoring setup (2) on IV pole
PA catheter (single, double, triple, or quadruple lumen)
Catheter introducer and guidewire
Cutdown tray
 Syringes and needles
 Scalpel
 4 × 4s
 Sterile basin
 Suture equipment
 Drapes
Xylocaine 1%
Black silk skin suture
Sterile gloves
Razor and soap
Iodophor solution
Iodophor ointment (optional)
Hypoallergenic tape
Fluoroscopy table and equipment (optional)
Lead aprons (if fluoroscopy is planned)
Defibrillator
Emergency cart and medications
Microprocessor for measuring S$\bar{v}$O$_2$ (optional)
Five-lumen fiberoptic PA catheter (optional; used to measure S$\bar{v}$O$_2$)

CLIENT/FAMILY TEACHING

- Answer questions about PA catheter insertion. Use a PA catheter and heart diagrams as necessary.
- Reassure the client that a local anesthetic will be given and that discomfort should be minimal.

IMPLEMENTATION PHASE

NURSING ACTIONS	RATIONALE/AMPLIFICATION
1. Obtain baseline vital signs.	Leave the blood pressure cuff on the client's arm during the procedure to record vital signs periodically.
2. Obtain clear ECG signal and baseline ECG recording.	Check that the electrodes will not interfere with the operative site and fluoroscopy.
3. Position client supine on fluoroscopy table.	
4. Balance and calibrate prepared transducers.	Positon the transducer at the level of the phlebostatic axis.
5. Shave operative site if necessary and prepare skin with iodophor solution.	Use 70% isopropyl alcohol if the client is allergic to iodophor.

* If a prepackaged percutaneous sheath introducer kit is available, instruments, drapes, and catheter introducer and guidewire will be included.

6. Open cutdown tray to provide sterile field. Open PA catheter on sterile field.

7. Submerge catheter tip in sterile saline and inflate balloon with .75 ml to 1.5 ml of air to test for leaks. Deflate balloon and prime lumens with saline.

The amount of air used to inflate the balloon depends on the size of the balloon. Balloons are available in .75-ml and 1.5-ml sizes.

8. Proximal end of PA catheter is passed off sterile field to be connected to flush solutions.

9. Connect proximal and distal ports to prepared transducers while flushing with fast-flush valve.

The proximal port will be situated in the RA and the distal port in the PA.

10. Physician administers local anesthetic, performs cutdown, and locates vein.

Reassure the client during the procedure and tell the client what to anticipate.

11. Catheter is moistened in saline to facilitate insertion.

12. Physician advances catheter until an RA waveform is observed on monitor (see Fig. 5-5).

Instruct the client to cough. The waveform will fluctuate if the catheter is in the thoracic cavity.

13. Inflate balloon to facilitate passage through right ventricle into PA wedge position.

Observe right ventricular, PA, and wedge waveforms on the monitor (see Fig. 5–5). Record the pressures. Placement may also be guided by fluoroscopy.

14. Observe ECG while catheter advances through ventricle. Prepare Xylocaine bolus (see ACLS in Chap. 3).

Advancement of the catheter may cause ventricular irritability. Count ectopic beats and other arrhythmias out loud.

15. Deflate balloon.

The physician will pull the catheter back 2 cm to 4 cm and suture it in place to prevent inadvertent advancement.

16. Dress insertion site with iodophor ointment (if used) and occlusive pressure dressing.

Record the date and time of insertion on the dressing.

17. Balance and recalibrate transducer, and record PA and PCW pressures.

If the client is unable to lie supine, note the angle at which these readings are recorded. Subsequent readings should be taken at this angle to ensure consistency.

18. Set monitor alarms 20 mm Hg above and below client's range.

Validate the position of the catheter with a chest film.

RELATED NURSING CARE

NURSING ACTIONS	RATIONALE/AMPLIFICATION
1. Monitor hemodynamic status. Record PA pressure hourly or as ordered.	The normal PA pressure range is 20 mm Hg to 30 mm Hg systolic and 8 mm Hg to 12 mm Hg diastolic. An elevated PA pressure may indicate LV failure, pulmonary hypertension, mitral stenosis, or left-to-right shunt.
2. Take PCW pressure every 2 hours to 4 hours by inflating balloon with .75 ml to 1.5 ml of air, depending on size of balloon.	The normal PCW pressure range is 4 mm Hg to 12 mm Hg. An elevated PCW pressure may indicate LV failure or problems with the mitral valve.
3. Integrate pressure readings with other hemodynamic parameters and clinical assessment of client.	Isolated readings are not as valuable as serial recordings. Notify the physician of significant changes so that the therapeutic regimen may be reassessed.
4. Observe correct procedures for balloon management.	Use a 1-ml tuberculin syringe for a .75-ml balloon, and a 2-ml syringe for a 1.5-ml balloon. Inflate the balloon only until a wedge waveform appears on the monitor. Remove the syringe when deflating the balloon. Deflating with the syringe in place can cause premature balloon rupture.

5. Evaluate for balloon rupture.

Inflation of the balloon is always associated with a feeling of resistance. If resistance is not felt and the balloon does not wedge, the balloon has ruptured. Discontinue inflations and label balloon with tape, noting that it has ruptured. Continued inflations may cause an air embolus. The catheter can still be used for PA pressures, COs, and mixed venous blood samples.

6. Ascertain that balloon does not remain inflated.

Necrosis of the pulmonary artery may occur if the balloon remains inflated. If the balloon remains in the wedge position, turn the client to the right side and instruct him to cough and breathe deeply. Move the client's arm. *Notify the physician immediately if the balloon remains wedged.*

7. Ascertain that balloon has not slipped into right ventricle.

Observe the monitor for an RV waveform. *Because of the risk of ventricular irritability resulting from trauma, notify the physician of an RV waveform immediately.*

8. RA port (proximal) may be used for IV infusion. Do not use PA port (distal) for IV infusions.

Pulmonary extravasation can occur.

9. Change dressing and pressure monitoring setup every 48 hours; change flush solution every 24 hours. Mark dressing, tubing, and IV bag with date and time of change.

These precautions prevent infection.

10. Rebalance and recalibrate transducer every 4 hours.

Barometric pressure and position changes in relation to the transducer affect calibration.

11. If fiberoptic PA catheter is used, measure and record continuous $S\bar{v}O_2$ concentration.

    a. Reassess client if $S\bar{v}O_2$ falls below 60% or if it varies ± 10% for 3 minutes or longer.

Changes in the $S\bar{v}O_2$ occur approximately 30 minutes before clinical symptoms appear.

    b. Keep hard copy rolling so that trends can be observed and recorded.

The hard copy runs at approximately 4 inches/hour.

    c. Check for accuracy by correlating with blood sample every 24 hours.

Obtain a blood sample from the PA distal port. Instruct the laboratory to determine oxygen concentration using a measured-sample technique rather than a calculated quantitative technique.

12. Assess circulation to extremities every 2 hours to 4 hours if catheter has been inserted in extremity.

13. To assist with removal of PA catheter, proceed as follows:

    a. Close stopcocks to client.

Have defibrillator, emergency cart, and medication on hand. Removal may cause ventricular irritability.

    b. Open transducer stopcock to air and disconnect it from monitor.

    c. Monitor client while physician clips suture and removes catheter.

Check the client's vital signs and circulation to extremities before removal of the catheter.

    d. Up to .5 ml of air will remain in balloon until withdrawal to RA from pulmonary artery.

Leaving a small amount of air in the balloon during withdrawal from the pulmonary artery protects intracardiac structures. The balloon will be deflated before removal from the atrium.

    e. Apply pressure to site until bleeding stops.

    f. Apply pressure dressing and iodophor ointment (if used).

Monitor the extremities for bleeding or circulatory problems.

g. Remove pressure dressing 8 hours after catheter is discontinued. Check site and redress.

EVALUATION PHASE

ANTICIPATED OUTCOMES	NURSING ACTIONS
1. Prevention of complications of PA pressure monitoring	Evaluate for balloon rupture and determine whether the catheter is in the wedge position. Evaluate for complications of PA pressure monitoring, including sepsis, emboli, arrhythmias, electromicroshock, hemothorax, cardiac tamponade, lung ischemia, PA rupture, or extravasation.
2. Adjustment in therapy according to hemodynamic parameters	Evaluate hemodynamic parameters for significant changes.

PRODUCT AVAILABILITY

SWAN–GANZ CATHETER

American Edwards Laboratories

PA CATHETERS

Electro-Catheter Corp.

PERCUTANEOUS SHEATH INTRODUCER KIT

Arrow International

Obtaining mixed venous sample from pulmonary artery catheter

Objective
To obtain a mixed venous blood sample for laboratory analysis

ASSESSMENT PHASE

• Is a mixed venous blood sample required, or are other routes available for obtaining the sample? A mixed venous sample will be required to determine the O_2 content of venous blood.

PLANNING PHASE

EQUIPMENT

6-ml syringe — 2
Sterile 4 × 4s
Blood-specimen tube or syringe

CLIENT/FAMILY TEACHING

• Explain to the client that a blood sample will be drawn from the catheter for laboratory analysis.
• Reassure the client that the procedure will not cause discomfort.

IMPLEMENTATION PHASE

NURSING ACTIONS	RATIONALE/AMPLIFICATION
1. Ascertain that balloon is deflated. If IV infusion is flowing into proximal port (RA), turn off IV while sample is drawn.	If the balloon remains inflated, the sample may be contaminated with arterial blood.
2. Connect syringe to stopcock between PA catheter and transducer.	

3. Open stopcock to syringe and distal port (PA) and close to transducer.

4. Aspirate to clear line of flush solution.

5. Turn stopcock to halfway position (Fig. 5–16). Remove and discard syringe.

Fig. 5–16 Turn stopcock to halfway position before removing syringe.

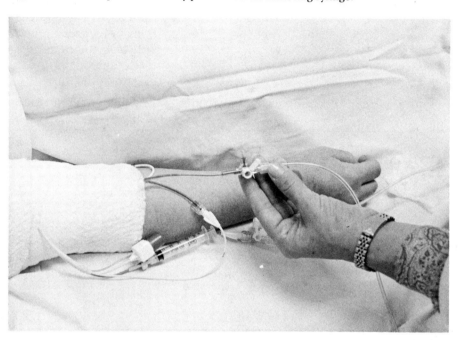

6. Connect sample syringe and draw sample.

7. Turn stopcock to halfway position. Remove sample syringe and cap, and insert sample into blood tube.

Turning the stopcock to the halfway position prevents entry of air into line and blood loss.

8. Open stopcock to continuous infusion device and close it to client.

9. Flush stopcock to clear. Prevent spillage with sterile 4 × 4.

10. Close and cap open stopcock port. Flush line to client.

Observe for the return of a PA pressure tracing. Restart the right atrial IV infusion if applicable.

EVALUATION PHASE

ANTICIPATED OUTCOME	NURSING ACTIONS
Prevention of complications	Evaluate for breaks in technique. Evaluate for sepsis, air embolus, clotting of catheter. Check the lines for correct stopcock positions to prevent accidental blood loss.

Central venous pressure

Objectives
To assess hemodynamic changes occurring in the right side of the heart
To administer fluids or medication directly into the RA
To obtain central venous blood samples

ASSESSMENT PHASE

- Why does the client require CVP monitoring (*e.g.*, bleeding, dehydration, vigorous diuresis)?

PLANNING PHASE

EQUIPMENT

Central venous catheter
Sterile stopcock
4 × 4
Hypoallergenic tape
Iodophor ointment (optional)
For intermittent CVP monitoring include the following:
     IV fluid (as ordered)
     IV administration set (microdrop)
     Volutrol (controlled volume administration) or IV pump/controller*
     CVP water manometer
     IV extension tubing (optional)
     Carpenter's level
For continuous CVP monitoring include the following:
     Prepared transducer and pressure-monitoring setup
     ECG and pressure module

CLIENT/FAMILY TEACHING

- Answer the client's questions about the purpose of the indwelling CVP catheter and the pressure readings. Use a CVP catheter and heart diagrams as necessary.
- Reassure the client and family about complex equipment and alarms if continuous CVP monitoring will be required.

IMPLEMENTATION PHASE

NURSING ACTIONS	RATIONALE/AMPLIFICATION

INTERMITTENT CVP MONITORING

1. If an IVAC 560 pump is used, connect special tubing to IV solution. Thread tubing through pump and prime tubing (Fig. 5–17).

2. If using water manometer, connect administration set to IV solution.

Use volutrol to prevent volume overload if a pump/controller is unavailable.

3. Connect manometer to IV tubing. Connect stopcock to manometer tubing. Prime tubing and flush stopcock ports. Close stopcock to manometer. Cap stopcock ports. Secure manometer to IV stand with zero on manometer positioned level with client's RA (Fig. 5–18).

Add an IV extension set between the manometer tubing and the client so that the setup will not restrict the client's activity (optional).

4. Assist physician with insertion of CVP catheter.

(See Chap. 18, Total Parenteral Nutrition.) Masks are optional for CVP catheter insertion. Respiratory flora should not present a problem in central venous catheterization.

5. Connect IV infusion to subclavian catheter when proximal end of catheter is passed off sterile field.

The physician will suture the catheter in place.

6. Start IV infusion at keep-open rate until position of catheter tip is confirmed by chest film.

7. Dress insertion site with iodophor ointment (if used) and occlusive dressing.

* If an IVAC 560 Pump (or similar device) is being used use special tubing with built-in pressure transducer. Omit volutrol and CVP water manometer.

Fig. 5-17 (*A*) Tubing primed with IV fluid and (*B*) connected to IVAC pump. (Courtesy IVAC Corporation, San Diego, CA)

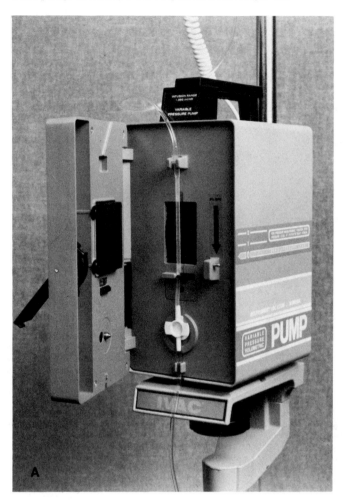

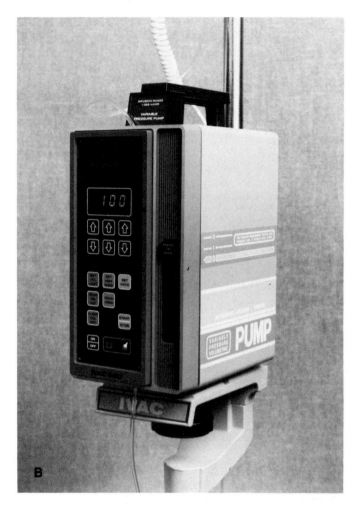

Fig. 5-18 Intermittent CVP setup using water manometer. Zero on manometer (*dashed line*) is level with client's right atrium.

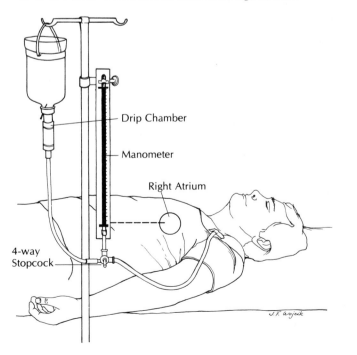

Drip Chamber

Manometer

Right Atrium

4-way Stopcock

8. Measure and record CVP.

   a. Place client supine.

If the client cannot tolerate the supine position, record the client's position when the reading is taken. Take subsequent readings with the client in the same position.

   b. Use carpenter's level to ascertain that zero on manometer is level with client's RA (see Fig. 5–2).

   c. Confirm patency of line by flushing IV tubing.

   d. Open three-way stopcock at base of manometer to IV solution and to manometer (Fig. 5–19A).

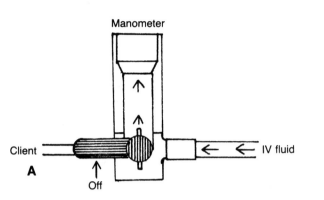

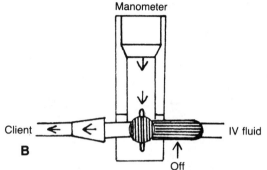

Fig. 5–19 (A) Stopcock position to fill manometer. (B) Stopcock position to measure CVP. (C) IV infusion open to CVP catheter.

   e. Allow manometer to fill three fourths, or 10 cm above anticipated reading.

   f. Open stopcock to manometer and to CVP catheter (Fig. 5–19B).

Change the mánometer setup if fluid accidentally contaminates the filter at the top of the manometer.

Observe for a decrease in the fluid level of the manometer as fluid drains into the line. The level should fluctuate with respirations and should drop approximately 1 cm with each pulse.

   g. Record reading when level stops falling.

The normal range for CVP is 2 mm Hg to 6 mm Hg (3 cm to 8 cm water pressure). If the client is on a ventilator, remove the ventilator briefly after the fluid level has stabilized. Record the level at which the fluid stops falling. If the client cannot breathe without the respirator, note that the reading was taken while the client was on the ventilator. Positive intrathoracic pressure will result in higher readings.

   h. Open stopcock to IV and CVP catheter and restart IV infusion (Fig. 5–19C).

9. If an IVAC 560 pump is used, depress pressure recording button and read CVP on display (Fig. 5–20). Be sure that transducer is level with phlebostatic axis.

Depress the conversion button to convert automatically to cm water pressure if required.

Fig. 5–20 Recording CVP on IVAC 560 pump. (Courtesy IVAC Corporation, San Diego, CA)

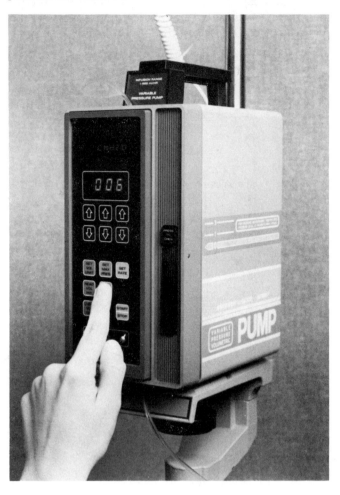

CONTINUOUS CVP MONITORING

1. When backflow from subclavian catheter is observed, connect catheter to prepared pressure-monitoring transducer setup while fast flushing.

This prevents the introduction of air into the catheter. Observe for a right atrial pressure tracing on the monitor.

2. Balance and calibrate transducer with air–fluid interface stopcock at level of phlebostatic axis.

(See Transducer Setup: Up to Two Pressures.) The physician will suture the catheter in place.

3. Record CVP.

Dress the insertion site.

RELATED NURSING CARE

NURSING ACTIONS	RATIONALE/AMPLIFICATION
1. Determine that connections are secure and that lines are free of air bubbles.	This prevents air embolism and accidental bleeding from the line.
2. Redress insertion site and change tubing/pressure-monitoring setup every 48 hours. Change IV solution/flush solution every 24 hours. Label IV bag, dressing, and tubing with date and time of change.	This precaution controls infection.
3. Monitor ECG for arrhythmias or left bundle branch block.	The catheter tip may slip into the RV, causing ventricular irritability.

4. Record CVP hourly or as required.

Integrate the readings with other hemodynamic parameters and the clinical status of the client. Report significant changes to the physician.

5. Obtain mixed venous blood sample by connecting 10-ml syringe to stopcock nearest to CVP catheter.

Refer to technique for obtaining mixed venous blood sample from PA catheter. Follow steps 2 through 10.

6. To remove CVP catheter, proceed as follows:

    a. Remove dressing aseptically.

Position the client supine.

    b. Close IV/pressure monitoring setup to client.

    c. Clip suture that secures catheter.

Culture the insertion site if infection is suspected.

    d. Remove catheter with one smooth motion while client performs Valsalva's maneuver.

This prevents air from entering through the catheter or the tract left by the catheter. Check the length of the CVP catheter and culture the catheter tip.

    e. Apply pressure until bleeding stops. Apply occlusive pressure dressing.

Monitor the site for hematoma or bleeding.

EVALUATION PHASE

ANTICIPATED OUTCOMES	NURSING ACTIONS
1. Prevention of complications of invasive vascular techniques	Evaluate for signs of sepsis, pulmonary emboli, arrhythmias, and electromicroshock.
2. Prevention of fluid overload	Take precautions to prevent accidental fluid overload (*e.g.*, microdrip, volutrol, and pump/controller).
3. Alteration of fluid and medication therapy according to hemodynamic parameters	Monitor serial CVP readings. Discuss significant trends with the physician.

PRODUCT AVAILABILITY   IV PUMP/CONTROLLER

    IVAC Corporation

Multi-Med subclavian catheter

Objectives
To administer different IV solutions directly into the RA at individual flow rates using a catheter inserted into the subclavian vein
To implement continuous monitoring of CVP
To obtain central venous blood samples

ASSESSMENT PHASE

- What medications (*e.g.*, Intropin, sodium nitroprusside, Xylocaine) will be administered using the Multi-Med catheter?
- What hemodynamic problems are present that require continuous CVP monitoring (*e.g.*, heart failure, open-heart surgery)?
- Will mixed venous blood samples be required to determine the O_2 content of venous blood?

PLANNING PHASE

EQUIPMENT*

Multi-Med catheter (Fig. 5–21)
8F introducer
Guidewire for catheter introduction
Cutdown tray

* If using a prepackaged percutaneous sheath introducer kit, omit the items that are included in kit.

Fig. 5–21 Multi-Med subclavian catheter. (*A*) Two-centimeter port extension (IV infusion). (*B*) distal port extension (IV infusion or pressure monitoring. (*C*) Five-centimeter port extension (IV infusion). (*D*) Adjustable suture loop. (Courtesy American Edwards Laboratories, Santa Ana, CA)

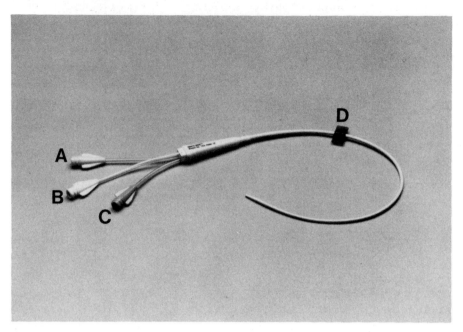

Sterile drapes
Needles and syringes
Scalpel
Suture equipment
Sterile basin
4 × 4s
Xylocaine 1%
Black silk skin suture on cutting needle
Sterile gloves
Iodophor solution
Iodophor ointment (if needed)
Hypoallergenic tape
Fluoroscopy (optional)
Lead aprons (if fluoroscopy is used)

CLIENT/FAMILY TEACHING

• Answer the client's questions about the purpose of CV catheter insertion. Use a demonstration catheter and heart diagrams as necessary.
• Reassure the client and family about the complex equipment and additional alarms that will be required.

IMPLEMENTATION PHASE

NURSING ACTIONS	RATIONALE/AMPLIFICATION
1. Prepare transducer and continuous flush system. Add another stopcock to attach distal-port extension of catheter directly to system.	(See Transducer Setup: Up to Two Pressures.) Place the client on the fluoroscopy table, if applicable.
2. Balance and calibrate system.	Position the air–fluid interface stopcock level with the RA (see Fig. 5–2).
3. When proximal end of catheter is passed off sterile field, connect it to pressure monitoring setup.	

4. Remain with client while physician locates vein and advances catheter into RA.

Observe the monitor for an RA waveform. Instruct the client to cough. Coughing produces fluctuations in the waveform if the catheter is in the thoracic cavity (see Fig. 5–5). The catheter may be advanced during fluoroscopy.

5. After physician sutures catheter in place, dress site with iodophor ointment (if used) and occlusive dressing.

6. Rebalance and recalibrate transducer. Record CVP.

The normal range for CVP is 2 mm Hg to 6 mm Hg (3 cm to 8 cm water pressure).

7. Connect prepared IV infusions to 2-cm and 5-cm ports of catheter.

Remove the protective cap from the port. Before connecting the IV infusion, aspirate with a syringe until blood is observed in the syringe. This prevents formation of air bubbles in the line.

8. Regulate IV infusions with a pump/controller.

This prevents accidental fluid overload. Flush the port with heparinized saline and recap if it is not required for IV infusion.

RELATED NURSING CARE   See previous section on Central Venous Pressure.

EVALUATION PHASE   See previous section on Central Venous Pressure.

PRODUCT AVAILABILITY
MULTI-MED CATHETER
American Edwards Laboratories

PERCUTANEOUS SHEATH INTRODUCER KIT
Arrow International, Inc.

Left atrial pressure

Objectives
To assess LVEDP indirectly (when mitral valve function is normal) using a catheter inserted directly into the LA
To assess hemodynamic changes in response to therapeutic intervention
To determine CVPs in the presence of low CO

ASSESSMENT PHASE
• Will the client return from the operating room with a LAP line in place? A LAP monitoring line is implanted during open-heart surgery for bedside monitoring.
• How many pressures will be monitored? Will a single- or a multiple-transducer setup be required?

PRECAUTIONS
• **LAP lines often are not used because of the danger of air or clots entering the left ventricle and becoming systemic emboli. Use an air filter near the LA catheter insertion site.**

PLANNING PHASE
EQUIPMENT
Pressure-monitoring module
Prepared transducer and flush setup
Air filter
Left atrial line

CLIENT/FAMILY TEACHING   See previous section on Transducer Setup: Up to Two Pressures.

IMPLEMENTATION
PHASE

NURSING ACTIONS	RATIONALE/AMPLIFICATION
1. Prepare transducer and pressure-monitoring setup. Add air filter near LAP catheter.	(See previous section on Transducer Setup: Up to Two Pressures.) Flush all lines and stopcock ports of air. LAP monitoring carries a high risk of air embolus.
2. Connect LAP line to prepared transducer.	
a. Open transducer to catheter.	
b. Observe for backflow from catheter.	
c. Connect pressure line to catheter while activating fast-flush valve.	This prevents air embolus.
d. Observe for LAP tracing.	The mean LAP range is 4 mm Hg to 12 mm Hg. Turn the monitor selector to "Mean." Systolic and diastolic pressures in the LA are not as significant as the mean pressure.
3. Rebalance and recalibrate transducer.	Position the air–fluid interface stopcock of the transducer level with the RA (see Fig. 5–2). Recalibrate every 4 hours, or when the client's position is changed in relation to the transducer.

RELATED NURSING CARE

NURSING ACTIONS	RATIONALE/AMPLIFICATION
1. Record LAP every hour or as ordered.	Notify the physician immediately if a good waveform is lost. The line may need to be removed.
2. Integrate LAP data with other hemodynamic parameters.	Report significant changes to the physician.
3. Maintain patency of line with continuous flush device.	Check for a flow rate of 3 ml to 4 ml/hour. Do not flush the line manually because of the risk of emboli.
4. Do not administer other IV infusions or medication through LA line.	
5. Redress site with occlusive dressing and change pressure-monitoring setup every 48 hours. Change flush solution every 24 hours. Label dressing, tubing, and flush solution with date and time of change.	These precautions prevent infection.
6. Assist with removal of LA line.	
a. Remove dressing aseptically.	Use sterile rubber gloves to prevent electromicroshock.
b. Monitor client while physician clips suture and removes line.	
c. Redress site.	Evaluate for increased drainage at the site and through chest tubes.
d. Obtain chest film 1 hour after removing line.	The chest tube should not be removed until the possibility of cardiac tamponade and hemothorax has been eliminated.

EVALUATION PHASE   See previous section on Transducer Setup: Up to Two Pressures.

Cardiac output

Objectives

To determine CO using the thermodilution method and a flow-directed PA catheter

To assess hemodynamic status and client response to therapeutic interventions

To compute CI using CO data

ASSESSMENT PHASE

Why are COs required for the client (*e.g.,* cardiogenic shock, open-heart surgery)?

- Is a thermodilution PA (Swan–Ganz) catheter *in situ*?
- Has a proper catheter position been verified? Observe for PA waveform on monitor. A PA waveform that is dampened or that shows a wedged position may indicate improper catheter position and will result in inaccurate CO measurements.

PRECAUTION

- **Observe for lethal arrhythmias during the CO procedure. Follow electric safety guidelines (see electrical safety techniques described in Chap. 33).**

PLANNING PHASE

EQUIPMENT*

10-ml syringe with cap—4

Refrigerated dextrose 5% in water (D_5W) (unless another injectate is used)

Ice bath

Plastic bag

CO computer

Thermodilution PA (Swan–Ganz) catheter

Emergency equipment and medication

CLIENT/FAMILY TEACHING

- Answer the client's questions about the reason for CO measurements. Use heart diagrams as appropriate.
- Reassure the client and family about additional equipment required to obtain CO.

IMPLEMENTATION PHASE

NURSING ACTIONS	RATIONALE/AMPLIFICATION
1. Fill four syringes with 10 ml of refrigerated D_5W and place in protective plastic bag.	The bag prevents contamination of the contents of the syringes with unsterile water and ice. Exactly 10 ml of injectate must be used. Control or spring-loaded syringes, if available, facilitate the speed of injection and minimize temperature changes, which occur through handling of the syringe barrel (Fig. 5–22).
2. Immerse syringes in prepared syringe bath of crushed ice. Connect injectate probe to computer and place a syringe of D_5W in bath. Plunger of syringe is replaced with probe, and syringe is recapped.	Allow the syringes to equilibrate for a minimum of 15 minutes. The temperature probe measures the temperature of the injectate. Alcohol may be added to the bath. Electric coolers are also available. Observe for freezing of the injectate if alcohol or an electric cooler is used.
Alternative: Use closed injectate delivery system with in-line temperature probe.	An in-line temperature probe measures the temperature of the injectate as it is injected.
3. Check that thermodilution catheter is positioned correctly in PA. Deflate balloon.	Observe for a PA waveform on the monitor. If a catheter introducer with a side-port extension is being used for IV infusion, close the IV line during the procedure. Measure CO with the client supine if the client can tolerate this position. Position changes will cause differences in CO.

* A closed delivery system may be substitued for the first four items.

Fig. 5-22 (*A*) Control syringe. (*B*) Spring-loaded syringe connected to proximal port of Swan–Ganz catheter. (Courtesy Becton Dickinson & Company, Paramus, NJ)

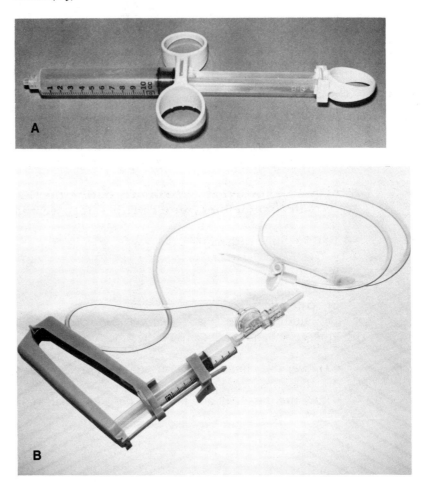

4. Turn on and calibrate CO computer according to manufacturer's instructions.

Enter the computation constant according to volume, temperature, and type of injectate being used.

5. Connect thermistor of PA catheter to computer.

Allow at least 5 minutes for computer to warm up. Check for proper functioning. Flush the system using the fast-flush valve.

6. Connect 10-ml syringe of injectate to three-way stopcock at proximal port (RA) of PA catheter.

Alternative method: If a closed system is used, release the IV clamp and aspirate 10 ml of injectate into the syringe. Close the IV clamp and adjust the syringe stopcock so that it is open to the PA catheter. The injectate should be cooled to between 0°C and 5°C. (Some authorities recommend that the injectate be kept at room temperature.)

7. Depress start button on computer, and rapidly and smoothly inject solution.

The injectate should be infused within 2 seconds to 4 seconds during the end-expiratory phase of expiration to avoid temperature changes.

8. Read CO from computer.

The computer calculates a temperature–time curve. The normal range for CO is 4 liters to 8 liters/minute (resting). Low COs may indicate congestive heart failure, valvular heart disease, myocarditis, or cardiac tamponade. High COs occur during septic shock, fever, and thyrotoxicosis.

9. Record average of three sequential CO determinations.

10. Remove syringe from proximal port of PA catheter and open stopcock from pressure-monitoring setup to PA catheter. Cap stopcock port and flush system.

11. Disconnect thermistor.

Disregard the first reading because the catheter is not primed with cold injectate. To ensure accuracy, measurements should be within .5 liter of each other.

Alternative method: Open the syringe stopcock to the infusion/pressure-monitoring setup and to the PA catheter.

RELATED NURSING CARE

NURSING ACTIONS	RATIONALE/AMPLIFICATION

1. Compute CI. If CO computer automatically computes CI, enter client's height and weight into computer and read CI.

Alternative method: Compute CI manually. Divide the CO by the BSA. The BSA is obtained from a nomogram (Fig. 5–23). On the nomogram, use a ruler to align the client's height and weight. Read the BSA in the middle column where the two points intersect. The normal range is 2.5 liters to 4 liters/minute/square meter. *Alternative method:* Input data into microcomputer. Use a hemodynamic parameter program to compute parameters.

Fig. 5–23 Dubois body surface area chart.

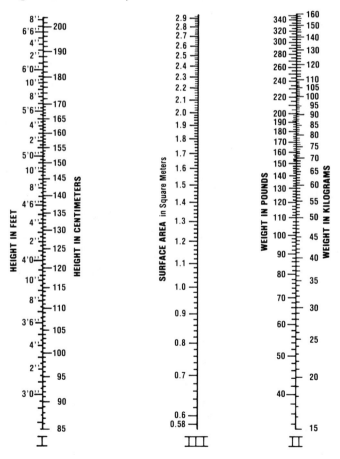

2. If volume overload presents problem, use 5 ml of injectate rather than 10 ml.

Take this into account when calibrating the computer. An automatic infusion device may be necessary for injectate volumes that are less than 5 ml.

EVALUATION PHASE

ANTICIPATED OUTCOMES	NURSING ACTIONS
1. Alteration of treatment plan in response to hemodynamic parameters	Evaluate CO in conjunction with other available hemodynamic measurements.
2. Generation of accurate CO measurements	Evaluate for sources of error in determining CO, such as low CO, intracardiac shunts, right-heart valve disease, thrombus formation on the thermistor, and arrhythmias. A catheter that is positioned incorrectly is also a source of error in determining CO. If the CO computer is equipped with a strip recorder, observe the thermodilution curve for smooth upstroke, peak, and smooth downstroke. Reject distorted curves, which can result from improper injection technique or catheter position (Fig. 5–24).

Fig. 5–24 (*A*) Accurate CO curve recorded on strip recorder. (*B*) Distorted CO curve.

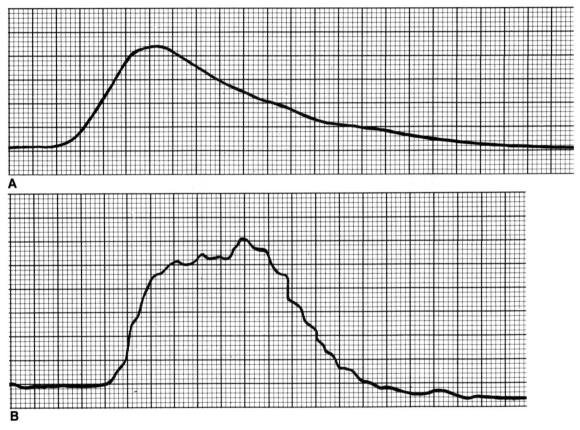

A

B

3. Prevention of complications of CO determination	Evaluate for possible complications such as sepsis, air embolus, arrhythmias, cardiac arrest, and electromicroshock.

PRODUCT AVAILABILITY CARDIAC OUTPUT COMPUTER

American Edwards Laboratories
Hewlett-Packard

CLOSED INJECTATE DELIVERY SYSTEM FOR COLD INJECTATE

American Edwards Laboratories

SWAN – GANZ THERMODILUTION CATHETER

American Edwards Laboratories

SELECTED REFERENCES

Daily EK, Schroeder JS: Techniques in Bedside Hemodynamic Monitoring, 2nd ed. St. Louis, CV Mosby, 1981

Hudak CM, Lohr T, Gallo BM: Critical Care Nursing, 3rd ed. Philadelphia, JB Lippincott, 1982

Jaquith S: The Oximetrix Opticath: What is it and how can it facilitate nursing management of the critically ill patient? Critical Care Nurse, May/June 1984, pp 55 – 58

Lalli SM: The complete Swan-Ganz. RN 41:64 – 77, 1978

Palmer PN: Advanced hemodynamic assessment. DCCN 1(3):139 – 144, 1982

Riedinger MS, Shellock FG: Technical aspects of the thermodilution method for measuring cardiac output. Heart and Lung 13(3):215 – 221, 1984

Runkel R, Burke L: Troubleshooting Swan – Ganz catheters. Heart and Lung 12(6):591 – 596, 1983

Sanderson RG, Kurth CL: The Cardiac Patient: A Comprehensive Approach. Philadelphia, WB Saunders, 1983

NONINVASIVE TECHNIQUES

BACKGROUND

A number of variables have been shown to influence the accuracy of blood pressure readings, including cuff size and measurement technique.

CUFF SIZE

Two factors influence the accuracy of cuff size: the length of the arterial segment that is compressed and the length of the inflatable bladder within the cuff, which surrounds the extremity that is being compressed. The width of the occluding cuff is determined by the size of the limb — by either the diameter or the circumference. The circumference is easier to measure than the diameter. The cuff width should be about 40% of the limb circumference in order to obtain an accurate reading. If the cuff width is too narrow, the indirect pressure reading will be much higher than it actually is. Conversely, if the cuff width is too wide, the pressure reading will be too low. The American Heart Association recommends that the inflatable bladder be 30 cm in length so that it nearly or completely encircles the limb, in order to avoid any risk of misapplication.

Most cuffs that are commercially available on the market today have a range of sizes (neonate to large adult) that come with sophisticated electronic monitoring devices. Separate arm and thigh cuff sizes are also available.

MEASUREMENT TECHNIQUE

The factors inherent in measuring blood pressure noninvasively include cuff placement, deflation rate, identification of systolic and diastolic points, and auscultatory apparatus. The cuff, including the inflatable bladder, should be placed directly over the artery to be compressed. Manufacturers often indicate the ideal site on the cuffs by an arrow or some other means. This is helpful because the inflatable bladder is inside the cuff and is not always readily identified (Fig. 5 – 25).

The rate of deflation of the cuff and the client's heart rate and systolic pressure are all related to the accommodation of venous congestion in the distal bed. To avoid this congestion a deflation rate of 2 mm Hg to 3 mm Hg per heartbeat is incorporated in the design of current automatic blood pressure measuring devices. (There has been some debate about the determination of diastolic pressure. It has been argued that a reliable diastolic pressure reading is obtained more consistently at the point of a muffled sound rather than at the point of no sound, which often persists well below the true diastolic pressure.)

Other factors that affect blood pressure measurement include the acuteness of the auditory system of the care-giver taking the blood pressure and the quality of the stethoscope.

When frequent blood pressure measurements are required in critically ill clients who are not candidates for invasive pressure monitoring, an automatic or semiauto-

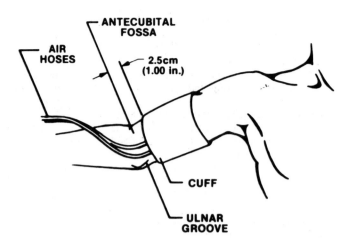

AIR HOSES

ANTECUBITAL FOSSA

2.5cm (1.00 in.)

CUFF

ULNAR GROOVE

Fig. 5-25 Recommended cuff monitoring site. (Dinamap Monitor Operation Manual. © CRITIKON, 1983. Reprinted with permission)

matic noninvasive blood pressure measuring device should be considered. These devices, if used correctly and in accordance with the manufacturer's instructions, can provide blood pressure readings with a higher level of accuracy than manual methods that depend on the variables already discussed. In addition, this method is less disturbing to the client, as well as more efficient, because each individual blood pressure does not have to be manually recorded by the care-giver. If a digital readout is provided by the equipment, it can be incorporated into the client's record, thereby decreasing the time required for charting.

Automatic blood pressure monitoring

Objectives

To measure systolic and diastolic blood pressure using a noninvasive automatic device

To correlate mean arterial (MA) pressure readings with heart rate in predetermined pressure frequencies

To provide a digital readout of blood pressure readings and heart rate

ASSESSMENT PHASE

- Is the client a candidate for noninvasive pressure monitoring rather than invasive monitoring? Postoperative clients usually are candidates for noninvasive monitoring.
- Is the client receiving medication that will alter cardiovascular status? This may dramatically affect the client's blood pressure readings.
- Has the equipment been checked for electric leakage in the last 6 months by the biomedical department?
- Is there adequate space to allow for heat dissipation from the equipment?
- Is the client experiencing convulsions or tremors? Automatic monitoring will be ineffective.
- Is the client connected to a heart–lung machine? If so, an automatic device cannot be used to measure blood pressure.
- Are there factors present during the determination cycles that may affect the accuracy of the recording (*e.g.*, talking, anxiety)?
- Are cardiac arrhythmias present? If so, the recorded blood pressure may be incorrect. Cardiac arrhythmias interfere with the equipment's ability to determine blood pressure parameters.
- Does the automatically recorded heart rate differ significantly from the heart rate recorded on the ECG monitor? The automatic blood pressure monitor measures actual peripheral pulses whereas the ECG monitor counts electric impulses. Not all electrical impulses result in a peripheral pulse wave.

PRECAUTIONS

- **Erroneous readings may be obtained if the proper cuff size is not selected or if the cuff is placed incorrectly.**
- **Place the monitored extremity on the same level as the heart to ensure correct readings.**
- **Do not use automatic blood pressure monitoring in the presence of flammable anesthetics.**

PLANNING PHASE

EQUIPMENT

Automatic blood pressure monitor
Tape (to measure extremity)
Appropriate blood pressure cuff
Stethoscope and sphygmomanometer (if calibration is needed)

CLIENT/FAMILY TEACHING

- Discuss the reasons for frequent blood pressure monitoring with the client and family.
- Reassure the client that the measurement is not painful. Tell the client to inform the nurse if any pain is experienced while the blood pressure cuff is in place.
- Tell the client to avoid rapid movement if possible. This may trigger the alarm system.
- Describe the alarm system to avoid any undue emotional stress for the client.

IMPLEMENTATION PHASE

NURSING ACTIONS	RATIONALE/AMPLIFICATION
1. Secure dual air hose to connections on rear of monitor.	
2. Measure extremity for proper size cuff and attach securely to dual connectors.	The cuff should be approximately 40% wider than the diameter of the limb. If the client is obese, the cuff may be transferred to a smaller extremity, for example, the ankle. Improper cuff size may produce erroneous readings. Check the operations manual to be sure that the cuff size is compatible with the hose size.
3. Squeeze air from cuff before wrapping it securely around extremity. Place cuff bladder correctly on major artery (Fig. 5–26).	An excessively tight cuff will cause venous congestion and limb discoloration.
4. Support extremity at heart level.	Do not place the cuff on an extremity that has an IV infusion.

Fig. 5–26 Recommended cuff placement sites. (Dinamap Monitor Operation Manual. © CRITIKON, 1983. Reprinted with permission)

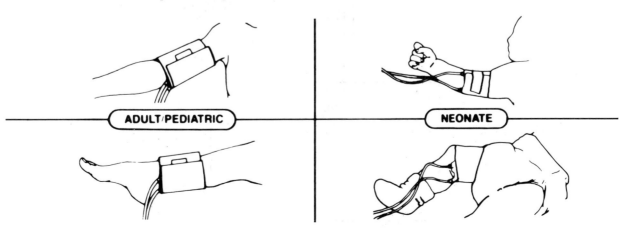

ADULT/PEDIATRIC   NEONATE

5. Arrange cuff hoses so that they are not obstructed during recording.

6. Adjust monitor so that it is level with heart.

7. Before operating monitor, place all switches in desired position.

    a. Turn off power until all switches are ready.

    b. Turn on alarm limits.

    c. Turn to "Auto" mode.

    d. Turn cycle time to "All down."

    e. Turn on power.

If the cuff is changed to another limb, check again to make sure that the cuff size and hose are compatible.

The audible alarm switch should always be turned on to avoid hazardous conditions.

In this position the monitor will automatically update readings at approximately 1-minute intervals. (See the operations manual if the readings should be increased.) Intervals may vary in different models.

Remove the locking screw on the bottom of the chassis (if applicable). Observe the warnings and caution labels. Check the power cord and pneumatic hoses.

Set the optional switches (*e.g.,* date, time, and alarm limits) if applicable.

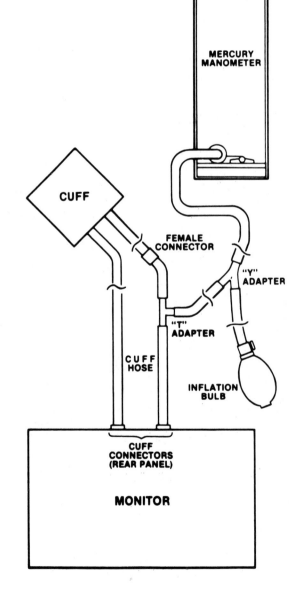

Fig. 5-27 Calibration check with mercury manometer. (Dinamap Monitor Operation Manual. © CRITIKON, 1983. Reprinted with permission)

8. Observe monitor for readings to be displayed. These include systolic and diastolic pressures, MA pressure, and heart rate, depending on capabilities of specific model.

In the automatic mode, the cuff will inflate within 5 seconds after the power is turned on. Between cycles there is a "wait" period in which the cuff is deflated to allow for venous return to the extremity.

RELATED NURSING CARE

NURSING ACTIONS	RATIONALE/AMPLIFICATION
1. Calibrate monitor at least monthly or if doubt about correct readings exists.	Consult the manufacturer's instructions. Verify the calibration with a mercury manometer (Fig. 5–27).
2. Adjust readings if monitored extremity is not at heart level.	To compensate for this hydrostatic effect, add 1.8 mm Hg for every 2.5 cm (1 inch) above the heart level, or subtract 1.8 mm Hg for every 2.5 cm below the heart level.
3. Observe for respiratory or vasomotor variations that may alter blood pressure during determination cycle.	

EVALUATION PHASE

ANTICIPATED OUTCOMES	NURSING ACTIONS
1. Accurate, noninvasive recording of hemodynamic parameters	Check frequently for correct cuff connections, unobstructed tubing, system leaks, or failure of the alarm system.
2. Prevention of complications of noninvasive automatic blood pressure monitoring	Evaluate for inaccurate pressure readings, electric shock, skin breakdown, or malfunction of the equipment.

PRODUCT AVAILABILITY   AUTOMATIC BLOOD PRESSURE MONITORS

Critikon Inc.
Datascope Corp.
Applied Medical Research
Roche
Omega
Physio Control

SELECTED REFERENCES   Kinney MR: Clinical Reference for Critical Care Nurses, pp 1002–1004. New York, McGraw-Hill, 1981

Seaman D. Should you trust automatic blood pressure monitors? Nursing '85, January 1985, pp 55–57

Monitoring blood pressure and peripheral pulses using Doppler ultrasound

BACKGROUND   Doppler ultrasound techniques can be used to amplify and assess peripheral blood flow. A variety of probes are available, including disks that are flat, pencil-shaped probes, or probes that are similar to a pocket stethoscope. Transmitting crystals in the probe emit ultrasound beams that collide with red blood cells moving through the blood vessel. The beam of sound is transmitted from the red blood cell to a receiver. The change in sound is converted into an audible sound that may be amplified to be heard. If the blood flow is less than 5 cm/second, is shielded by bone, or is located deep below the skin's surface, it cannot be heard.

Objectives
To assess blood flow in peripheral vessels
To diagnose peripheral vascular disorders
To amplify the blood pressure when it cannot be auscultated using traditional methods

ASSESSMENT PHASE

• Has the peripheral circulation been assessed using conventional methods? Check the extremities for color, temperature, venous return, hair distribution, and the condition of the nail beds.
• Is the client scheduled for vascular surgery? Obtain a baseline assessment of peripheral vascular blood flow.

PRECAUTIONS

• **Avoid using the Doppler probe near the client's eyes because this may damage delicate nerve tissue.**
• **In critically ill clients, the diastolic pressure may be difficult to ascertain.**

PLANNING PHASE

EQUIPMENT

Doppler probe with amplifier
Ultrasound conductive gel
Alcohol-soaked wipes
Flow sheet (to record results)

CLIENT/FAMILY TEACHING

• Reassure the client that the examination is relatively painless. Pressure will be felt from the cuff, and the conductive gel will be cool. A peripheral vascular examination takes approximately 10 minutes to 15 minutes.
• Describe or demonstrate the amplified sounds the client may hear. Demonstrate these sounds before vascular surgery if applicable.

IMPLEMENTATION PHASE

NURSING ACTIONS	RATIONALE/AMPLIFICATION
1. To assess arterial flow, proceed as follows:	
a. Apply conductive gel to faceplate of probe.	Conductive gel improves the transmission of sound to the receiver.
b. Turn on the Doppler probe and insert stethoscope earpieces.	
c. Place probe over vessel and tilt slightly against direction of flow.	This position improves sound transmission. Too much pressure on the probe will obliterate the pulse.
d. Adjust volume control as necessary.	Three basic signals may be heard:
	a. A triphasic or multiphasic sound is normally two long sounds with a short whipping sound (recorded as $\mathcal{N}$).
	b. A biphasic sound occurs or decreased vessel elasticity and includes two long lower pitched sounds (recorded as $\mathcal{\Lambda}$).
	c. A monophasic signal occurs with severely reduced blood flow and consists of one long sound that is low in pitch and volume (recorded as /).
	An arterial sound consists of a high-pitched systolic sound followed by one or more low-pitched diastolic sounds. Venous flow may be distinguished from arterial flow because the sound changes with the respiratory cycle.
e. Record results on a flow sheet.	Pulses may be graded on a five-point scale in which 4/4 means bounding, 3/4 means readily palpable, 2/4

means faintly palpable, 1/4 means barely palpable, and 0/4 means not palpable.

f. Mark pulse location with magic marker. Compare blood flow bilaterally.

2. To obtain blood pressure measurement using Doppler ultrasound, proceed as follows:

a. Take blood pressure in usual manner, substituting prelubricated Doppler probe for stethoscope (Fig. 5–28).

Standard arterial locations are brachial, radial, femoral, popliteal, dorsalis pedis, or posterior tibial.

Fig. 5–28 Ankle pressure is determined by placing Doppler probe over posterior tibial artery.

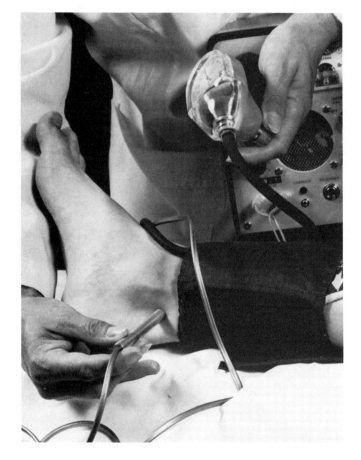

b. Inflate blood pressure cuff until arterial sound is no longer heard.

c. Deflate cuff slowly, listening for systolic and diastolic pressures.

d. Clean gel from client's skin using alcohol-soaked sponges. Clean faceplate of Doppler probe according to manufacturer's directions.

Avoid using alcohol on the faceplate of the probe because it may damage the faceplate.

RELATED NURSING CARE

NURSING ACTIONS	RATIONALE/AMPLIFICATION
1. Check extremities frequently for warmth and color as well as for blood flow.	This is particularly important after vascular surgery. The extremity may be warm and pink, but a fresh clot may be present and blood flow decreased.

2. Evaluate effectiveness of CPR compressions using Doppler ultrasound if appropriate.

EVALUATION PHASE

ANTICIPATED OUTCOMES	NURSING ACTIONS
1. Detection of decreased peripheral blood flow	Integrate Doppler findings with other assessments of peripheral blood flow.
2. Accurate determination of blood pressure in critically ill clients	Integrate serial readings with other hemodynamic parameters.

PRODUCT AVAILABILITY

ULTRASONIC DOPPLER FLOW DETECTOR

Parks Medical Electronics
Medsonics Inc.

SELECTED REFERENCES

Cudworth–Bergin K: Detecting arterial problems with a Doppler probe. RN, January 1984, pp 38–41

Durbin N: The Application of Doppler Techniques in Critical Care. Focus on Critical Care, 10(3):44–46, June 1983

6

Circulatory assist techniques

INVASIVE TECHNIQUES

BACKGROUND

The intra-aortic balloon pump (IABP) is a counterpulsation device that was developed in the 1960s in an attempt to reduce disease and death associated with left ventricular failure. The counterpulsation system consists of a balloon-tipped catheter that is advanced into the thoracic aorta, and a power console that rapidly inflates and deflates the balloon during diastole with helium or carbon dioxide gas. The power console is equipped with a monitoring system that senses the R wave from the client's ECG and permits synchronization of balloon action with the cardiac cycle. Balloon timing is refined by referring to the arterial tracing. The console also incorporates a pneumatic system that controls inflation and deflation of the balloon, as well as automatic alarms and safety features that prevent inflation during systole. The client can be transported by switching from wall current to battery power.

BALLOON CATHETERS

Several balloon configurations are available. They fall into two general types according to the inflation pattern. The unidirectional balloon has two chambers: a distal cylindric chamber and a proximal spheric chamber. The proximal chamber is inflated first, occluding the aorta, followed by inflation of the distal chamber. This inflation sequence promotes retrograde unidirectional flow and perfusion of the coronary arteries (Fig. 6–1). Omnidirectional balloons are elliptic and inflate from the center, allowing both retrograde flow into the coronary arteries and forward flow into the peripheral vascular system (Fig. 6–2).

Balloons are available with or without a central lumen. The double-lumen balloon allows guidewire insertion if vascular lesions are a problem. Arterial pressure can be

Fig. 6–1 Unidirectional balloon.

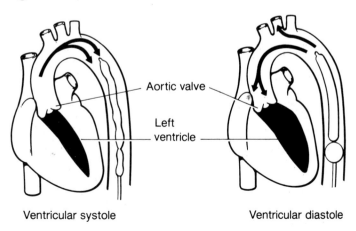

Ventricular systole   Ventricular diastole

Fig. 6-2 Omnidirectional balloon.

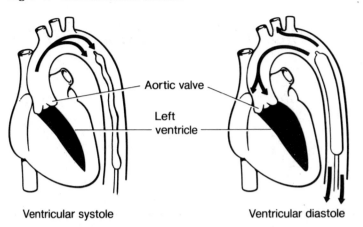

Ventricular systole   Ventricular diastole

monitored using the central lumen, making a separate arterial line for balloon timing unnecessary. The distal balloon is connected to semiflexible tubing, which connects the balloon to the console.

BALLOON INSERTION

The balloon is most commonly inserted percutaneously into the common femoral artery, with the client under local anesthesia. It is advanced into the aorta just distal to the left subclavian artery and proximal to the renal arteries. Before insertion the required length is estimated by measuring the catheter length from Louis' angle to the entry point. To facilitate insertion the balloon is wrapped and threaded through a sheath into the artery (Fig. 6-3). The balloon is unwrapped in the thoracic aorta, and the position is confirmed by fluoroscopy or chest film.

Alternatively, the balloon may be inserted surgically through a common femoral artery cutdown with the client under local anesthesia. A temporary side-arm vascular graft is used to accommodate the balloon catheter. The balloon is implanted surgically in the operating room, catheterization lab, or the critical care unit, as long as surgical asepsis is maintained. The balloon may also be inserted directly into the thoracic aorta after cardiac surgery.

PHYSIOLOGICAL PRINCIPLES OF IABP

The primary effects of counterpulsation with the IABP are reduction of afterload (the pressure against which the ventricle ejects) and the improvement of cerebral, renal, and coronary artery perfusion. Deflation of the balloon, just before ventricular systole, lowers the aortic end-diastolic pressure, thus facilitating ventricular unloading in the succeeding cardiac cycle (reduction of afterload). Inflation of the balloon during diastole boosts coronary-bed and peripheral perfusion by increasing the diastolic pressure. Eighty percent of coronary artery perfusion occurs during diastole. These effects of counterpulsation result in decreased myocardial oxygen demand and improved contractility.

The primary indications for IABP are cardiogenic shock after acute myocardial infarction (MI) and left ventricular failure after open-heart surgery. IABP may also benefit clients with severe unstable angina and post-MI angina, and those with refractory ventricular arrhythmias. IABP is contraindicated in the presence of severe peripheral vascular occlusive disease, previous femoral grafts, aortic aneurysm, and aortic-valve incompetence.

Intra-aortic balloon pump

Objective
To decrease cardiac afterload and improve cardiac and renal circulation through counterpulsation

Fig. 6-3 Percutaneous balloon threaded through sheath into femoral artery. (Courtesy Datascope Corp, Paramus, NJ)

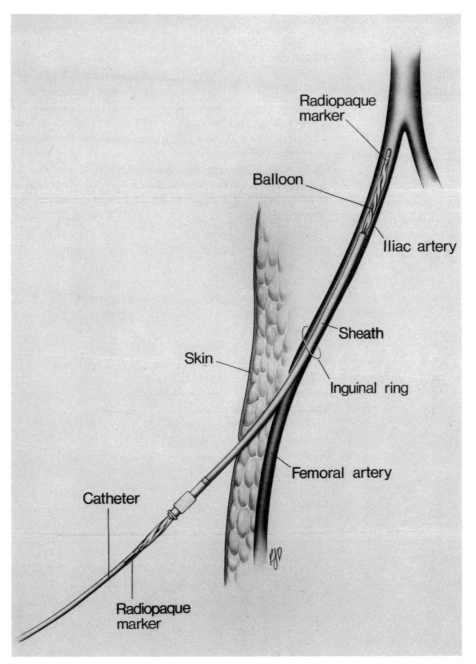

ASSESSMENT PHASE

- Why does the client require IABP (*e.g.*, cardiogenic shock or left ventricular failure that is unresponsive to medical therapy, or septic shock)?
- Are a pulmonary artery (PA) catheter and arterial line *in situ?* PA and pulmonary capillary wedge (PCW) pressures and mean arterial (MA) pressure will be indicators of hemodynamic status during IABP. The timing of the IABP requires an arterial tracing.
- Is a Foley catheter in place? Close monitoring of urine output will indicate improvement in renal perfusion with IABP.
- What are the baseline assessments of peripheral pulses, skin color and perfusion, and mental status?
- Is a hematologic profile available? The IABP can damage red blood cells. Heparinization may be required during and after insertion.

- Has blood been typed, crossmatched, and placed on hold during insertion? Arterial trauma and inadvertent blood loss will require transfusion.
- Are peripheral pulses adequate? Mark pulses with a magic marker to facilitate evaluation after balloon insertion. The IABP can obstruct circulation to the lower extremities. If the position of the balloon in the aorta occludes the left subclavian artery, the left radial pulse rate will be decreased.

PRECAUTIONS

- **Never resterilize or reuse balloons. Balloon integrity may be impaired.**
- **Protect the balloon surface from contact with metal objects or glove powder. Damage to the antithrombogenic surface may result.**
- **Inspect the balloon for imperfections before insertion by inflating it with a 50-ml syringe.**
- **If insertion is temporarily interrupted and the balloon is removed, rinse with sterile heparinized saline to prevent thrombus formation.**

PLANNING PHASE

EQUIPMENT

IABP catheter
IABP console
Arterial line (or prepared transducer/pressure-monitoring setup)
Iodophor solution
Xylocaine 1%
2-ml syringe and needles (for local anesthesia)
Sterile dressing
Hypoallergenic tape
Advanced cardiac life-support (ACLS) equipment
Multichannel cardiac monitor
Heparin bolus
Rheomacrodex infusion (if ordered)
IV antibiotic (if ordered)
Continuous suction outlets—2
Fluoroscopy table (optional)
Lead aprons (if fluoroscopy is used)
Operating light
Sterile drapes and gowns
Masks
Sterile gloves
For percutaneous insertion include the following:
    Percutaneous insertion kit
        60 cm × 0.035 inch stainless steel "J" guidewire
        145 cm × 0.035 inch Teflon-coated medium floppy "J" guidewire
        18-gauge thin-walled Potts–Cournand needle
        8F dilator
        12F dilator sheath assembly
        Skin suture
For surgical insertion include the following:
    Surgical vascular instrument set
        Syringes and needles
        50-ml syringe
        Sterile suction tip
        Sterile suction tubing
        Lap sponges
        4 × 4
        145 cm × 0.035 inch Teflon-coated floppy "J" guidewire
        10-mm woven Dacron side-arm graft
        Suture

CLIENT/FAMILY TEACHING

- Answer the client's questions about the reasons for using an IABP. Use a balloon catheter and diagrams as necessary.

- Reassure the client and family about additional complex equipment required for the IABP.
- Reassure the client and family about alarms associated with the balloon console.
- Discuss with the client sensations associated with IABP insertion (*e.g.*, discomfort associated with fluoroscopy table).
- Reassure the client that the procedure will not be painful and that a local anesthetic will be administered, as well as a sedative if necessary.
- Discuss precautions associated with heparinization (if applicable).

IMPLEMENTATION PHASE

NURSING ACTIONS	RATIONALE/AMPLIFICATION
1. Prepare transducer and pressure-monitoring setup (see Transducer Setup: Up to Two Pressures in Chap. 5).	This setup will be required only if the central lumen of the balloon will be used to monitor arterial pressure. Place client on fluoroscopy table, if required.
2. Turn on balloon console and check functioning and gas volume (Fig. 6–4).	Calibrate pressure channels and adjust the setting to zero.

Fig. 6–4 Balloon console. (Courtesy Datascope Corp., Paramus, NJ)

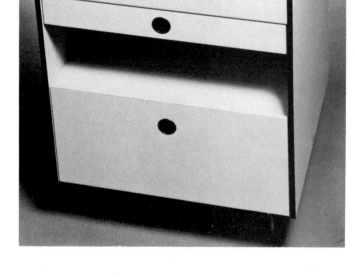

3. Establish direct ECG using console ECG cable.	The ECG signal drives the console. Establishing dual sources of an ECG signal minimizes the interruption of pumping if the signal is lost.

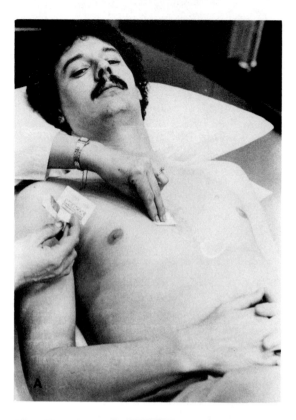

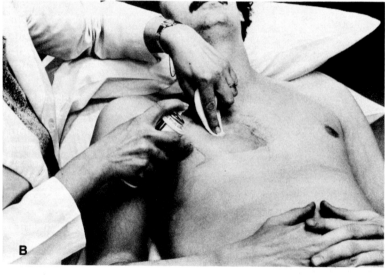

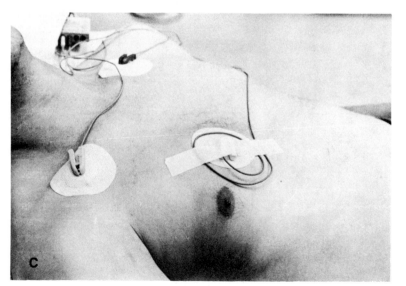

4. Establish indirect ECG from bedside monitor to console.

Locate the lead that maximizes the R wave and minimizes other waves or pacemaker artifacts that may be sensed by the console and cause the disruption of pumping. Consoles require a positive (upright) R wave to trigger the balloon. Use the switch on the console that inverts the signal to obtain a positive spike if necessary. Determine that the ECG trigger light flashes once with each R wave. (See Fig. 6–5 for method of securing ECG electrodes.)

5. Obtain baseline data, including vital signs, PA and PCW pressures, if available, and 12-lead ECG.

A 12-lead ECG can be used to locate the lead with the best R wave to trigger the console.

6. Make preliminary adjustments of inflation and deflation timing controls by

Select trigger logic if it is required for the specific balloon console being used.

a. Positioning inflation marker on peak of T wave

Observe the position of inflation and deflation markers on the oscilloscope.

b. Positioning deflation marker between P wave and R wave (Fig. 6–6).

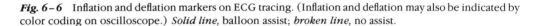

Fig. 6–6 Inflation and deflation markers on ECG tracing. (Inflation and deflation may also be indicated by color coding on oscilloscope.) *Solid line,* balloon assist; *broken line,* no assist.

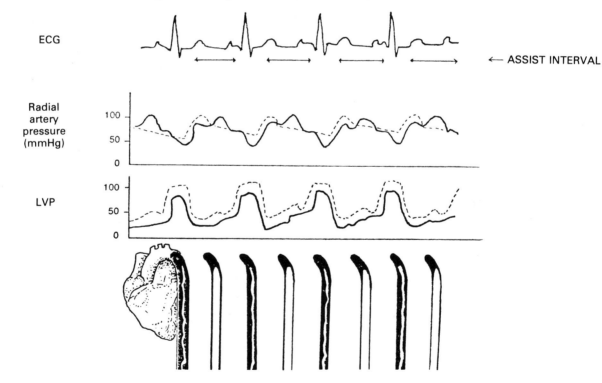

7. Select 1 : 1 balloon pumping ratio.

When the console is set on 1 : 1 ratio, the balloon is inflated following each ventricular contraction. The balloon inflates following every second heart beat if the setting is 1 : 2.

8. Adjust gas displacement control to one-half volume.

9. Initiate antibiotic coverage as ordered.

Allow sufficient time for the blood level to be established.

10. Assist surgical team with masks, caps, and gowns.

Masks and caps should be worn by all persons in the immediate area.

11. Shave both groin areas.

12. Assist with preparation of sterile field.

    a. Open sterile packages on sterile field.

    b. Help physician to drape operative site after preparing skin with iodophor solution.

Maintain access to IV lines.

    c. Adjust operative light.

    d. Assist with administration of local anesthetic.

13. Monitor client's baseline vital signs and hemodynamic parameters during insertion.

14. Notify physician of significant changes in clinical status during procedure.

Severe back pain can indicate aortic dissection. Angina can be controlled with medication prescribed to prevent myocardial infarction. For percutaneous insertion the physician will insert the balloon using a guidewire and sheath to introduce the balloon into the femoral artery (Seldinger technique). After the balloon is wrapped, a vacuum is created with a 50-ml syringe or wall suction to prevent unwrapping. The balloon unwraps automatically when pumping begins.

15. Administer heparin bolus as ordered before arteriotomy.

For surgical insertion the balloon is inserted by a cutdown and side-arm graft into the femoral artery. A vacuum is created with a 50-ml syringe or wall suction to facilitate insertion.

16. If safety chamber is used, proceed as follows:

Balloon consoles are available with or without a safety chamber that connects the balloon to the console.

    a. Use "Auto-fill" to preload safety chamber/IABP circuit with CO_2.

    b. Extend and attach circuit securely to balloon when proximal end is passed off sterile field.

    c. Secure connections.

17. If a safety chamber is not used, proceed as follows:

    a. Connect balloon plug to console when proximal end is passed off sterile field.

    b. Purge gas lines with helium and fill balloon using appropriate controls.

The rubber sleeve is moved away from the balloon catheter vent to allow air to escape during purging.

18. If balloon has central lumen for monitoring arterial pressure, connect arterial port to pressure-monitoring setup.

If the console displays an arterial tracing, connect output from the arterial pressure monitor to the console. Calibrate the arterial pressure tracing according to the manufacturer's instructions.

19. Begin pumping at half volume.

20. Refine timing using arterial pressure tracing.

Timing can be adjusted using a peripheral arterial tracing or an arterial tracing directly from the central lumen of the balloon. (See previous section IABP Timing.)

21. Evaluate balloon function.

Observe the safety chamber or the balloon pressure curve. Assess for hemodynamic deterioration. Determine PA, PCW, and MA pressures.

22. Fill balloon to full volume.

23. Recheck timing and correct balloon function.

24. Activate console alarms.

Conditions that interfere with pumping activate an audible alarm and display an alarm message. If this occurs, correct the problem and restart pumping.

25. Dress site using a dry, sterile, occlusive dressing.

26. Evaluate peripheral pulses.

27. Obtain chest film to verify balloon position unless fluoroscopy is used during insertion.

RELATED NURSING CARE

NURSING ACTIONS

RATIONALE/AMPLIFICATION

1. Assess circulation to extremities hourly and record on flow sheet. Check peripheral pulses and skin temperature and color.

The balloon may obstruct peripheral blood flow. Use Doppler ultrasound to assess weak pulses. Notify the physician of inadequate circulation.

2. Change dressing using sterile technique every 24 hours to 48 hours.

Observe the insertion site for signs of infection.

3. Monitor hemodynamic and clinical status every 15 minutes to 60 minutes.

4. Recheck balloon timing every hour and correct as necessary (see previous section on IABP Timing).

Unsafe timing can cause hemodynamic deterioration. Adjust timing for maximum effectiveness.

5. Continue antibiotic coverage 24 hours to 48 hours after insertion as ordered.

6. Continue anticoagulation regimen if ordered.

Anticoagulation drugs may be prescribed to prevent venous thrombosis. Some physicians order low molecular weight dextran 500 ml/24 hours to discourage platelet aggregation on the balloon catheter. Monitor partial thromboplastin time (PTT) and prothrombin time and observe for spontaneous bleeding.

7. Maintain head of bed no higher than 30 degrees and instruct client not to bend leg in which balloon is inserted.

This protects the balloon catheter from damage. If the balloon catheter cracks, reinforce it with electrician's tape.

8. Rapidly inflate and deflate balloon with 50-ml syringe several times every 10 minutes if console malfunctions.

This prevents thrombus formation in balloon folds. Exchange consoles or consider removing the balloon if the console cannot be repaired within 30 minutes.

9. To assist with balloon removal, proceed as follows:

    a. Begin weaning procedure by gradually reducing pumping ratio from 1:1 to 1:8.

Closely monitor hemodynamic and clinical status during weaning.

    b. Turn off console as ordered.

    c. Recreate insertion environment.

10. To assist with removal of percutaneous balloon, proceed as follows:

    a. Aspirate balloon to deflate before removal.

The physician will remove the suture and withdraw the balloon.

    b. Apply manual pressure to insertion site for 20 minutes.

    c. Apply sterile pressure dressing.

A sandbag may be placed over the insertion site.

d. Evaluate site for hematoma or bleeding every 15 minutes until client is stable. Evaluate periodically for 24 hours.

If bleeding is observed, apply digital pressure just above the site for 20 minutes, or until the physician arrives, to reestablish hemostasis.

11. To assist with removal of surgical balloon, proceed as follows:

a. Aspirate balloon to deflate before removal.

Initiate antibiotic coverage if ordered. The surgeon will reopen the cutdown, remove the balloon, and repair the artery.

b. Apply sterile dressing after wound is sutured.

c. Evaluate for bleeding or hematoma in 15 minutes, and periodically for 24 hours.

EVALUATION PHASE

ANTICIPATED OUTCOMES	NURSING ACTIONS
1. Support of failing left ventricle through counterpulsation	Evaluate hemodynamic parameters every 15 minutes to 60 minutes. Indications for weaning from IABP include a cardiac index (CI) greater than 2 liters/minute, a PCW pressure less than 20 mm Hg, and a systolic blood pressure reading greater than 100 mm Hg.
2. Improvement of coronary circulation	Evaluate cardiac rhythm and cardiac output (CO).
3. Improvement of peripheral circulation	Evaluate cognition to determine whether the cerebral circulation has improved. Evaluate urine output every hour. Improved urine output indicates increased renal perfusion.
4. Prevention of complications of IABP insertion	Evaluate for correct console function. Evaluate for balloon rupture or leak, which can cause gas embolism. Assess hematologic profile for a decrease in platelet and red blood cell counts caused by balloon function. Assess the peripheral circulation for circulatory insufficiency.

PRODUCT AVAILABILITY   FULL RANGE OF BALLOONS, BALLOON INSERTION KITS, AND BALLOON PUMPS

Datascope Corp.
Kontron Cardiovascular Inc.

Intra-aortic balloon pump timing

Objectives

To achieve maximum afterload reduction through correct timing of inflation and deflation of the IABP

To increase aortic pressure and volume through displacement

To increase mean systemic arterial-perfusion pressure

ASSESSMENT PHASE   • Is an arterial tracing available for balloon timing? The arterial tracing may be obtained directly from the balloon, if the balloon has a central lumen, or a radial or femoral arterial tracing may be used.

PRECAUTION   • **Observe the arterial tracing and clinical status for signs of incorrect or dangerous timing.**

PLANNING PHASE   IABP

EQUIPMENT   Intra-aortic balloon (in place)
Arterial tracing

IMPLEMENTATION PHASE

NURSING ACTIONS	RATIONALE/AMPLIFICATION
1. Turn pump to 1 : 2 assist ratio.	The balloon will inflate during every other cardiac cycle. Most clients tolerate this for a brief period. If the arterial pressure drops significantly, run a strip recording or "freeze" the tracing on the console. Timing may then be analyzed while the client is returned to a 1 : 1 ratio.
2. Identify timing landmarks on arterial tracing (Fig. 6–7).	

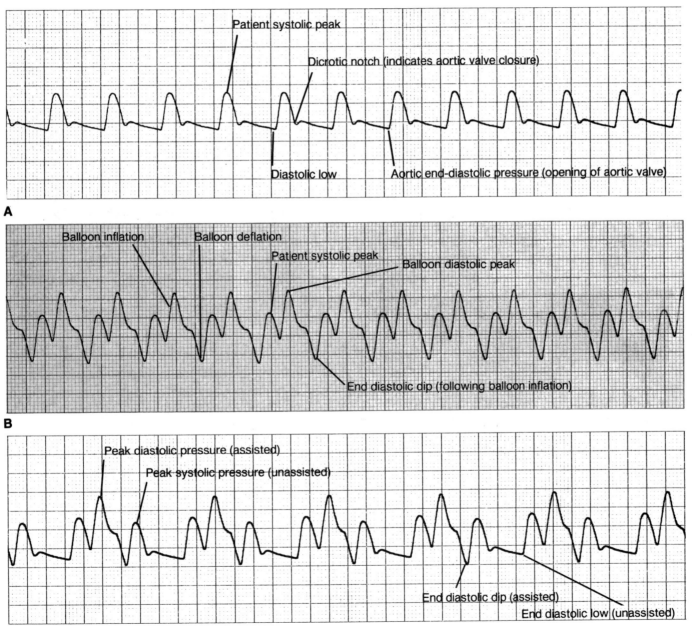

Fig. 6–7 Arterial tracing. (*A*) Normal arterial pressure tracing. (*B*) Arterial tracing with 1 : 1 balloon augmentation ratio. (*C*) Arterial tracing with 1 : 2 balloon augmentation ratio.

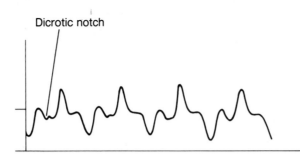

Dicrotic notch

Fig. 6–8 Adjustment of inflation control (1 : 2 ratio). Note gradual disappearance of dicrotic notch.

3. Adjust inflation controls.

a. Move inflation control left until balloon is inflating at dicrotic notch.

The dicrotic notch will disappear on the arterial tracing (Fig. 6–8).

b. If peripheral arterial line is used, continue to move inflation control left until optimal arterial tracing is obtained. This tracing indicates that balloon is inflating immediately following aortic-valve closure (Fig. 6–9).

Pressures that are obtained with a radial or femoral arterial line are slightly delayed representations of events occurring at the aortic root.

c. Observe for increase in diastolic peak.

As timing improves, diastolic augmentation will improve. Diastolic augmentation should equal or exceed the client's systolic pressure.

4. Adjust deflation controls.

a. Slowly move deflation control right (longer inflation) and observe for decrease in depth of end-di-

The end-diastolic dip should be 10 mm to 15 mm below the diastolic low (without balloon augmentation). The

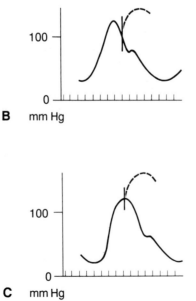

A   mm Hg

B   mm Hg

C   mm Hg

Fig. 6–9 Optimal arterial pressure waveforms with diastolic augmentation (balloon inflation). (*A*) Aortic root waveform. Inflation occurs on the dicrotic notch. (*B*) Radial artery waveform. Inflation occurs 40 to 50 msec before the dicrotic notch. (*C*) Femoral artery waveform. Inflation occurs 120 msec before the dicrotic notch.

Fig. 6-10 Adjustment of deflation control (1 : 2 ratio). Note progressive reduction in depth of end-diastolic dip and decline in height of systolic peak after balloon augmentation. (*1*) Maximal reduction in height of systolic peak (unassisted) demonstrates effect of reduced afterload. (*2*) End-diastolic dip (after balloon inflation) equal to or 10 mm to 15 mm below level of diastolic low.

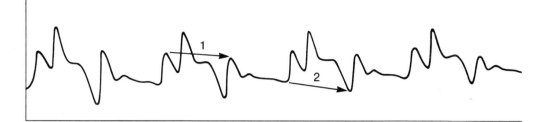

astolic dip and for height of systolic peak after balloon augmentation (Fig. 6-10).

height of the systolic peak after balloon augmentation will gradually decline relative to the systolic peak, which is unaffected by balloon action.

5. Observe for the following signs of dangerous timing:

a. Early inflation, beginning before aortic-valve closure

The ventricle must unload against the inflating balloon, causing increased afterload and myocardial oxygen demand.

b. Late deflation encroaching on client systole

The ventricle must unload against the balloon, which remains inflated.

6. Observe balloon pressure tracing for correct balloon action.

Observe the action of the safety chamber if one is being used.

EVALUATION PHASE

ANTICIPATED OUTCOMES	NURSING ACTIONS
1. Improvement of left ventricular function	Evaluate for the following improvements in hemodynamic and clinical status: **a.** Normalization of cardiac parameters such as increased MA pressure, decreased PCW pressure and heart rate, increased CO, decreased arrhythmias and chest pain, and absence of S_3 (ventricular) and S_4 (atrial) gallops **b.** Normalization of respiratory parameters such as rate, ABGs, clearing rales, and interstitial edema, which can be seen on chest film **c.** Normalization of urinary parameters such as urinary output ($>$30 ml/hour), and decreased specific gravity and blood urea nitrogen (BUN) **d.** Improved sensorium **e.** Improved circulation to extremities
2. Avoidance of effects of dangerous or incorrect timing	Evaluate for signs of increased afterload or increased myocardial oxygen demand, including changes in the arterial tracing, arrhythmias, and hemodynamic deterioration. Evaluate for signs of clinical deterioration such as clouded sensorium, decreased urinary output, pulmonary edema, and loss of peripheral pulses.

Evaluation of IABP action on arterial waveform

Inflation occurs at the dicrotic notch.
The diastolic peak (balloon action) is greater than or equal to the preceding systolic peak.
The end-diastolic dip after balloon action is

10 mm to 15 mm lower than the diastolic low.
The systolic peak after balloon action is lower than the systolic peak without preceding balloon action.

SELECTED REFERENCES

Haak SW: Intra-aortic balloon pump techniques. DCCN 2(4):196–204, July–August 1983
Hudak CM, Lohr T, Gallo BM: Critical Care Nursing, 3rd ed. Philadelphia, JB Lippincott, 1982
Purcell JA, Pipin L, Mitchell M: Intra-aortic balloon pump therapy. Am J Nurs 83(5):775–790, May 1983
Quaal SJ: Comprehensive Intra-Aortic Balloon Pumping. St. Louis, CV Mosby, 1984

NONINVASIVE TECHNIQUES

BACKGROUND

EXTERNAL PRESSURE CIRCULATORY ASSIST DEVICE

The antigravity suit is a noninvasive circulatory assist device. It is called by several names: G suit, military antishock trousers (MAST), or antishock airpants. The antigravity suit is valuable in emergency situations in caring for multitrauma victims or clients in hypovolemic shock resulting from other causes. The suit is made of nylon, and it is waterproof, flame resistant, and radiolucent, with three separate chambers. It inflates to a maximum pressure of 104 mm Hg, and features pop-off valves to prevent overinflation and in-line gauges to measure pressures in each chamber. Adult and pediatric sizes are available. The suit has several openings. A perineal opening allows for bladder catheterization, and foot openings allow for assessment of pedal pulses, electrode placement, and venous cutdown.

Antigravity suits merely assist in the initial stabilization of the hypotensive client and are not considered a definitive therapy. The suit can be applied in approximately 60 seconds while another care-giver is starting an IV line or while waiting for blood to arrive.

Antigravity suit

Objectives

To redistribute available blood volume proximally to the general circulation to maintain perfusion of the vital organs
To apply direct pressure to the lower extremities to reduce blood loss and immobilize injuries
To distend upper limb veins to facilitate initiation of IV therapy
To increase intra-abdominal pressure to tamponade bleeding sites in the abdomen and pelvic regions
To facilitate oxygen transport through autotransfused blood

ASSESSMENT PHASE

- Is the client severely hypotensive with a systolic blood pressure of less than 60 mm Hg? Regardless of the cause of hypotension, use of the antigravity suit should be considered.
- Are there contraindications to the use of the suit? Severe flexion contracture, protruding bone fragments, or an impaling object such as glass or rock are contraindications, and the risks of applying the suit with or without these complications should be weighed.
- Is the client's size compatible with the suit? For clients under 105 cm (3 feet, 6 inches) and very thin or obese clients, it is difficult to use the suit. If the client is

thin, both legs may fit into one chamber of the antigravity suit. If the client is obese, use the suit in the usual way, using tape instead of Velcro to fasten it.

- Does the client have wounds or possible abdominal injuries? Assess wounds and abdominal signs carefully because these will be obliterated once the suit is in place.
- Are intrathoracic bleeding injuries present? The inflated suit will cause further bleeding. It still may be advantageous to increase the blood in the central circulation with pooled blood from the lower extremities.
- Is the client at risk of increased intracranial pressure (ICP) (*e.g.,* resulting from head injuries)? The suit will increase ICP, but it may be necessary to elevate the client's blood pressure and to provide circulatory support.
- Is electromechanical dissociation (EMD) present? The antigravity suit may be used with EMD that is caused by hypovolemic shock.
- Is the client pregnant? The effect of the antigravity suit on fetal circulation is unknown, but if the mother is severely hypotensive, the conduction of the fetus will be compromised. Consider the inflation of the leg units only, and, with severe hypovolemia, consider inflating the entire suit.
- Has a baseline respiratory physical assessment been performed? Once the suit is inflated, the respiratory assessment will be used to determine possible respiratory distress.
- Is the ventilatory capacity decreased, and is the client severely hypotensive? If so, only the leg units should be inflated.
- Will transportation of the client be required? Obtain a portable tank of noncombustible gas.
- Will the client be transported by air? The antigravity suit may be used in unpressurized cabins with pressures above 104 mm Hg escaping through bleed-off valves. Check the client's blood pressure during descent.

PRECAUTIONS

- **Avoid perforation of the suit with sharp objects.**
- **Never position the antigravity suit above the xiphoid area. This will interfere with ventilation.**
- **Avoid abrupt deflation of the antigravity suit, which may cause severe hypotension.**
- **Prevent kinking or blocking of the pop-off valves. This will allow excess pressure to bleed off.**

PLANNING PHASE

EQUIPMENT

Antigravity suit
Attachment for foot pump
Compressed air
Abdominal (ABD) pads and Kerlix (optional)
Lanolin (optional)

CLIENT/FAMILY TEACHING

- Discuss the rationale for the use of the suit with the client (if the client's condition permits) and family.
- Reassure the client and family that this procedure is not painful.
- Discuss the discomfort the client may experience (*i.e.,* nausea or vomiting, or feelings of the need to urinate or defecate because of abdominal pressure and pressure on the diaphragm).

IMPLEMENTATION PHASE

NURSING ACTIONS	RATIONALE/AMPLIFICATION
1. Assess lower extremities and abdomen for foreign objects or wounds.	
2. Remove client's belt and shoes and check trouser pockets for any sharp objects.	Sharp objects may puncture the antigravity suit.

3. Unfold suit. Open stopcock valves and attach foot pump.

4. Logroll client onto suit.

5. Wrap and fasten trouser legs, and then fasten abdominal straps. If pressure tubing is color coded, match it with tubing of same color on suit (Fig. 6–11).

If the suit is being used in a controlled environment, apply lanolin to the skin and protect the bony prominences with ABD dressings and Kerlix.

If one is available, the client may be wrapped in a bath blanket before using the trousers to further protect the skin. Be sure the bath blanket is free of wrinkles.

Wrap the abdominal straps below the xiphoid area. Another care-giver may initiate an IV line. Wrap only the leg areas if respiratory distress is evident. Keep the blood pressure cuff attached to the client's arm to take serial readings throughout the procedure.

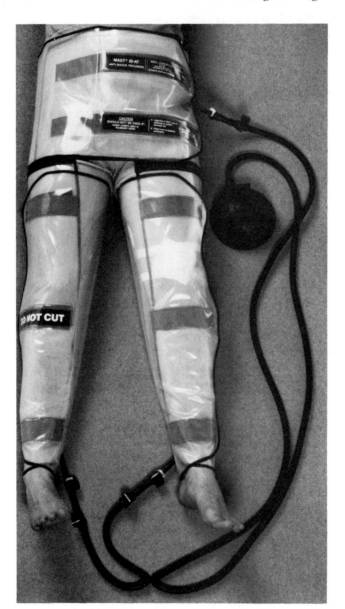

Fig. 6–11 Antigravity trousers.

6. Inflate suit to approximately 20 mm Hg to 30 mm Hg, or as ordered.

Any or all chambers may be inflated. When one chamber is being inflated, the stopcocks of the other two chambers must be closed. Limit the inflation pressure to 40 mm Hg. The degree of inflation may be determined by observing when air begins to escape from the stopcocks or when the client's systolic blood pressure rises to an acceptable level (100 mm Hg). While one care-giver is inflating the suit, a second care-giver checks the client's blood pressure every 15 seconds.

7. Check to see that stopcocks are closed. Disconnect pump.

RELATED NURSING CARE

NURSING ACTIONS	RATIONALE/AMPLIFICATION
1. Monitor vital signs every 5 minutes to 15 minutes.	This will help to evaluate the client's hemodynamic response.
2. Assess for signs of respiratory distress.	Respiratory distress warns of impending fluid overload.
3. If client is intubated, assess for changes in ventilatory function, especially inspiratory and expiratory volumes.	These changes suggest changes in lung compliance.
4. Order laboratory work to measure lactate level and ABGs.	These analyses reflect the effects of the suit's compression and the degree of hypovolemic compromise.
5. To transport client, obtain portable tank of noncombustible gas. Do not clamp valves for transportation.	Do not use oxygen for inflation.
6. Deflate suit only when client is stabilized or when admitted to surgical unit or operating room.	When necessary, as in the case of severe abdominal bleeding, the suit may be removed in the operating room. The optional inflation time for the suit is 2 hours, although it can be used for many days at low pressure.
7. Deflate suit when appropriate.	
a. Deflate one chamber at a time *starting with abdominal chamber.*	
b. Deflate gradually while second care-giver checks blood pressure every 15 seconds.	If the client's blood pressure drops 5 mm Hg, stop deflating. Reinflate the section that was being deflated when the client's blood pressure dropped, and increase the rate of IV fluids. Wait until the blood pressure stabilizes before proceeding.
c. Continue with deflation sequence from abdominal chamber to individual leg chambers.	The leg sections are *never* deflated before the abdominal section because this section acts as a tourniquet for the pooling of large volumes of blood in the legs.
d. Remove trousers when they are loose enough to be removed easily.	Be sure that the blood pressure is stabilized before removing the suit.

EVALUATION PHASE

ANTICIPATED OUTCOMES	NURSING ACTIONS
1. Stabilization of hemodynamic parameters until definitive therapy can be initiated	
2. Stabilization of client's blood pressure until bleeding in abdomen or lower extremities has slowed considerably or stopped	
3. Effective perfusion of vital organs in presence of severe hypotension	

4. Prevention of complications resulting from use of antigravity suit

Evaluate for atelectasis or pneumonia that is secondary to reduced pressure on the diaphragm and reduced vital capacity. Assess for pulmonary edema when fluid from the extremities is redistributed. Assess for thromboemboli and skin breakdown caused by pressure.

PRODUCT AVAILABILITY

MEDICAL ANTISHOCK TROUSERS (MAST)

Armstrong Industries Inc.

JOBST GLADIATOR ANTISHOCK AIRPANTS

The Jobst Institute Inc.

SELECTED REFERENCES

Budassi S, Barber JM: Emergency Nursing: Principles and Practice, pp 247–249. St. Louis, CV Mosby, 1981

McIntyre K, Lewis AJ (eds): Textbook of Advanced Cardiac Life Support, pp v, 2–3. Dallas, American Heart Association, 1981

Nursing Now Shock. Nursing '84, 1984, pp 39–40

7

Artificial pacemakers

BACKGROUND

Artificial pacemakers have been in use since the early 1950s. Although the sophistication of pacemaker models has expanded dramatically since then, the purpose of an artificial pacemaker has remained the same—to cause the heart to beat.

The working cells of the myocardium depolarize and subsequently contract when stimulated by an electric potential of sufficient amplitude (strength). In a normal heart, this is accomplished when an electric impulse reaches the myocardial cells through the conduction system (Fig. 7–1). When the conduction system is diseased and therefore unreliable or nonfunctional, an artificial pacemaker may be indicated. Pacemakers may be used in sick sinus syndrome, high degree heart block, extreme bradycardia, or asystole.

Fig. 7–1 Normal conduction system. *SA*, sinoatrial; *AV*, atrioventricular.

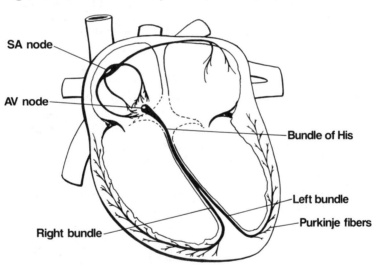

PACEMAKER COMPONENTS

A pacemaker consists of an electric generator, an electric lead, and one or two electrodes (Fig. 7–2). The generator can be programmed for the amount of energy delivered, the rate of delivery, and the degree of sensitivity to the client's intrinsic (natural) rhythm. There are various types of electric leads available that aid in the insertion and location of the pacemaker in different areas of the heart. A lead may be unipolar (one electrode) or bipolar (two electrodes). With both types there is the complete negative-to-positive current flow that is essential for pacing. The electrodes must be in contact with a viable myocardium to conduct the electric impulse and to depolarize myocardial cells.

CLASSIFICATION OF PACEMAKERS

Pacing leads can be placed in the atrium, the ventricle, or both. If the lead is located in both, the pacemaker is called an *atrioventricular* (AV) *sequential* pacemaker. Atrial

Fig. 7-2 Temporary pacemaker components. (*A*) Temporary generator. (*B*) Bridging cable. (*C*) Bipolar pacing lead.

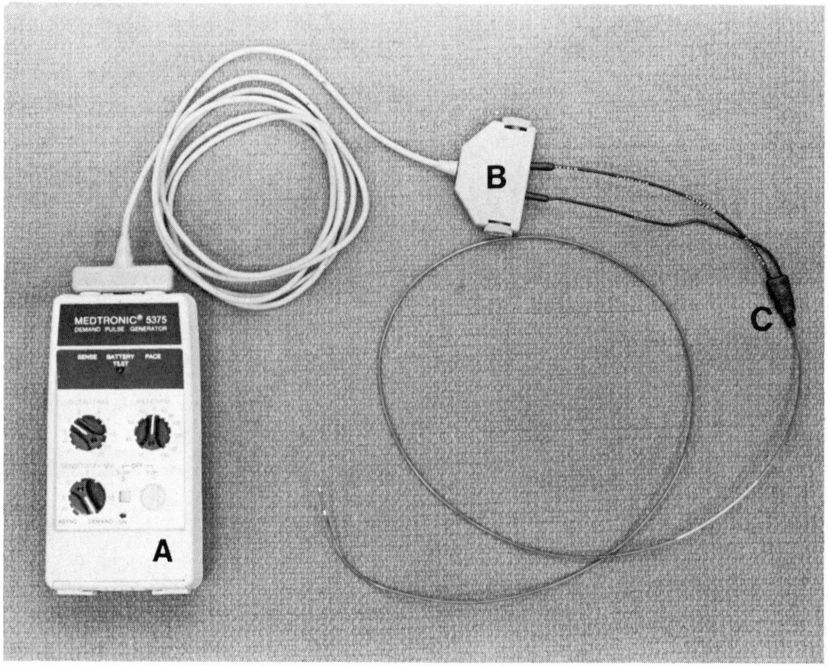

pacing, either alone or in sequence with the ventricles, preserves the atrial kick. The *atrial kick* is the contraction of the atrium in late ventricular diastole that is responsible for 20% to 30% of the ventricular filling pressure. If the ventricles only are paced, the atrial kick is lost. This can significantly affect cardiac output (CO) in some diseased hearts.

A pacemaker may be temporary or permanent. Temporary generators remain external; permanent generators are implanted subcutaneously. For transvenous pacing, the lead is guided into the right side of the heart through a vein. The electrodes are positioned in the trabeculae carneae of the endocardium. Alternatively, the permanent pacemaker may be epicardial. Epicardial pacemakers require a thoracotomy because the electrodes are implanted directly on the epicardium.

An artificial pacemaker may be programmed to function on demand, that is, only when the client's intrinsic rate falls below a predetermined limit, or it may be a fixed rate pacemaker, which functions as programmed regardless of intrinsic rhythms. This is also called *asynchronous* pacing.

If the pacemaker is functioning on demand, it "senses" the client's intrinsic rhythm. The generator is programmed to interpret the incoming signal and to respond in one of two ways. The mode of response may be inhibition or triggering. If it is inhibited, the generator will not release its next expected output and will recycle from the time of the intrinsic beat. If the mode of response to a sensed impulse is triggering, the pacemaker will release its output with the intrinsic beat.

A three-letter identification code was developed in 1974 to simplify the nomenclature used to describe implantable permanent pacemakers. The authors of the original code expanded it to five letters in 1981. Position IV describes programming functions and position V describes special antiarrhythmic features. Position III was revised to include a code for reverse functions, such as the pacemaker is silent at slow rates and activated by fast rates (Table 7-1).

Examples of currently available pacemakers using the five-letter code include the following:

VVI pacemakers feature ventricular pacing and sensing and inhibitory mode. They are nonprogrammable and have no special antiarrhythmic functions. Therefore letters present in the IV-V positions do not apply.

Table 7–1
Five-position identification code for permanent pacemakers

Position	Category	Letters Used
I	Chamber paced	V—ventricle A—atrium D—double
II	Chamber sensed	V—ventricle A—atrium D—double O—none
III	Mode of response	T—triggered I—inhibited D—double O—none R—reverse
IV	Programming functions	P—single programming (rate and output) M—multiprogrammability O—none
V	Antiarrhythmic functions	B—bursts N—normal rate E—external If none, position is left blank.

(From Parsonnet V, Furman S, Smyth NPD: A revised code for pacemaker identification. PACE 4(4):400–403, July 1981)

AAR, ON pacemakers are used for rapid atrial pacing for termination of rapid supraventricular tachycardias. They feature atrial pacing and sensing, have a reverse mode of response, and are nonprogrammable and normal-rate competitive.

PACEMAKER TERMINOLOGY

Pacemakers function by delivering a predetermined amount of energy to the myocardium. This is known as the *output* and is measured in milliamperes (mA). When a pacemaker fires, a spike or pacemaker artifact is seen on the electrocardiogram (ECG). The pacemaker captures when the spike is followed by myocardial depolarization. A P wave on the ECG is evidence of atrial depolarization and should follow atrial pacing spikes. A QRS complex on the ECG indicates ventricular depolarization and should follow ventricular pacing spikes.

Ventricular pacing bypasses the normal conduction system. Therefore, ventricular-paced beats characteristically have a wide QRS complex (*i.e.*, 0.12 seconds or greater). If an intrinsic beat occurs at the same time as the paced beat, a fusion beat results. The QRS-complex morphology of a fusion beat is a mixture of that of the intrinsic beat and the paced beat. These beats are not dangerous (Fig. 7–3).

Fig. 7–3 Fusion beat. *PB*, pacemaker beat; *IB*, intrinsic beat; *FB*, fusion beat.

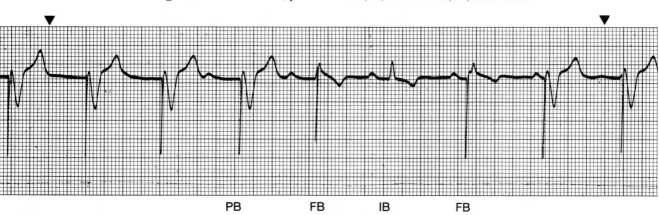

PB   FB   IB   FB

The amount of time a pacemaker waits to sense the client's rhythm before it fires is called the *escape interval* and can be measured on the ECG as the time between an intrinsic beat and a subsequent paced beat. The pacemaker will continue to fire at a given rate as long as the client's rate is inadequate. The *automatic interval* is the time between two consecutively paced beats (Fig. 7–4).

Fig. 7–4 Demand pacing. Escape interval is equal to automatic interval. *PB*, pacemaker beat; *IB*, intrinsic beat.

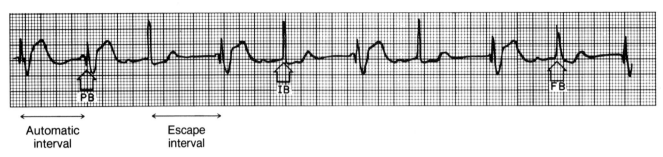

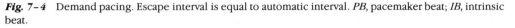

Usually the escape and automatic intervals are the same. However, because ventricular pacing eliminates the atrial kick, artificially paced beats may have a lower cardiac output (CO) than intrinsic beats do. Some pacemaker models can be programmed such that the escape interval is longer than the automatic interval. This allows the client's intrinsic rhythm, augmented by the atrial kick, to fall to a lower rate than is required when pacing. The paced rate, defined by the automatic interval, will be faster than the lowest intrinsic rate in order to maintain an adequate CO without the atrial kick. This phenomenon is known as *hysteresis* (Fig. 7–5).

Fig. 7–5 Hysteresis. Escape interval is significantly longer than automatic interval. *PB*, pacemaker beat; *IB*, intrinsic beat; *FB*, fusion beat.

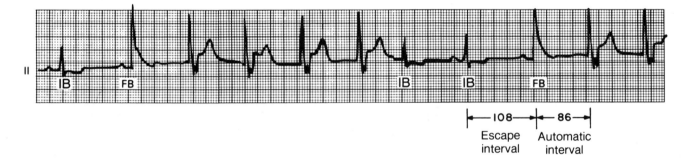

ASSESSING PACEMAKER FUNCTION

Most modern permanent pacemaker generators are accompanied by a special magnet that is specific to the model of pacemaker. This magnet can be used to assess battery life and, in some cases, the sensing ability and threshold of the pacemaker. Generally, when the magnet is placed over the permanent generator, it converts the pacemaker to a fixed mode at a specified rate. The fixed rate may be higher or lower than the programmed rate, depending on the model.

Pacemaker function is described in terms of sensing, firing, and capture. *Failure to sense* means that the pacemaker has fired inappropriately because it has not detected the client's intrinsic rhythm (Fig. 7–6). The most frequent causes of failure to sense include a displaced pacemaker lead (*i.e.*, one that is not in direct contact with the myocardium) or fixed rate pacing, which occurs when the sensitivity of the generator has been decreased. Corrective measures include increasing the generator's sensitivity setting or turning the client to the left lateral recumbent position. It may be possible to turn off the generator, leaving it in place should pacing be required.

Failure to fire means that the pacemaker generator does not deliver its energy to the myocardium when the intrinsic rate falls below the limit defined by the escape

Fig. 7-6 Pacemaker sensing incorrectly. *PB*, paced beat; *IB*, intrinsic beat; *IB₁*, sensed; *IB₂*, not sensed.

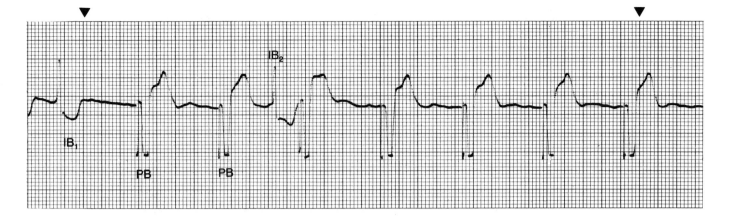

interval. No pacer artifacts will appear on the ECG. This may be caused by generator or battery failure, loose connections between the lead and generator, or inhibition of the pacemaker generator by an extraneous signal. Corrective measures include checking for any loose connections and replacing the battery or generator. If the pacemaker is being inhibited by electromagnetic interference, it may require reprogramming or elimination of the interference.

Failure to capture appears on the ECG as a pacer spike that is not followed by evidence of depolarization, that is, either a P wave or QRS complex (Fig. 7-7). Possible causes of failure to capture include inadequate electric output or a pacemaker electrode that is not in contact with a viable myocardium. Corrective measures include increasing the pacer output to 20 mA and turning the client to the left lateral recumbent position. The lead may need to be repositioned.

Fig. 7-7 Ventricular pacing with failure to capture.

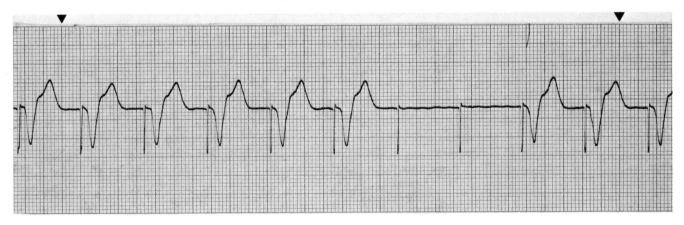

Runaway pacemaker is a term used to describe a rare pacemaker malfunction. On the ECG, pacemaker spikes will be seen at a rate of 100 times to 400 times per minute, but the rate can be as high as 1000 beats per minute with intermittent capture. Capture may mimic true ventricular tachycardia or appear as ventricular fibrillation. The problem may be intermittent, but it indicates a component failure and requires replacement of the generator. It may be necessary to externally inhibit a permanent pacemaker if the client is symptomatic and immediate generator replacement is not feasible.

OVERDRIVE PACING

In addition to protecting the client from extremely slow rates, a pacemaker can be used to cardiovert rapid atrial and ventricular rhythms. Cardioversion is achieved by overdrive pacing, which occurs when the pacemaker fires at a rate above that of the tachyarrhythmia. By stimulating the myocardium briefly at an overdrive rate, the abnormal electric conduction causing the tachyarrhythmia may be terminated, and function of the client's normal conduction system can be restored.

TRANSCUTANEOUS PACING

The myocardium may be stimulated to depolarize by an electric impulse that is applied to the skin, if the electric energy of the impulse is high enough. The first pacemakers designed in the 1950s used this principle, but the painful skin and muscle stimulation associated with the pacemakers caused them to be abandoned. Generators are now capable of delivering outputs up to 200 mA over a period of 20 msec to 40 msec. The prolonged impulse duration allows lower outputs to be used and thus causes less skin and muscle stimulation, but very effective cardiac-muscle stimulation.

The external pacing device may be programmed to function on demand or at a fixed rate, depending on the model. Output and rate can be adjusted for the client's needs. The pacing stimulus is delivered through two large skin electrodes placed anteriorly and posteriorly on the thorax. Transcutaneous pacing can be rapidly instituted without the considerable skill required for invasive methods. There is no danger of inducing ventricular fibrillation or tachycardia with transcutaneous pacing, even during asynchronous pacing, because ventricular fibrillation requires seven times the threshold stimulus, and the generator will not deliver this amount of output.

Temporary transvenous pacemaker

Objective
To stimulate the myocardium to depolarize at a rate sufficient to maintain adequate CO until definitive treatment can be instituted

ASSESSMENT PHASE

- Why does the client require temporary pacing (*e.g.*, transient bradyarrhythmias following an inferior myocardial infarction (MI), extreme bradycardia or high-degree heart block due to drug toxicity, or to stabilize the client before permanent pacemaker implantation)?
- Which approach is planned (*i.e.*, antecubital vein, subclavian or jugular vein, or femoral vein)?

PRECAUTIONS

- **Advanced cardiac life support (ACLS) equipment and medications should be kept at the bedside during insertion.**
- **Be prepared to defibrillate the client if ventricular fibrillation or ventricular tachycardia occurs during insertion.**
- **Keep all equipment in the client's room grounded and monitored for stray current to protect the client from microshock.**

PLANNING PHASE

EQUIPMENT

Temporary pacemaker generator
New 10-volt battery
Bridging cable
Pacing lead
Cardiac monitor
ACLS drugs and equipment
Sterile towels and drapes
Sterile gowns
Sterile gloves
Masks
4 × 4s
Skin-preparation supplies
    Soap
    Razor
    Acetone or alcohol
    Iodophor solution

Xylocaine 1%, with sterile needle and syringe
Cutdown tray (for antecubital-vein insertion)
Insertion kit with dilator-sheath assembly (for jugular- or subclavian-vein insertion)
Skin suture or sterile tape
Benzoin (optional)
Tape
Sterile dressing
Fluoroscopy equipment (optional)

CLIENT/FAMILY TEACHING
- Reinforce the physician's explanation of the indications, benefits, and risks of temporary pacemaker therapy if the client's condition permits.
- Explain the limitations on activity that accompany temporary pacemaker insertion. These limitations are necessary to maintain proper pacemaker function.
- Explain pacemaker function using diagrams as appropriate.

IMPLEMENTATION PHASE

NURSING ACTIONS	RATIONALE/AMPLIFICATION
1. Prepare external generator.	
a. Insert new battery.	Align the positive and negative poles.
b. Set output, rate, and sensitivity as ordered by physician.	Sensitivity is usually set in demand mode.
c. Turn on generator and assess for battery function.	Check the battery test light on the generator.
d. Connect bridging cable to generator.	The cable allows for slack between the generator and the lead to prevent tension on the lead after insertion.
2. Prepare client.	
a. Position client supine on fluoroscopy table if applicable.	If the subclavian approach is used, place a rolled towel between the client's shoulders and place the bed in Trendelenburg's position.
b. Obtain baseline vital signs and assess level of consciousness.	
c. Shave site if necessary.	
d. Prepare skin with acetone or alcohol and allow to dry.	
e. Paint site with iodophor using sterile gloves and 4 × 4s.	Preparation may be done by the physician after scrubbing.
3. Assist physician with mask, sterile gown, and gloves.	
4. Help physician to drape client and to give local anesthetic at insertion site.	Hold Xylocaine 1% while the physician draws the anesthetic into a sterile syringe.
5. Open sterile supplies and place on sterile field.	The open wrapper of the cutdown tray provides a sterile field.
6. Monitor client's tolerance of procedure and reassure as necessary.	The physician will inject Xylocaine 1% and will locate the vein to be used for insertion of the lead.
7. Monitor and record vital signs every 5 minutes during procedure.	
8. Watch ECG for arrhythmias during lead insertion.	Call out the number of premature ventricular contractions (PVCs), runs of ventricular tachycardia, or extreme bradycardia.

Fig. 7-8 Pressure dressing applied to pacemaker insertion site. Looping lead outside dressing prevents undue tension on lead.

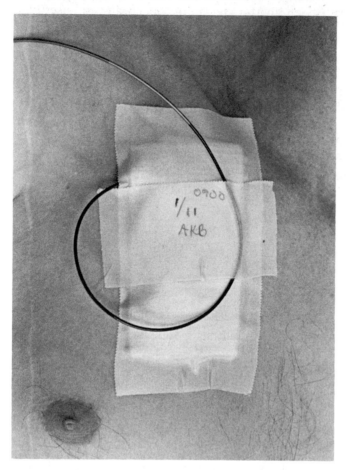

9. Attach pacemaker leads to generator bridging cable.

10. Adjust settings on generator as requested by physician.

Initially, the rate will be set above the client's intrinsic rate, and the output will be increased until capture is seen. Chart this as the threshold potential. The output is then generally set at a rate that is 2.5 times higher than the threshold. The rate is adjusted according to the client's condition.

11. Assess client for hemodynamic response.

Check the client's vital signs, urine output, and level of consciousness.

12. Analyze ECG for proper pacemaker function.

13. Apply pressure dressing to insertion site. Secure lead by looping and taping the lead wire outside the dressing (Fig. 7-8).

The physician will suture the lead in place. If the lead is not sutured in place, paint the skin with benzoin and secure the lead wire with sterile tape using the Chevron technique.

RELATED NURSING CARE

NURSING ACTIONS

RATIONALE/AMPLIFICATION

1. Maintain continuous ECG monitoring.

The ECG provides a record of pacemaker function.

2. Limit client's activity to bed rest and sitting in chair to avoid lead displacement.

If the lead is inserted in the antecubital vein, apply an armboard and instruct the client to restrict arm movement. If the lead is inserted in the subclavian or jugular vein, limit movement of the arm on the affected side. If the lead is placed in the femoral vein, the head of the bed should not be raised above 30 degrees to prevent fracture of the pacemaker lead.

3. Check all connections at least every 8 hours.

4. Protect client from microshock.

   a. Wear rubber gloves when handling generator or leads.

   b. Be sure all equipment is grounded and checked by biomedical engineer for safe operation.

   c. Do not handle other electric equipment while holding pacemaker.

   d. Enclose any noninsulated part of generator or lead in rubber glove.

   e. Do not allow client to use electric equipment.

EVALUATION PHASE

ANTICIPATED OUTCOMES	NURSING ACTIONS
1. Prevention of complications of temporary transvenous pacing	Assess for complications related to insertion, including hemothorax; pneumothorax; myocardial perforation, which results in cardiac tamponade; and myocardial irritability, which causes ectopic beats; microshock; and infection.
2. Maintenance of satisfactory CO	Monitor the client's hemodynamic status by checking vital signs, urine output, and mentation.
3. Maintenance of proper functioning of artificial pacemaker	Evaluate for signs of generator failure or displacement of electrodes. Observe ECG for failure to fire, capture, or sense (see previous section on Assessing Pacemaker Function).

PRODUCT AVAILABILITY

TEMPORARY GENERATORS

American Pacemaker Corp.
Biotronik Sales Inc.
Cordis Corp.
Medtronic Inc.
Pacesetter Systems Inc.
Telectronics

TEMPORARY ENDOCARDIAL PACEMAKER LEADS

American Edwards Laboratories
Cordis Corp.
Electro-Catheter Corp.
MediDyne Instrument Inc.

PACEMAKER LEAD INTRODUCER KITS WITH DILATOR SHEATH ASSEMBLIES

Cordis Corp.
Arrow
American Edwards Laboratories
Medtronic Inc.

Emergency transthoracic pacemaker

Objectives

To insert a pacing electrode percutaneously into the right ventricle

To stimulate the myocardium to depolarize at a rate sufficient to maintain CO in an emergency situation

ASSESSMENT PHASE

- Why does the client require emergency myocardial pacing (*e.g.*, asystole, third-degree AV block, or extreme bradycardia requiring ACLS)?
- Is there time to insert an artificial pacemaker transvenously and thus decrease the client's risk? Is a transcutaneous pacemaker available?
- Have the appropriate drugs (*e.g.*, atropine, epinephrine, or isoproterenol) been ineffective?

PRECAUTIONS

- **Cardiopulmonary resuscitation (CPR) will have to be stopped during insertion. Have all equipment and supplies ready for a rapid procedure.**
- **Continuing CPR after insertion can dislodge leads.**

PLANNING PHASE

EQUIPMENT

Sterile towels
Sterile gloves
Iodophor solution
Sterile 4 × 4s
Skin suture or sterile tape
ECG monitor
ACLS equipment and medication
Temporary pacemaker generator
10-volt battery
Transthoracic pacemaker kit (Fig. 7–9)*

Fig. 7–9 Transthoracic pacemaker kit. (Courtesy Electro-Catheter Corp., Rahway, NJ)

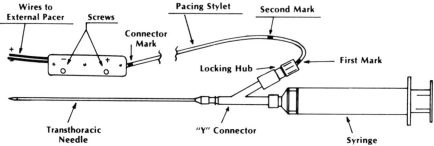

CLIENT/FAMILY TEACHING

- Explain the function and appearance of the artificial pacemaker to the client and family when the emergency situation is resolved.
- Explain that the transthoracic pacemaker will be replaced with a transvenous or permanent pacemaker when the client's condition permits.

IMPLEMENTATION PHASE

NURSING ACTIONS	RATIONALE/AMPLIFICATION
1. Prepare external generator.	
a. Insert new battery.	Align the positive and negative poles.
b. Set output as requested by physician.	Output is usually set at 20 mA at onset.

* A transthoracic pacemaker lead and a 10-ml syringe with a transthoracic needle (sterile) can be used in place of a transthoracic pacemaker kit.

c. Set rate.

Rate is usually 60 to 80 impulses per minute according to anticipated client need.

d. Set sensitivity.

The sensitivity setting is usually placed in demand mode.

e. Turn on generator and assess for battery function.

There is a battery test light on the generator to test battery function.

f. Connect bridging cable to generator.

Bridging cable is not essential to pacemaker insertion but it allows more slack between the heavy generator and the transthoracic lead to avoid dislodging the lead.

2. Prepare client for insertion.

a. Position client supine.

Continue CPR until all equipment is prepared and the physician is ready to prepare the client's skin and insert the pacemaker lead.

b. Provide sterile gloves and towels for draping.

Maintain sterility as much as possible because of the invasive nature of the procedure.

c. Reconfirm functional ECG monitoring.

3. Attach transthoracic pacemaker leads to generator or bridging cable before insertion (Fig. 7–10).

Align the positive and negative poles.

Fig. 7–10 Transthoracic pacing leads attached to bridging cable.

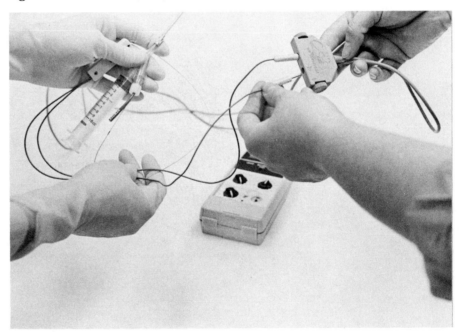

4. Stop external cardiac compressions and prepare skin using iodophor solution and sterile gloves.

The physician will insert a transthoracic needle into the right ventricle using a subxiphoid approach. The lead will be threaded through the transthoracic needle (Fig. 7–11).

5. Observe for correct pacemaker function.

Observe the ECG for a pacemaker spike followed by a QRS complex or an appropriately sensed intrinsic rhythm.

6. Assess for hemodynamic response to pacing.

Check vital signs. The client may exhibit electromechanical dissociation (EMD) in which there is a good ECG tracing but no associated perfusion. If EMD is present, resume CPR.

Fig. 7–11 Transthoracic pacing lead is threaded into right ventricle by a transthoracic needle. (*A*) Anterior view. (*B*) Lateral view. (Courtesy Electro-Catheter Corp., Rahway, NJ)

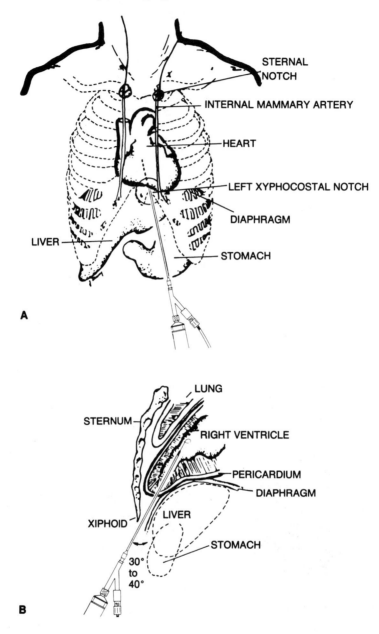

RELATED NURSING CARE

NURSING ACTIONS	RATIONALE/AMPLIFICATION
1. Maintain continuous ECG monitoring.	
2. Continue ACLS as indicated.	A well-oxygenated myocardium is essential for electromechanical coupling.
3. Prepare client for insertion of transvenous pacemaker if client's condition warrants.	
4. Protect client from microshock by grounding all electric equipment and by handling pacemaker and leads with rubber gloves.	

EVALUATION PHASE

ANTICIPATED OUTCOMES	NURSING ACTIONS
1. Temporary maintenance of CO	Evaluate for improved hemodynamic status, as indicated by a systolic blood pressure greater than 80 mm Hg, a urine output of 30 ml/hour, and an increased level of consciousness. Titrate IV drugs as required and evaluate the client's response.
2. Prevention of complications of transthoracic pacing	Monitor for potential complications such as cardiac tamponade, pneumothorax, and infection.
3. Maintenance of proper function of artificial pacemaker	Monitor for signs of generator failure or lead displacement. Observe the ECG for failure to fire, capture, or sense.

PRODUCT AVAILABILITY

EMERGENCY TRANSTHORACIC PACING AND INTRACARDIAC INJECTION KIT

Electro-Catheter Corp. (Pace-Jector)
Cordis Corp.
R2 Corp.
USCI Cardiology and Radiology Products

EXTERNAL PACEMAKER GENERATOR

American Pacemaker Corp.
Cardiac Resuscitation Corp.
Cordis Corp.
Medtronic Inc.
Siemens–Elema Pacemaker Systems
Teletronics

Temporary transcutaneous pacing

Objectives
To stimulate the myocardium to depolarize through the skin
To maintain adequate CO until definitive treatment can be implemented

ASSESSMENT PHASE
- Why does the client require temporary pacing (*e.g.*, transient bradyarrhythmias after an inferior MI, extreme bradycardia or high-degree heart block, prophylaxis in the presence of bifascicular block, emergency treatment for asystole or extreme bradycardia, or a malfunctioning permanent pacemaker)?
- Has the client had appropriate first-line therapy (*i.e.*, CPR and ACLS) for asystole or extreme bradycardia?

PRECAUTIONS
- **Transcutaneous pacing is not effective in the presence of severe hypoxia and acidosis. CPR and ACLS are essential.**
- **If defibrillation is required, disconnect the pacing electrodes from the generator to avoid disabling the generator.**

PLANNING PHASE

EQUIPMENT
Transcutaneous pacing generator
Transcutaneous pacing electrodes
ECG monitoring equipment
Scissors or razor

CLIENT/FAMILY TEACHING
- Explain the appearance and function of the external pacemaker to the client and family.

- Explain the reasons for possible muscle twitching or a thumping sensation in the chest, and tell the client that pain medication or a sedative will be given.
- Reassure the family and visitors that the client is not an electric hazard and that contact will not result in a shock.

IMPLEMENTATION PHASE

NURSING ACTIONS	RATIONALE/AMPLIFICATION
1. Establish ECG monitoring.	If the generator operates in demand mode, connect an ECG cable to the generator.
2. Shave or clip excess hair on left anterior chest.	If the skin is moist or oily, it should be cleaned and dried to enhance electrode contact.
3. Position electrode marked "apex" or "positive" on anterior chest, centering it at fourth intercostal space left of sternum (Fig. 7–12).	Avoid placing the electrode over the large pectoral muscle, because this will increase the client's discomfort from muscle stimulation.
4. Position second electrode on client's back in left subscapular region (Fig. 7–13).	
5. Connect electrodes to transcutaneous pacing generator.	

Fig. 7–12 Position of apex (positive) electrode for transcutaneous pacing on anterior chest left of sternum (V₃ position).

Fig. 7–13 Position of posterior electrode for transcutaneous pacing in left subscapular region.

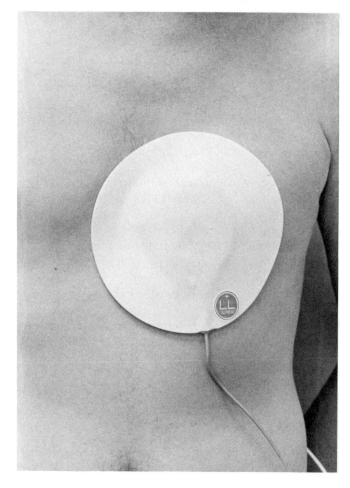

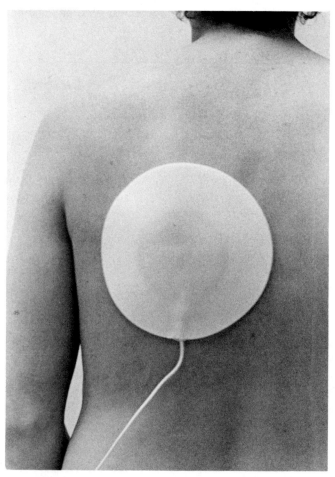

6. Set pacemaker parameters.

Follow the manufacturer's instruction manual.

7. Turn on unit.

Follow the manufacturer's instruction manual.

8. Assess ECG for evidence of pacemaker capture.

The high output levels required will produce a large pacemaker artifact, which will not be distinguishable from the QRS complex. Criteria for identifying successful capture include the following:

a. Pacing artifact and QRS complex greater than 0.14 seconds

b. T wave present after pacing artifact and the QRS complex

c. Elimination of underlying rhythms (Fig. 7–14)

Fig. 7–14 Transcutaneous pacing. (*A*) Idioventricular rhythm at 30 beats per minute. (*B*) *Open arrow* indicates beginning of external stimulation. (*C*) External pacing at 100 beats per minute (half standardization; recording polarity altered). (*D*) Effect of reducing stimulation current below threshold *(closed arrow)*. Pacing ceases and underlying bradycardia is seen. Stimulation mode is nondemand. *R*, intrinsic QRS complex; *St*, pacemaker stimulus, *T*, repolarization (T wave of paced beat). (Falk RH, Loll P, Zoll R: Safety and efficacy of noninvasive cardiac pacing. N Engl J Med 309: 1166–1168, 1983)

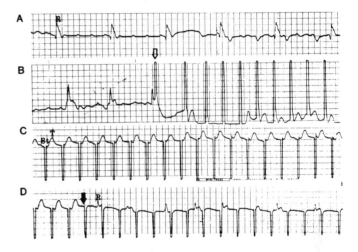

9. Increase output in increments of 10 mA until capture is seen.

Usually 75 mA to 90 mA will produce capture. Acidotic or ischemic hearts require high outputs and may not respond at all.

10. Assess hemodynamic response to pacing.

Palpate for a carotid or femoral pulse. Be careful to distinguish between actual pulse and the "shock wave" effect caused by muscle and skin stimulation. If a pulse is present, take blood pressure reading.

RELATED NURSING CARE

NURSING ACTIONS	RATIONALE/AMPLIFICATION
1. Maintain continuous ECG monitoring.	
2. Administer and monitor effects of any necessary adjunct treatment.	The client may require ventilatory support or vasoactive drugs.
3. Monitor continuously for perfusion and hemodynamic stability.	Check pulse rates and blood pressure every 15 minutes.

EVALUATION PHASE

ANTICIPATED OUTCOMES	NURSING ACTIONS
1. Maintenance of captured rhythm and hemodynamic stability	Monitor ECG and hemodynamic parameters.
2. Client tolerance of transcutaneous pacing	If muscle stimulation is excessive and painful, consider moving the electrode further away from the large pectoral muscle. Sedate the client as necessary.

PRODUCT AVAILABILITY

EXTERNAL NONINVASIVE CARDIAC PACEMAKERS

Cardiac Resuscitation Corp. (Pace Aid)

EXTERNAL NONINVASIVE PACING ELECTRODES

Micromedical Devices Inc.

Pacemaker inhibition

Objectives

To inhibit permanent pacemaker function through stimulation of the chest wall
To assess the pacemaker generator for an intact sensing circuit
To assess the client's intrinsic rhythm
To temporarily disable the permanent generator

ASSESSMENT PHASE

- Does the client have an intrinsic rhythm that is compatible with hemodynamic stability?
- Is the pacemaker unipolar or bipolar? Electrode placement differs for each type of pacemaker.

PRECAUTIONS

- **If the client is pacemaker dependent, prepare ACLS equipment (see Advanced Cardiac Life Support in Chap. 3).**
- **Monitor client's ECG continuously.**

PLANNING PHASE

EQUIPMENT

External temporary pacemaker
Cup electrodes — 2
Alligator-clip cables — 2
Conductive gel

CLIENT/FAMILY TEACHING

- Explain the purpose and the expected duration of the procedure to the client and family.
- Tell the client that slight chest-wall muscle twitching may be sensed, but that it is not dangerous.

IMPLEMENTATION PHASE

NURSING ACTIONS	RATIONALE/AMPLIFICATION
1. Place cup electrodes on skin over approximate location of internal lead electrodes. Use conductive gel to decrease resistance.	If the client has a unipolar pacemaker, place one electrode over the right ventricular apex and one electrode over the implanted generator. If the pacemaker is bipolar, place one electrode over the right ventricular apex and the second electrode approximately 2.5 cm (1 inch) above and to the right of the first electrode (Fig. 7–15).

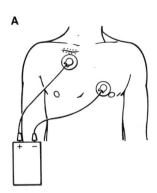

A **B**

Fig. 7-15 Correct position of electrodes on chest wall for pacemaker inhibition. (*A*) Unipolar pacer. (*B*) Bipolar pacer.

2. Connect electrodes to external generator using alligator cables.

Connect the electrode over the right ventricular apex to the negative (−) terminal, and the second electrode to the positive (+) terminal.

3. Adjust settings on external generator as indicated by physician.

Set the rate above that of the permanent pacemaker, set the pacemaker in the asynchronous mode, and set output at 4 mA initially.

4. Turn on generator and increase number of mA until permanent pacemaker is inhibited.

Observe the ECG for inhibition of the permanent pacemaker and for the appearance of the client's intrinsic rhythm. Inhibition of the permanent generator by chest-wall stimulation suggests that the sensing circuit is intact. If the generator is not inhibited, this does not necessarily mean that the sensing circuit is faulty.

5. Document client's intrinsic rhythm and tolerance of pacemaker inhibition.

The client's intrinsic rhythm can be assessed during pacemaker inhibition and documented with a 12-lead ECG or rhythm strip.

EVALUATION PHASE

ANTICIPATED OUTCOME	NURSING ACTION
Inhibition of pacemaker function	Document pacemaker inhibition with a 12-lead ECG.

PRODUCT AVAILABILITY EXTERNAL PACEMAKER GENERATORS

See previous section on Temporary Transvenous Pacemaker.

Pacemaker reprogramming

Objective
To alter the pacing parameters of an operational permanent pacemaker system noninvasively

ASSESSMENT PHASE
- Does the client have a programmable pacemaker?
- Is the client pacemaker dependent?
- Why are program changes indicated, and what is the expected response (*e.g.*, to decrease output or pulse width and thus prolong battery life, to increase rate to overdrive a tachydysrhythmia or to augment CO, or to decrease rate to allow intrinsic rhythm to dominate)?

PRECAUTIONS
- **Be sure that the programmer is functioning properly.**
- **Monitor the client closely for hemodynamic changes during reprogramming.**

> • **Be prepared to administer BLS and ACLS to a pacemaker-dependent client should programming error cause pacing to be lost.**

PLANNING PHASE

EQUIPMENT

Programmer with current operating instructions
ECG monitoring equipment
ACLS equipment and medication

CLIENT/FAMILY TEACHING

• Answer the client's questions about the reasons for reprogramming the pacemaker and any potential problems.
• Reassure the client that the reprogramming procedure will not cause pain and that close monitoring will be maintained.
• Explain any changes in pacemaker function that have been made.
• Teach the client and family to assess for proper pacemaker function (*e.g.*, by checking pulse rate).

IMPLEMENTATION PHASE

NURSING ACTIONS	RATIONALE/AMPLIFICATION
1. Prepare programmer (Fig. 7–16).	Follow the manufacturer's instructions and ensure that a reliable power source is available.

Fig. 7–16 Programmer and electromagnet.

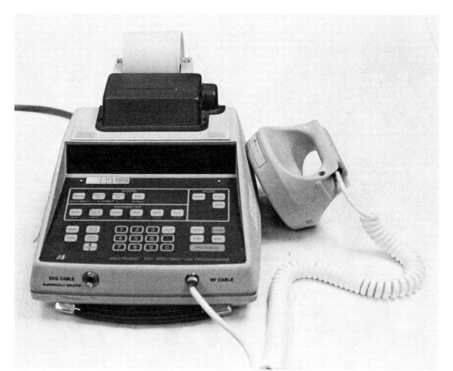

NURSING ACTIONS	RATIONALE/AMPLIFICATION
2. Establish ECG monitoring.	Choose the lead that shows pacemaker artifacts as well as good depolarization waveforms (usually lead II or MCL_1). (See Hard-Wire Monitoring in Chap. 1.)
3. Establish baseline vital signs.	Document rhythm with an ECG strip, and check pulse rate, blood pressure, and level of consciousness.
4. Assist physician as necessary in making program changes.	The physician will position the electromagnet over the generator and use the key pads on the programmer to make the desired changes (Fig. 7–17).
5. Monitor client's response. Document rhythm with ECG.	Check pulse rate, blood pressure, and level of consciousness.

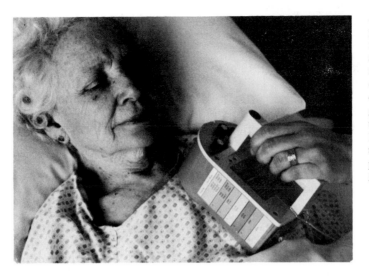

Fig. 7–17 Programmer is placed over skin covering permanent pacemaker to adjust settings such as sensitivity, rate, and AV delay. This client's generator is located on the left. More commonly generators are positioned on the right. (Shirley D, Littrel K: Troubleshooting malfunctions of the dual-chambered pacemaker. DCCN, Vol. 4, No. 3, May/June 1985)

6. Communicate program changes to client.

7. Notify personnel of program changes.

Making personnel aware of program changes is essential to correct interpretation of pacemaker function.

RELATED NURSING CARE

NURSING ACTION	RATIONALE/AMPLIFICATION
Monitor client's response to program changes until homeostasis is ensured.	The degree of monitoring will be determined by the changes that are made in pacemaker function.

EVALUATION PHASE

ANTICIPATED OUTCOMES	NURSING ACTIONS
1. Establishment of satisfactory hemodynamic function during and after reprogramming procedure	Monitor for signs of hemodynamic instability such as falling blood pressure, loss of consciousness, and cool clammy skin.
2. Establishment of effective pacemaker function	Evaluate the client's ECG rhythm for pacing function.
3. Development of client knowledge about changes in pacemaker function and how to assess function	Allow the client to verbalize understanding and to demonstrate an ability to assess pacemaker function. Make necessary changes on client's pacemaker ID card.

PRODUCT AVAILABILITY   PACEMAKER FUNCTION ANALYZERS AND PROGRAMMERS

American Pacemaker Corp.
Cardiac Pacemakers Inc.
Cordis Corp.
Medtronic Inc.
Pacesetter System Inc.
Siemens–Elema Pacemaker Systems Division

Permanent transvenous pacemaker

Objectives
To provide a permanent and reliable source of electric stimulation for the heart using a surgically implanted generator
To depolarize the myocardium at a rate to maintain adequate CO

ASSESSMENT PHASE

- Has the client developed a dysrhythmia or conduction system disease that requires artificial pacing (*e.g.*, bradydysrhythmia that requires temporary pacing and has not resolved after 7 days, complete AV heart block, bifascicular block, or sick sinus syndrome)?
- What symptoms did the client experience with the conduction disorder? Recurrence of these symptoms may indicate pacemaker malfunction later.
- What mode of pacing is indicated (*e.g.*, AV sequential, ventricular, bipolar, or unipolar)? Generally, the physician makes this decision based on an evaluation of the client's conduction system, hemodynamic function, and environmental factors.
- Is the client normally exposed to any potential sources of electromagnetic interference (*e.g.*, arc welding equipment, industrial magnets, or ignition systems)? A bipolar pacemaker may be indicated, or the client may be advised to avoid such interference.
- Does the client participate in sports such as bowling or shooting, which use the right arm? The pacemaker generator is usually positioned on the right shoulder. If necessary, the generator may be positioned on the left shoulder or on the abdomen.
- Will the pacemaker be inserted in the operating room, catheterization laboratory, or special procedures room? The operating room is preferred for pacemaker insertion.
- Assess the ability and willingness of the client and family to assume responsibility for pacemaker care. Education is very important to facilitate psychological wellness.

PRECAUTIONS

- **Restrict activity in the affected extremity for 24 hours to 48 hours to prevent lead displacement.**
- **If the client requires defibrillation, place the paddles as far from the pulse generator as possible and perpendicular to the current flow through the generator and leads (see Defibrillation in Chap. 2).**
- **Verify that the pacemaker is functioning properly after defibrillation.**

PLANNING PHASE

EQUIPMENT

ECG monitoring equipment
Fluoroscopy equipment
Lead aprons
Sterile gowns and gloves
Masks
Sterile drapes and towels
Sterile sponges and 4 × 4s
Razor
Iodophor solution
Xylocaine 1% or 2%
Cutdown tray
Lead introducer for subclavian or external jugular vein (as indicated)
Lead (unipolar or bipolar, ventricular or atrial, as indicated)
Pacemaker generator
Pacing-system analyzer
Programming equipment
Skin suture
Elastic tape
ACLS medication and equipment

CLIENT/FAMILY TEACHING

- Reinforce the physician's explanation of the benefits and risks of permanent pacing. Answer any questions that the client or family may have.
- Explain the procedure to the client and family. Include information about the use of local anesthesia and cardiac monitoring throughout the procedure.
- Emphasize the need to restrict the activity of the affected arm for the first 24 hours to 48 hours after the pacemaker is inserted to prevent lead displacement. Instruct the client to remain passive while being transferred to different beds.

- Warn the client who is scheduled to receive a ventricular pacemaker that the heartbeat may be more noticeable and that the "kicking in" and "kicking out" of the pacemaker may be sensed. This should resolve after the first month.
- Arrange a visit from a member of the American Heart Associations' Mended Heart program if possible.
- Inform the client and family of follow-up care and stress the importance of keeping follow-up appointments.
- Give the client an ID card that includes the following pacemaker information: manufacturer, type, date of implantation, and program parameters (see sample card). Emphasize the importance of carrying this card at all times.

CARDIAC PACEMAKER PATIENT
P.O. Box 43079•St. Paul, MN 55164•Tel. 612-631-3000

Patient **MR. JOHN SMITH**
100 Oak Street
Mainville, MN 55444
Phone **612-555-5555**
Implant Date **4/1/80** Model **0623** S/N **PG000000**
Lead **CPI 4110 LC 000000**
Dr. **M. Smith**   Phone **555-5551**
Hospital **Mainville Hospital**
Mainville, MN
Initial Setting: Rate **72** Pulse Width **.6**

Cardiac pacemaker client ID card. (Cardiac Pacemakers Inc., St. Paul, MN. Reprinted with permission)

- If transmission of the client's ECG to a pacemaker clinic or physician's office is available, instruct the client and family in how to place the electrodes and transmit by telephone. Arrange a schedule for transmission and discuss the procedure to follow in an emergency.
- Teach the client and family to take the client's pulse rate and assess pacing function.
- Teach the client and family to recognize and report to the physician signs and symptoms of the following:
  Pacemaker malfunction, for example, recurrence of symptoms experienced before pacemaker insertion
  Infection, for example, swelling or redness at pocket site, and fever
  Power-source failure, for example, slowing or acceleration of pulse rate, and recurrence of symptoms experienced before pacemaker insertion
- Teach the client about electromagnetic interference. Diathermy and the use of electrocautery within 3 inches of the pulse generator are contraindicated. Advise the client to remain 3 feet away from an operating microwave oven and not to use linear-power amplifiers. Electric razors or other electric tools and appliances are safe if they do not come in contact with the skin that is directly over the pulse generator.

IMPLEMENTATION PHASE

NURSING ACTIONS	RATIONALE/AMPLIFICATION
1. Begin ECG monitoring.	
2. Start IV line.	Stimulation of the endocardium during lead placement may precipitate ventricular ectopia, which may require ACLS.
3. Position client on radiolucent table or bed.	A fluoroscope is essential to satisfactory lead placement.
4. Shave operative site if necessary.	
5. Prepare operative site with iodophor scrub.	Usually the right subclavian area is used for first-time implantation.

6. Open cutdown tray. Open sterile packages on sterile field.

The inside of the wrapper will serve as the sterile field.

7. Assist physician and assistants with masks, sterile surgical gowns, and gloves.

Strict asepsis is imperative when implanting a permanent foreign object in the body.

8. Help physician to drape client and to draw up local anesthetic.

9. Establish baseline vital signs and ECG rhythm.

10. Remain with client during procedure and monitor ECG, vital signs (every 5 minutes), and tolerance of procedure.

The physician will usually make an incision on the right side of the chest. The incision is approximately 15 cm long and runs transversely from the deltopectoral groove. The cephalic vein is isolated, and the lead is passed through this vein. Alternative veins are the external jugular or subclavian vein, which require a percutaneous introducer. If two leads are being positioned, one of these veins will be used for the second lead.

11. Inform physician of repetitive ventricular ectopia. Be prepared to defibrillate or medicate client if ectopia persists.

Once the vein is isolated, the lead is positioned in the right atrium or ventricle using fluoroscopy. Premature ventricular beats commonly occur at this time and are likely to terminate spontaneously when lead manipulation is stopped.

12. Assist physician to obtain intracavity ECG and determine myocardial threshold.

Follow the instructions that accompany each manufacturer's pacing-system analyzer.

13. Assess for diaphragmatic pacing by palpating for muscle contractions over diaphragm.

The muscle contractions will correspond with pacemaker output. If contractions are present, the lead will have to be repositioned.

14. Assist physician with pacemaker programming.

The physician will attach the lead to the generator and suture the generator in the subcutaneous pocket.

15. Monitor ECG for pacemaker function while pocket is being closed.

Document pacemaker function with an ECG strip if possible. Any malfunction may indicate that lead placement should be reassessed.

16. Apply sterile pressure dressing to prevent hematoma formation in pocket.

Cut a small square in the tape to allow for assessment of bleeding.

RELATED NURSING CARE

NURSING ACTIONS	RATIONALE/AMPLIFICATION
1. Keep affected arm immobile for 24 hours to 48 hours after the procedure.	Time is required for the lead to be fixed securely in the myocardium. Tension on the lead will impede fixation.
2. Monitor ECG continously for 24 hours to 48 hours.	
3. Medicate client as indicated for pain at incision site.	

EVALUATION PHASE

ANTICIPATED OUTCOMES	NURSING ACTIONS
1. Prevention of complications of transvenous pacemaker insertion	Monitor for complications such as infection in the pocket; bacteremia; lead fracture, which causes chest muscle contraction; myocardial perforation, which causes diaphragmatic stimulation; and electromagnetic interference, which causes pacemaker malfunction.

2. Establishment of hemodynamic stability that is compatible with client's quality of life

Monitor hemodynamic response to pacing and assist with reprogramming as indicated (see previous section on Pacemaker Reprogramming).

PRODUCT AVAILABILITY   PACEMAKER GENERATORS, LEADS, PACEMAKER SYSTEM ANALYZERS AND PROGRAMMERS

Medtronic Inc.
Siemens – Elema Pacemaker Siptems Division
Cordis Corp.
Teletronics
Cardiac Pacemakers Inc.

SELECTED REFERENCES   Dreifus LS (ed): Pacemaker therapy. Cardiovascular Clinics 14(2):31–44, 97–147, 1983

Falk RH, Zoll PM: Safety and efficacy of noninvasive cardiac pacing. N Engl J Med 309:1166–1168, November 1983

Hoffman SJ: Artificial cardiac pacing. In Hudak CM, Lohr T, Gallo BM: Critical Care Nursing, 3rd ed, pp 81–93. Philadelphia, JB Lippincott, 1982

Owen PM: The effects of external defibrillation on permanent pacemakers. Heart and Lung, 12(3):277–280, May 1983

Parsonnet V, Furman S, Smyth NPD: Implantable cardiac pacemaker status report and resource guideline. Circulation 50:A21–A35, October 1974

Sagar DP: The person requiring cardiac pacing. In Guzzetta CE, Dossey BM: Cardiovascular Nursing Bodymind Tapestry, pp 357–417. St. Louis, CV Mosby, 1984

Slusarczyk SM, Hicks FD: Helping your patient to live with a permanent pacemaker. Nursing '83, 13(1):58–64, April 1983

8 *Rotating tourniquets*

Rotating tourniquets are used for the client who is experiencing pulmonary edema or severe congestive heart failure. With this technique tourniquets are systematically rotated on the extremities to temporarily remove a volume of blood from the central circulation. This decreases the venous return to the heart until other interventions, such as phlebotomy, pharmacologic therapy (diuretics, morphine, nitrates, and digitalis), and oxygenation measures, are initiated to relieve the fluid overload.

Inflatable cuffs are applied to the extremities and rotated sequentially, either manually or using a device that automatically inflates and deflates the tourniquets according to a specified schedule. One extremity remains unconstricted at all times.

Nursing intervention is directed toward assessing the client's clinical response during therapy, monitoring for circulatory problems, and discontinuing rotating tourniquets correctly to avoid a sudden increase in the volume. of circulating blood.

Objective
To temporarily decrease the volume of circulating blood by restricting venous return from the extremities until definitive therapy is initiated to correct fluid overload

ASSESSMENT PHASE

- Why does the client require rotating tourniquets (*e.g.*, acute pulmonary edema)?
- Does the client have any existing peripheral vascular disease that will compromise circulation? If peripheral vascular disease is present, the rotation schedule may need to be shortened.
- Has an assessment of the client's peripheral pulse rates been completed? Mark peripheral pulses with a magic marker.
- Has a baseline blood pressure reading been obtained? This is required to determine the inflation pressure of the cuffs.
- Will a subclavian IV infusion be required? Tourniquets will interfere with peripheral IV lines.
- Will a Foley catheter be used to monitor the client's response to therapy?
- Is emergency equipment on standby?

PRECAUTIONS

- **Maintain the cuff pressure just above the diastolic pressure to prevent the interruption of arterial flow.**
- **At the conclusion of therapy, remove the cuffs one at a time as the prescribed inflation sequence is completed. Removal of all the cuffs at the same time may precipitate pulmonary edema.**
- **The application of rotating tourniquets may precipitate hypotension in some clients.**

PLANNING PHASE

EQUIPMENT

4 soft pads or towels
Automatic rotating tourniquet equipment
For manual rotating tourniquets, include the following:
    4 sphygmomanometer cuffs (or 4 wide, soft rubber tourniquets)
    Stopwatch
    Flow sheet (for recording inflation and deflation)

CLIENT/FAMILY TEACHING
- Discuss the reasons for using rotating tourniquets.
- Describe the effect of the tourniquets, if the client's condition permits.
- Tell the client and family that the client's extremities will become discolored during the procedure.
- Reassure the client and family that the tourniquets are a temporary measure.
- Remain with the client and provide reassurance. The client will be fearful and will have difficulty breathing.

IMPLEMENTATION PHASE

NURSING ACTIONS	RATIONALE/AMPLIFICATION
1. Position client in semi-Fowler's position. Record vital signs.	This position assists respiration.
2. Apply cuffs or tourniquets high on each extremity over soft towel (Fig. 8–1).	A towel protects the skin under the cuff.

Fig. 8–1 Sphygmomanometer cuffs applied to extremities. Soft towels protect skin of extremities.

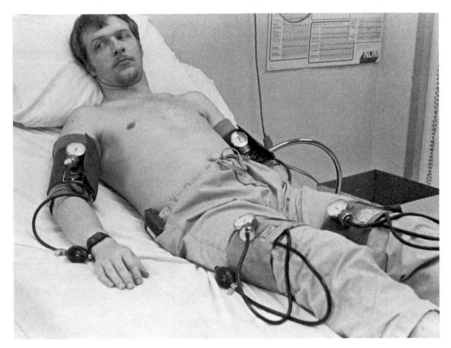

3. For manual rotating tourniquets, proceed as follows:	
a. Inflate three cuffs to pressure just above client's diastolic pressure.	This prevents the interruption of arterial flow. If a soft rubber tourniquet is used, monitor the arterial pulse rates in the extremities to be certain that arterial flow is not impeded.
b. Release one tourniquet every 15 minutes.	Follow this schedule unless a different time cycle is ordered by the physician.
c. Inflate cuff on another extremity.	No cuff should be inflated for more than 45 minutes (15 minutes × 3 inflations) (Fig. 8–2).
d. Rotate tourniquets in clockwise sequence.	
e. Maintain rotation flow sheet.	

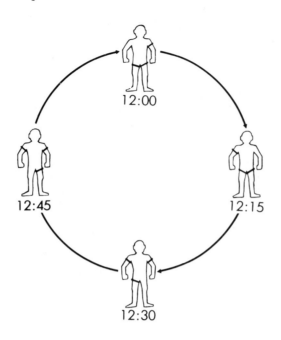

Fig. 8–2 Fifteen-minute rotation sequence. (Brunner LS, Suddarth DS: The Lippincott Manual of Nursing Practice, 4th ed. Philadelphia, JB Lippincott, 1986)

4. For automatic rotating tourniquets proceed as follows:

    a. Secure cuffs to valves located on automatic rotation device.

    b. Clamp all outlet valves.

    c. Set automatic inflation timer to required cycle length (Fig. 8–3).

Set automatic inflation timer every 15 minutes unless ordered otherwise by the physician.

Fig. 8–3 Automatic rotating tourniquets. Machine maintains inflation of three cuffs. Rotation occurs automatically according to preset cycle.

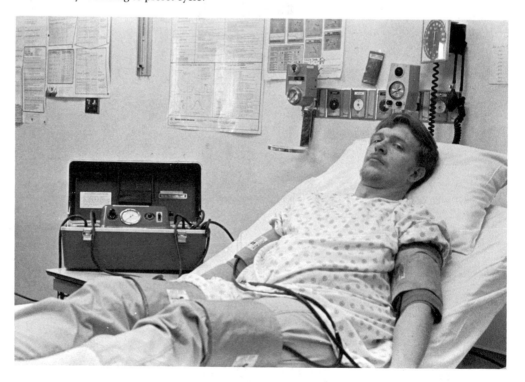

d. Set cuff pressure just above client's diastolic blood pressure.

e. Set alarm system.

The alarm system will sound if the cuffs are not inflating correctly.

f. Open valves one at a time.

The machine will begin cycling. Evaluate the client's condition for signs of hypotension.

5. Discontinue therapy.

a. Remove cuffs one at a time during deflation cycle.

Removal of cuffs one at a time prevents circulatory overload caused by a sudden increase in venous return to the heart.

b. Close valve and disconnect from equipment after cuff is removed.

RELATED NURSING CARE

NURSING ACTIONS	RATIONALE/AMPLIFICATION
1. Monitor blood pressure every 5 minutes to 15 minutes.	Frequent blood pressure recordings monitor the effect of the rotating tourniquets on the client's vascular system.
a. Close valve to deflated arm cuff.	
b. Attach aneroid sphygmomanometer to obtain blood pressure reading.	
c. Reconnect to cycling device and open valve.	
d. If manual tourniquets are used obtain blood pressure reading on uncuffed extremity.	
2. Assess extremities every 15 minutes for arterial pulse rate, color, and temperature.	Limbs will be cool and discolored when the cuff is inflated.
3. Assess skin integrity every 45 minutes as cuff deflates on one extremity.	
4. Administer pharmacologic therapy as ordered by physician.	

EVALUATION PHASE

ANTICIPATED OUTCOMES	NURSING ACTIONS
1. Improvement in hemodynamic status	Evaluate blood pressure, pulmonary artery and pulmonary wedge pressures, cardiac rate and rhythm, and urinary output.
2. Prevention of complications of rotating tourniquets	Evaluate for skin integrity, peripheral ischemia, and hypotension.

PRODUCT AVAILABILITY   ROTATING TOURNIQUETS
Kidd
Scherer

SELECTED REFERENCES   Hudak CM, Lohr T, Gallo BM: Critical Care Nursing, 3rd ed, pp 72–75. Philadelphia, JB Lippincott, 1982

9 *Pericardiocentesis*

Pericardiocentesis is the aspiration of fluid or blood from the pericardial sac using a needle. Fluid, blood, or exudate collects in the pericardial sac as a result of chest trauma, cardiac surgery, pericarditis, or malignant neoplasm. Performed by a physician for diagnostic and therapeutic reasons, pericardiocentesis relieves cardiac tamponade or compression of the heart, thereby restoring cardiac function. Pericardiocentesis may be performed in an extreme emergency if fluid in the pericardial sac embarrasses cardiac function and decreases cardiac output (CO) and venous return. The removal of as little as 15 ml to 20 ml of blood or fluid may be sufficient to restore cardiac function and normal blood pressure. Advanced cardiac life support (ACLS) equipment should be readily available during pericardiocentesis.

Objectives

To drain blood or fluid from the pericardial sac
To relieve cardiac tamponade and restore cardiac function
To obtain fluid or exudate from the pericardial sac for laboratory analysis or cytology
To instill medication directly into the pericardial sac

ASSESSMENT PHASE

- Does the client's history include chest trauma, cardiac surgery, recent infection, or malignancies?
- Are heart sounds muffled? Muffled heart sounds may indicate cardiac tamponade and impaired cardiac function.
- Do hemodynamic assessments indicate cardiac tamponade? Check for the following signs: increasing venous pressure, decreasing arterial pressure, narrowing pulse pressure, abnormal decrease in systolic arterial pressure during inspiration (paradoxical pulse), distended neck veins, or an inspiratory increase in venous pressure.
- Does the client sit up and lean forward? This is the characteristic position for a person with cardiac tamponade.
- Is the client tachypneic, apprehensive, or cyanotic? As blood circulation is compromised, hypoxia increases.

PRECAUTIONS

- **Maintain continuous cardiac monitoring during the procedure.**
- **Have ACLS equipment readily available.**

PLANNING PHASE

EQUIPMENT

Sterile pericardiocentesis tray
    Sterile drapes
    50-ml Luer-Lok syringe
    Three-way stopcock
    Suture instruments
    Sterile specimen container
    4 × 4s
    Intracardiac or spinal needles
Iodophor solution

Sterile gloves
Xylocaine 1% or 2%
For continuous drainage include the following:
    Intra-cath intravenous (IV) cannula
    Sterile tubing
    Sterile drainage bottle

CLIENT/FAMILY TEACHING

- If time allows, explain the procedure to the client and family.
- Assist the physician in obtaining an informed consent.
- If the client is alert, explain that pressure will be felt as the needle is inserted. Reassure the client that a local anesthetic will be given.
- Stress that absolute immobility will be necessary to avoid damage to surrounding tissue.

IMPLEMENTATION PHASE

NURSING ACTIONS	RATIONALE/AMPLIFICATION
1. Obtain baseline vital signs. Administer premedication if ordered.	This serves as a basis for evaluating client status during and after the procedure. Premedication may be ordered to encourage relaxation. Absolute immobility is required during the procedure.
2. Connect cardiac monitor if monitoring has not been started. Obtain baseline rhythm strip.	
3. If IV line is not in place, start IV infusion using large-bore cannula.	Perforation of the myocardium or surrounding tissue may necessitate rapid blood replacement.
4. Place client in comfortable position with head of bed raised 60 degrees.	This position facilitates needle insertion.
5. Wash your hands.	Handwashing before opening the sterile equipment reduces contamination.
6. Open pericardiocentesis tray on bedside table to provide sterile field. Open sterile equipment on sterile field.	
7. Assist physician in preparing operative site with iodophor solution (Fig. 9–1), administering local anesthetic, and draping client with sterile drapes.	A large area is prepared because a thoracotomy to suture an inadvertent tear of the myocardium may be necessary.
8. Monitor vital signs and ECG pattern during insertion of needle into pericardial sac.	The physician assembles the 50-ml syringe, three-way stopcock, and intracardiac needle. The needle is inserted and advanced slowly until blood or fluid returns. A hemostat is attached to the needle at the chest wall when the needle is in the pericardial sac to prevent accidental displacement. Blood or fluid is aspirated slowly, using the three-way stopcock to prevent the entry of air into the pericardial sac.
9. Monitor client for cardiac arrhythmias or pattern changes.	If the needle is in contact with the ventricle, the ST segment (end of S wave to beginning of T wave) increases and ventricular ectopic beats may occur. Prepare a bolus of Xylocaine for IV administration and keep on standby (see ACLS technique in Chap. 3). If the needle touches the atrium, the P–R segment (end of P wave to beginning of QRS complex) is elevated. Large, erratic QRS complexes with progressive cardiac disturbances may occur if the myocardium is penetrated.

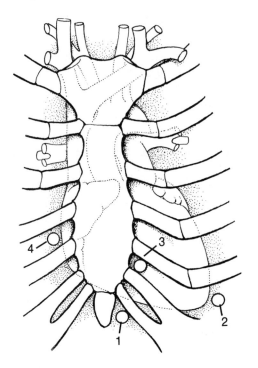

Fig. 9–1 Operative sites for pericardiocentesis. (Brunner LS, Suddarth DS: The Lippincott Manual of Nursing Practice, 4th ed. Philadelphia, JB Lippincott, 1986)

10. If large amount of fluid or blood must be drained, the physician may insert intra-cath and leave in pericardial sac. Attach intra-cath to drainage tubing and collection bottle or bag to drain remaining fluid by gravity.

Continual drainage prevents accumulation of additional fluid in the pericardial sac.

11. When needle or intra-cath is removed, place sterile 4 × 4 over site and tape.

RELATED NURSING CARE

NURSING ACTIONS	RATIONALE/AMPLIFICATION
1. Monitor client's vital signs every 5 minutes to 15 minutes during procedure, and every 15 minutes for 4 hours to 8 hours after procedure.	
2. Document any clotting of aspirated blood.	The presence of clotted blood signals puncture or laceration of the myocardium. Blood that remains in the pericardial sac for an extended time will not clot because it has been defibrinated by the heart.
3. Note color, consistency, odor, and amount of fluid drained.	An accurate description of the fluid aids diagnosis and future treatment.
4. Correctly label any specimens obtained and forward them to laboratory.	Laboratory analysis may include bacteriology studies, cytology, and protein and clotting studies.

EVALUATION PHASE

ANTICIPATED OUTCOMES	NURSING ACTIONS
1. Removal of pericardial fluid	Monitor hemodynamic parameters for recurrence of the pericardial effusion.
2. Prevention of the following complications, which result from pericardiocentesis:	

a. Laceration or puncture of myocardium or coronary artery, with resulting hemorrhage

Monitor the client for movement during the procedure. Monitor the continuous ECG pattern. Observe aspirated fluid for clotting.

b. Cardiac arrhythmias

Evaluate continuous ECG rhythm strip during the procedure. Keep an IV line open for the emergency administration of drugs. Have ACLS equipment and temporary pacing equipment on standby.

c. Perforation of lungs, liver, or stomach

Observe for sudden, unexplained chest or epigastric pain, dyspnea, decreasing blood pressure, tachycardia without other arrhythmias, anxiety or restlessness, nausea, or hematemesis.

d. Infection

Observe sterile technique during the procedure.

e. Recurring cardiac tamponade

Monitor hemodynamic parameters for signs of pericardial effusion.

PRODUCT AVAILABILITY   DISPOSABLE PERICARDIOCENTESIS KIT

Abbott Laboratories
Travenol Laboratories Inc.
Pharmaseal Inc.

SELECTED REFERENCES   Kaye W: Invasive therapeutic techniques: Emergency cardiac pacing, pericardiocentesis, intracardiac injections, and emergency treatment of tension pneumothorax. Heart and Lung 12(3):300–319, May 1983

King TE, Stelzner TJ, Sahn SA: Cardiac tamponade complicating the postpericardiotomy syndrome. Chest 83(3):500–503, March 1983
Pursley P: Acute cardiac tamponade. Am J Nurs 83(10):1414–1418, October 1983

10 *Blood/blood component administration*

Blood and blood product administration have become an integral part of therapy in the care of the critically ill client. The safe administration of whole blood, or of the components of whole blood, has become the responsibility of the critical care nurse. Therapy is prescribed by monitoring the hematologic values of the individual client. The values of the complete blood count and the results of clotting studies indicate the type of blood component that is needed. The comparatively recent advance in separating blood components from whole blood and the lengthening of the storage time of blood and blood components have made blood-replacement therapy more available than in the past.

Currently, whole blood is infused less often than are packed red cells, or plasma. Single-donor plasma is used less commonly than fresh frozen plasma. If whole blood is required, the nurse may be responsible for mixing the plasma and the red blood cells.

BLOOD COMPONENTS

Component therapy includes the use of one or more blood products. The components are separated from whole blood in the blood bank, stored, and used as needed. The use of blood and blood components is regulated by the federal government. Guidelines for the collection, labeling, storage, and administration of blood and blood products are approved by the Food and Drug Administration, the American Association of Blood Banks, and the American Red Cross. Components that are currently used include whole blood, plasma, packed red blood cells, packed red blood cells with the leukocytes removed, washed red blood cells, cryoprecipitated clotting factor VIII, platelets, and, less commonly, granulocytes and clotting factors II, VII, IX, and X (Table 10–1).

Table 10–1
Blood factors

Name	Factor	Use
Whole blood	All factors present	Volume replacement
Packed red blood cells	Red blood cells	Increase oxygen-carrying capability without as much increase in volume
Packed red blood cells	Most of plasma removed	Decrease chance of febrile reaction to antibodies contained in plasma
Washed red blood cells	No plasma present	Decrease chance of reaction
Leukocyte-poor red blood cells	Leukocytes removed	Decrease chance of reaction
Clotting factors VIII, II, IX, VII, and platelets	Clotting factors removed by cryoprecipitation	Replacement therapy
Granulocytes	Specific white blood cells	Replacement therapy in immunosuppression states

BLOOD TYPING

The administration of blood or blood components requires typing for A, B, AB, and O compatibility and Rh factor matching. This is done in the blood bank, as are tests for the presence of antibodies. When red blood cells are thawed for use, the plasma sent with them from the blood bank may or may not be of the same A, B, or O type as the red blood cells. The compatibility of the plasma and the red blood cells depends on the antibodies that are present in the plasma. It is always recommended that red blood cells and plasma be of the same A, B, or O type if possible. If this is not possible, be aware of potential incompatibilities (Table 10–2).

Table 10–2
*Blood–plasma compatibilities**

Blood type	Plasma type	Compatible
O	O	Yes
O	A	No
O	B	No
O	AB	Yes
A	A	Yes
A	O	No
A	B	No
A	AB	Yes
B	B	Yes
B	O	No
B	A	No
B	AB	Yes
AB	Any	Yes

* If there is any doubt about compatibility, check with the blood bank.

EXPERIMENTAL TECHNIQUES AND AUTOTRANSFUSION

Recently developed experimental techniques in blood administration include the administration of an artificial substitute for human blood and autotransfusion. Artificial substitutes are chemical substances that are capable of volume replacement and have the ability to transport oxygen. Artificial substitutes are intended for use in extreme emergencies. Autotransfusion is used when there are antibody incompatibilities or when religious principles prevent the acceptance of human blood. Autotransfusion is accomplished by one of two methods.

The first method is used in cases in which the need for autotransfusion is anticipated. With this method the client donates blood to the blood bank before an anticipated need, and this blood is then frozen and stored until needed.

The second method is more commonly used in an emergency. With this method the client's blood is filtered, or both filtered and washed, and is retransfused as needed after recovery from chest tubes or other suction site. This method is used in the event of trauma or surgery.

TRANSFUSION OF UNCROSSMATCHED BLOOD

Transfusion of uncrossmatched blood, or *in vivo* transfusion, is used when there are incompatibilities that the blood bank cannot match. Approximately 30 ml to 50 ml of uncrossmatched blood is transfused. After 20 minutes a hemoglobin sample is drawn and checked for lysis of the recipient's red blood cells. If lysis has not occurred, the transfusion is completed. This method is also used in emergency situations.

BLOOD WARMING TECHNIQUES

Blood warming techniques are used because the administration of large amounts of cold blood or components is contraindicated. The technique of running the tubing through a bath of warm water in a basin is not recommended. Hypothermia and transfusion reactions can be reduced by the use of blood warmers. Blood warmers that accurately control the temperature of the blood are available commercially.

DISEASES TRANSMITTED
THROUGH BLOOD
TRANSFUSION

Donor blood is checked for hepatitis A, hepatitis B, syphilis, and Acquired Immune Deficiency Syndrome (AIDS). At present there are no tests for hepatitis non-A and non-B. These are diseases that are known to be transmitted by blood transfusion.

WHOLE BLOOD ADMINISTRATION

Objectives
To provide volume replacement
To increase the oxygen- and nutrient-carrying capacity of the circulating blood volume

ASSESSMENT PHASE

- Is there an existing intravenous (IV) line with a gauge that will allow the infusion of cellular components?
- Is there a signed consent form?
- Has the client previously had transfusions?
- Were there any unpleasant effects?
- Have typing and crossmatching been completed?
- Has correct identification of the client and blood been completed according to institution policy?

PRECAUTIONS

- **Administer blood components within 30 minutes after removal from the controlled temperature of the blood bank or they will have to be discarded.**
- **Carefully monitor fluid balance for clients who have the potential for fluid overload.**
- **Check typing, crossmatching, and client identification with a second registered nurse and document according to hospital policy.**

PLANNING PHASE

EQUIPMENT

Blood administration set
IV catheter (at least 20 gauge)
Normal saline
Tape and dressing
Tourniquet
Armboard or restraint (optional)
IV stand

CLIENT/FAMILY TEACHING

- Discuss the reason for the administration of blood.
- Explain the reason for an IV access line.
- Explain the procedure for starting the IV line.
- Instruct the client to report any feelings of rising temperature. Fever is a common reaction to blood transfusion.
- Other signs of reaction to the blood transfusion are chest or back pain located over the flank, pruritus, urticaria, chills and fever, and dyspnea. These symptoms generally occur near the end of the transfusion. Instruct the client to report them immediately.

**IMPLEMENTATION
PHASE**

NURSING ACTIONS	RATIONALE/AMPLIFICATION
1. Spike normal saline with one of three tails of blood administration set, making sure that two remaining lines are clamped (Fig. 10–1).	Normal saline is the prefered solution because of its isotonicity. Dextrose 5% in water (D₅W), lactated Ringer's, or saline solutions other than normal saline should not be used.

Fig. 10-1 Spike normal saline solution with one line of blood administration set.

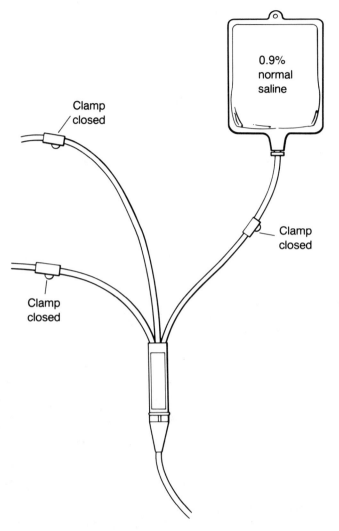

0.9% normal saline

Clamp closed

Clamp closed

Clamp closed

2. Flush line with normal saline.

Remove air from the entire line at this time.

3. Spike red blood cells and plasma with remaining tails of three-tail set.

4. Close clamp on saline.

5. Invert red blood cells and open clamp. Open clamp on plasma (Fig. 10-2).

6. Allow plasma to flow into red blood cells. Close clamp on plasma. Gently mix blood.

This mixing reconstitutes the whole blood from the two components. Gentle mixing prevents damage to the red blood cells.

7. Check vital signs before starting infusion and again 10 to 15 minutes after transfusion begins. Remain with client during first 20 minutes. Check vital signs every 15 minutes during procedure.

Frequent checks of the vital signs detect febrile reaction, shock, or circulatory reaction.

8. Open clamp on whole blood.

9. Begin blood flow at 4 drops to 6 drops/minute, and increase to 10 drops to 20 drops/minute after 50 ml has been infused.

The slower rate allows for observation of the client for reaction during the first 20 minutes of the procedure.

Fig. 10–2 Invert red cells to reconstitute with plasma.

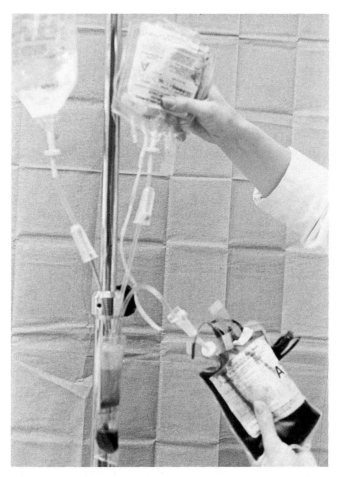

RELATED NURSING CARE

NURSING ACTIONS	RATIONALE/AMPLIFICATION
1. Ensure proper flow to maintain patency of line.	Observe for client comfort; fever is not uncommon and must be assessed to differentiate from reaction.
2. Monitor client for adverse reactions.	
3. Treat hemolytic reaction or incompatibility immediately.	Hemolytic reaction or incompatibility is indicated by signs of shock and severe allergic reaction.
a. Stop transfusion.	
b. Maintain IV line with normal saline.	
c. Treat for shock and hypovolemia.	
d. Prepare to administer mannitol or other diuretic and sodium bicarbonate intravenously.	
e. Insert indwelling Foley catheter.	
f. Obtain blood and urine specimens and send to laboratory for testing for presence of hemoglobin, which indicates hemolysis.	
g. Recrossmatch client's blood immediately. Further transfusion may be required.	
h. Return remaining blood and blood administration set to laboratory.	

EVALUATION PHASE

ANTICIPATED OUTCOMES	NURSING ACTIONS
1. Prevention of complications of blood transfusion	
a. Microemboli	Always ensure that there is a functioning micropore filter in line.
b. Febrile reaction	Stop the transfusion. Maintain the IV line with the normal saline. Notify the physician. Obtain cultures of the client's blood as ordered and send the remaining blood and tubing to the laboratory.
c. Hemolytic reaction or incompatibility	Check blood type, crossmatch, and client identification before the administration of blood. Monitor the client for symptoms of shock and severe allergic reaction.
d. Fluid overload	Monitor respiratory status and cental venous or pulmonary artery pressures along with other vital signs.
2. Improved hemodynamic status	Evaluate for increased hematologic values, improved skin color, decreased pulse rate, and increased arterial blood pressure.

BLOOD COMPONENT ADMINISTRATION

Objective

To replace one or more of the factors present in whole blood when the use of whole blood is not required or is contraindicated

ASSESSMENT PHASE

- Is there an existing order for the specific factor to be administered?
- Has the client received blood-factor therapy in the past?
- Did any reaction occur?
- If an existing IV line will be used, is the needle or catheter gauge adequate for the component ordered?
- Are typing and crossmatching necessary? Both procedures are necessary if cellular-containing components will be administered.
- Have the necessary laboratory tests been performed?
- Has proper identification of the client and the blood factor been performed according to institution policy?

PRECAUTIONS

- **Factor VIII, antihemophilic factor (AHF), and factor IX, plasma thromboplastin component (PTC), have a much higher change of transmitting hepatitis than single-donor products do. Be especially careful when handling contaminated needles and syringes and used vials.**
- **If a care-giver is punctured with a contaminated needle, follow institution policy for incident reporting. The incident report should include the manufacturer's name and the lot number of the vial from which the factor was taken.**

PLANNING PHASE

EQUIPMENT

IV access*
Component administration set (Fig. 10–3)
IV tubing and normal saline starter solution

* Either an existing line with the proper access gauge and a compatible starter solution or a new IV line may be used.

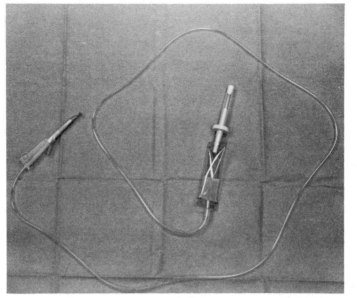

Fig. 10–3   Blood component administration set.

IV stand
Armboard (optional)
IV catheter (19 gauge or larger)
Dressings and tape
Tourniquet
Blood component infusion set with filter (for platelets or cryoprecipitate) (Fig. 10–4)
10-, 35-, and 50-ml syringes (for platelets or cryoprecipitate)
    30-ml syringe filled with sterile saline for injection
    18-gauge needle (for platelets or cryoprecipitate)

CLIENT/FAMILY TEACHING

- Common reactions to component therapy are fever, chills, pruritus, and urticaria.
- If the client has experienced a reaction with previous therapy, the chance of reaction to subsequent therapy is high.
- Reactions to factor VIII and factor IX are rare.
- Risk of hepatitis transmission with factor VIII and factor IX is high. Instruct the client and family to report signs and symptoms of disease such as malaise, fatigue, listlessness, nausea and vomiting, anorexia, joint and muscle pain, changes in senses of taste and smell, fever, jaundice, dark urine, and clay-colored stools.

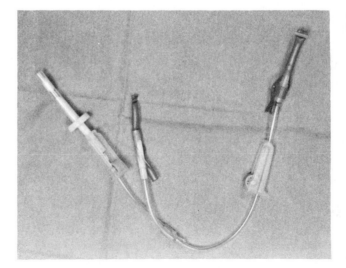

Fig. 10–4   Blood component infusion set.

- Explain the reason for IV needle insertion.
- Discuss the procedure for the insertion of the IV needle.

Red blood cell transfusion

**IMPLEMENTATION
PHASE**

NURSING ACTIONS	RATIONALE/AMPLIFICATION
1. Make sure all clamps are closed on blood administration set. Spike normal saline with one side of the blood administration set (see Fig. 10–1).	Normal saline is the solution of choice for starter solutions. Do not use lactated Ringer's or D_5W solution because they will cause hemolysis of the cells.
2. Open clamps on two tubings to saline and spike tubing through which red blood cells will be infused. Allow saline to fill both sides of tubing. Close clamp to tubing to be used for red blood cells.	If only red blood cells are to be transfused, a "Y"-type blood administration set can be used.
3. Squeeze drip chamber until it is one-third to one-half full.	
4. Flush line with saline.	Remove air from the entire line at this time.
5. Spike red blood cells with other line of "Y" tubing.	
6. Close clamp to saline and open clamp to red blood cells.	
7. Squeeze drip chamber until filter is completely full (Fig. 10–5).	Do not allow the red blood cells to drip directly on the filter. This will damage the cells and cause hemolysis.

Fig. 10–5 Squeeze drip chamber until filter chamber is completely full.

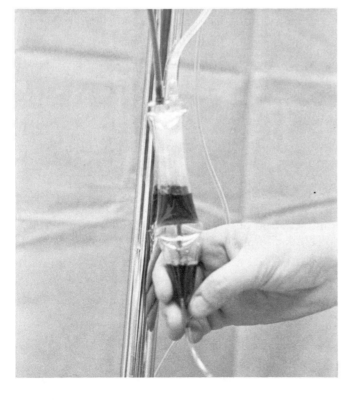

8. Regulate flow of red blood cells (see previous section on Whole Blood Administration).

9. Monitor client (see previous section on Whole Blood Administration).

RELATED NURSING CARE

NURSING ACTION	RATIONALE/AMPLIFICATION
Observe client closely for reaction (see previous section on Whole Blood Administration).	

EVALUATION PHASE

ANTICIPATED OUTCOMES	NURSING ACTIONS
1. Prevention of complications of red blood cell administration	
a. Microemboli	Always ensure that a micropore filter is in line.
b. Febrile reaction, incompatibility, or hemolysis	Proper identification of blood type and client is imperative. Monitor vital signs (see previous section on Whole Blood Administration).
2. Increase oxygen-carrying capacity of blood	Monitor the client's hemoglobin level, hematocrit, and hemodynamic status.

Plasma infusion

ASSESSMENT PHASE

- Determine why the plasma is being administered. The flow rate will be determined in part by the reason for administration.
- If the plasma is being administered for clotting-factor replacement, the rate of infusion will be as fast as the client can tolerate, but preferably not longer than 1 to 2 hours.
- If the plasma is being given for volume replacement, it can be given over a period of up to 4 hours.

IMPLEMENTATION PHASE

NURSING ACTIONS	RATIONALE/AMPLIFICATION
1. Start IV line of normal saline using 24- to 20-gauge needle.	Use the normal saline to maintain the patency of the IV line. A needle with a smaller gauge than that used for the administration of red blood cells can be used because no cellular components are present in plasma.
2. Identify client (see previous section on Whole Blood Administration).	Plasma should be of same type (A, B, O).
3. Spike plasma with one line of blood component administration set	The blood component administration set contains a filter to remove any clots.
4. Open clamp and fill filter chamber and tubing. Close clamp.	Remove air from the tubing.
5. Piggyback plasma into IV line.	

6. Stop saline infusion and open clamp on plasma.

7. Regulate drip rate.

If the plasma is being given to replace volume, it can be given within 4 hours. If the plasma is being given to provide clotting factors, it should be given within 1 hour to 2 hours.

8. Monitor vital signs as needed before and after transfusion.

Vital signs will detect febrile reaction, shock, or circulatory overload.

RELATED NURSING CARE

NURSING ACTION	RATIONALE/AMPLIFICATION
Maintain IV line with normal saline after infusion is completed.	An IV line provides venous access should more plasma need to be given.

EVALUATION PHASE

ANTICIPATED OUTCOMES	NURSING ACTIONS
1. Prevention of complications of plasma infusion	
a. Microemboli	Make sure that an in-line blood filter is in place.
b. Febrile reaction	Monitor vital signs as indicated.
c. Circulatory overload	Monitor respiratory status and vital signs.
d. Allergic reaction	Assess client for urticaria and pruritus.
2. Increase in circulating volume	Monitor for an increase in arterial blood pressure, a decrease in heart rate, and changes in respirations.

Platelet infusion

IMPLEMENTATION PHASE

NURSING ACTIONS	RATIONALE/AMPLIFICATION
1. Obtain platelets from blood bank.	Blood type (A, B, AB, O) and Rh factor will not necessarily match that of the client.
2. Check unit for clumps or aggregates.	If aggregates are found, knead the unit gently until the clumps disappear. If the platelets cannot be resuspended, return the unit to the blood bank.
3. Start IV line with normal saline using straight infusion set.	
4. Spike platelets with blood component administration set and fill tubing.	This set contains a filter that removes microaggregates (see Fig. 10–3).
5. Piggyback platelets into normal saline line as close to needle insertion site as possible (Fig. 10–6).	This reduces the distance that the platelets have to travel through the tubing. The platelets will adhere to the plastic tubing.
6. Close clamp on saline line. Open clamp on platelets.	
7. Infuse platelets rapidly over period of 1 minute to 10 minutes.	Platelets lose viability rapidly.

Fig. 10–6 Piggyback platelets into normal saline solution as close to needle insertion site as possible.

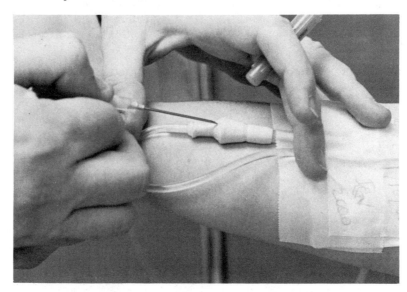

Fig. 10–7 Spike platelets with one lead of blood component infusion set.

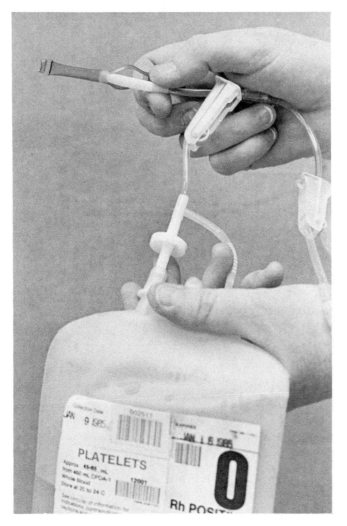

8. Observe client for reactions.

Febrile or allergic reactions may occur. If a reaction occurs, stop the infusion and restart the normal saline at a keep-open rate. Notify the physician.

9. When infusion is finished, invert bag and open saline. Fill bag with 30 ml to 50 ml of normal saline.

Platelets adhere to the plastic bag and to the filter. Flushing the bag, filter, and tubing will ensure that the client receives all of the platelets.

10. Close clamp on saline and rehang platelet bag.

11. Open clamp on platelet bag and flush line, filter, and tubing with normal saline.

The following alternative method may be used for platelet infusion:

1. Spike platelets with one line of blood component infusion set, making sure that all clamps are closed (Fig. 10-7).

The blood component set contains a clot filter that removes possible emboli.

2. Attach 35-ml syringe to female port of "Y" tubing (Fig. 10-8). Open clamps above "Y" connection.

Use aseptic technique to reduce the risk of contamination.

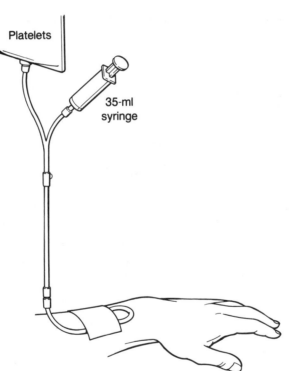

Fig. 10-8 Attach syringe to female outlet port of infusion set.

3. Withdraw platelets from platelet bag into syringe. Close clamp to platelets.

4. Open clamp below "Y" connection. Depress plunger, filling "Y" and short tubing to male connector.

This will fill the short tubing and remove air from the line.

5. Connect 18-gauge needle to male adapter and piggyback into starter saline line as close to needle insertion site as possible.

This will reduce the amount of tubing through which the platelets must travel.

6. Inject platelets at rate of 10 ml/minute. Maintain steady pressure on syringe plunger.

Observe the insertion site continuously for signs of infiltration.

RELATED NURSING CARE

NURSING ACTION	RATIONALE/AMPLIFICATION
If more than one unit is to be given, maintain patency of IV line with normal saline.	Usually, multiple units of platelets are ordered.

EVALUATION PHASE

ANTICIPATED OUTCOMES	NURSING ACTIONS
1. Prevention of complications of platelet administration	
a. Chills, fever, or allergic reactions	Monitor the client throughout the administration of the platelets.
2. Increase in platelet count	Usually the platelet counts are checked 1 to 3 hours after the infusion and again 18 to 24 hours later. Units are given until the client's platelet count is raised 50,000 mm/l.

Leukocyte infusion

IMPLEMENTATION PHASE

NURSING ACTIONS	RATIONALE/AMPLIFICATION
1. Follow procedure described for beginning administration of whole blood (see previous section on Whole Blood Administration). Use blood component administration set (see Fig. 10–3).	Leukocytes must be type (A, B, O) and Rh compatible with the client.
2. Check leukocyte expiration date and time.	Leukocytes become inactive 24 hours after collection.
3. Spike white blood cells with one line of blood component administration set. Fill tubing and filter chamber.	Remove air from the tubing.
4. Piggyback leukocytes into starter IV line.	If the client develops a reaction, give the white blood cells in divided doses. Use the starter IV line to maintain the patency of the venous access line.
5. Monitor client's vital signs every 15 minutes during infusion.	A febrile reaction commonly occurs with white blood cell administration. If the client's temperature is elevated above 104°F, stop the infusion and notify the physician.
6. Have meperidine hydrochloride and diphenhydramine hydrochloride available for use before and during leukocyte administration.	The client may be premedicated to reduce the severity of reactions.
7. Flush infusion set with saline.	Ensure that all of the white blood cells are administered.

RELATED NURSING CARE

NURSING ACTIONS	RATIONALE/AMPLIFICATION
1. Maintain client comfort.	Check premedication orders.

2. Stay with client during infusion.	Observe the client for a febrile reaction, pulmonary distress, and changes in blood pressure. *Caution:* If the client is receiving amphotericin B therapy, there is a high risk of pulmonary toxicity.

EVALUATION PHASE

ANTICIPATED OUTCOMES	NURSING ACTIONS
1. Prevention of complications of white blood cell infusion	
a. Microemboli	Use a blood administration set or a blood component administration set with a clot filter.
b. Febrile reaction	Monitor the client's temperature and observe for chills every 15 minutes during the infusion. Check for type (A, B, O) and Rh compatibility before the infusion is started.
2. Reduction or prevention of infection	Monitor the client's temperature and vital signs every 2 hours to 4 hours between doses. Units are usually given daily until the infection clears.

Cryoprecipitate infusion

IMPLEMENTATION PHASE

NURSING ACTIONS	RATIONALE/AMPLIFICATION
1. Obtain cryoprecipitate or commercially prepared clotting factor solution from blood bank or pharmacy.	Cryoprecipitate should be refrigerated only until use. Infuse cryoprecipitate at room temperature.
2. Spike cryoprecipitate with cryoprecipitate infusion set, or draw up commercially prepared clotting factor solution with filter needle after dilution with sterile diluent (Fig. 10–9).	Use the filter needle that is supplied by the manufacturer of commercially prepared clotting factor complexes. *Caution:* Do not use bacteriostatic sterile water for dilution of commercially prepared clotting factor complexes. The use of sterile water for injection may be harmful to the client who has coagulation deficiency disease. Sterile water is not isotonic and can cause hemolysis.
3. Close all clamps of cryoprecipitate infusion set. Spike cryoprecipitate with one lead of cryoprecipitate infusion set.	Use aseptic technique to reduce the risk of contamination. The cryoprecipitate set contains a filter that reduces the risk of embolus.
4. Attach 35-ml syringe to female port above "Y" connection.	
5. Withdraw cryoprecipitate into syringe. Close clamp to cryoprecipitate and open clamp below "Y" connection.	
6. Fill short tubing below "Y" connection by depressing plunger of syringe.	Remove air from the tubing.
7. Perform venipuncture with 23- to 25-gauge scalp vein set.	The use of the small-gauge needle decreases trauma to the vein and the risk of postinfusion hemorrhage at the venipuncture site.

Fig. 10–9 Spike cryoprecipitate using cryoprecipitate infusion set.

Fig. 10–10 Inject cryoprecipitate slowly, at a rate of 10 ml/minute.

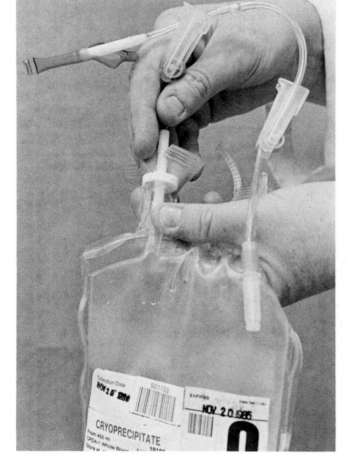

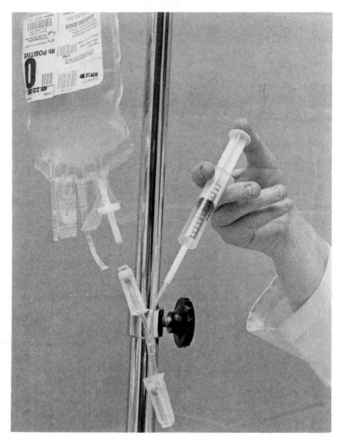

8. Attach short tubing of cryoprecipitate infusion set to scalp vein set.

9. Inject cryoprecipitate or clotting factor complex at rate of 10 ml/minute (Fig. 10–10).

Slow rates of infusion decrease the risk of reaction.

10. Remove 35-ml syringe from scalp vein needle and replace it with 10-ml syringe filled with sterile saline. Flush cryoprecipitate tubing, filter, and scalp vein set with saline.

Ensure that the client receives all of the clotting factor complex.

11. Commercially prepared clotting factors can be given by intravenous push (IVP).

Flush the tubing in the manner described for leukocytes (see previous section on Leukocyte Infusion).

RELATED NURSING CARE

NURSING ACTIONS	RATIONALE/AMPLIFICATION
1. Observe for hemorrhage or hematoma formation at needle insertion site during infusion.	The use of a small-gauge needle reduces the risk of trauma. A large-gauge needle is not necessary because there are no cellular components in cryoprecipitate.
2. Record lot number of commercially prepared clotting factor complexes.	If the client develops hepatitis, the lot number will be used to trace the infected donor.

3. Use good handwashing technique and treat contaminated equipment with caution to prevent risk of contracting infections transmitted through blood inoculation.

Pooled donor preparations increase the risk of hepatitis infection.

4. Observe for signs of intravascular clotting or febrile reaction.

Signs of intravascular clotting or a febrile reaction include chest or back pain, changes in vital signs, dyspnea, or coughing. Monitor the client's vital signs during the infusion.

EVALUATION PHASE

ANTICIPATED OUTCOMES	NURSING ACTIONS
1. Prevention of complications of cryoprecipitate infusion	
a. Hemolytic reactions	Do not use bacteriostatic water as a diluent.
b. Loss of factor VIII	Use only a plastic syringe because factor VIII may bind to the surface of a glass syringe.
c. Emboli	Avoid rapid administration of the cryoprecipitate.
2. Decrease in clotting times	Evaluate the client's laboratory values. Assess for decreases of hematoma, ecchymosis, epistaxis, bleeding gums, or other signs of hemorrhage.

AUTOLOGOUS TRANSFUSION

Objectives

To provide blood replacement using blood that was donated before the need arose or was reclaimed during emergency procedures

To reduce the likelihood of transfusion reactions in clients with blood typing and crossmatching problems

To provide volume replacement and to increase the oxygen- and nutrient-carrying capacity of the circulating blood volume

ASSESSMENT PHASE

• Why does the client need transfusions of whole blood (*e.g.*, open-heart surgery or trauma)?
• Has a signed consent form been obtained?
• What type of autologous transfusion will be used?
• Is the equipment necessary for autologous transfusion ready for use?

PLANNING PHASE

EQUIPMENT

Haemonetics Cell Saver (or other autologous blood recovery system)
Disposable Harvey Reservoir H, 700F
Open Heart Pack 8618
Aspiration and Anticoagulation Assembly 7452
IV access line with 18-gauge catheter
1000 ml normal saline — 3 bags
Heparin, 30,000 units to 60,000 units
Blood administration set with filter
Suction source with pressure regulation

CLIENT/FAMILY TEACHING

• Discuss with the client the reason for the autologous transfusion.
• Instruct the client to report reactions as for whole blood administration.

**IMPLEMENTATION
PHASE**

NURSING ACTIONS	RATIONALE/AMPLIFICATION
1. Follow manufacturer's instructions for setting up Cell Saver machine (Fig. 10–11).	The tubing used for the recovery of the client's blood is color coded to make the setup process easier.
2. When volume of shed blood reaches 400 ml to 500 ml, press "Fill" button. Fill until blood reaches top curve of centrifuge.	If the flow of lost blood is steady, the "Fill" button may be pressed when the volume reaches the 100-ml mark.

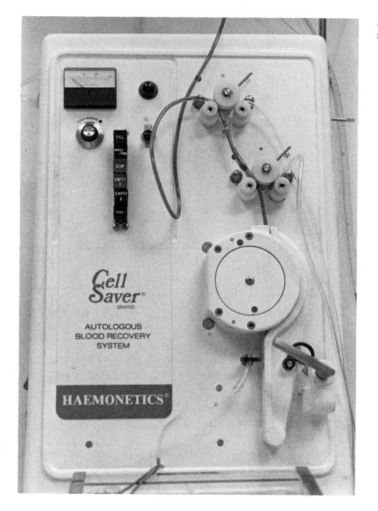

Fig. 10–11 The Haemonetics Cell Saver.

3. Adjust centrifuge speed to 200 ml/minute.

4. Press "Stop" button and set dial at zero.

5. Press "Wash" button.

6. Adjust centrifuge speed to 200 ml/minute. Wash recovered blood with 700 ml heparinized saline.	Each 500 ml of recovered blood will contain approximately 50 units of heparin, with a mixture of 60,000 units of heparin in 1000 ml of normal saline.
7. Press "Stop" button and set speed dial to zero.	Allow centrifuge to stop before proceeding further. This allows the last of the wash solution to empty into the waste bag.
8. Press "Empty-2" button and turn speed dial to 300 ml/minute.	Allow all the air in tubing to empty into the waste bag.

Fig. 10–12 Pall Micropore Filter.

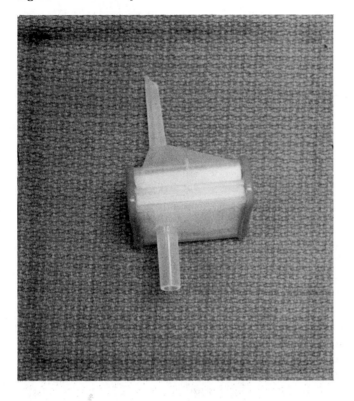

9. Press "Stop" and set dial to zero.

10. Use filter to attach blood administration set to recovery bag (Fig. 10–12).

Infuse blood through a micropore filter to reduce the possibility of emboli.

RELATED NURSING CARE

NURSING ACTIONS	RATIONALE/AMPLIFICATION
1. Monitor client continuously for signs of shock.	This procedure is usually performed during periods when the client is at high risk of circulatory depletion.
2. Monitor client for reaction to transfusion.	Microorganisms that cause febrile reactions may be introduced during the procedure. Reaction to the blood is unlikely.

EVALUATION PHASE

ANTICIPATED OUTCOMES	NURSING ACTIONS
1. Prevention of microemboli complications caused by autologous transfusion	Always ensure that a functioning micropore filter is in line in the transfusion set.
2. Increase in circulating volume	Evaluate for an increase in arterial blood pressure and oxygenation of tissue.

SELECTED REFERENCES   Heustis DW, Bove JR, Busch S: Practical Blood Transfusion. Boston, Little, Brown & Co. 1969

Luckman J, Sorenson KC: Medical–Surgical Nursing, 2nd ed. Philadelphia, WB Saunders, 1980

Tucker, SM et al: Patient Care Standards, 3rd ed. St. Louis, CV Mosby, 1984

11 *Phlebotomy*

Objectives

To perform a venesection to remove up to 500 ml of blood
To decrease the circulating blood volume in acute pulmonary edema
To decrease the red blood cell mass
To collect blood for potential autotransfusion

ASSESSMENT PHASE

- Is the client experiencing acute pulmonary edema? Phlebotomy can be used in conjunction with rotating tourniquets, diuretic therapy, and respiratory therapy.
- Does the client have polycythemia, a chronic respiratory problem, or other condition that causes an increase in the red blood cell mass?
- Will the client require blood transfusions in the immediate future? Is there a reason that blood from the blood bank cannot be infused (*e.g.*, rare blood group, religious restriction)?
- Have baseline vital signs been obtained?
- If the procedure is elective, have baseline determinations of hemoglobin level and hematocrit been obtained?

PRECAUTIONS

- **Removing more than 500 ml of blood at one time can cause syncope.**
- **Establish a keep-open intravenous (IV) line for emergency use before the phlebotomy begins.**

PLANNING PHASE

EQUIPMENT

Vacuum collection bag or bottle (with anticoagulant)
Blood labels
Phlebotomy tubing
Large-bore needle (16 gauge to 19 gauge)
Tourniquet
Iodophor solution
4 × 4s
Tape
Iodophor ointment (optional)
Band-Aid

CLIENT/FAMILY TEACHING

- Reinforce the physician's explanation of the procedure. Answer any questions about phlebotomy and the expected outcomes.
- Reassure the client that the procedure is not excessively painful. It should be similar to the procedure that is used to start an IV line.
- Tell the client that bed rest will be required for at least 1 hour after the procedure to prevent syncope.

IMPLEMENTATION PHASE

NURSING ACTIONS	RATIONALE/AMPLIFICATION
1. Prepare vacuum bottle or bag.	
a. Check collection bag for integrity.	
b. Close tubing clamp and insert tubing into collection bag.	Closing the clamp retains the vacuum.
c. Place collection bag 15 cm to 30 cm (6 inches to 12 inches) below level of venipuncture.	This position decreases the risk of air embolism. Gravity will facilitate flow.
d. Place large-bore venipuncture needle on tubing.	Leave the protective cap in place to prevent contamination. Use a large-bore needle to prevent red blood cell lysis if blood is required for autotransfusion.
2. Place client supine. Wash your hands.	Make sure that the client is comfortable.
3. Prepare selected venipuncture site with iodophor solution. Apply tourniquet and perform venipuncture (see Venipuncture in Chap. 4).	Ask the client to open and close fist. This will facilitate venous engorgement. Do not make the venipuncture above an existing IV line to prevent withdrawing IV fluid with the blood.
4. Observe for backflow of blood into tubing.	Backflow indicates vein entry.
5. Open tubing clamp and begin phlebotomy (Fig. 11–1).	Gently rotate the collection bag periodically to mix the blood with the anticoagulant solution.
6. Dress and tape venipuncture site.	

Fig. 11–1 Therapeutic phlebotomy.

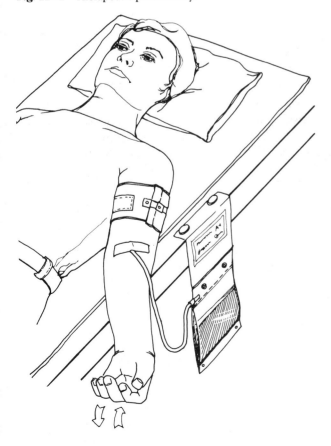

7. Monitor client's hemodynamic status during phlebotomy. Monitor vital signs every 15 minutes.

The rate of flow may be controlled with the clamp if necessary. If the phlebotomy is elective, control the flow at a slower rate than in an emergency.

8. When prescribed amount of blood has been withdrawn, clamp tubing and remove needle from vein.

Do not contaminate the collection system when the needle is withdrawn from the vein.

9. Apply digital pressure at venipuncture site until bleeding stops. Dress with iodophor ointment and Band-Aid.

RELATED NURSING CARE

NURSING ACTIONS	RATIONALE/AMPLIFICATION
1. Label blood and send to blood bank immediately.	Blood may be required for autotransfusion, and refrigeration and storage of the blood must begin immediately. If blood is withdrawn for reasons other than for autotransfusion, the blood bank may accept the blood for transfusion if it meets the bank's standards.
2. Observe venipuncture site after phlebotomy for hematoma formation.	
3. Check vital signs every 15 minutes after procedure until they are stable.	
4. Place client on bed rest for at least 1 hour after phlebotomy.	Bed rest prevents syncope.
5. Encourage client to drink fluids after phlebotomy unless fluids are contraindicated by client's condition.	Fluids help to replenish the circulating blood volume.

EVALUATION PHASE

ANTICIPATED OUTCOMES	NURSING ACTIONS
1. Removal of up to 500 ml of blood	Monitor the client's hemodynamic status.
2. Prevention of complications of phlebotomy	Monitor for syncope, hematoma, cardiorespiratory arrest, hypovolemia, convulsions, and vagal response (*i.e.*, nausea, vomiting). Monitor infection-control techniques (see Infection-Control Protocol for Blood/Body Fluid Precautions in Chap. 4).

PRODUCT AVAILABILITY   VACUUM PHLEBOTOMY BOTTLES
Travenol Laboratories, Inc.

Heart transplantation

BACKGROUND

The first human heart transplant was performed in December 1967 by Dr. Christian Barnard in South Africa. This important clinical event precipitated an increase in the number of transplantation centers around the world. By 1968 there were 64 transplant teams in 22 countries performing heart transplants. Unfortunately, few of these early recipients survived, and it became evident that the complexity of heart transplantation was not in the surgical procedure but in the postoperative medical and nursing care of the immunosuppressed client, who is at risk of infection and rejection. As a result, few transplantation centers continued to be active after 1970.

In recent years, there has been a dramatic improvement in the survival figures of heart transplant patients. Between 1968 and 1984 the one-year survival rate increased from 22% to 84%. Over 50% of recipients survive more than 5 years. This improvement in survival figures can be attributed to a refinement in recipient selection criteria and to postoperative management advances, such as the endomyocardial biopsy, immunologic monitoring, and the development of new antirejection immunosuppressive agents such as cyclosporine A (CyA). As a result, there has been a resurgence of interest in heart transplantation. The protocols and techniques outlined in this chapter may be adapted by nurses to design a program of care for heart transplant recipients in their center.

Presurgical cardiac recipient protocol

Objectives

To prepare the potential recipient both physically and emotionally for the heart transplant procedure and the postoperative course

ASSESSMENT PHASE

- Does the potential recipient meet the selection criteria (*i.e.*, end-stage heart disease with less than 6 months to live, no other medical therapy would benefit the client)?
- Is the recipient younger than 55 years of age?
- Are any of the following contraindications to transplantation present?
  Systemic disease that would limit recovery or survival
  Pulmonary hypertension that is unresponsive to vasodilators
  Liver or kidney dysfunction unrelated to low cardiac output (CO)
  Severe peripheral or cerebrovascular disease
  Active infection (The candidate will be temporarily removed from the waiting list because this predisposes the recipient to potentially fatal infectious complications after the transplant.)
  Pulmonary infarction, which predisposes the recipient to pulmonary infections after the transplant
- Are there psychosocial contraindications to transplantation (*e.g.*, drug or alcohol abuse or dependence, mental illness or severe emotional instability, absence of family/friend social support system)?

PLANNING PHASE

CLIENT/FAMILY TEACHING

- Answer questions about the operative procedure and immediate postoperative care using photographs or diagrams.
- Discuss the implications of the endotracheal tube, ventilator, monitors, chest tubes, bleeding, pacemaker wires, pain medication, and family visiting hours.
- Describe the nursing care specific to transplantation once the recipient is extubated.
- Explain reverse isolation and its purpose.
- Describe immunosuppressive drugs.
- Discuss 1:1 client/nurse ratio and primary-care nursing.
- If possible, arrange for the primary-care nurse to meet with the recipient and family before the transplant.
- Conduct a tour of the intensive care unit (ICU) and transplant isolation room with the client and family before the transplant. This allows the recipient and family to acquire some familiarity with the nurses and the unit.
- Answer questions about the length of the waiting period for a cardiac donor in the local area.
- Explain how the recipient's beeper will sound when a donor call is received. Tell the client where to report in the hospital.

IMPLEMENTATION PHASE

NURSING ACTIONS	RATIONALE/AMPLIFICATION
1. Obtain baseline vital signs and weight.	
2. Ask client to take nothing by mouth (except medications) from admission to surgery.	NPO (*non per os,* nothing by mouth) is routine preparation for any surgical procedure.
3. Ensure that consent forms are completed. This may include consent form for transplantation as experimental procedure.	The potential risks and benefits of heart transplantation should be explained to the client by the surgeon.
4. Order immediate chest film.	A chest film will provide baseline data for this hospitalization.
5. If transport to radiology department is necessary, provide a wheelchair.	Recipients are severely debilitated as a result of end-stage heart disease.
6. Draw routine admission laboratory work.	Laboratory work provides baseline data for this hospitalization.
7. Draw blood to type and crossmatch 10 units of whole blood.	Bleeding is always a potential risk with open-heart surgery.
8. Collect routine sputum and urine samples.	These provide baseline data for fungal and bacterial studies.
9. Culture throat and urine samples for cytomegalovirus (CMV).	These provide baseline data for CMV studies.
10. Draw anaerobic and aerobic blood cultures.	These provide baseline data for infection.
11. Draw blood for toxoplasmosis titer, CMV titer, and legionella.	These are viral infections that are potentially harmful after the transplant.
12. Arrange for surgical preparation shave from chin to knees.	Shaving reduces the risk of bacterial contamination from body hair.
13. After shaving, help client to scrub entire body with pHisoHex for 10 minutes.	Scrubbing reduces the risk of contamination from skin bacteria.
14. Administer 1 unit to 2 units of fresh frozen plasma if prescribed.	Severe right-sided heart failure with back pressure to the liver will prolong coagulation times. Rarely, vitamin K (aquaMEPHYTON) may also be given.

15. Administer preoperative immunosuppressive medications as ordered (usually CyA and methylprednisolone).

The recipient is immunosuppressed before the transplant to prevent rejection. Drugs are prescribed according to body weight. Arm bands identify the client and warn of drug allergies.

EVALUATION PHASE

ANTICIPATED OUTCOME	NURSING ACTION
Completion of nursing actions outlined above within 2 hours	Completing the preparation of the client within 2 hours allows the donor heart to be transplanted as quickly as possible.

Cardiac donor protocol

BACKGROUND

Nurses are actively involved in transplantation programs, not only in large medical centers that support a transplant program but throughout the country wherever a donor may become available. The typical donor at Stanford University Hospital is frequently a young man in his early twenties who has been involved in a traumatic motor accident or other catastrophe. A brain-dead donor may have few other physical injuries, and nurses caring for such clients require much peer support to comfortably care for a young victim and support the family. If the hospital has a transplant coordinator, this person is often experienced in helping family and staff deal with a potential emotional crisis. This is especially true if the client has been in the ICU for any length of time before being declared brain dead. Once the brain-dead person is identified as a potential donor, the heart is normally transplanted within 12 hours. The transplant team will come to a hospital to recover the heart only, or to transport the donor, depending on the wishes of the family, the coroner, and the physicians involved.

The following protocols describe the care of the cardiac donor. Today most donors are multiorgan donors, and the nurse may receive conflicting medical orders from several transplant teams. A transplant coordinator may help to establish a compromise between the needs of different medical teams and organ systems.

Objective

To stabilize the brain-dead donor to preserve the heart and other organs for transplantation

ASSESSMENT PHASE

- Does the potential donor meet all of the following selection criteria?

Under 35 years of age. There is a greater risk of coronary artery disease with increasing age.

No active infection that may be exacerbated by the immunosuppressive drug regimen after the transplant

No severe chest trauma that may have damaged the donor heart

No prolonged cardiac arrest that would have depleted the myocardial cellular energy supplies or damaged the myocardium

Hemodynamically stable without high-dose inotropic support. High doses of dopamine or epinephrine also deplete myocardial glucose supplies.

No history of previous heart disease. Normal electrocardiogram (ECG) without Q waves or ST-segment changes, which signify ischemic damage.

Two flat electroencephalograms (EEGs), certified brain dead by two physicians who are *not* associated with the transplant program, and a negative toxicology screen to eliminate the possibility of a drug overdose mimicking brain death

- Have the following recipient–donor matching criteria been met?

ABO blood group compatibility

Negative crossmatch of donor and recipient white blood cells to prevent hyperacute rejection postoperatively

Compatible heart-size match

PLANNING PHASE

CLIENT/FAMILY TEACHING

- Provide nursing support for the family of the donor. Family members will be experiencing the first stages of the grief process.
- Answer any questions from the donor family about the procedure. Explain that there will be no medical costs to the family for organ procurement.

IMPLEMENTATION PHASE

NURSING ACTIONS	RATIONALE/AMPLIFICATION
1. Monitor neurologic vital signs.	Neurologic vital signs establish an important baseline. The donor will be flaccid and unresponsive to stimuli as a result of brain stem damage. The pupils will be fixed, dilated, and unresponsive to light.
2. Maintain mean arterial pressure (MAP) between 70 mm Hg and 80 mm Hg or cuff systolic pressure above 100 mm Hg.	Damage to the vasomotor center in the brain causes loss of vascular tone. This leads to vasodilation, peripheral pooling of blood, and lowered circulating volume. Rehydration with crystalloid or colloid solution is essential to prevent cardiac collapse. Use blood if hematocrit is below 30%.
3. Maintain central venous pressure (CVP) between 5 cm and 12 cm of water (cm H_2O).	Damage to the vasomotor center also results in the loss of venous vascular tone and the peripheral pooling of blood. Several liters of intravenous (IV) fluids may be required to correct hypovolemia and to achieve an adequate CO.
4. Correct hypotension (MAP > 60 mm Hg) with CVP *below* 5 cm H_2O (CVP of 4 mm Hg) by volume replacement.	The circulating volume is inadequate. Give a 1-liter bolus of fluid (*e.g.*, lactated Ringer's solution or D_5.2NS [dextrose 5% and .2% normal saline] with 20 mEq potassium/liter) over 30 minutes and reevaluate.
5. Correct hypotension (MAP > 60 mm Hg) with CVP *above* 10 cm H_2O (CVP of 8 mm Hg) using inotropic support.	The circulating volume is adequate. It may be necessary to increase cardiac contractility with low-dose inotropic support (*e.g.*, dopamine 2 mcg/kg/minute). Check arterial blood gases (ABGs) because both acidosis and hypoxia may decrease contractility and thus lower CO.
6. Auscultate chest every 2 hours.	The development of rales and rhonci may indicate pulmonary edema. Decreased breath sounds may indicate consolidation, effusion, or collapse. The cardiac transplant donor is at risk of several of the following pulmonary complications:
	a. Hypervolemic pulmonary edema due to excessive IV fluid replacement
	b. Neurogenic pulmonary edema as a result of brain death and raised intracranial pressure. Treatment for both conditions includes diuretics and increased positive end-expiratory pressure (PEEP) using a ventilator.
	c. Atelectasis and lobar collapse as a result of immobility and loss of respiratory clearance mechanisms such as the cough and gag reflexes.
7. Keep donor intubated on volume-cycled ventilator (10 ml to 15 ml/kg tidal volume).	Large tidal volumes decrease the risk of atelectasis.

8. Set ventilator for PEEP of 3 cm H_2O to 10 cm H_2O.

PEEP will keep alveolar sacs open at end expiration to decrease alveolar collapse and pulmonary complications.

9. Maintain arterial oxygen partial pressure (paO_2) between 80 mm Hg and 100 mm Hg with low inspired oxygen concentration (*e.g.*, 40% to 60%).

These parameters ensure adequate systemic oxygenation. If the donor requires high inspired O_2 concentrations, pulmonary damage may have occurred.

10. Maintain normal *p*H between 7.35 and 7.45.

This is the physiologic range for optimal body metabolism.

11. Draw ABGs every 2 hours.

ABGs are part of the respiratory assessment. They allow the nurse to evaluate ventilation and, if needed, to make ventilator changes. CO_2 reflects ventilation and the suitability of the tidal volume and ventilator rate. PaO_2 reflects the adequacy of O_2 delivered to the tissues. *p*H reflects acid–base balance.

12. Suction endotracheal tube hourly or as indicated by quantity of secretions.

Removal of secretions prevents the development of pneumonias and mucous plugs that cause lobar collapse.

13. Suction oropharynx hourly or as required.

Oral secretions must be cleared because these clients do not have a gag reflex and will aspirate secretions into the lung, causing bacterial pneumonias.

14. Turn and reposition client every 2 hours.

Immobility results in pooling of pulmonary secretions, atelectasis, alveolar collapse, and pneumonia. Pulmonary infections may mean that the heart cannot be transplanted.

15. Insert nasogastric (NG) tube and connect to low wall suction.

The absence of a gag reflex potentiates aspiration of gastric contents. Use of an NG tube connected to low suction and raising the head of the bed to a 30-degree angle minimize the risk of this complication.

16. Record accurate intake and output. Replace urine output each hour, and add 50 ml to 100 ml of IV fluids. (Lactated Ringer's solution or D_5.2NS with 20 mEq potassium/liter). Give IV infusion of Pitressin, or antidiuretic hormone (ADH), as ordered.

Damage to the pituitary gland results in diabetes insipidus or the production of an excessive volume of dilute urine. In brain-dead clients ADH is no longer released from the posterior pituitary gland and urine is not reabsorbed from the distal tubules of the kidney. Treatment includes hydration and replacement of lost urine volume. For a urine output that is greater than 200 ml/hour, give aqueous Pitressin (ADH) 5 units to 10 units intramuscularly (IM) every 2 hours.

17. Monitor electrolytes, especially potassium (K^+), every 4 hours.

Potassium is lost in the urine as a result of diabetes insipidus.

18. Replace K^+ as necessary and as prescribed to maintain serum potassium level between 4.5 mEq to 5 mEq/liter.

Hypokalemia will potentiate cardiac arrhythmias and cardiac arrest.

19. Monitor serum glucose level every 4 hours.

Damage to the hypothalamus results in hyperglycemia, which may require an IV infusion of insulin. Hyperglycemia also produces osmotic diuresis and loss of K^+.

20. Give IV infusion of insulin for elevated blood sugar as required and prescribed.

21. Monitor heart rate and rhythm.

Arrhythmias are rare in the cardiac donor, except in hypokalemic states.

22. Maintain donor's body temperature between 34°C and 36°C and monitor continuously with rectal thermometer.

Brain death causes malfunction of the hypothalamus, which controls temperature regulation in the body. This results in a low body temperature. A body temperature below 30°C may potentiate ventricular fibrillation.

23. Place donor on warming blanket. Note any temperature spikes.	A sudden rise in temperature may indicate active infection.
24. Collect routine samples, including endotracheal aspirate, urine, and blood, for culturing.	Bacterial, fungal, and viral cultures are obtained before broad-spectrum antibiotic coverage is initiated.
25. Administer prophylactic antibiotic coverage as prescribed.	Nafcillin, Mandol, and chloramphenicol are examples of antibiotics used for a donor drug regimen.
26. Apply sterile dressings to any open wounds.	Sterile dressing of wounds reduces the risk of sepsis before the transplant.

EVALUATION PHASE

ANTICIPATED OUTCOMES	NURSING ACTIONS
1. Successful transplantation of donor heart	Monitor the donor's physiological parameters.
2. Successful transplantation of other organs, such as kidneys, corneas, liver, pancreas, or skin	Follow appropriate protocols of transplant teams for transplantation of other organ systems.

Heart transplant protocol (immediate postoperative period)

BACKGROUND   A knowledge of how heart transplant surgery is performed is essential to understand the rationale for much of the postoperative nursing care of the recipient. A description of the operative procedure follows.

1. The recipient and donor are placed in adjoining operating rooms, each staffed by a full surgical team. If the heart has been harvested from a distant donor, the second operating room is unnecessary.
2. The surgery is performed using a median sternotomy incision.
3. The recipient's body temperature is cooled to below 34°C and the intracardiac temperature is cooled to below 10°C. Hypothermia is necessary to reduce the body's metabolic demands during surgery. Postoperatively, the rapid rewarming of the recipient accounts for much of the hemodynamic instability.
4. The recipient is placed on cardiopulmonary bypass (CPB).
5. The disabled heart is removed, leaving only the posterior walls of the atria, which contain the orifices of the pulmonary veins and vena cava. Thus the donor heart will not have to be anastomosed to each vessel individually.
6. The new donor heart is implanted with the following three major anatomoses: the atria, the aorta, and the pulmonary artery (Fig. 12–1).
7. When the donor and recipient atria are sutured together, great care is taken to preserve the sinoatrial (SA) node in the donor right atrium. The new heart no longer receives impulses from the body's autonomic nervous system, and protection of the donor heart's electric conduction system is essential.
8. Two epicardial pacing wires are placed in the right atrium. The pacing wires will be used in the event of bradycardia in the denervated heart.
9. The recipient is removed from CPB. The donor heart should now be beating in normal sinus rhythm.
10. An isoproterenol (Isuprel) drip is started to increase heart rate to 100 beats per minute and thus increase CO. This is necessary for the first 2 to 4 postoperative days because the heart no longer has a direct nerve supply.
11. A low-dose dopamine drip (2 mcg/kg/minute) may be started to increase contractility. Because the heart has been manipulated, has had a period of ischemia, and has been cooled and anesthetized, CO may be depressed.
12. A low-dose sodium nitroprusside drip (2 mcg/kg/minute) may be started to decrease systemic vascular resistance to cardiac ejection and to facilitate rewarming.

Fig. 12-1 Surgical technique of cardiac implantation. (*A*) Initiation of anastomosis at left atrium. (*B*) Right atrium opened and anastomosis begun. (*C*) Aortic anastomosis and expurgation of air by way of atrial catheterization. (*D*) Pulmonary artery anastomosis. (*E*) Epicardial pacing wires inserted on right atrium. (Reproduced with permission from Baumgartner WA et al: Cardiac homotransplantation. In Ravitch MM et al (eds): Current Problems in Surgery. Copyright © 1979 by Year Book Medical Publishers, Inc., Chicago)

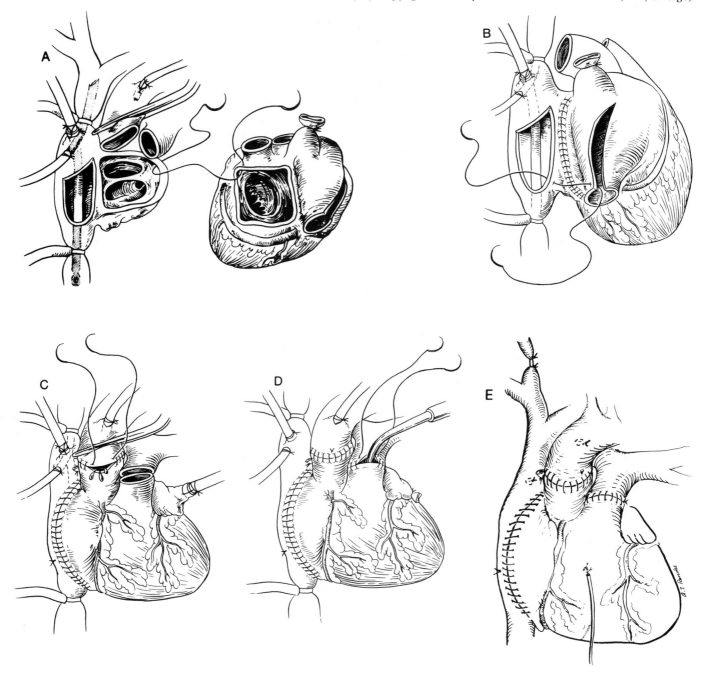

13. Mediastinal chest tubes are inserted, and the chest is closed.
14. The recipient is returned to the cardiovascular ICU, accompanied by the surgeon and anesthesiologist.

PREPARATION OF THE
ISOLATION ROOM IN THE
INTENSIVE CARE UNIT

The transplant room is cleared of all supplies and is cleaned with a bactericidal agent by the housekeeping staff. The room is restocked with sterile, disposable supplies when possible. Nondisposable supplies are cleaned with a bactericidal agent or a gas autoclave.

Objectives
To stabilize the recipient hemodynamically
To wean the client from ventilator support in the immediate postoperative period

ASSESSMENT PHASE

• Was the heart transplant recipient stable during surgery?
  Ask the anesthesiologist or surgeon whether the recipient was hemodynamically stable and whether any IV drips are running, such as isoproterenol, dopamine, or sodium nitroprusside.
  Was there any ventricular irritability or signs of heart block?
  Are pacemaker wires *in situ?*
  Are chest ECG leads connected to the monitor to allow assessment of heart rhythm?
  Is the recipient bleeding? What are the results of coagulation studies?
• Are all of the invasive lines and tubes in place and functioning? Invasive lines include an arterial line and a CVP line. Swan–Ganz and left atrial lines are not usually necessary because the donor heart is healthy and the CVP is used to monitor volume status.
• Is the endotracheal tube correctly positioned? Obtain a chest film to confirm position. Auscultate the chest to verify that the recipient is being ventilated in both lung fields.
• Are chest tubes patent and connected to low suction?
• Is an NG tube in position and connected to low suction?
• Is a suprapubic (or Foley) catheter *in situ* and draining clear urine? Hematuria indicates trauma from cardiopulmonary bypass. A suprapubic urinary catheter may be used to minimize the risk of urinary tract infection.
• Can the heart transplant recipient's CO be adequately assessed without the aid of a Swan–Ganz catheter?
  Use clinical assessment to evaluate CO. As the recipient's body temperature increases, the peripheral pedal pulses change from barely palpable to full and bounding. This indicates normal CO. With rewarming, the peripheral (foot) skin temperature changes from cold to warm. Skin color will change from white and vasoconstricted to pink and vasodilated. If nailbeds are cyanotic, assess ABGs. With rewarming, the capillary refill time will return to normal. This is tested by gently squeezing the nailbed until it blanches. When released, it becomes pink immediately if peripheral blood flow is adequate. This indicates normal CO.
  Urine output of at least 30 ml/hour or 0.5 ml/hour/kg indicates adequate renal perfusion and CO.
  MAP remains between 70 mm Hg and 90 mm Hg and CVP between 8 mm Hg and 12 mm Hg. If pulsus paradoxus is present, the recipient may be hypovolemic. This is seen as an arterial waveform that fluctuates more than 10 mm Hg with the ventilator respiratory cycle. CO may not be adequate.
• Is a 1:1 nurse to client ratio available during the acute period?

PRECAUTIONS

• **No person with an active infection (*e.g.,* influenza, herpes lesions) should enter the isolation room. The immunosuppressed recipient is extremely vulnerable to infection.**
• **No pregnant women should enter the isolation room. Immunosuppressed clients may have active CMV or toxoplasmosis. Rarely, these conditions have been associated with fetal malformations.**

PLANNING PHASE

CLIENT/FAMILY TEACHING

• Encourage the family to visit as soon as the client is stable after surgery (approximately 45 minutes).
• Explain the purpose of the isolation room. Help the family to put on face masks and to wash their hands thoroughly with pHisoHex.
• Answer any questions the family may have about the transplant procedure or the client's condition.

**IMPLEMENTATION
PHASE**

NURSING ACTIONS	RATIONALE/AMPLIFICATION
1. Monitor cardiac status and maintain heart rate between 100 beats and 110 beats per minute with isoproterenol (Isuprel).	The denervated heart requires a fast heart rate to optimize CO.
2. Monitor cardiac rhythm for arrhythmias.	Isoproterenol causes ventricular irritability, which is seen as PVCs.
3. Check serum K^+ if premature ventricular contractions (PVCs) are present.	Excessive diuresis after surgery as a result of post-CPB diuretics depletes serum K^+. Hypokalemia causes ventricular irritability and PVCs.
4. Monitor cardiac rhythm for bradycardia. If client is bradycardic, increase Isuprel drip and connect pacing wires to pacemaker.	Myocardial edema and manipulation of the heart during surgery increase the risk of bradycardia in the denervated heart.
5. Maintain MAP between 70 mm Hg and 90 mm Hg.	Excessive diuresis, bleeding, and vasodilation secondary to rewarming predispose the recipient to hypotension.
6. Maintain CVP between 8 mm Hg and 12 mm Hg.	The denervated heart depends on a large stroke volume to stretch the myocardial fibers and to produce a strong contraction (Frank–Starling mechanism).
7. Correct hypovolemic hypotension (MAP < 60 mm Hg with CVP *below* 8 mm Hg [11 cm H_2O]).	The circulating volume is inadequate. As the recipient's body temperature increases and the vessels vasodilate, relative hypovolemia results. Replace fluid with crystalloid or colloid IV solutions. Use blood if hematocrit is below 28%.
8. Correct hypotension secondary to decreased contractility (MAP < 60 mm Hg with an adequate CVP of at least 10 mm Hg).	The circulating volume is adequate. Increase inotropic support to increase contractility. Increase dopamine to 3 mcg to 5 mcg/kg/minute.
9. Monitor for cardiac tamponade which is indicated by rising CVP (> 15 mm Hg), falling MAP (< 55 mm Hg), decreased peripheral perfusion, decreased urine output, decreased chest tube output, and muffled heart sounds.	Postoperative bleeding is a major risk after heart transplantation. Tamponade occurs when blood is not evacuated through the chest tubes and compresses the heart. Clinically, this will increase CVP, decrease MAP, and decrease peripheral perfusion.
10. Monitor for bleeding of more than 50 ml/hour from chest tubes. Order coagulation studies and replace chest tube output with blood. Inform surgeon.	Preoperative right-sided heart failure causes back pressure on the liver and may lengthen coagulation times. CPB also lengthens coagulation times. If coagulation times are abnormally long, fresh frozen plasma may be administered.
11. Monitor for bleeding of over 100 ml to 200 ml/hour from chest tubes over several hours. Inform surgeon.	If coagulation studies are normal, the recipient may be returned to the operating room for hemostasis.
12. Check ABGs frequently as recipient's body temperature increases to assess for metabolic acidosis.	When cold body tissue is rewarmed, acidotic waste products are released. This is seen as an increase in CO_2 on ABGs.
13. As recipient warms and CO_2 is released, increase ventilator rate.	The ventilator rate is increased to eliminate CO_2 and to maintain a normal pH in the body.
14. Maintain recipient on volume-cycled ventilator (10 ml to 15 ml/kg tidal volume) with PEEP of 5 cm H_2O until recipient is hemodynamically stable and rewarmed.	Large tidal volumes and PEEP decrease the risk of postsurgical atelectasis, especially in the left lower lobe.

15. Wean recipient from ventilator 6 hours to 12 hours after transplant when warm, alert, and hemodynamically stable.

Weaning involves decreasing the inspired O_2 content and decreasing the ventilator rate in response to ABGs and recipient over breathing.

16. Suction endotracheal tube every 2 hours or as indicated by quantity of secretions.

Excellent pulmonary toilet is essential to prevent pulmonary infections.

17. Assess recipient for readiness for extubation.

Assessment includes cardiac, respiratory, neurologic, and renal functions.

18. Following extubation, place client on 40% O_2 using face mask and draw ABGs.

Assessment of ABGs and clinical assessment will reflect whether respiratory function is adequate.

EVALUATION PHASE

ANTICIPATED OUTCOMES	NURSING ACTIONS
Recipient is awake and alert after extubation and has stable cardiac status	Answer any questions that the recipient or family may have. Most recipients are euphoric at this stage with the knowledge that they have survived the procedure. Continue to monitor physiological parameters.

Immunosuppressed heart transplant recipient protocol

BACKGROUND

IMMUNE SYSTEM

Immunosuppressive medications are routinely given after heart transplantation to suppress the body's ability to recognize and to reject foreign tissue. The immune system is composed of two principal parts: the phagocytic white blood cells that are part of the nonspecific immune response and the lymphocytic white blood cells that have memory and a specific immune reaction that enables lymphocytes to reject transplanted organs. Lymphocytes make up 30% of white blood cells and include two specific groups: T cells and B cells. T cells are derived from the thymus gland and protect the body from viral, fungal, and protozoan infections. It is the T cells that cause acute rejection in transplanted organs. The T-cell system is also responsible for cellular immunity because it fights infections inside the cell rather than in the bloodstream. B cells are believed to be produced in the fetal liver and in Peyer's patches in the gut. They protect the body against bacterial infections by producing immunoglobulins (IgM, IgG, IgA, IgD, IgE) in the bloodstream or in other body fluids. B-cell immunoglobulins are responsible for hyperacute rejection if the heart is not ABO compatible. The B-cell system is also known as humoral immunity and requires a functioning T-cell system to work effectively. B and T cells working together are believed to be responsible for chronic cardiac rejection (Table 12–1).

IMMUNOSUPPRESSIVE DRUGS

There are four principal immunosuppressive agents that are used in varying combinations to prevent rejection of the transplanted heart. These include corticosteroids, azathioprine, Cyclosporine A (CyA) and antithymocyte globulin (ATG).

Table 12–1
Types of rejection and immune response

Rejection	Time	Immune response
Hyperacute	Immediate	B-cell immunoglobulins
Accelerated	24 hours to 36 hours	B-cell immunoglobulins
Acute	1 week to 3 months	T cells
Chronic	3 months to years	B cells and T cells

Corticosteroids (prednisone) were the first immunosuppressive agents used to prevent rejection. They act by stabilizing the cell wall and suppressing the body's inflammatory response to foreign proteins, such as a transplanted heart. Corticosteroids remain an integral part of the transplant protocol, although today they are prescribed at lower dosages than previously. The initial dosage of 1 mg/kg/day that is given at the time of transplant is tapered down to a long-term dosage of 0.2 mg/kg/day to minimize the many side-effects. These side-effects include increased risk of infection, diabetes, osteoporosis, fragile skin, redistribution of body fat, muscle wasting with thin extremities, accumulation of fluid secondary to sodium retention and loss of potassium, gastric irritation and ulceration, and emotional instability with mood swings. Many nursing interventions are used to mitigate these side-effects.

In the event of rejection of the transplanted heart, which is diagnosed by the endomyocardial biopsy, the first line of treatment is to increase IV corticosteroids. The recipient remains in isolation, and the biopsy is repeated 4 days to 7 days later.

Azathioprine (Imuran) acts by interfering with purine (protein) synthesis and prevents replication of active B and T cells. Recipient dosage varies according to platelet and white blood cell counts and ranges from 1.5 mg to 2 mg/kg/day. It has many toxic side-effects, including bone marrow suppression, which in turn causes leukopenia; thrombocytopenia; anemia; and hepatic dysfunction, which causes uremic jaundice, diarrhea, and vomiting.

CyA is a new immunosuppressive agent approved by the Food and Drug Administration for use in organ transplantation in 1983. It acts specifically against the production of T cells to prevent rejection of the transplanted heart. CyA has greatly improved early survival statistics, but initial enthusiasm has been tempered by its side-effects of hypertension and progressive nephrotoxicity. The major clinical advantage of CyA is that although episodes of rejection and infection occur just as frequently as with other immunosuppressive agents, these episodes are not as severe and are easier to treat. This has resulted in decreased mortality for the heart transplant recipient. The initial dosage varies greatly from 5 mcg to 16 mcg/kg/day, depending on the protocol used. It is then gradually tapered to lower dosages.

Antithymocyte globulin (ATG) acts specifically against T cells by coating them (which marks them as foreign) so that they will be digested in the recipient's lymphatic system. ATG is prepared by injecting T cells into an animal (horse, rabbit, or goat), producing antiserum against the human T cells. The ATG serum is then purified and injected into the cardiac recipient to prevent or treat rejection. At Stanford University Hospital, IV injections of equine ATG are given during the first postoperative days to prevent rejection and to decrease the levels of circulating T cells to below 5% of normal. Acute rejection episodes that do not respond to increased corticosteroids are treated with IM injections of rabbit ATG given over 3 days. Side-effects include anaphylactic reaction to the serum, pain at the IM injection site, and lymphoma, especially when used with high-dose CyA. All four of these immunosuppressive drugs are used in combination to prevent rejection of the transplanted heart. An example of this drug regimen is shown in Table 12–2.

MONITORING FOR REJECTION

In the first 2 weeks after transplantation, circulating T cells are reduced to 5% of their normal volume by a combination of immunosuppressive drugs. Many transplant centers around the world are using different combinations of these drugs to determine optimal immunosuppression for their clients. With current knowledge there is no right or wrong protocol, although all of the centers use combinations of the drugs described above.

Circulating T cells are measured by the sheep e-rosette test. In this test 10 ml of blood from the recipient is mixed with sheep erythrocytes. The T cell binds the sheep erythrocytes around itself in a rosette pattern. This allows the T cell lymphocytes to be identified and counted, and the immunosuppressive drugs to be increased or decreased depending on the percentage recorded. In recipients on the prednisone/Imuran protocol, a rise in T cells indicates an episode of acute rejection. In recipients

Table 12–2
Heart transplantation—adult

Immunosuppression	Loading dose	Maintenance dose	Laboratory work*	Biopsy	Acute rejection (first and second episodes)	Ongoing rejection
Solu-Medrol	500 mg IV after cardiopulmonary bypass 125 mg IV q12—3 doses	See Prednisone.			1 g IV for 3 days with biopsy on days 5–7 after rejection episode	1 g IV for 3 days (+ RATG) and rebiopsy (if rejection does not resolve, retransplant)
Prednisone		0.2 mg/kg; taper by 1 mg–2 mg/day until 0.1 mg/kg is reached *after* discharge			Prednisone held at current patient dosage during 3 days of Solu-Medrol IV	Increase Prednisone dosage after Solu-Medrol
Cyclosporine A	16 mg/kg preoperatively 12 mg/kg/day preoperatively for renal insufficiency	9 mg/kg/day (until result of measurement of cyclosporine level)	Measure cyclosporine level qMon/Wed/Fri 200 ng–300 ng/ml (trough) for 1–30 days 50 ng–150 ng/ml (trough) for > 30 days	Weekly and prn for increased temperature	No change	No change
ATG (either rabbit or horse; not both together)	Horse ATG IV 10 mg/kg/day for 7 days		E-rosette count daily Circulating T lymphocytes < 5%, differential count after T-cell recovery		Not given for first or second rejection episodes	Rabbit ATG 2.5 mg/kg/day IM for 3 days (individualized)
Imuran (Azathioprine)	4 mg/kg preoperatively	2 mg/kg	WBC and platelet counts daily until stable, then Mon/Wed/Fri (WBC differential only if indicated)		No change in dosage	No change in dosage

* Additional tests for all transplant recipients include the following: creatinine/BUN, daily; 12° creatinine clearance, twice a week; ECG, once a week; CMV blood titer, complement fixation titer, IgG, IgM, once a week; CMV throat culture and urine culture, once a week; sputum and urine for culture and sensitivity, once a week and prn; toxoplasmosis titer, legionella titer, pretransplant, pretransplant, 2 weeks after transplant and at hospital discharge.

on the CyA protocol, a rise in T cells does not occur early enough to predict rejection or initiate treatment.

The endomyocardial biopsy remains the gold standard for monitoring acute rejection because it allows direct examination of a piece of the myocardium. Acute rejection episodes are expected to occur within the first 6 weeks after transplantation. An endomyocardial biopsy is performed 1 week after the transplant, and weekly thereafter. Biopsies will be performed more frequently than weekly if the clinical condition of the recipient changes (*e.g.,* fever spike) and depending on the results of previous biopsies.

The endomyocardial biopsy resembles a right-sided cardiac catheterization and is performed with the client under local anesthesia in the cardiac catheterization laboratory (Fig. 12–2). The endomyocardial biotome is inserted through the right jugular vein to the right ventricle, where three specimens are taken from the right septal wall. These specimens are examined by an experienced pathologist, and results are available within 24 hours. Recipients are treated for rejection only if the biopsy shows myocyte necrosis with hemorrhage. Lymphocyte infiltration alone is not treated in recipients on CyA.

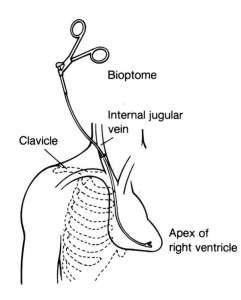

Fig. *12-2* Endomyocardial biopsy technique. (After Griep RB, Stinson EB, Shumway NE: Transplantation of the heart. Surg Ann 8:47–62, 1976)

Bioptome

Internal jugular vein

Clavicle

Apex of right ventricle

If CyA is used as the principal immunosuppressive agent, the endomyocardial biopsy is the only reliable means of monitoring rejection. Currently, researchers are searching for noninvasive methods of monitoring rejection in CyA patients. Using the echocardiogram to look at changes in diastolic function has shown promise in young children who are too small for biopsy. In these cases the echocardiogram has not replaced the biopsy, because it is not sufficiently reliable in identifying rejection. However, it has reduced the number of biopsies performed on young children after heart transplantation.

If corticosteroids (prednisone) and azathioprine (Imuran) are used as the principal immunosuppressive agents, noninvasive methods of diagnosing rejection are well established. On the routine ECG, a decrease in QRS complex (beginning of Q wave to end of S wave) voltage of more than 20% from the recipient's normal voltage indicates acute rejection. The QRS complex is measured in millimeters from top to bottom, and the total of leads I, II, III, V_1, and V_6 are added. The recipient's voltage is normally consistent from day to day as long as the ECG leads are placed in identical positions each time. Therefore a drop in voltage of more than 20% may be considered significant. A decrease in voltage and the appearance of a third or fourth heart sound occur because of the myocardial edema that accompanies prednisone/Imuran rejection. Table 12–3 compares the differences in diagnosis of rejection between the cyclosporine group and prednisone/Imuran group.

Table 12–3
Diagnosis of rejection in cardiac transplant recipients with different immunosuppressive drug protocols: cyclosporine A and prednisone/Imuran (azathioprine)*

Action	Cyclosporine A and low-dose prednisone	Prednisone/Imuran
Monitor daily T-cell levels (by e-rosette method).	No change in level of circulating T cells.	T-cell levels rise before an acute rejection episode.
Measure ECG voltage in leads I, II, III, V_1; and V_6.	No change in ECG voltage.	A fall in voltage of over 20% indicates acute rejection.
Monitor clinical signs and symptoms of early rejection.	No early clinical signs or symptoms are apparent.	Development of third or fourth heart sound and atrial arrhythmias indicate early rejection.
Monitor clinical signs and symptoms of late rejection.	CHF progresses slowly to biventicular heart failure and is easy to control.	CHF progresses rapidly to biventricular heart failure and can be difficult to control.
Monitor endomyocardial biopsy to detect early rejection.	Mild rejection or "infiltrate" of white cells into the area is not treated. Rebiopsy in 4 days.	Mild rejection or "infiltrate" of white blood cells is treated with increased corticosteroids. Rebiopsy in 4 days to 7 days.
Obtain endomyocardial biopsy to detect moderate or severe rejection.	Moderate to severe rejection is classified as myocyte necrosis and hemorrhage. Increase corticosteroids and rebiopsy in 4 days.	Use rabbit ATG to combat myocyte necrosis and hemorrhage. Rebiopsy in 4 days.
Obtain endomyocardial biopsy to detect ongoing rejection.	Use rabbit ATG to fight rejection. Rebiopsy in 4 days. If intractable rejection continues, consider retransplantation.	Continue to give rabbit ATG. Rebiopsy in 4 days. If intractable rejection continues, consider retransplantation.

* Various combinations of these drugs are used to obtain optimal immunosuppression with the lowest possible dosage.

CLINICAL SIGNS AND SYMPTOMS OF REJECTION

Early rejection is well tolerated by recipients on the CyA protocol. There are no early signs and symptoms of rejection, which is why the endomyocardial biopsy is so important. Moderate to severe rejection is associated with a third heart sound, atrial arrhythmias, and signs and symptoms of congestive heart failure. Late or severe rejection shows all the signs of advanced pump failure, decrease in CO with decreased blood pressure, decreased urine output, decreased peripheral perfusion, increased CVP or pulmonary capillary wedge (PCW) pressure, rales, decrease in arterial O_2 content, and increased temperature.

Objective

To prevent rejection and destruction of the transplanted heart by the recipient's immune system without leaving the recipient vulnerable to massive infections

ASSESSMENT PHASE

• Are the recipient's vital signs stable? An increase in body temperature above 37.5°C indicates infection. Corticosteroids decrease normal body temperature to approximately 36.5°C so that temperatures above 37°C should be investigated. Atrial arrhythmias, a third heart sound or decrease in blood pressure, fatigue, and breathlessness also may indicate rejection.

• Is there any change in the assessment of the recipient's physical condition?

The development of rales may indicate congestive heart failure (CHF) and rejection.

The development of rhonci and copious sputum often indicates infection. The lungs are the most frequent site of infection after cardiac transplantation.

Redness or induration at the incision site indicates infection.

Herpes simplex lesions will present as a red irritant rash.

The mouth is the potential site for fungal infections such as *candida albicans* (thrush), which is seen as a white rash.

Burning during urination indicates a urinary tract infection.

PRECAUTIONS

- Use an isolation room, mask, and good handwashing technique for the first weeks after transplantation when recipients are maximally immunosuppressed.
- Pregnant women or persons with active infections should not enter the isolation room.
- Unpeeled fruit or flowers should not be allowed in the isolation room. Fruits such as oranges or lemons carry mold in the crevices of the skin.
- Thoroughly clean all equipment that enters the isolation room, such as a radio or tape recorder brought from home.

PLANNING PHASE

CLIENT/FAMILY TEACHING

- Teaching after the transplant is a three-step process. Step one is recognition. Once the recipient is extubated, awake, and alert, the names and actions of the drugs are repeated and emphasized. Step two is participation. The recipient will pour all of the medications (immunosuppressive and cardiac) and be aware of the action, dosage, and side-effects of the medications. Step three is independence. The recipient knows the times when medications are to be taken, keeps an independent record of medications, and pours them without supervision.
- To facilitate this learning process, place a large medication chart on the wall of the isolation room that includes the names, actions, dosages, and side-effects of the cardiac and immunosuppressive drugs (Table 12–4).
- Document the client's progress in learning medication protocols.
- Teach the client to keep an accurate record of intake, output, and daily weight.
- If the client is being given prednisone, teach the client urine testing for sugar and acetone and to use guaiac to test stool samples (see example of heart transplantation flowsheet).

Heart transplantation teaching flow sheet used at Stanford University Hospital.

Please check appropriate box and include date.

John X: Heart Transplant 11/3

Tests	Nurse	Patient With Assistance	Patient	Comments
Measure Output	12/1	12/5	12/13	12/13
Specific Gravity	12/5	12/7	12/13	John recognizes and
Sugar and Acetone	12/5	12/7	12/13	pours all of his own
Hematest Stool	12/8	12/10	12/13	meds. He likes a nurse to
Specimens	**Nurse**	**Patient With Assistance**	**Patient**	check the prednisone
Urine	12/1	12/7	12/13	dosage because it is
Sputum	12/1	12/7	12/13	still being weaned down.
Diet	**Nurse**	**Patient With Assistance**	**Patient**	
Menu Selection	12/1	12/3	12/5	John has his own schedule
Measure Intake	12/1	12/5	12/10	for specimens, urine testing, etc.

Medications	Recognizes	Pours	Dosage	Action	Side-Effects
Persantine	12/3	12/5	12/10	12/9	12/10
Prednisone	12/3	12/5	12/11	12/5	12/11 ✔ dosage
Cyclosporine	12/3	12/5	12/10	12/5	12/10
Mycostatin	12/3	12/7	12/10	12/10	12/12
Mouthwash (TNHC)	12/3	12/7	12/10	12/10	12/12
Titralac	12/3	12/7	12/10	12/10	12/12
Potassium	12/6	12/8	12/10	12/10	12/10
Lasix	12/6	12/8	12/10	12/10	12/10
Tylenol	12/5				PRN only
Benadryl					PRN with ATG

Table 12–4
Medication chart for client teaching

Medication	Dosage	Action	Side-effects
Persantine (25- and 75-mg tablets)	75 mg qid (9 AM, 1 PM, 5 PM, 9 PM)	Persantine prevents platelet aggregation and development of atherosclerosis	Stomach irritation, dizziness, headache, flushing, skin rash, and bruising
Titralac	1 tsp p̄c and hs (9 AM, 1 PM, 5 PM, 9 PM)	Titralac is an antacid that prevents ulcers and relieves heartburn by neutralizing increased gastric acids, which are caused by Prednisone and cyclosporine. It also acts as a calcium supplement.	Constipation and nausea
TNHC mouthwash (gargle and rinse), 30 ml	30 ml p̄c and hs (9 AM, 1 PM, 5 PM, 9 PM)	Tetracycline–Nystatin–hydrocortisone–Chlor-Trimeton mouthwash protects against development of bacterial and fungal mouth infections.	None
Mycostatin suppository (dissolves in mouth)	1 lozenge p̄ and hs following TNHC mouthwash	Mycostatin suppository protects against development of fungal mouth infections	None
Colace (100-mg capsules)	100 mg bid prn (9 AM, 6 PM)	Colace softens the stool.	Abdominal cramps (rare) and diarrhea
Lasix (40-mg tablets)	Varies. Check medicine card daily.	Lasix is a diuretic necessary for promoting the excretion of water and counterbalancing the salt-retaining effects of prednisone.	Loss of K^+, decrease in blood pressure, nausea, vomiting, blurred vision, and loss of hearing (reversible)
K-Lor (potassium chloride)	20 mEq bid (9 AM, 6 PM)	K-Lor replaces the potassium that is lost with the administration of Lasix.	Stomach upset, stomach irritation.
Prednisone (1-, 5-, 20-mg tablets)	Varies. Check medicine card daily.	Prednisone is an immunosuppressant that suppresses cell reactions to prevent rejection of the heart.	Diabetes mellitus (rare), increased risk of infection, increased risk of bone fractures, increased appetite, sodium and water retention, peptic ulcers, skin rash, loss of muscle mass, redistribution of body fat—"moon face" and large abdomen, and mood swings—euphoria to depression
Cyclosporine A	Varies. Check medicine card daily. Mix with juice or chocolate milk.	Cyclosporine A is an immunosuppressant that inhibits rejection of the heart.	Renal dysfunction, liver dysfunction, hypertension, and increased risk of infection
Mannitol	12.5 g IV bid (9 AM, 6 PM) (given by RN)	Mannitol is a diuretic used to prevent renal failure, which may be caused by cyclosporine A. It "flushes" the kidneys.	Dry mouth, thirst, nausea, and vomiting
Imuran (Azathioprine)	Varies. Check medicine card daily.	Imuran is an immunosuppressant that inhibits rejection of the heart.	Increased risk of infection, decreased white blood cell count, decreased platelet count.
Antithymocyte globulin (ATG)	Varies (given by RN). IV horse ATG is given for prevention; IM rabbit ATG is given for rejection.	ATG is an immunosuppressant that prevents rejection of the heart.	Pain and burning at injection site in thigh (IM), chills, and fever.

IMPLEMENTATION PHASE

NURSING ACTIONS	RATIONALE/AMPLIFICATION
1. Implement cardiac transplant isolation protocols.	
a. Wash your hands and put on mask before entering isolation room.	The lung is the most common site of infection after heart transplantation.
b. Recipient may leave isolation room after first negative biopsy. Make sure client wears mask.	The immunosuppressive drugs are gradually tapered, and the risk of infection lessens. The recipient wears a mask because he is still highly immunosuppressed and requires protection from infections in the hospital.
c. Ensure that housekeeping staff cleans isolation room thoroughly using bactericidal cleaning agent.	The hospital environment is kept as clean as possible to limit nosocomial infections.
d. Limit visitors to immediate family, primary-care nurses, and treating physicians.	Minimizing the number of extra visitors to the isolation room decreases the risk of infection.
e. Plan diversional activities to pass time for recipient while in reverse isolation.	If the client is feeling well, time can pass slowly with limited company. Encourage the client to watch television, telephone friends, read, and play board games.
f. Use calendar to chart progress.	This record of personal milestones can be a morale booster for the client.
2. Implement routine immunosuppressive drug protocols.	
a. Administer prednisone as prescribed. Taper daily dosage until maintenance level of 0.2 mg/kg is reached.	Prednisone is a powerful immunosuppressant and anti-inflammatory agent that is used to prevent acute rejection.
b. Administer CyA in prescribed dose of 5 mg to 15 mg/kg, depending on protocol used and CyA blood levels.	CyA is a powerful immunosuppressant with a specific action against T cells. It is used to prevent acute rejection.
c. Administer Imuran as prescribed. Dose varies from 2 mg to 4 mg/kg and is tapered to reach maintenance level.	Powerful immunosuppressant used to prevent acute rejection.
d. Administer IV infusion of equine ATG. Dosage varies with protocol used; typical dosage is 10 mg/kg for 7 days.	Equine ATG is a powerful immunosuppressant that is used to prevent rejection. It has a specific action against T cells.
e. Premedicate with IV infusion of Benadryl 25 mg to 50 mg and Tylenol 650 mg PO every 30 minutes before equine ATG administration.	Some recipients experience fever and chills because of sensitization to the animal serum.
3. Monitor immunosuppression protocols.	
a. Draw daily white blood cell count.	Imuran may decrease white blood cell counts and decrease platelet levels. Maintain white blood cell count between 3000/μl and 5000/μl. A rising white blood cell count may signify infection.
b. Draw CyA level 3 times per week.	The dosage of CyA is calculated after CyA blood levels have been determined. Maintain levels between 200 ng and 300 ng/ml in the acute period, 150 ng and 200 ng/ml long term (trough levels).
c. Draw daily T-cell count (by e-rosette method).	T cells are suppressed by CyA to prevent rejection of the transplanted heart. ATG also depresses T cells.
d. Evaluate results of CyA blood level and T-cell rosette counts.	If CyA is the principal immunosuppressive drug used, T cells do not rise before acute rejection. High CyA blood levels precipitate acute renal failure.

e. Evaluate results of T-cell rosette counts in recipients on the prednisone/Imuran protocol.

The level of the circulating T cells will rise before an acute rejection episode if the principal immunosuppressive drugs are prednisone/Imuran.

f. Calculate summed voltage of leads I, II, III, V_1, and V_6 to determine ECG voltage in prednisone/Imuran recipients at least 3 times per week.

In recipients who are primarily immunosuppressed with prednisone and Imuran, rejection causes myocardial cellular edema, which decreases ECG voltage.

g. Prepare for endomyocardial biopsy on seventh postoperative day and every 4 days to 7 days following, as indicated by previous biopsy results and clinical condition. The biopsy is performed with client under local anesthesia in cardiac catheterization laboratory.

Endomyocardial biopsy monitors the presence or lack of rejection in the cardiac muscle.

4. Give daily bath and inspect skin.

The skin becomes thin and fragile because of prednisone therapy. Wound healing is also delayed. Recipients are at risk of small cuts and bruises because of the antiplatelet inhibitor therapy (aspirin and Persantine).

5. Inspect lymph nodes in axilla and groin weekly.

Lymphoma is a known side-effect of CyA therapy. The incidence of all types of cancer increases with the use of immunosuppressive drugs.

6. Give mouth care after every meal and before bedtime. Use medicated mouthwash. Medicated mouthwash used at Stanford University Hospital consists of 62.5 mg of tetracycline, 60,000 units of Nystatin, and 2.3 mg of hydrocortisone. Chlor-Trimeton, an antihistamine solution, is added to above medications for total of 5 ml.

Immunosuppressed individuals are at risk of opportunistic infections in the mouth and gastrointestinal tract.

7. Collect biweekly 12-hour urine sample for creatinine clearance.

CyA causes interstitial renal fibrosis and decreased glomerular filtration. This is seen clinically as a decreased creatinine clearance, increased blood creatinine, urea, and nitrogen (BUN).

8. Administer IV infusion of 12.5 g of mannitol with each CyA dose.

Mannitol is an osmotic diuretic that is used to diminish the risk of renal insufficiency.

9. Monitor blood pressure.

CyA produces severe hypertension often within 1 to 2 weeks of the transplant.

10. Dilute CyA 1 : 10 before oral intake.

Dilute to decrease the potential toxicity. Use chocolate milk or orange or cranberry juice to disguise the taste of the olive oil base.

11. If recipient is being given prednisone, test urine for sugar and acetone.

Prednisone alters carbohydrate metabolism by stimulating glucose production in the liver. Blood glucose rises and response to insulin decreases, causing a "spill" of glucose into the urine.

12. Administer antacids with meals and at night.

Prednisone causes gastric irritation and bleeding.

13. Test all stool samples with guaiac.

These tests will reveal gastric bleeding secondary to prednisone.

14. Maintain accurate record of intake, output, and daily weight.

Prednisone causes fluid and sodium retention. Increased weight may also indicate decreased renal function (secondary to CyA) or development of CHF.

15. Administer calcium supplements and explain reasons for their use.

Prednisone causes leaching of calcium from the bones, leading to osteoporosis.

16. Support recipient and family during periods of emotional instability and mood swings.

Explain that emotional instability is related to the use of prednisone because prednisone causes labile mood swings. This can be especially problematic during rejection episodes, when corticosteroid dosage is augmented.

17. Diminish risk of infection after transplant.

    a. Change all invasive-line tubing and IV fluids every 24 hours.

Changing of tubing and fluids reduces the risk of systemic infection.

    b. Change dressings every 24 hours.

Change dressings to reduce the risk of infection from the wound or the pacemaker wire.

    c. Obtain weekly sputum culture or more frequent specimens if recipient develops productive cough or fever spike.

The lungs are the most common site of infection after cardiac transplantation.

    d. Monitor color and quantity of sputum, especially if recipient's body temperature is over 37.5°C.

If pulmonary infection is suspected, the physician may collect a sterile specimen by transtracheal aspiration.

    e. Ensure that daily chest film is obtained.

Monitor the client's pulmonary status.

    f. Auscultate chest every 4 hours.

The nurse is often the first person to note a change in the recipient's pulmonary status.

    g. Obtain weekly sterile urine culture, or more frequently if recipient's temperature spikes.

Monitor for urinary tract infections.

    h. If oral temperature is over 37.5°C, obtain aerobic and anaerobic sterile blood cultures.

Monitor for systemic infections. The client's body temperature is lowered to approximately 36.5°C by corticosteroids.

    i. Obtain sputum, urine, and blood samples weekly to test for CMV.

CMV may be carried by the immunosuppressed recipient without any symptoms, or it may cause fever, malaise, and pulmonary infections. CMV may be associated with congenital defects if a pregnant woman is exposed to the virus.

18. Implement transplant antibiotic protocols.

    a. Administer prophylactic antibiotics.

Cefamandole 1 g every 4 hours for 3 days is an example of a prophylactic regimen.

    b. Before major invasive procedure such as endomyocardial biopsy, administer prophylactic antibiotics.

Cefamandole 1 g or Nafcilin 1 g may be prescribed to reduce the risk of major infection.

    c. Administer prescribed antibiotics when infection is documented.

Infection is an almost inevitable complication of massive immunosuppression. Bacterial infections are the most common. Those that are difficult to treat are viral, fungal, and protozoan infections, which are normally eliminated by T cells. CyA depresses T-cell levels.

19. Implement nursing protocols during acute rejection episodes.

    a. If acute rejection is diagnosed by endomyocardial biopsy, administer IV infusion of methylprednisolone 1 g/day for 3 days. Maintain CyA dose at same level.

Acute rejection is expected in the first 6 weeks after the transplant. While CyA is effective in preventing rejection, it is less effective once rejection is established. High-dose corticosteroids are potent against active rejection.

    b. Recipient should remain in isolation room during acute rejection episode.

With augmented immunosuppression, the risk of infection increases.

    c. If acute rejection continues, administer IM infusion of rabbit antithymocyte globulin (RATG) 2.5 mg/kg for 3 days.

RATG is a powerful antithymocyte cell immunosuppressant used as a second line of defense against rejection. (Equine ATG is a less potent form that is used to prevent rejection.)

d. Thirty minutes before IM injection of RATG, premedicate with IV infusion of Benadryl 25 mg to 50 mg PO and Tylenol 650 mg PO as indicated.

An IM infusion of RATG causes intense pain and burning at the injection site. Some recipients experience fever and chills from sensitization to the animal serum.

e. Use heating pad and massage over injection site (thigh) before and after RATG administration.

A heating pad and massage are used to decrease pain and discomfort. Some recipients also benefit from relaxation exercises.

f. Divide doses among four syringes and add local anesthetic (3 ml of RATG and 0.5 ml of Marcaine 0.5%).

Divide doses to decrease pain and burning at the injection site.

g. Use deep Z-track injection in anterior thigh (Fig. 12–3).

Z-track injections limit pain and inflammation.

Fig. 12–3   Technique of Z-track injection for administration of IM antithymocyte globlin (ATG). (*A*) Move skin to side with firm hand pressure *(arrow)*. (*B*) Insert needle of ATG syringe. Aspirate needle, if blood appears, select new site. Inject slowly and smoothly. (*C*) Withdraw needle and release skin. This creates "Z" pattern that blocks infiltration of ATG into subcutaneous tissue and limits pain and inflammation.

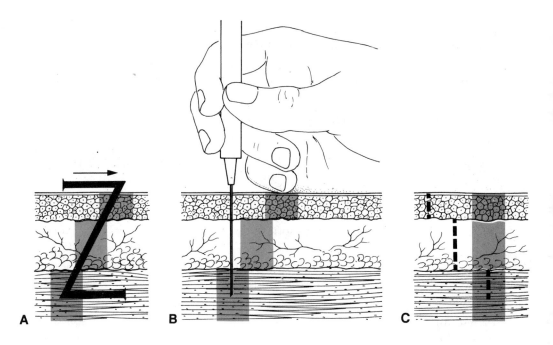

20. Prevent long-term rejection and cardiac complications.

a. Administer antiplatelet inhibitor medications (aspirin and Persantine) and explain rationale to recipient.

Chronic rejection of the transplanted heart takes the form of proliferative deposition of platelets in the coronary arteries.

b. Counsel recipient to eat low-fat, low-sodium diet at home.

Serum triglyceride and cholesterol levels may be increased with prednisone.

EVALUATION PHASE

ANTICIPATED OUTCOMES	NURSING ACTIONS
1. Prevention of rejection of transplanted heart	
2. Prevention of secondary infection	

Exercise protocol after heart transplantation

BACKGROUND

PHYSIOLOGY OF THE
TRANSPLANTED HEART

After heart transplantation the new donor heart does not receive sympathetic or parasympathetic input from the recipient's autonomic nervous system. To achieve an optimal CO, the denervated heart depends on an adequate stroke volume returned to the right side of the heart to stretch the myocardial fibers, circulating catecholamines from the adrenal glands, and the donor heart's intrinsic conduction system. Occasionally, P waves from both the donor SA node and the residual SA node can be seen on the ECG (Fig. 12–4). This has no hemodynamic significance for the recipient because the electric conduction does not cross the atrial suture line.

Fig. 12–4 ECG from heart transplant recipient showing extra P waves.

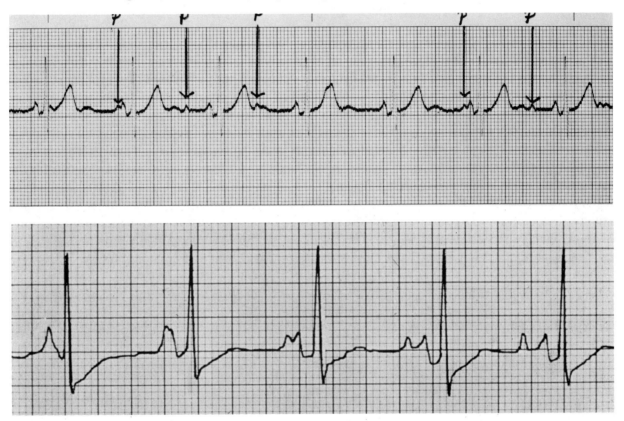

EXERCISE AND THE
TRANSPLANTED HEART

For approximately the first 5 minutes of exercise, the heart rate is unchanged. Heart rate then increases in response to increased stroke volume returned to the heart by physical leg movement, increased circulating catecholamines, and increased body temperature. After exercise is finished, the heart rate remains above control values for up to 20 minutes. Therefore, recipients are taught to monitor their exercise tolerance by assessing their respiratory rate—not their heart rate—and to do warm-up exercises.

Objective

To allow the recipient to increase levels of physical endurance before discharge and to be aware of how to exercise safely within the physiological limits of the denervated heart

ASSESSMENT PHASE

- Is the client cachexic or debilitated because of end-stage cardiac disease before the transplant?
- Does the recipient understand the physiology of the transplanted heart?

PRECAUTIONS	• **During episodes of acute rejection, the recipient may feel weak and fatigued. Do not increase the exercise level at this time.** • **If the recipient has had IM injections of rabbit ATG, leg exercises will be painful. Be gentle when exercising the client's legs.**
PLANNING PHASE	EARLY EXERCISE (FIRST WEEK)
EQUIPMENT	No equipment is necessary.
	INTERMEDIATE EXERCISE (SECOND WEEK)
	Stationary bicycle in room
	PREDISCHARGE EXERCISE
	Stationary bicycle with increased resistance. Client may go to gym with physical therapist.
CLIENT/FAMILY TEACHING	• Describe the physiology of the transplanted heart with relation to exercise. • Explain the importance of monitoring the respiratory rate for effort. • Explain that the exercise program will help offset the peripheral muscle wasting caused by prednisone.

IMPLEMENTATION PHASE

NURSING ACTIONS	RATIONALE/AMPLIFICATION
1. During first week teach recipient to do warm-up exercises such as hip–knee flexion, arm circles, and backward and forward bends.	Many recipients are quite debilitated because of their end-stage cardiac disease before the transplant and need to increase their exercise tolerance slowly.
2. During second week after negative endomyocardial biopsy, increase exercise intensity to include stationary bicycle in isolation room.	Increased strength and increased appetite allow a greater exercise tolerance.
3. Use low-level unrestricted pedaling and increase bicycling from 5 minutes to 20 minutes in five-minute increments each day if there are no contraindications.	An active exercise program helps to prevent the muscle atrophy and osteoporosis caused by prednisone.
4. In preparation for discharge, increase resistance on bicycle.	If necessary, cycling time may be decreased initially.
5. Reemphasize importance of warm-up exercises and importance of monitoring respiratory rate.	Heart rate does not increase with exercise until after approximately 5 minutes. Some recipients may become breathless if they attempt vigorous exercise without warming up because the respiratory rate increases immediately.

EVALUATION PHASE

ANTICIPATED OUTCOMES	NURSING ACTIONS
Increase in physical conditioning within individual tolerance level	

SELECTED REFERENCES

Barnhart GR, Hastillo A, Goldman MH, Katz MR et al: A prospective randomized trial of pretransfusion/azathioprine/ATG/prednisone immunosuppression versus cyclosporin/prednisone immunosuppression in cardiac transplantation: Progress report. Heart Transplantation (Supp) 4(2):115, 1985

Baumgartner WA: Infection in cardiac transplantation. Heart Transplantation 3(4):75–80, 1983

Bolman RM, Elick B, Olivari MT, Ring WS, Arentzen CE: Improved immunosuppression for heart transplantation. Heart Transplantation 4(3):315–318, 1985

Cardin S, Clark S: A nursing diagnosis approach to the patient awaiting cardiac transplantation. Heart and Lung 14(5):499–504, 1985

Copeland JC: Facts to be considered prior to undertaking a heart transplantation program. Heart Transplantation 3(4):275–277, 1984

Dawkins KD, Oldershaw PJ, Billingham ME, Hunt SA et al: Changes in diastolic function as a non-invasive marker of cardiac allograft rejection. Heart Transplantation 3(4):286–294, 1984

Evans RW, Manninen DL, Gersh BJ, Hart LG, Rodin J: The need for and supply of donor hearts for transplantation. Heart Transplantation 4(1):57–59, 1984

Grady KL: Development of a cardiac transplantation program: Role of the clinical nurse specialist. Heart and Lung 14(5):490–494, 1985

Griepp MB, Egrin MA: The history of experimental heart transplantation. Heart Transplantation 3(2):145–151, 1984

Gunderson L: Teaching the transplant recipient. Heart Transplantation 4(2):226–227, 1985

Hakim M, Wregitt TG, English TA, Stovin PG et al: Significance of donor transmitted disease in cardiac transplantation. Heart Transplantation 4(3):302–306

Hoyt G, Golin G, Billingham M, Miller DC, Jamieson SW: Effects of anti-platelet regimens in combination with cyclosporin on heart allograft vessel disease. Heart Transplantation 4(1):54–56, 1984

Hunt SA: Complications of heart transplantation. Heart Transplantation 3(1):70–74, 1983

Kaye MP: The international heart transplantation registry—The 1984 report. Heart Transplantation 4(3):290–292, 1985

McGregor CG, Jamieson JW, Oyer PE, Baldwin JC et al: Heart transplantation at Stanford University. Heart Transplantation 4(1):31–32, 1984

McKelvey SA: Effects of denervation in the cardiac transplant recipient. In Douglas MK, Shinn JA (eds): Advances in Cardiovascular nursing. Rockville, MD, Aspen Systems Corporation, 1985

Mersch J: End-stage cardiac disease: Cardiomyopathy. In Douglas MK, Shinn JA (eds): Advances in Cardiovascular nursing. Rockville, MD, Aspen Systems Corporation, 1985

Moran M, Tomlanovich S, Myers BD: Cyclosporin-induced nephropathy in human recipients of cardiac allografts. Transplantation Proceedings (Suppl 1) 17(4):185–190, 1985

Myers BD, Ross J, Newton L, Luetscher J, Perlroth M: Cyclosporin-associated chronic nephrotoxicity. N Engl J Med 311(11):699–705, 1984

Sadowsky HS, Fries K: Introduction to the treatment of cardiac and cardiopulmonary transplant patients. Stanford, CA, Stanford University Hospital: Department of Physical and Occupational Therapy, 1984

Shinn JA: Cardiac transplantation and the artificial heart. New York, Appleton–Century–Crofts, 1980

Thompson ME: Selection of candidates for cardiac transplantation. Heart Transplantation 3(1):65–69, 1983

Thornby DC: Cardiac transplantation: Nursing during the acute period. DCCN 2(4):212–224, 1983

Yusuf S, Theodoropoulos S, Dhalla N, Mathias C, Yacoub M: Effect of beta blockade on dynamic exercise in human heart transplant recipients. Heart Transplantation 4(3):312–313, 1985

II   *Gastrointestinal techniques*

13 *Gastrointestinal intubation*

BACKGROUND

Acute gastric distention, severe upper gastrointestinal (GI) bleeding, and ingestion of toxic or caustic substances are conditions that frequently require nasogastric (NG) or esophageal intubation. Distention results from an adynamic ileus, which is caused by a disease process such as cancer or by a mechanical trauma such as surgery. Causes of sudden upper GI bleeding include ruptured esophageal varices, erosive gastritis, duodenal or gastric ulcers, tumors, and esophageal tears that result from prolonged retching and vomiting. Ingestion of toxic or caustic substances includes both accidental and intentional poisonings. The insertion of an NG or esophageal tube provides emergency access to the compromised tissue, relieves or provides increased pressure, allows the collection of gastric samples for diagnostic purposes, and delivers medication and solutions directly to the GI tract.

TYPES OF NASOGASTRIC TUBES

Polyvinyl unweighted single-lumen tubes without air vents (Levin tubes) are frequently placed for temporary instillation of irrigation fluids, medications, or nutritional supplements. Because the tubes lack a venting system, connection to suction for decompression may result in mucosal damage. However, small samples for gastric analysis or culturing are easily obtained without damage to gastric tissue.

Unweighted, radiopaque, clear plastic, double-lumen (Salem-sump) tubes are used for irrigation, decompression, monitoring, and temporary instillation of medications, solution, and nourishment into the GI tract. The small blue air vent, if patent, prevents the adherence of the NG tube to the gastric mucosa because of an increased vacuum. The large lumen acts as the port for aspiration of gastric contents and instillation of fluids and other substances (Fig. 13–1).

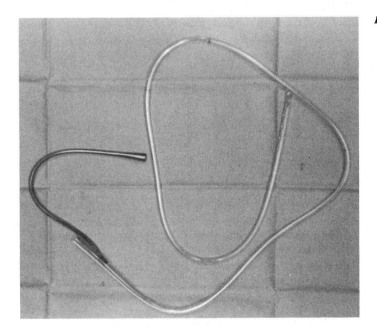

Fig. 13–1 Salem-sump tube.

COMPLICATIONS OF
NASOGASTRIC TUBE USE

Prolonged use of single- and double-lumen NG tubes risks complications such as inflammation or necrosis of the nares, sinusitis, gastric ulceration, and incompetence of the gastroesophageal sphincter. Without frequent and correct maintenance of double-lumen NG tubes, gastric contents may leak through the air vent. Inadequate care of single- and double-lumen tubes also results in an accumulation of mucous plugs in the primary lumen, decreased or insufficient suction, and adherence of the tube to gastric tissue. Because of the potential complications and the frequent maintenance required with large-bore single- and double-lumen tubes, small-bore weighted tubes are recommended when extended nutritional feedings are required (see Chap. 17, "Enteral Hyperalimentation").

CONDITIONS REQUIRING
ESOPHAGEAL TUBES

Certain emergency situations dictate the use of esophageal tubes. These tubes are inserted as a temporary tamponade to control severe intraesophageal or intragastric bleeding. They are usually used for 24 hours to 48 hours or until the source of the bleeding is found and other measures planned for controlling it. Use of an esophageal tube for more than 48 hours can result in pressure necrosis and further hemorrhage or perforation. Other methods of controlling bleeding, such as iced saline lavage or vasopressors, are usually used in conjunction with esophageal tubes to shorten their usage time and to decrease the risk of complications.

TYPES OF ESOPHAGEAL
TUBES

Several types of esophageal tubes are available. The selection of a specific type of tube is determined by the site and amount of hemorrhage, the need for gastric or esophageal suction, and the physician's preference. Esophageal tubes contain three or four lumens and single or double balloons.

The Sengstaken–Blakemore tube, one of the most commonly used esophageal tubes, is a three-lumen, double-balloon tube. It has an esophageal balloon for compressing esophageal varices and an intragastric balloon for decreasing venous circulation in the cardia of the stomach, thereby reducing blood flow to the bleeding esophageal varices. It also has a gastric-aspiration lumen that removes gastric contents below the gastric balloon and instills medications and solutions directly into the stomach. The Blakemore–Sengstaken tube does not include a lumen for esophageal suction. A

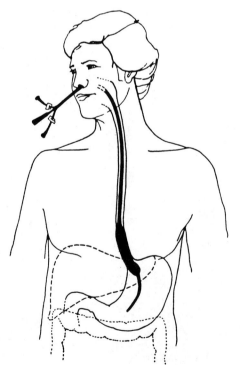

Fig. 13-2 The compressing balloon (Sengstaken–Blakemore) tube is in place in the stomach and the lower esophagus, but is not inflated.

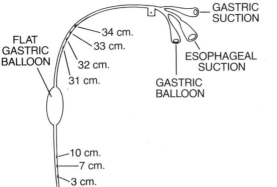

Fig. 13–3   Linton tube. (Courtesy Davol Inc.)

single-lumen NG tube is frequently used concurrently with the Blakemore–Sengstaken tube for esophageal suction. Connecting a blood pressure manometer and a "Y" connector to the esophageal balloon inflation lumen adds the capability of varying balloon pressures (Fig. 13–2).

The Linton tube, which is also commonly used, is a three-lumen, single-balloon esophageal tube (Fig. 13–3). It includes a gastric balloon only, thereby reducing the risk of esophageal necrosis. The large-capacity balloon of the Linton tube compresses venous flow in the cardia of the stomach. The lumens are used for gastric suction below the balloon, for esophageal suction above the balloon, and for inflation of the gastric balloon.

A third esophageal tube is the Minnesota esophagogastric tamponade tube. This four-lumen, double-balloon tube provides esophageal and gastric aspiration, esophageal and gastric compression, and variable compression capabilities for both balloons (Fig. 13–4). Use of the pressure-monitoring ports in the Minnesota tube allows both balloon pressures to be increased or decreased, depending on bleeding control. Continuous or intermittent gastric lavage through the ports indicates the extent of bleeding control. This permits the esophageal balloon pressure to be maintained at the lowest pressure required to stop bleeding, thus reducing the risk of esophageal necrosis.

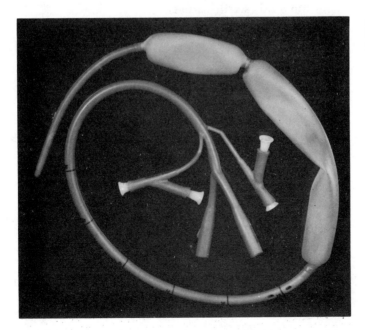

Fig. 13–4 Minnesota four-lumen esophageal tamponade tube.

Nasogastric tube insertion

Objectives

To relieve nausea or vomiting

To alleviate distention by removing fluid and gas from the upper GI tract (decompression)

To remove gastric samples for diagnostic testing

To administer medications, solutions, or nutritional feedings directly into the GI tract

ASSESSMENT PHASE

- Has the client had previous experience with NG intubation?
- Is the client able to follow instructions and assist with intubation?
- Are any of the following contraindications present: gastroesophageal surgery or trauma, basal skull fracture, fractures of the nose or face, or recent nasopharyngeal surgery?
- Does the client have a history of fractures of the nose, a deviated septum, or corrective surgery? Previous fractures, structural defects, or corrective surgery may result in obstructed or narrowed posterior nares.

PRECAUTIONS

- **An endotracheal tube that is already in place tends to guide an NG tube into the trachea.**
- **The placement of an NG tube in clients with basal skull fractures risks introduction of the tube into the cranium. The physician will insert the NG tube with fluoroscopy in these cases.**
- **Wear gloves when intubating clients with possible herpetic lesions of the mouth to avoid contracting herpetic whitlow, a painful, viral infection of the pulp space of the finger.**

PLANNING PHASE

EQUIPMENT

Disposable NG tube (either Levin or Salem-sump, size 12F to 18F for adults)

Water-soluble lubricant

Basin of ice or warm water (as needed)

Towel and washcloth or tissues

Emesis basin

Glass of water and straw

Irrigation kit with 30-ml syringe

Irrigation fluid (sterile saline)

Stethoscope

Hypoallergenic tape

Safety pin

Suction apparatus (if indicated)

CLIENT/FAMILY TEACHING

- Explain the purpose of tube insertion.
- Describe the procedure and probable sensations. Alert the client to the gag reflex, which occurs when the tube reaches a certain point in the pharynx. Use diagrams as necessary.
- Involve the client in the procedure by allowing the client to hold and inspect the tube. Ask the client to hold pieces of equipment, such as the emesis basin, glass of water and straw, or syringe.
- Rehearse with the client the initial steps of insertion and the point at which swallowing is indicated.
- Agree on a hand signal for the client to use when he has difficulty breathing or needs a pause in the procedure.
- Discuss any dietary restrictions that accompany the placement of the NG tube.
- Describe any activity restrictions. Emphasize activities that can be maintained and encourage the client to be as autonomous as possible.
- Answer any questions and elicit cooperation.

IMPLEMENTATION PHASE

NURSING ACTIONS	RATIONALE/AMPLIFICATION
1. Place client in sitting position. Support head and shoulders with pillow. Raise bed to comfortable working height.	The sitting position facilitates passage of the tube. A position that is comfortable for the client promotes relaxation. Raising the bed prevents undue back strain and allows the client to maintain eye contact with the caregiver.
2. Cover client with towel and place emesis basin within reach.	When the tube reaches the nasopharynx, emesis may be stimulated.
3. Determine patency of each nostril by asking client to breathe through one nostril while other nostril is occluded.	Use the nostril with the largest lumen to facilitate initial insertion. When changing an NG tube, insert the tube in the unused nostril to allow healing of inflammation in the previously used nostril.
4. Measure tube to determine approximate length of insertion. Mark NEX point (distance from tip of *n*ose to earlobe and from there to *x*iphoid process) with tape (see Weighted Feeding Tube Insertion in Chap. 17).	The NEX measurement approximates the internal distance to the upper portion of the stomach.
5. Coil approximately 15 cm (6 inches) of end of tube tightly around your index finger.	A curved tube simulates the inner structure of the nasal cavity.
6. If tube is excessively stiff, place it in basin of warm water until limber. If tube is too limber, stiffen it in warm water.	Excessively stiff tubes may cause tissue injury on insertion. A tube that is too soft is difficult to insert.
7. Lubricate approximately 10 cm (4 inches) of end of tube with water-soluble jelly.	If the tube travels into the trachea or bronchi, oil-aspiration pneumonia may be prevented by the use of water-soluble lubricant.
8. Ask client to breathe through mouth and to hyperextend head.	Hyperextending the head promotes relaxation and provides an easier angle of insertion.
9. With curved end pointed downward, insert tube about 12 cm to 14 cm (5 inches) along floor of nasal cavity. Aim tube downward toward client's ear.	To avoid hitting the nasal turbinates, aim downward toward the ear and not up the nose.
10. After tube passes posterior naris, ask client to flex head.	By flexing the head, the client helps to guide insertion into the esophagus rather than into the trachea.
11. Rotate tube 180° and continue insertion.	Rotation of the tube prevents insertion of a curved-tip tube into the trachea.
12. When tube reaches posterior naspoharynx or client begins to gag, instruct client to swallow water repeatedly. If tube inadvertently travels into trachea, pull it back to nasopharynx and reinsert.	Swallowing forces the epiglottis to close the trachea and helps guide the tube into the esophagus. Unrelieved coughing or gasping signals tracheal insertion.
13. With client swallowing repeatedly, advance tube smoothly and continuously until NEX mark is reached.	The flow of water past the oropharynx and down the esophagus lubricates the tissue and carries the tube smoothly into the cardia portion of the stomach.
14. Check placement by rapidly injecting 10 ml to 20 ml of air into primary lumen with syringe while auscultating just below costal margin of upper left abdomen.	Due to the cavernous structure of the stomach, the sound of a sudden bolus of air can be heard in the stomach. This sound is not heard when air is introduced into the esophagus.
15. Recheck for placement of tube in stomach by aspirating gently with syringe.	Aspiration of large amounts of gastric contents indicates location in the stomach.
16. If gastric contents are not returned, turn client to left lateral position.	Failure to aspirate gastric contents initially could result from a small amount of gastric contents in the stomach.

17. Aspirate again. If gastric contents are still not returned, insert tube another 5 cm (2 inches) and aspirate again.

Turning the client to the left pools gastric contents in the greater curvature of the stomach.
Insertion of the tube past the NEX point introduces the tip below the fluid level.

18. When proper placement has been ensured, secure tube to side of client's face. Avoid exerting pressure on nares (see Weighted Feeding Tube Insertion in Chap. 17). Use washcloth to remove any traces of water-soluble lubricant from nares.

Tissue necrosis can result from excessive or prolonged pressure. Cleaning the skin with alcohol removes dirt, oil, and perspiration, which interfere with tape adherence. Application of tincture of benzoin protects the skin and promotes tape adherence.

19. Attach tube to suction, if indicated.

The large lumen of a Salem-sump tube is attached to continuous (30 mm Hg) or intermittent (80 mm Hg to 120 mm Hg) suction.

20. If suction is sluggish initially, instill 30 ml of air into small blue lumen.

Obstruction of the airway by water-soluble lubricant or gastric contents may have occurred during insertion.

21. If suction remains sluggish, irrigate large lumen with 30 ml of sterile saline.

Irrigation of the primary lumen will clear any obstruction and allow adequate suction.

22. Secure tube approximately 25 cm (10 inches) from client's nose with tape and use safety pin to attach it to client's gown or robe.

Securing the NG tube relieves pressure on the nares, acts as a safeguard against sudden dislodgement of the tube, and affords good head movement.

RELATED NURSING CARE

NURSING ACTIONS	RATIONALE/AMPLIFICATION
1. Position blue airway of the Salem-sump tube above level of client's stomach.	Gravity may cause gastric leakage when the airway hangs below the client's stomach.
2. Irrigate both lumens of Salem-sump tube every 2 hours. Instill 30 ml of sterile saline into large lumen and 30 ml of air into air vent.	Frequent irrigation prevents mucosal sucking. Instillation of fluid instead of air into the air vent can cause fluid leakage through the air vent at a later time.
3. Check placement before instillation of any fluid, medication, or feeding.	Instillation of fluid into a dislodged tube can result in aspiration pneumonia.
4. Rotate tube daily.	Rotation prevents adherence of the tube to mucous membranes.
5. Provide frequent nose and mouth care while tube is in place.	Mouth breathing dries mucous membranes.
6. Observe tube patency, amount and color of aspirated contents, and adequacy of suction hourly.	Mucous plugs can obstruct the tube and decrease suction.
7. Record intake and output every 8 hours.	Constant gastric suction can cause dehydration.
8. To remove tube, untape it and pull with one quick, constant motion. Give nose care after removal.	A quick, constant motion reduces gagging.
9. Empty or change gastric collection bottles or bags every 8 hours.	Frequent disposal of gastric contents prevents bacterial growth and offensive odors in the collection container.

EVALUATION PHASE

ANTICIPATED OUTCOMES	NURSING ACTIONS
1. Prevention of nausea and vomiting and alleviation of gastric distention	Maintain the patency of the tube and maintain suction.

2. Prevention of complications of NG tube use

a. Aspiration pneumonia	Check tube placement before instilling any fluid, medication, or feeding.
b. Necrosis of nares	Secure the tube to the side of the client's face. Observe the skin every 8 hours for signs of inflammation. Alternate nostrils when changing NG tubes.
c. Incompetence of gastroesophageal sphincter	Maintain adequate suction, thereby preventing gastric distention. Elevate the head of the bed 30° to 45°. Remove NG tubes as soon as possible.
d. Mucosal damage	Maintain suction at the appropriate levels. Prevent mucosal sucking by irrigating the primary lumen every 2 hours. Maintain the airway of the Salem-sump tube.

PRODUCT AVAILABILITY

STOMACH TUBE (LEVIN TYPE)

Cutter Resiflex
Seamless Hospital Products Company

SALEM-SUMP TUBE

Argyle Company

SELECTED REFERENCES

Beck ML: What to do when they call for inserting gastrointestinal tubes. Nursing '81 11:74, 76, March 1981

Gastric lavage for removal of toxic substances

Objective
To remove or dilute unabsorbed poison after ingestion of noncorrosive toxic substances

ASSESSMENT PHASE

• Is the client comatose, having seizures, lacking the gag reflex, or experiencing extreme sedation? Is unconsciousness imminent? Clients exhibiting profound effects on the central nervous system (CNS) are at significant risk of aspiration during gastric lavage.
• Does the client have a history of cardiac arrhythmias? Vagal stimulation during passage of the tube through the posterior pharynx induces bradyrhythmias.
• Did the client ingest acids, alkalis, hydrocarbons, petroleum distillates, or other corrosive agents? Ingestion of corrosive substances increases the risk of perforation of the esophagus during tube insertion, thereby contraindicating gastric lavage for these clients.

PRECAUTIONS

• **Because the risk of aspiration of irrigation fluid is substantial, have immediate suction available.**
• **If client restraint is necessary, secure all four extremities on the same side of the stretcher to reduce the possibility of aspirating vomitus and to aid in suctioning.**
• **In clients with CNS depression or an inadequate gag reflex, insert an endotracheal tube and inflate the cuff before inserting the tube.**
• **Constant cardiac monitoring is essential to detect arrhythmias during the procedure.**

Fig. 13-5 Ewald tube.

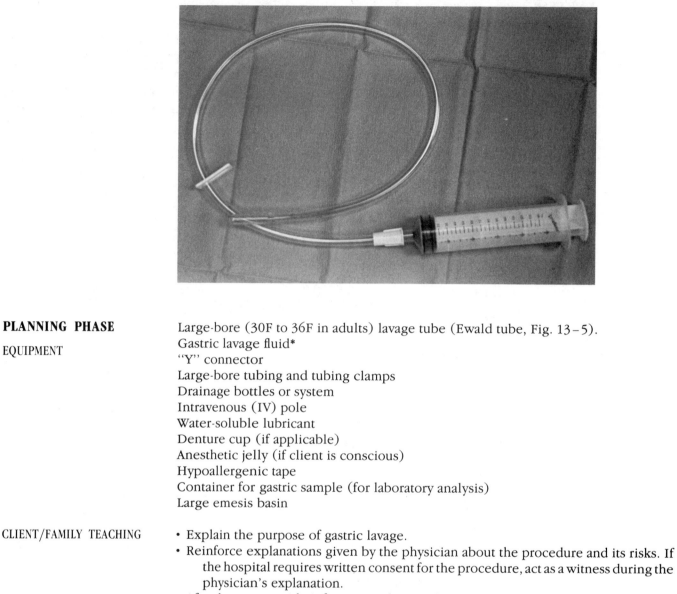

PLANNING PHASE	Large-bore (30F to 36F in adults) lavage tube (Ewald tube, Fig. 13–5).
EQUIPMENT	Gastric lavage fluid*
	"Y" connector
	Large-bore tubing and tubing clamps
	Drainage bottles or system
	Intravenous (IV) pole
	Water-soluble lubricant
	Denture cup (if applicable)
	Anesthetic jelly (if client is conscious)
	Hypoallergenic tape
	Container for gastric sample (for laboratory analysis)
	Large emesis basin

CLIENT/FAMILY TEACHING

- Explain the purpose of gastric lavage.
- Reinforce explanations given by the physician about the procedure and its risks. If the hospital requires written consent for the procedure, act as a witness during the physician's explanation.
- After lavage, provide information designed to prevent accidental poisonings in the future. Psychiatric evaluation is indicated for clients who intentionally ingest toxic substances. Community support systems for the client and family may be recommended.

IMPLEMENTATION PHASE

NURSING ACTIONS	RATIONALE/AMPLIFICATION
1. Place client in high Fowler's or sitting position. Remove dentures if applicable.	The sitting position facilitates passage of the tube.
2. Measure target point of insertion (NEX measurement) (see Weighted Feeding Tube Insertion in Chap. 17).	The NEX measurement is particularly helpful when inserting large-bore tubes.

* Large volumes (3 liters to 5 liters) of room temperature and warmed (46°C) gastric lavage fluid (normal saline, 0.45% sodium chloride, or tap water) will be needed.

3. Liberally lubricate tube with water-soluble jelly. Apply anesthetic jelly if client is responsive.

Anesthetic jelly makes insertion more comfortable.

4. Insert tube with slow and gentle motion into nose or mouth to target point. Have immediate suction ready.

Excessive force can result in epistaxis and tissue injury. Emesis is stimulated during the passage of the tube through the posterior pharynx.

5. Check placement of tube by aspirating gastric contents.

Free-flowing gastric contents are needed to remove large chunks of the unabsorbed substance. Inadvertent pulmonary insertion and lavage may result in death.

6. Obtain 20-ml to 40-ml sample of gastric contents for toxicology analysis.

7. Tape tube securely. Insert bite-block if tube is inserted orally.

The bite-block prevents the client from constricting the tube and the flow of fluid.

8. Position client in left lateral recumbent position, with knees flexed and head in Trendelenburg's position (Fig. 13–6).

This position inhibits the normal flow of gastric contents into the duodenum and prevents aspiration during vomiting.

Fig. 13-6 Left lateral Trendelenburg's position for gastric lavage using Ewald tube.

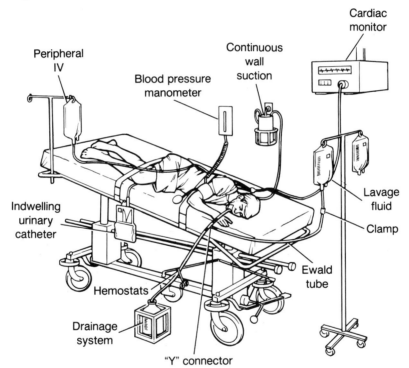

9. Connect tube to "Y" connector, to lavage fluid, and to drainage system.

A closed system allows gastric lavage to be completed by one nurse.

10. Begin phase-1 lavage by clamping drainage tubing and instilling 200 ml to 300 ml of room temperature lavage fluid. Observe client's tolerance of fluid instillation.

Instillation of more than 500 ml of lavage fluid encourages pyloric reflux. Lavage should be stopped temporarily if the client shows signs of intolerance. Signs of intolerance include tachycardia and vomiting.

11. Clamp lavage-fluid tubing and unclamp drainage tubing, allowing contents to drain.

Note the amount of drainage fluid. A significant difference between the instilled volume and the drainage volume may indicate poor tube position in the stomach.

12. Continue phase-1 lavage until return is clear, saving all fluid for possible analysis.

Phase-1 lavage removes suspended substances. Three liters to 5 liters of fluid are used in phase-1 lavage.

13. Begin phase-2 lavage by instilling 500 ml of warmed lavage fluid.

Phase-2 lavage removes undigested chunks and pieces of the toxic substance. Use of a large volume of fluid stretches the stomach rugae, thereby freeing trapped pieces of medication. Warmed fluid prevents hypothermia, increases dissolution of the ingested substance, and decreases the flow of the substance through the pylorus by decreasing gastric peristalsis.

14. Apply external massage to epigastric area during drainage.	Repetitive pressure aids in breaking up large chunks and in suspending particles in fluid for easy removal.
15. Continue phase-2 lavage until contents of drainage are consistently clear.	As contents break up and dissolve, the solution may appear cloudy. Three liters to 5 liters of warmed fluid are used during phase-2 lavage.
16. When lavage is completed, maintain tube in stomach for instillation of antidote or cathartic, if ordered.	Instillation of the cathartic or antidote through the tube increases the rate of absorption. Cathartics increase peristalsis and subsequent excretion of the substance.
17. To remove tube, pinch it off and pull gently and constantly. Keep suction available.	Pinching the tube prevents aspiration of fluid remaining in the tube. Removal of the tube may prompt vomiting.

RELATED NURSING CARE

NURSING ACTIONS	RATIONALE/AMPLIFICATION
1. Suction frequently if tube is inserted orally.	Oral secretions are increased with oral insertion.
2. Record total instilled and drainage volumes. Notify physician of any significant differences.	A large discrepancy may indicate pyloric reflux or aspiration of fluid.
3. Evaluate vital signs, cardiac rhythm, urine output, neurologic function, and level of consciousness.	Frequent client evaluation aids in preventing complications.
4. Keep drainage fluid obtained early in lavage separate from drainage fluid obtained later.	Toxicology analysis may be desired on both samples.
5. If gut lavage is ordered, warmed electrolyte solution is pumped into stomach through lavage tube by peristaltic pump at rate of 75 ml/minute.	Although not routinely used, gut lavage may be indicated after stomach lavage for some clients and substances.

EVALUATION PHASE

ANTICIPATED OUTCOMES	NURSING ACTIONS
1. Prevention of aspiration of lavage fluid or emesis	Place the client in Trendelenburg's and left lateral recumbent positions, and have immediate suction available. Maintain an inflated cuff on the endotracheal tube during the procedure. Check the position of the tube before beginning lavage.
2. Prevention of pyloric reflux	Instill a maximum of 500 ml of fluid at each washing. Maintain Trendelenburg's and left lateral recumbent positions.
3. Maximum removal of toxic substance	Use warmed solution and epigastric massage during phase-2 lavage.

PRODUCT AVAILABILITY GASTRIC LAVAGE EQUIPMENT

Davol Incorporated (Ewald Tube)
Sherwood Medical (Monoject Edlich gastric lavage kit)

SELECTED REFERENCES McDougal CB, Maclean MA: Modifications in the technique of gastric lavage. Ann Emerg Med (10):514–516, October 1981

14

Upper gastrointestinal bleeding

Objectives

To control intraesophageal or intragastric bleeding caused by esophageal or gastric varices

To prevent the pooling of blood in the gastrointestinal (GI) tract and subsequent ammonia intoxication after decomposition of blood

ASSESSMENT PHASE

- Does the client have a history of alcohol abuse, hepatitis, cirrhosis, or symptoms of portal hypertension? Liver damage results in increased coagulopathy and potential bleeding after tube removal.
- How actively is the client bleeding? A client with orthostatic hypotension of 10 mm Hg or more and symptoms of nausea, thirst, light-headedness, diaphoresis, and syncope has lost 20% or more of the circulating blood volume. Shock, oliguria, tachycardia, and stupor signal a 40% loss of blood volume. Depending on the amount and rate of bleeding, an esophageal tube may be indicated for stabilization before surgery or endoscopy.

PRECAUTIONS

- **This procedure is reserved for clients with confirmed bleeding esophageal varices. Other causes of GI bleeding such as ulcers or tumors require other methods of control.**
- **Vomiting with an inflated esophageal balloon in place may result in pulmonary aspiration. A single-lumen nasogastric (NG) tube may be inserted above the esophageal balloon concurrently with the Sengstaken–Blakemore tube to provide intermittent or standby suction. The Minnesota esophagogastric tamponade tube and the Linton tube contain esophageal-suction capabilities.**
- **Pressure necrosis of the esophagus or stomach cardia is possible with the use of esophageal tubes. Sudden chest pain or sudden, unexplained resumption of bleeding may signal esophageal or gastric rupture.**
- **Dislodgement of the gastric balloon from the cardia or rupture of the gastric balloon may result in obstruction of the trachea by the esophageal balloon. Constant attendance of a client with an esophageal tube is imperative. Tape a pair of scissors to the head of the bed for emergency deflation of the balloons.**
- **The placement of an endotracheal tube and inflation of the cuff is indicated before the insertion of an esophageal tube in clients who have an increased risk of aspiration if vomiting occurs.**

PLANNING PHASE

EQUIPMENT

Esophageal tube (Sengstaken–Blakemore, Linton, or Minnesota esophagogastric tamponade tube)

18F single-lumen NG (Levin) tube (for Sengstaken–Blakemore tube)

Anesthetic nasal spray

Water-soluble lubricant

Cup of water and straw

Large basin of water
Stethoscope
Waterproof pen
Oral bite-block (if inserted orally)
Sponge-rubber nasal cuff
1.3-cm ($\frac{1}{2}$-inch) tape
Disposable irrigation set with 50-ml syringe
Iced normal saline irrigation solution—1 liter
Basin of ice
"Y" connector
Intermittent or continuous suction setup—2
Blood pressure manometer (mercury manometer is used for Minnesota tube)
Approximately 75 cm ($2\frac{1}{2}$ feet) of rubber tubing (size and quality used on blood pressure equipment)
Rubber-shod clamps (3 for Sengstaken–Blakemore tube, 2 for Linton tube, and 2 clamps and 2 plastic plugs for Minnesota tube)
Scissors
Traction equipment (football helmet or basic frame with pulleys and 0.5-kg (1-pound) weight

CLIENT/FAMILY TEACHING

- Explain the use of the equipment and the purpose of the procedure to the client and family.
- Describe the initial sensations of pressure caused by the tube in the nose and throat during insertion. Explain the sensations of pressure and distention after balloon inflation. Inform the client that the discomfort will decrease after the tube has been in place for a while.
- Explain the need for a quiet environment and emotional calm to the client and family.
- If the client is conscious, enlist cooperation by rehearsing the mouth breathing and swallowing that will facilitate insertion.
- Inform the client of the need for strict bed rest and continuous gastric traction during use of an esophageal tube.
- Inform the client about dietary restrictions during use of the esophageal tube. An NPO (*non per os,* nothing by mouth) status is maintained until the tube is removed or until the physician orders a diet or tube feeding.

IMPLEMENTATION PHASE

NURSING ACTIONS	RATIONALE/AMPLIFICATION
1. Attach traction equipment to bed and prepare it for attachment to tube after insertion. Prepare football helmet if it will be used instead of basic traction.	Traction is applied to the tube to prevent the gastric balloon from floating in the stomach.
2. Prepare suction machines for connection after tube insertion. Have continuous suction on standby during tube insertion.	Esophageal suction prevents tracheal aspiration while the esophageal balloon is inflated. Gastric suction decreases distention, prevents gastroesophageal reflux, and monitors bleeding. Tube insertion prompts emesis, which may require suctioning of the pharynx.
3. Prepare manometer for connection to tube.	Balloon pressures are varied to provide optimal tamponade pressure with a decreased risk of pressure necrosis.
4. Test balloons for air leaks. Inflate balloons and submerge them in basin of water.	Continuous air bubbles surfacing from the submerged, inflated balloons indicate a leak.
5. If Minnesota tube is used, attach mercury manometer to gastric-pressure–monitoring outlet. Inflate gas-	The pressures of the gastric balloon during inflation (after insertion) are compared with the preinsertion

Fig. 14–1 Minnesota four-lumen esophageal tamponade tube connected to a manometer. (Courtesy Davol Inc.)

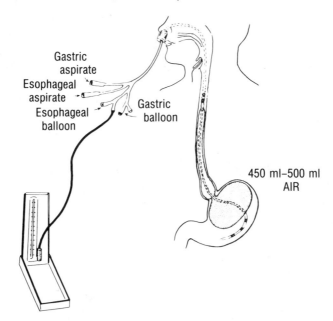

Gastric aspirate

Esophageal aspirate

Esophageal balloon

Gastric balloon

450 ml–500 ml AIR

tric balloon with 100 ml, 200 ml, 300 ml, 400 ml, and 500 ml of air. Note pressure at each volume (Fig. 14–1).

6. Remove balloons from water and deflate them. Clamp lumens.

7. Test patency of aspiration lumens by aspirating water. When patency is ensured, remove all water from aspiration lumens by forcing 50 ml of air through each.

8. Carefully label all ports and lumens with waterproof pen.

9. Place tube in basin of ice to stiffen it.

10. Place client in semi-Fowler's position.

11. Mark NEX (distance from tip of *n*ose to *e*arlobe and from there to *x*iphoid process) point (see Weighted Feeding Tube Insertion in Chap. 17).

12. Physician will anesthetize posterior pharynx.

13. Lubricate tube with water-soluble lubricant.

14. Physician will insert tube into client's nose.

15. When tube reaches posterior pharynx, physician will ask client to flex head and swallow.

16. Physician will insert tube to point that is 1.3 cm ($\frac{1}{2}$ inch) past NEX mark.

17. Physician will check tube placement by aspirating gastric contents with 50-ml syringe and auscultating bolus of air (see Nasogastric Tube Insertion in Chap. 13).

18. Physician will inflate gastric balloon with 20 ml of air.

pressures. A difference of 15 mm Hg or more signals placement in the esophagus rather than the stomach.

Clamping the balloon inflation ports ensures deflation during insertion.

Water that remains in the lumens may be aspirated into the lungs during insertion.

Labeling prevents inadvertent deflation of a balloon or irrigation through the esophageal aspiration lumen.

A stiff tube is easier to insert than a limber one.

This position helps to empty the stomach and prevents aspiration. If a Minnesota tube is used, insertion is done with fluoroscopy.

The NEX point should approximate the 50-cm mark on the tube.

This reduces discomfort and gagging during insertion.

Lubrication reduces friction during insertion.

The physician determines nasal patency. Oral insertion is performed if severe nasal deformities or injuries exist.

Flexing the head prevents passage of the tube into the trachea.

Insertion of the tube past the NEX mark ensures proper placement.

An improperly placed tube can result in pulmonary aspiration, rupture of the esophagus during balloon inflation, or tracheal obstruction after balloon inflation.

A small amount of air holds the balloon in place but does not present the danger of esophageal rupture.

19.   Abdominal film is used to determine proper placement.

20.   With proper placement verified, physician will inflate gastric balloon with air (200 ml to 250 ml for Sengstaken–Blakemore tube, 700 ml to 800 ml for Linton tube, and 450 ml to 500 ml for Minnesota tube).

Inflation of the gastric balloon in the esophagus can result in esophageal rupture.

Before inflating the Minnesota balloon, the physician will connect the pressure-monitoring port of the gastric balloon to the mercury manometer. The gastric balloon is inflated in 100-ml increments, with concurrent monitoring of the intragastric balloon pressure. If the pressure varies 15 mm Hg or more from the preinsertion pressures at the corresponding volume, the balloon is deflated and inserted until it is completely inside the stomach.

21.   When Minnesota gastric balloon is fully inflated, physician will ligate or clamp inflation and pressure-monitoring ports of gastric balloon.

Clamping the inflation and pressure-monitoring ports maintains correct inflation volume.

22.   Physician will pull on tube until resistance is felt.

The gastric balloon exerts pressure on the cardia of the stomach.

23.   While maintaining tension on tube, tape sponge-rubber cuff to tube at nostril (see Fig. 14–1).

The sponge-rubber cuff guards the nostril from pressure necrosis.

24.   Physician will attach traction to tube using pulleys and 0.5-kg (1-pound) weight, or football helmet with face guard and chin strap (Fig. 14–2).

Gentle traction is applied to the venous circulation in the cardia of the stomach.

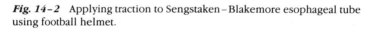

Fig. 14–2   Applying traction to Sengstaken–Blakemore esophageal tube using football helmet.

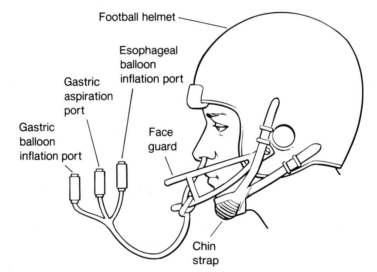

25.   Lavage stomach with iced normal saline using gastric aspiration port until contents are consistently clear.

Iced lavage promotes topical vasoconstriction. Emptying the stomach provides a baseline for the determination of further bleeding and removes blood, which is broken down into ammonia later.

26.   If bleeding continues, physician will inflate esophageal balloon on Sengstaken–Blakemore tube by connecting esophageal balloon lumen to "Y" connector and a sphygmomanometer inflation bulb and manometer. Esophageal pressure-monitoring port of Minnesota tube is connected directly to mercury manometer.

The esophageal balloon is inflated to 35 mm Hg to 45 mm Hg. Balloon pressure varies with respirations and esophageal contractions. Brief peak pressures of up to 70 mm Hg may be seen.

27.   When desired esophageal pressure is attained, clamp tubing.

The tubing is clamped to prevent air leaks.

28. Establish esophageal suction by connecting esophageal aspiration port of Minnesota tube to 120 mm Hg to 200 mm Hg of continuous suction. If single-lumen NG tube was sutured to Sengstaken–Blakemore tube and inserted simultaneously, connect to intermittent suction. Attach esophageal suction lumen of Linton tube to continuous suction.

The client is unable to swallow secretions when the balloon is inflated and is at risk of tracheal aspiration from fluids in the esophagus.

29. Attach gastric aspiration port to intermittent suction at 60 mm Hg to 120 mm Hg.

Intermittent suctioning of the stomach prevents mucosal sucking.

RELATED NURSING CARE

NURSING ACTIONS	RATIONALE/AMPLIFICATION
1. Constantly observe for signs of esophageal rupture when esophageal balloon is inflated.	Signs and symptoms of shock, such as increased bleeding or sudden, unexplained bleeding, and sudden, unexplained chest pain may indicate esophageal rupture.
2. Constantly observe for signs of respiratory distress when using esophageal tubes.	A dislodged balloon may cause tracheal obstruction and asphyxiation.
3. Keep scissors taped to head of bed at all times.	If respiratory distress occurs, the balloons may be quickly deflated and removed by cutting the tube.
4. If ordered, deflate esophageal balloon for 5 minutes every 8 hours to 12 hours. Reinflate immediately if massive bleeding resumes. *Caution:* Do not deflate the gastric balloon.	Brief deflation reduces esophageal necrosis.
5. Observe and document amount of air initially injected into balloons (Sengstaken–Blakemore, Linton).	This volume of air will be removed on extubation.
6. Observe and document esophageal balloon pressure (Sengstaken–Blakemore, Minnesota), gastric balloon pressure (Minnesota), and control of bleeding when balloon is first inflated and every 15 minutes after inflation.	A changing esophageal pressure may indicate leakage or dislodgement. Documentation of the point at which bleeding is controlled is important to maintain the lowest possible esophageal balloon pressure.
7. Irrigate gastric aspiration port with 50 ml of warm water every 15 minutes and document color of fluid returned.	Frequent irrigation of the tube prevents obstruction by blood clots or mucus.
8. Maintain appropriate suction on gastric and esophageal aspiration lumens.	The accumulation of gastric contents prompts vomiting, and the collection of esophageal fluid risks pulmonary aspiration.
9. Suspend traction weights from foot of bed at all times.	A reduction in the amount of traction may dislodge the tube and cause bleeding to resume.
10. Maintain client in semi-Fowler's position.	Semi-Fowler's position counterbalances traction weight and maintains tube stability.
11. Monitor vital signs every 15 minutes.	Frequent monitoring of vital signs allows early detection of hemorrhage.
12. Monitor intake and output.	Gastric suction promotes dehydration.
13. Provide nose care every 8 hours.	Nose care prevents necrosis. Avoid using Vaseline if using red rubber tubes.
14. Give mouth care frequently.	Mouth care removes the taste of blood and decreases the drying of mucous membranes caused by mouth breathing.

15.   Gently suction mouth with 12F catheter as needed. Provide tissues and basin to collect oral secretions.

Due to the client's inability to swallow when the esophageal balloon is inflated, oral secretions must be suctioned or spit out.

16.   Provide emotional support. Reassure client about feeling of distention during inflation of esophageal balloon. Give sedatives as needed.

The client may feel pressure in the chest when the esophageal balloon is inflated.

17.   Maintain bed rest.

Excessive movement may cause tube dislodgement.

18.   If iced saline lavage is ordered, pour 0.9% sodium chloride solution into irrigation basin. Chill irrigation basin in container of ice. Instill 50 ml of iced saline into gastric aspiration lumen with syringe. Aspirate stomach contents immediately with syringe. Continue instillation and aspiration until contents return consistently clear.

Lavaging with iced fluid encourages vasoconstriction of venous circulation in the gastric submucosa. Normal saline is an isotonic solution that reduces electrolyte imbalances.

19.   If ordered, 2 ampules of levarterenol (Levophed) may be mixed with 1 liter of iced normal saline and used to lavage stomach.

Levarterenol causes topical vasoconstriction of gastric venous circulation. It is metabolized in the liver immediately after gastric absorption and therefore does not cause systemic vasoconstriction.

20.   If ordered, topical thrombin may be instilled into stomach.

Thrombin combines with fibrinogen at the site of bleeding to form clots.

    a.   Empty stomach by aspirating with syringe through gastric aspiration lumen.

Intragastric thrombin is used to speed clotting.

    b.   Instill 60 ml (2 ounces) of buffer solution and clamp lumen for 5 minutes.

Diluted gastric acid interferes with thrombin.

    c.   Instill 100,000 units of topical thrombin in 60 ml of buffer solution and clamp lumen for 30 minutes.

The speed of clotting depends on the thrombin concentration.

    d.   Aspirate stomach.

    e.   If fresh blood does not return, instill 60 ml of buffer solution and clamp lumen.

Neutralized stomach *p*H is necessary for thrombin to work.

    f.   Instill 60 ml of buffer solution every 1 hour to 2 hours for 24 hours to 48 hours.

    g.   If fresh blood returns on aspiration, repeat procedure until bleeding is controlled.

Topical thrombin does not produce systemic clotting.

    h.   Document amount of fluid instilled and amount aspirated.

The buffer solution is absorbed.

21.   If ordered, give intravenous (IV) infusion of vasopressin (Pitressin) concurrently to control bleeding. Infuse 250 ml of dextrose 5% in water (D_5W) with 20 units to 50 units of Pitressin over 30 minutes to 40 minutes (0.2 units/minute).

A Pitressin IV infusion causes temporary systemic vasoconstriction and reduced portal pressure. Bradycardia and coronary insufficiency are potential complications of Pitressin IV therapy.

22.   After selective arteriography, start intra-arterial infusion of vasopressin at rate of 0.05 units to 0.1 units/minute by infusion pump into superior mesenteric artery.

An infusion of more than 0.4 units/minute can cause total vascular collapse.

23.   If physician orders gastric feeding, instill 100 ml to 150 ml of formula in gastric aspiration lumen every hour or as ordered. Follow formula with 30 ml of water.

Flushing the tube with water after the formula has been administered prevents clogging in the tube.

24.   Check stomach for residual formula before each feeding.

Aspiration of stomach contents prevents gastric distention and detects bleeding.

25. Do not instill milk of magnesia or barium in esophageal tube.

These substances will clog the lumen.

26. Relax gastric traction on Linton tube 12 hours to 24 hours before extubation.

If bleeding recurs, the gastric balloon should be reinflated.

27. To remove esophageal tube, physician will deflate esophageal balloon by aspirating air with syringe or cutting across tube with scissors approximately 7.6 cm (3 inches) from nostril. *Caution:* If you are cutting tube with scissors, be sure to grasp tube firmly at nostril.

The severed tube may fall back into the esophagus if it is not held firmly.

28. Linton gastric balloon should remain inflated for no longer than 48 hours.

Inflation for longer than 48 hours causes necrosis of the gastric mucosa.

29. Sengstaken–Blakemore and Minnesota tubes may remain inflated for 2 days to 4 days.

Periodic deflation of the esophageal balloon reduces necrosis. Minimal traction and a gastric balloon volume that is smaller than that of the Linton tube allow longer periods of inflation before the development of tissue necrosis.

EVALUATION PHASE

ANTICIPATED OUTCOMES	NURSING ACTIONS
1. Control of bleeding	Maintain the esophageal and gastric balloon pressures as ordered. Maintain the gastric traction. Initiate iced saline lavage as needed. Irrigate the client's stomach frequently to detect bleeding.
2. Prevention of complications associated with esophageal tube	
a. Esophageal rupture	Maintain the least amount of esophageal pressure needed to control bleeding. Keep the head of the bed elevated and the client inactive to prevent dislodgement of the gastric balloon. Observe the client's condition for chest pain and changes in vital signs.
b. Asphyxiation due to tracheal obstruction	Maintain gastric traction to prevent tube dislodgement. Keep scissors taped to the head of the bed at all times for emergency transection of the tube and deflation of the balloons. *Caution:* Avoid accidental aspiration of the gastric balloon inflation lumen.
c. Tissue necrosis	Avoid taping the tube to the nares by using a sponge-rubber nasal cuff. Esophageal necrosis can be avoided by periodically deflating and reinflating the esophageal balloon. Remove the esophageal tube as soon as possible.

PRODUCT AVAILABILITY ESOPHAGEAL AND NASOGASTRIC TUBES

Davol Incorporated

SELECTED REFERENCES
Busby HC, Seiffert W: Acute gastrointestinal bleeding. In Hudak CM, Gallo BM (eds): Critical Care Nursing, 3rd ed. Philadelphia, JB Lippincott, 1982

Cohee WR: Intra-arterial vasopressin in the treatment of upper gastrointestinal hemorrhage: A focus on bradycardia. Am J Intravenous Therapy and Clin Nutr, 9(6):25–32, June 1982

Larson EL: Gastrointestinal bleeding. In Larson EL, Vasquez M (eds): Critical Care Nursing. Philadelphia, WB Saunders, 1983

15 *Abdominal paracentesis*

BACKGROUND

Abdominal paracentesis is the aspiration or drainage of fluid or blood from the peritoneal space using a needle or trocar. The procedure is performed by a physician. The critical care nurse assesses the client's condition, assists with the procedure, monitors the client for the type and amount of drainage and for complications, and provides emotional support to the client.

Objectives

To remove fluid from the peritoneal space

To relieve pressure on the diaphragm, abdominal organs, and abdominal vasculature, which is caused by fluid accumulation in the peritoneal space (ascites)

To obtain specimens of peritoneal fluid for laboratory analysis

To detect abdominal bleeding after blunt abdominal trauma

ASSESSMENT PHASE

• Does the client have a history of liver disease, alcoholism, or bleeding tendencies? Liver pathology may result in deficiencies of the clotting factors, which increase the risk of bleeding during or after the procedure.

• Are the client's vital signs stable? Changes in the hemodynamic parameters can occur with intra-abdominal bleeding.

• Does the client have a large abdominal tumor? Perforation of the tumor and subsequent bleeding is possible. Pregnancy creates an additional risk during paracentesis.

• Is the client able to assist with the procedure by remaining still during trocar insertion?

PRECAUTIONS

• **The client's bladder should be emptied before the procedure to reduce the risk of perforation of the bladder.**

• **If more than 1500 ml of peritoneal fluid is removed at one time, salt-poor human albumin is given to replace aspirated fluid and to prevent hypovolemia.**

PLANNING PHASE

EQUIPMENT

Sterile paracentesis tray
    Sterile gloves
    Sterile drapes
    Antiseptic solution
    5-ml syringe with 21- or 25-gauge needle
    Scalpel
    Needle holder and suture
    Scissors
    Hemostat
    10- to 24-gauge trocar and cannula*
    Three-way stopcock

* A 16- to 24-gauge spinal needle with a 50-ml Luer-Lok syringe may be substituted.

> Drainage tubing
> Sterile gauze 4 × 4s
> Local anesthetic
> 1000-ml (or larger) sterile drainage bottle
> Sterile specimen containers and labels
> Sterile dressing and tape

CLIENT/FAMILY TEACHING
- Reinforce the physician's explanation of the procedure and the expected benefits. Help the physician to obtain an informed consent if necessary.
- Inform the client to expect to feel pressure when the trocar is inserted and that a local anesthetic will be provided.
- Advise the client to remain still during the procedure.

IMPLEMENTATION PHASE

NURSING ACTIONS	RATIONALE/AMPLIFICATION
1. Obtain baseline vital signs, weight, and abdominal girth at umbilicus.	These measurements will be used to monitor the client's status during and after the procedure. Mark the abdomen with a magic marker to show where the tape was placed to obtain the abdominal girth.
2. Ask client to void or insert indwelling bladder catheter if ordered.	Emptying the bladder reduces the risk of perforation.
3. Place client in Fowler's position or in sitting position.	This position encourages the collection of peritoneal fluid in the lower abdomen and facilitates drainage.
4. Expose abdomen from diaphragm to pubis.	
5. Wash your hands. Open paracentesis tray on bedside table to provide sterile field. Open sterile supplies on field.	
6. Assist physician in preparing abdomen with iodophor solution and in draping operative site with sterile drapes. Assist with administration of local anesthetic.	
7. Monitor client and record vital signs during procedure.	The physician will make a small incision 3 cm to 4 cm below the umbilicus to tap pooled fluid and avoid major abdominal organs. The trocar is inserted through the incision into the peritoneal space, and it is connected to a three-way stopcock, drainage tubing, and a collection bottle (Fig. 15–1). Fluid can also be removed using a three-way stopcock and 50-ml syringe setup.
8. Assist in specimen collection. Label specimens and send to laboratory.	When drainage is completed, the physician will remove the trocar and suture the incision.
9. Apply sterile pressure dressing to incision. Measure drainage and record amount on intake and output record.	

RELATED NURSING CARE

NURSING ACTIONS	RATIONALE/AMPLIFICATION
1. Monitor client's vital signs every 15 minutes during procedure.	Hypovolemic shock may occur if the fluid is removed too rapidly or if too much fluid is drained at one time. Assess for diaphoresis, tachycardia, dizziness, faintness, increased anxiety, and hypotension.

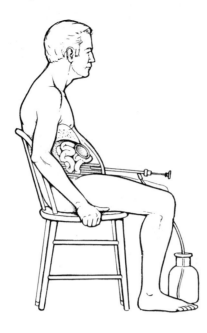

Fig. 15–1 Abdominal paracentesis. The sitting position is preferred because the intestines will float away from the site of paracentesis. (Brunner LS, Suddarth DS: Textbook of Medical–Surgical Nursing, 5th ed. Philadelphia, JB Lippincott, 1984)

2. After procedure check vital signs every 15 minutes for 1 hour. As client's condition improves, decrease frequency of monitoring.

3. Measure abdominal girth and weigh client after drainage of fluid is completed.

Comparisons are made between pre- and postparacentesis measurements.

4. Obtain daily weight and measurement of abdominal girth.

Daily weight and abdominal girth measurement monitor the recurrence of ascites.

5. Note color, consistency, amount, and odor of peritoneal fluid.

An accurate description of the fluid aids diagnosis and future treatment.

6. If needle or cannula is left in place for period to facilitate drainage, place light, dry sterile dressing at entry site. Regulate speed and amount of drainage to prevent hypovolemic shock.

EVALUATION PHASE

ANTICIPATED OUTCOMES	NURSING ACTIONS
1. Relief of ascites	Monitor the amount of fluid drained and observe for hypovolemia. Maintain the client in Fowler's position to facilitate drainage.
	Evaluate serial recordings of the daily weight and the abdominal girth measurement. Evaluate for recurrence of ascites.
	Assess the client's respiratory status for relief of pressure on the diaphragm. Assess urinary drainage and bowel movements for relief of pressure on the abdominal organs.
2. Prevention of complications of abdominal paracentesis	
a. Hypovolemic shock	Monitor the client's vital signs and the rate of drainage.

b. Perforation of abdominal organs

Palpate the bladder before the procedure. Help the client to remain still during the procedure.

c. Peritonitis

Monitor aseptic technique. Observe for signs of infection after the procedure and monitor serial temperature readings.

PRODUCT AVAILABILITY

DISPOSABLE ABDOMINAL PARACENTESIS KIT

Abbott Laboratories
Travenol Laboratories Inc.
Pharmaseal Inc.

SELECTED REFERENCES

Rubin W: The spectrum of cirrhosis. Emergency Medicine 15(13):28–58, July 1983

16

Infection control for gastrointestinal techniques (enteric precautions)

BACKGROUND

Critical care clients and care-givers are at risk for infections that are transmitted by contact with feces. Many clients in critical care units require a total-care approach, which frequently includes assistance with body hygiene after the use of the bedpan or after episodes of incontinence. In addition the client's condition or treatments may predispose the client to diarrheal illness such as *Clostridium difficile* enterocolitis, which can result from antibiotics and enteral feedings. Diarrhea can increase the potential for contamination with infectious material.

The use of enteric precautions will prevent the spread of the pathogens that are spread through feces. However, it is prudent professional practice to use enteric precautions in all exposures to feces; the unknown carrier or asymptomatic person is the greatest risk to others in a crowded critical care unit.

Objective

To prevent cross-infection of diseases that are transmitted by direct or indirect contact with feces

ASSESSMENT PHASE

• Is the client debilitated or unable to practice good body hygiene?
• Is the client receiving medications that alter gastrointestinal (GI) tract flora?
• Does the client have a communicable disease known to be transmitted by contact with feces? (See list of diseases requiring enteric precautions.)

PLANNING PHASE

EQUIPMENT

Private room (if client hygiene is poor)
Infection-control cart

    Gloves
    Gowns
    Enteric precautions isolation sign (brown)

CLIENT/FAMILY TEACHING

• Discuss with the client and family the need for enteric precautions. They will find it easier to comply with instructions if they understand the reasons for them.
• Stress the importance of good hygiene, especially handwashing
• Assure the client and family that it is the infectious agent — not the client — that is being isolated.

IMPLEMENTATION PHASE

NURSING ACTIONS	RATIONALE/AMPLIFICATION
1. Place "Enteric Precautions" sign on bed or door.	This is a ready reference for the client, family, and personnel.
2. Label interdepartmental communications such as laboratory slips or x-ray film requests "Enteric Precautions." Label cover of client's record "Enteric Precautions."	Labeling provides interdepartmental communication about enteric precautions.

3. Follow specifications on front of Centers for Communicable Disease (CDC) precautions sign (see list of enteric precautions).

EVALUATION PHASE

ANTICIPATED OUTCOME	NURSING ACTION
Prevention of transmission of infection through contact with feces	Monitor client, family, and personnel compliance with CDC guidelines for enteric precautions.

PRODUCT AVAILABILITY	ISOLATION CARDS National Technical Information Service (NTIS), United States Department of Commerce
SELECTED REFERENCES	CDC Guidelines for Isolation Precautions in Hospitals. Atlanta, United States Department of Health and Human Services (HHS Publication No. (CDC) 83-8314) 1983

Diseases requiring enteric precautions *

Amebic dysentery
Cholera
Coxsackievirus disease
Diarrhea, acute illness with suspected
   infectious etiology
Echovirus disease
Encephalitis (unless known not to be caused
   by enteroviruses)
Enterocolitis caused by *Clostridium*
   difficile or *Staphylococcus aureus*
Enteroviral infection
Gastroenteritis caused by
   Campylobacter species
   Cryptosporidium species
   Dientamoeba fragilis
   Escherichia coli (enterotoxic, enteropath-
     ogenic, or enteroinvasive)
   Giardia lamblia
   Salmonella species
   Shigella species
   Vibrio parahaemolyticus
   Viruses — including Norwalk agent and
     rotavirus

Yersinia enterocolitica
Unknown etiology but presumed to be an
   infectious agent
Hand, foot, and mouth disease
Hepatitis, viral, type A
Herpangina
Meningitis, viral (unless known not to be
   caused by enteroviruses)
Necrotizing enterocolitis
Pleurodynia
Poliomyelitis
Typhoid fever *(Salmonella typhi)*
Viral pericarditis, myocarditis, or meningitis
   (unless known not to be caused by
   enteroviruses)

* A private room is indicated for enteric precautions if patient hygiene is poor. A patient with poor hygiene does not wash hands after touching infective material, contaminates the environment with infective material, or shares contaminated articles with other patients. In general, patients infected with the same organism may share a room.

Enteric precautions

VISITORS — REPORT TO NURSES' STATION BEFORE ENTERING ROOM

1. Masks are not indicated.
2. Gowns are indicated if soiling is likely.
3. Gloves are indicated for touching infective material.
4. HANDS MUST BE WASHED AFTER TOUCHING THE PATIENT OR POTENTIALLY CONTAMINATED ARTICLES AND BEFORE TAKING CARE OF ANOTHER PATIENT.
5. Articles contaminated with infective material should be discarded or bagged and labeled before being sent for decontamination and reprocessing.

III   *Nutritional support techniques*

17 *Enteral hyperalimentation*

BACKGROUND

Severe protein-calorie malnutrition occurs in up to 60% of clients on general medical and surgical units. Its causes include anorexia and malabsorptive or hypermetabolic conditions. Malnutrition leads to impaired cell-mediated immunity, delayed wound healing, and an increased chance of infection. For clients who need nutritional support, tube feeding is a more physiologic, safer, simpler, and comparatively economic alternative to total parenteral nutrition (TPN).

FEEDING TUBE SELECTION

Before the development of pliable, fine-bore weighted feeding tubes, rubber or polyvinyl feeding tubes (16F to 18F) were the only option for enteral feeding. Although contraindicated for feeding purposes, these tubes are still commonly used. Large-bore feeding tubes are irritating to the gastrointestinal (GI) tract and cause pressure necrosis, particularly in critically ill clients with artificial airways. They deteriorate when exposed to gastric juice and therefore require frequent replacement. Furthermore, the large bore tends to cause incompetence of the gastroesophageal sphincter, thus increasing the chance of esophageal reflux and aspiration.

Several fine-bore weighted feeding tubes are available (Fig. 17–1). Depending on the length of the tube inserted, they may be used for nasogastric feeding, which requires a 90-cm (36-inch) tube, or nasoenteric feeding, which requires a 108-cm (43-inch) tube. The bolus weight aids passage of the tube into the intestine and also helps to anchor the tube after placement is confirmed. The tube selected for enteral feeding should be the smallest size through which the feeding will flow. Smaller tubes (5F or 6F) and viscous formulas require a feeding pump to maintain tube patency.

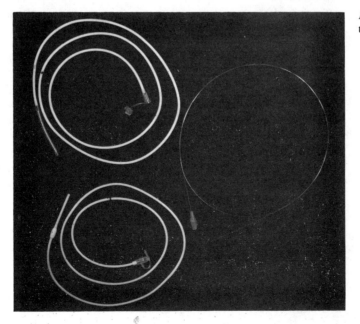

Fig. 17–1 Weighted feeding tubes.

Intubation using fine-bore feeding tubes may be difficult. The tubes are available with a stainless steel or plastic stylet to stiffen the tube during insertion. Polyurethane intravenous (IV) catheters have been adapted for enteral feeding. The risk of trauma to the GI tract by the makeshift guidewires that are used to insert these tubes makes them undesirable for enteral feeding. Levin tubes (16F) have been used as carriers to place small-bore feeding tubes whose tips are encased in a gelatin capsule. This practice risks tracheal delivery of the gelatin capsule and trauma to the upper GI tract.

ADMINISTRATION OF ENTERAL FEEDINGS

Formula may be delivered by either gravity or an enteral feeding pump, which may be either volumetric or peristaltic. Continuous drip administration with a feeding pump provides optimum utilization of formula and avoids the complications associated with obsolete bolus feeding methods, that is, GI upset and aspiration of formula. Continuous administration at a constant rate is mandatory when predigested nutrients are infused directly into the intestine. This prevents the infusion of a bolus of hypertonic solution, which would result in diarrhea and potential dehydration caused by an osmotic reaction.

Once the client is stabilized on continuous feedings, the regimen may progress to intermittent gravity drip administration (300 ml to 400 ml of formula every 4 hours to 6 hours) or to cyclic feeding in which the client is removed from the feeding program for a period each day, for example, 12 hours on and 12 hours off. This goal is an appropriate one for planning a feeding program.

ENTERAL FEEDING FORMULAS

The following are several categories of commercially available formulas: blenderized, milk based, lactose free, complete formulas with predigested nutrients; special formulas for clients with liver or renal disorders; and modular feedings, which can be used to individualize feedings. The small intestine is more sensitive than the stomach to both the volume and osmolality of formula. Enteric feedings are delivered by a continuous drip and, ideally, are low in osmolality. The osmolality of the feeding varies when concentrated or special formulas are used, which is often the case in critical care units. Isotonic formulas are more easily tolerated than hypertonic formulas and do not have to be diluted as much. Obtain specific formula information from the individual supplier.

Weighted feeding tube insertion

Objective
To provide an alternative nutritional source when the absorptive surface of the gut is intact, but oral intake is contraindicated or insufficient

ASSESSMENT PHASE

• Is the client able to follow instructions and to maintain desired positions to assist with intubation?
• Has the client had previous experience with nasogastric intubation?

PRECAUTIONS

• **The presence of an endotracheal tube tends to guide the feeding tube into the trachea.**
• **Refer clients with head injury and possible fracture of the cribriform plate to the physician for placement of the GI tube under direct vision or with fluoroscopy. The danger of placing the tube into the cranium exists.**
• **Use gloves when intubating clients with possible herpes lesions of the mouth to avoid contracting herpetic whitlow, a painful, viral infection of the pulp space of the finger.**

PLANNING PHASE

EQUIPMENT

Weighted feeding tube with stylet (7F to 8F)
Hypoallergenic tape (1.5 cm, ½ inch)
Water-soluble lubricant (if tube is not prelubricated)
Glass of water (if tube is prelubricated)

Mineral oil (if gelatin stylet is used)
Safety pin
Glass of water with straw or ice chips (if permitted)
Linen protector
Stethoscope
Irrigation set (asepto syringe and emesis basin)
Litmus paper (optional)
If the tube will be inserted without a stylet, include the following items:
    Basin of ice chips
    Cotton swab
Gloves (optional)

CLIENT/FAMILY TEACHING

- Discuss the reason for the tube insertion.
- Describe the procedure and possible sensations, such as a feeling of choking when the tube is passed through the pharynx. Use diagrams and a sample tube as appropriate.
- Agree on a predetermined hand signal that the client can use to show that he is having difficulty breathing. This may indicate that the tube has been inserted in the trachea.
- Promote active or passive exercise while the tube is in place. Reassure the client that this will not dislodge the tube.

IMPLEMENTATION PHASE

NURSING ACTIONS	RATIONALE/AMPLIFICATION
1. Place client in high Fowler's or sitting position. Wash your hands.	
2. For gastric placement, determine approximate length for insertion. Measure distance from tip of *n*ose to *e*arlobe, and from there to *x*iphoid process (NEX measurement).	*Alternative method:* Mark the 50-cm point on the tube. The insertion length is midway between the 50-cm point and the NEX measurement. For enteric placement, add approximately 22.5 cm (9 inches) to the NEX measurement.
3. Mark this point on tube with tape, or note closest mark on tube.	
4. If stylet with prelubricated tube is being used, activate lubricant inside tube by flushing with water. Insert stylet, making sure it is locked in place behind weighted tip.	Prelubricated tubes are lubricated at the tip as well as within the lumen to facilitate withdrawal of the stylet.
5. Activate lubricant on weighted tip of tube by dipping in water. If tube is not prelubricated, apply water-soluble lubricant to first 10 cm (4 inches) of tube.	If a gelatin stylet is being used, a small amount of mineral oil may be used to lubricate the stylet, which tends to become sticky with water. *Caution:* Aspiration of mineral oil can result in granulomatous pneumonia.
6. Determine preferred nostril by having client breathe through each nostril alternately.	Insert the tube into the most patent nostril.
7. Flex client's neck. Pass lubricated tip through nostril and into nasopharynx.	This anatomic position facilitates passage of the tube.
8. Rotate tube 180° and encourage client to swallow.	Giving small amounts of water through a straw or asking the client to chew and swallow ice chips may assist the passage of the tube. Stroking the throat may stimulate reflex swallowing in the unconscious client.
9. Pass tube until premeasured length is inserted.	Do not force the tube against resistance. Pull the tube back a few centimeters and try to pass it again, or remove the tube and report the problem.

10. If tube accidentally enters trachea, pull it back to nasopharynx and attempt to reinsert it.

Accidental placement in the trachea usually causes choking and coughing. This may not be as apparent with small-diameter tubes. The client will be unable to speak if the tube is inserted in the larynx. For the alert client a prearranged hand signal may be helpful to indicate breathing difficulty.

11. Ascertain proper position of tube in stomach by injecting bolus of air into tube while auscultating left upper quadrant of abdomen with stethoscope.

If a "flow-through" stylet is being used, a Luer-Lok type of syringe may be attached directly to the stylet connector. If an occlusive stylet is used, it will have to be removed before the position of the tube can be checked.

Correct positioning of the tube is indicated by auscultating a whooshing sound as the air is injected. If stomach contents can be withdrawn with a small-bore tube, test with litmus paper to determine that the contents are acidic.

12. Prepare skin benzoin. Tape tube to nose, avoiding pressure on naris. Attach tube to client's gown with safety pin and tape tab.

Tear a slit in a 5-cm (2-inch) piece of tape to form a "Y." Tape the stem of the "Y" to the client's nose. Secure the tube with the arms of the "Y" in a spiral fashion.

13. Remove stylet. Be careful not to remove tube simultaneously.

Caution: Do not reinsert the stylet when the tube is *in situ*. The stylet may exit through the terminal exit holes, damaging the GI tract.

14. If enteric placement is desired, place client on right side in semi-Fowler's position to encourage migration of bolus weight into duodenum.

Spontaneous transpyloric passage of the weighted tip usually occurs in 24 hours to 48 hours. Tape tube loosely to allow migration.

15. Continue to insert tube slowly over number of hours until correct length has been inserted.

If it is not contraindicated, an infusion of feeding solution may be started before the transpyloric passage of the tip.

16. Confirm placement by x-ray film.

17. Connect feeding tube to prepared feeding apparatus.

18. To insert tube without stylet, proceed as follows:

a. Place tube on ice to stiffen it.

Leave the tube on ice until you are ready to use it. The tube will remain stiff for a short period only.

b. Place uncovered end of cotton swab into distal eye of tube.

c. Use swab to stabilize tube and to aid in passing it into nasopharynx (Fig. 17–2).

d. Remove swab.

When the mercury bolus falls behind the soft palate, the tube may be easily passed into the stomach.

EVALUATION PHASE

ANTICIPATED OUTCOME	NURSING ACTION
Prevention of aspiration	Recheck tube placement every 8 hours or when a new or intermittent feeding is initiated.

PRODUCT AVAILABILITY

FEEDING TUBES

Biosearch Medical Products, Inc. (Hydromer–Dobbhoff feeding tube; Entriflex nasogastric feeding tube)
Corpak Co. (Keofeed feeding tube)

Fig. 17-2 Stabilizing feeding tube using cotton swab.

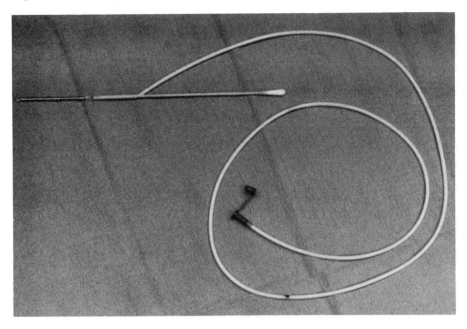

Enteral feeding pump

Objective

To provide gastric or enteric feeding formulas at a controlled rate

ASSESSMENT PHASE

- Is an appropriate feeding tube in place? A sump tube may need to be replaced with a fine-bore feeding tube.
- Which risk factors that are associated with poor nutritional status are present (*e.g.,* NPO [*non per os,* nothing by mouth] for 10 days or more, anorexia, alcohol abuse, burns)?
- Is there a history of lactose intolerance or renal or liver disorders, which require special formulas?

PRECAUTIONS

- **Use an infusion pump specifically designed for enteral feeding. IV pumps can provide pressures greater than 40 pounds per square inch (psi), which can damage the tube (*e.g.,* IVAC 500 and 530 series).**

PLANNING PHASE

EQUIPMENT

Enteral feeding pump
Formula bag and administration set
IV pole
Ice (if feeding bag has ice pouch)

CLIENT/FAMILY TEACHING

- Explain the goals of the feeding regimen to the client and family.
- Inform the client of dietary restrictions. Oral intake may be permitted.
- Explain the importance of maintaining physical activity (active or passive) while on the feeding program. Exercise will encourage anabolism (tissue building) as well as prevent complications of bed rest. Reassure the client that exercise will not dislodge the tube.
- Tell the client that the frequency of bowel movements may decrease because of the low residue content of the feeding. Keep in mind that many critically ill patients develop diarrhea. Diarrhea may be a problem until the feeding regimen is adjusted for the client's requirements.
- Encourage the involvement of the client and family in all aspects of the feeding program.

**IMPLEMENTATION
PHASE**

1. Assemble administration tubing and feeding bag. Clamp tubing.

Label the administration set and feeding bag with the date.

2. Fill feeding bag with enough formula for 4 hours and hang feeding bag on IV stand.

Formula should not be left in the bag for more than 4 hours to discourage bacterial growth.

3. Insert tubing into pump mechanism according to manufacturer's directions (Fig. 17–3).

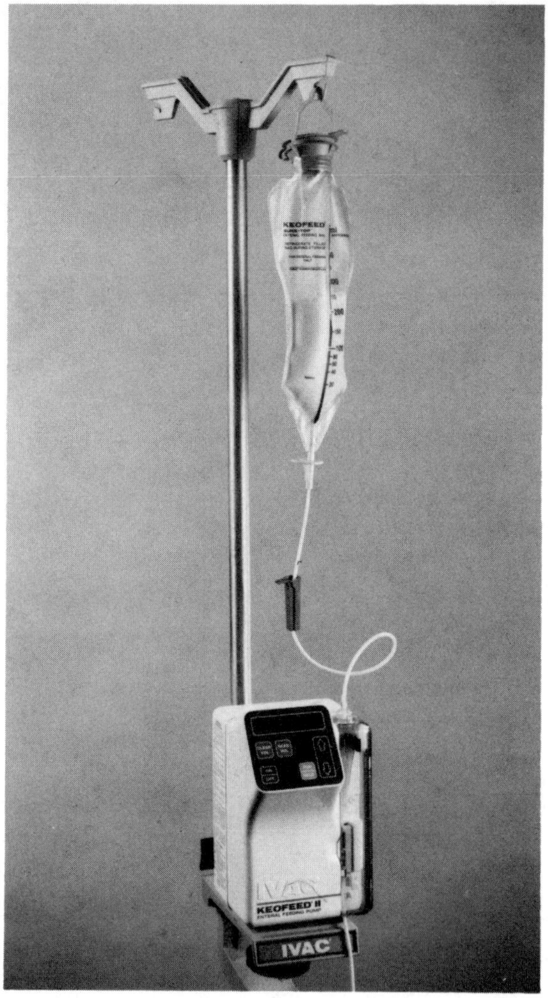

Fig. 17–3 IVAC Keofeed II enteral feeding pump. (Courtesy IVAC Corporation, San Diego, CA)

4. Prime administration set with formula and connect it to feeding tube.

Label the enteral tubing distinctively to avoid confusion with IV lines.

5. Set pump rate to begin infusion slowly at 50 ml/ hour, at one-half to one-third strength formula.

The client who has been NPO for a period requires time to adapt to refeeding.

6. Increase rate 25 ml to 50 ml/hour/day while monitoring client's condition until prescribed infusion rate is reached.

Assess for nausea, vomiting, diarrhea, and glycosuria to determine tolerance.

7. When final infusion rate is reached, increase strength of formula as tolerated.

If the feeding is not tolerated, decrease the rate and strength of the feeding. Gradually increase the rate and

8. Irrigate feeding tube with 20 ml to 25 ml of water as follows:

    a. Every 3 hours to 4 hours when not using continuous drip, or every 6 hours when using continuous drip

    b. Each time feeding container is changed

    c. Whenever feeding is interrupted

9. Maintain client in semi-Fowler's position or place head of bed on 15-cm (6-inch) blocks.

strength, allowing the client time to adjust to enteral feeding. Avoid altering both the rate and the strength at the same time.

Use a 50-ml syringe to irrigate the tube and to clear blockages. Smaller syringes generate higher pressures, which can damage the tube.

Elevating the client's head reduces the chance of regurgitation or aspiration.

RELATED NURSING CARE

NURSING ACTIONS	RATIONALE/AMPLIFICATION
1. Change bag and administration set every 24 hours and label with date.	This is an infection-control precaution.
2. Do not add fresh formula to formula remaining in bag.	This deters bacterial growth.
3. If bag has ice compartment, check periodically and keep filled.	This deters bacterial growth.
4. Check urine sugar and acetone levels every 4 hours.	Glycosuria can result from the added glucose load provided by the formula until insulin production increases accordingly. Urine checks may be discontinued in non-diabetic clients after 48 hours if the results are consistently negative.
5. Check pump rate every hour.	
6. Check residual feeding every 4 hours until regimen is established; then check during every shift.	Aspirate the residual feeding from the tube. If the volume is less than 100 ml, reinstill the feeding, flush the tube, and resume the feedings. If the volume is greater than 100 ml, reinstill the feeding, flush the tube, and hold the feeding for 1 hour. Recheck the residual feeding. If the volume of the residual feeding remains over 100 ml, consider possible reasons for delayed gastric emptying and notify the physician. (The residual feeding may be difficult to obtain with a small-bore feeding tube.)

EVALUATION PHASE

ANTICIPATED OUTCOMES	NURSING ACTIONS
1. Avoidance of complications of enteral feeding	
a. Pneumonia due to aspiration of formula	Confirm the placement of the tube each time formula is added to the bag. Elevate the head of the bed at least 30°. Food coloring may be added to the formula to alert the nurse if aspiration occurs.

b. Diarrhea due to feeding-or nonfeeding-related causes	Evaluate the client's condition for possible causes of diarrhea. Nonfeeding-related causes include antibiotic therapy, low serum albumin, lactose intolerance, and fecal impaction. Feeding-related causes include bacterial contamination and osmolar overload.
c. Constipation due to low-residue feedings	Add residue to the feeding if appropriate. Administer medications or enemas as ordered.
d. Fluid and electrolyte disturbances due to high protein-to-water ratio or high glucose content of feeding	Record accurate intake and output measurements. Monitor serum electrolyte levels, blood urea nitrogen (BUN), hematocrit, and urine specific gravity. Monitor blood glucose levels and glycosuria to prevent osmotic diuresis.
e. Gastric distention or rupture due to paralytic ileus	Monitor the residual feeding. Assess for increasing abdominal girth. Auscultate bowel sounds during each shift.
2. Attainment of nutritional goals	Monitor the client's weight daily and request laboratory work as ordered (*e.g.,* nitrogen balance studies, blood counts and chemistries).

PRODUCT AVAILABILITY

ENTERAL FEEDING PUMPS AND FORMULAS

Biosearch Medical Products, Inc. (Dobbhoff enteric feeding bag, enteral feeding pump)

Ross Laboratories (Flexiflo Flexitainer feeding bag, enteral feeding formulas)

Chesebrough–Ponds, Inc. (Kangaroo tube-feeding set, Kangaroo 220 enteral feeding pump)

Abbott Laboratories (Life Care Pump)

IVAC Corporation (Enteral feeding pump)

SELECTED REFERENCES

Cataldo CB, Smith L: Tube Feedings: Clinical Applications, Columbus, OH, Ross Laboratories, 1980

Griggs BA, Hoppe MC: Nasogastric tube feeding. Am J Nurs 79(3):481–488, March 1979

Murphy LM, Hostetler C: Tube feeding reconsidered. NITA 4(6):409–413, November/December 1981

Persons C: Why risk TPN when tube feeding will do? RN 44(1)35–41, January 1981

Persons CB: Enteral nutrition: State of the art. In Zschoske D (ed): Mosby's Comprehensive Review of Critical Care. St. Louis, CV Mosby, In press

18 *Total parenteral nutrition*

Many hospitalized clients are nutritionally depleted, yet an infusion of 1000 ml of dextrose 5% contains only 170 calories. If oral intake is impossible or insufficient, and enteral hyperalimentation is not an option, total parenteral nutrition (TPN) may be used to meet the client's nutritional needs. TPN solutions consist of a nitrogen source (protein), hypertonic dextrose, and supplementary vitamins and minerals and are infused into a central vein. TPN is prescribed to provide an amount of nitrogen that exceeds the amount required to maintain nutritional equilibrium, to promote protein synthesis and weight gain.

Because hypertonic solutions cause sclerosis of peripheral veins, TPN is infused into a central vein, typically the subclavian, where high blood flow rapidly dilutes the solution. At present right atrial (RA) catheters specifically developed for long-term use are being inserted for TPN. Clients may be allowed to have a home TPN program with indwelling RA catheters. Hickman, Broviac, and Centracil catheters are the RA catheters that are most commonly used (Fig. 18–1). The Hickman and Broviac catheters are similar in design, except that the lumen of the Broviac catheter is smaller than that of the Hickman. A double-lumen Hickman catheter is also available. It provides a route for continuous infusion and a second lumen for intermittent infusion of medications or concurrent lipid administration.

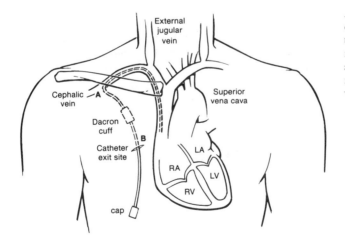

Fig. 18–1 Cuffed right atrial catheter placed in right atrium and threaded through subcutaneous tunnel. A Dacron cuff stabilizes catheter and provides barrier to infection. *RA*, right atrium; *LA*, left atrium; *RV*, right ventricle; *LV*, left ventricle.

The Hickman and Broviac catheters are placed percutaneously in the operating room or by cutdown. The catheter is advanced through a long subcutaneous tunnel into the superior vena cava or RA. The catheter design is similiar to that of the Tenckhoff catheter, which is used for home peritoneal dialysis, and features a Dacron-mesh cuff that assists in stabilizing the catheter in the subcutaneous tissue. Eventually, fibrous tissue will infiltrate the cuff. The location of the exit site away from the surgical insertion site decreases the risk of infection of the vascular system. The Centracil catheter does not have a cuff. Catheter lumens that are not used for continuous infusion are heparinized periodically to prevent clotting. Strict sterile technique is mandatory when changing the dressing or the injection cap to prevent infection and septicemia.

MEETING NUTRITIONAL
NEEDS WITH TPN

Unless an adequate number of calories (fats and carbohydrates) is supplied in addition to a nitrogen source, a negative nitrogen balance cannot be corrected. Intravenous (IV) delivery of fats appears to be ideal for supplying calories, because fats contain a higher number of calories per gram than glucose. However, no more than 60% of the total number of calories should be supplied by fats. The body requires some carbohydrate intake as well. Recent trends include the use of fats as a preferred calorie source in stressed and septic clients and the use of fats on a daily basis as a calorie source when low dextrose concentrations are used.

Protein is supplied in the form of crystalline amino acids that contain essential and nonessential amino acids. The ratio of calories to nitrogen that will ensure protein synthesis is approximately 150 calories to 200 calories to 1 gram of nitrogen. Amino acids can also be administered in dextrose 5% as a protein-sparing measure.

Electrolytes (*e.g.,* sodium, chloride, potassium, phosphate, calcium, and magnesium) are added to the TPN solution according to the client's specific needs. Fat- and water-soluble vitamins are added to infusions daily. Clients who are maintained on hyperalimentation for more than 1 month usually receive essential fatty acids and trace elements such as zinc through the infusion of whole blood or plasma biweekly. Essential fatty acids may be supplied through IV lipids, two to three bottles (500 ml) weekly. Vitamin B_{12}, vitamin K, and folic acid are administered intramuscularly or in the TPN solution.

TPN has disadvantages. Complications that are encountered relate to subclavian catheter insertion, sepsis, and metabolic disturbances. Clients who are stressed by surgery, sepsis, or steroid therapy will require exogenous insulin. The insulin may be added to the infusion or administered by a sliding scale according to urine or blood glucose levels (see Bedside Blood Glucose Monitoring in Chap. 34). To minimize metabolic problems in clients undergoing surgery, the TPN solution may be replaced with a 10% dextrose infusion immediately pre- and postoperatively. Diabetics or prediabetics require exogenous insulin. Clients with cardiac, renal, or liver problems require adjustments in TPN therapy, both in volume and in composition.

The maintenance of strict TPN protocols regarding catheter maintenance and solution preparation and administration is necessary to administer TPN safely. Ideally, a 24-hour supply of TPN solution should be prepared by the pharmacist under a laminar flow hood. If a laminar flow hood is not available, the solution should be prepared by a qualified nurse in an area that is reserved for admixtures.

Right atrial catheters (Intra-cath, Hickman, Broviac, Centracil)

Objective
To correct negative nitrogen balance when oral intake is insufficient or contraindicated by administering nutrients parenterally

ASSESSMENT PHASE

- Has a complete nutritional assessment been obtained?
- What are the client's baseline values, serum electrolyte levels, serum osmolality, complete blood count, fasting blood glucose levels, blood urea nitrogen (BUN), serum protein, and weight? Evaluate the results of urinalysis, chest films, and ECG.
- Is the client adequately hydrated? Cannulation of the subclavian vein is more difficult in a dehydrated client, and the risk of nonketotic hyperosmolar coma is increased.

• Are any potential sources of contamination of the TPN catheter present (*e.g.,* tracheostomy or draining wound)?

PRECAUTIONS

• **Maintain absolute aseptic technique in all aspects of TPN care.**
• **Do not administer routine medications, withdraw blood samples, or measure central venous pressure (CVP) using the TPN "lifeline."**
• **Avoid using piggyback IV infusions, extra IV extensions, and stopcocks. These are contamination hazards.**
• **Do not administer blood through the TPN line. This interrupts the TPN program and causes fibrin buildup in the catheter.**

PLANNING PHASE

EQUIPMENT

Skin preparation supplies (soap, razor, acetone, iodine, alcohol)
Rolled towel
Xylocaine 1%
Cutdown tray
Black silk skin suture
Subclavian catheter set, Intra-cath (8 inch) or Centracil catheter (Fig. 18–2)*
Sterile gowns, gloves, and masks
Nonallergenic tape
Benzoin
Acetone or alcohol
Isotonic IV solution
Regular IV tubing
In-line bacterial filter
TPN solution
IV pump/controller

Fig. 18–2 Subclavian catheter set with plastic clip to protect catheter from damage by needle tip; catheter is in sterile protective sleeve. 14-gauge needle and syringe are provided for venous puncture.

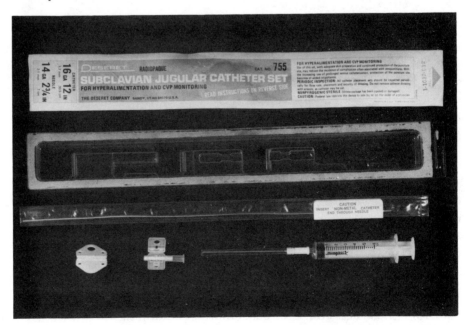

CLIENT/FAMILY TEACHING

• Reinforce the physician's explanation of the benefits and risks of TPN therapy.
• Discuss the importance of ambulation/exercise during the TPN program. Exercise minimizes the breakdown of muscle tissue and encourages the development of lean muscle mass. Reassure the client that the TPN catheter will not be dislodged during exercise.

* Hickman and Broviac catheters are placed in the operating room using a minor-procedure instrument set.

IMPLEMENTATION PHASE

NURSING ACTIONS	RATIONALE/AMPLIFICATION
1. Connect IV tubing and in-line filter to isotonic IV solution. Prime and clamp tubing.	
2. Shave insertion site.	
3. Swab skin with acetone or alcohol.	If acetone is unavailable, substitute alcohol. Note that acetone can damage some catheters.
4. Prepare site with iodine, followed by alcohol after iodine dries.	Begin in the center of the site and work in widening concentric circles. If the client is allergic to iodine, substitute iodophor or chlorhexidine. If iodophor is substituted for iodine, do not remove iodophor with alcohol, because its effectiveness is derived from the slow release of iodine.
5. Position client supine with rolled towel under shoulders.	This position facilitates location of the subclavian vein by elevating the clavicle.
6. Place bed in Trendelenburg's position.	This position allows the subclavian vein to fill.
7. Assist physician with sterile gown and gloves after scrub is completed. Provide masks for other staff members.	A mask is not necessary for the client. Turn the client's head away from the site to prevent contamination (Fig. 18–3*A*).

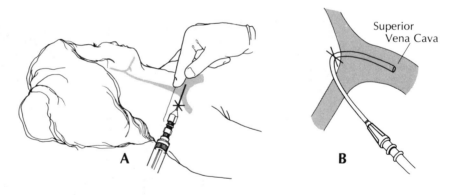

Fig. 18–3 Subclavian insertion procedure. (*A*) The client's face is turned away from sterile field while physician locates vein. (*B*) The syringe is removed from needle, and catheter is threaded into superior vena cava.

8. Open cutdown tray on bedside table to provide sterile field.	
9. Assist physician in drawing up Xylocaine for local anesthetic and applying sterile drapes.	
10. Adjust supplementary lights if necessary.	
11. Remain with client and give reassurance during subclavian insertion procedure.	Tell the client what to expect as the local anesthetic is given and as the procedure progresses. The physician will locate the vein by inserting a 14-gauge needle and syringe beneath the clavicle toward the suprasternal notch.
12. Return blood flow in syringe indicates entry into vein. Instruct client to perform Valsalva's maneuver (hold breath and bear down).	While the client performs Valsalva's maneuver, the physician will remove the syringe from the needle and thread the catheter into the superior vena cava (Fig. 18–3*B*). The needle is withdrawn through the skin, and

13. Connect IV setup to catheter when it is passed off sterile field by physician.

14. Start IV infusion at keep-open rate until position of catheter is confirmed by chest film.

15. Physician will paint skin with benzoin and apply antiseptic ointment (if used) to insertion site.

16. Occlusive dressing of sterile 4 × 4s and tape is applied. Loop IV tubing over outside of dressing to prevent accidental withdrawal of catheter.

17. When catheter position is verified by chest film, discontinue isotonic IV infusion and add first bottle of TPN.

18. Connect IV pump and set rate according to physician's order. Apply tape with time written on it to TPN bottle to check pump accuracy.

19. Maintain rate within 10% of desired rate. Do not attempt to "catch up on" infusion by temporarily increasing the rate.

the catheter is protected from the needle tip by a guard, which prevents air embolism.

The physician will suture the catheter in place.

Alternative method: A transparent dressing may be applied directly over the site after antiseptic ointment is applied.

Allow TPN to warm to room temperature before the infusion. The infusion of cold solutions decreases body temperature and causes venospasm.

Because of the high glucose content of TPN, the rate of administration is usually gradually increased during a stabilization period (2 days to 4 days) until the desired rate is reached. For example, 1000 ml of TPN may be ordered for the first 24 hours, with the remaining fluid requirements made up with dextrose 5%. This allows insulin production to increase accordingly.

If the infusion is too slow, consider recalculating the rate to administer the remaining TPN at a constant rate for the remainder of the 24 hours. This prevents sudden shifts in the blood glucose level and serum osmolality.

RELATED NURSING CARE

NURSING ACTIONS	RATIONALE/AMPLIFICATION
1. Check urine sugar and acetone levels every 6 hours. Report glycosuria values greater than 2+.	A sliding-scale insulin may be ordered by the physician to cover increases in blood glucose. Use a reagent strip to check blood glucose levels periodically if stabilization is a problem. Sudden glucose intolerance in a previously stabilized client can indicate catheter sepsis.
2. Monitor blood glucose levels daily until stabilized, and at least weekly thereafter.	Blood glucose levels should stabilize under 200 mg/dl. The critically ill client may require blood glucose determinations more frequently than weekly.
3. Monitor client's temperature every 6 hours.	An elevated temperature (*i.e.*, low grade, daily temperature spikes, or dramatic spikes accompanied by symptoms of septicemia) may be a sign of sepsis. Remove the bottle and tubing and send them to the laboratory for culturing if a sudden temperature spike occurs after the addition of a new bottle of TPN.
4. Change site dressing every 48 hours, or immediately if it becomes soiled.	Remove the soiled dressing aseptically. Prepare the skin and the catheter with acetone, iodine, and alcohol (see steps 3 and 4 under Implementation Phase). Reapply the dressing (see steps 15 and 16 under Implementation Phase). Use a mask and sterile gloves for the procedure. Record the date and the time of the dressing change on the dressing.
5. Make cloth dressing waterproof with plastic, self-adhering drape (Steridrape) if contamination may be a problem.	A waterproof drape is useful for clients with tracheostomies, draining wounds, nasogastric tubes, or high-humidity oxygen apparatus.

6. Change IV tubing and in-line filter every 24 hours to 48 hours using aseptic technique.

The IV tubing and in-line filter should be changed when the dressing is changed if possible. Record the date and time of the tubing change on the tubing with tape. Place the client supine during the procedure and instruct the client in performing Valsalva's maneuver. The high intrathoracic pressure that this produces prevents air embolism.

7. Weigh client daily.

Weigh the client at the same time each day on the same scales. Make sure that the client wears the same clothing while being weighed.

8. Before discontinuing TPN, wean client gradually.

Gradual weaning prevents rebound hypoglycemia. Dextrose 10% may be ordered when TPN is discontinued to complete the weaning process.

9. Before removal of subclavian catheter, prepare skin as for dressing changes. Withdraw slowly while client performs Valsalva's maneuver. Determine that catheter has been recovered completely. Clip catheter tip with sterile scissors and place in culture tube. Redress site (see steps 15 and 16 under Implementation Phase).

Request that the laboratory perform a semiquantitative culture, which uses a sheep-blood agar plate. Remove the Hickman or Broviac catheter using the same technique. Control the minimal amount of bleeding at the insertion site using manual pressure and a 4 × 4.

10. Repair damaged Hickman or Broviac catheter.

11. If sterilized repair kit is not immediately available, proceed as follows:

   a. Place piece of tape on catheter near chest wall and clamp catheter.

   b. Insert 14-gauge IV angiocath into damaged catheter and remove sytlet. Tape angiocath securely and flush it with heparin solution.

The catheter can be used while the repair kit is obtained, or the flush syringe can be left in place.

12. Catheters damaged more than 4 cm from chest wall can be repaired as follows:

   a. Flush catheter with heparin solution. Clamp catheter near chest wall over piece of tape.

The tape protects the catheter from damage from the clamps.

   b. Create sterile field using sterile towel. Open sterile 4 × 4s, alcohol- and iodophor-soaked wipes, sterile scissors or scalpel, and new injection cap on sterile field.

   c. Wear mask and sterile surgical gloves.

   d. Clean catheter with alcohol wipes, followed by iodophor.

   e. Change to another pair of sterile gloves and remove powder from gloves with sterile alcohol-soaked wipe.

Glove powder weakens the adhesive that is used for catheter repair.

   f. Load syringe barrel with 1 ml of adhesive and insert plunger into barrel. Attach blunted needle to syringe. Set aside for later use.

   g. Using scalpel or scissors, cut catheter just proximal to damaged section. Trim replacement tubing to required length (Fig. 18–4*A*).

When the catheter is repaired, it should extend no more than 15 cm to 20 cm from the chest wall.

   h. Connect damaged catheter and replacement tubing using connector (Fig. 18–4*B*).

Insert the connector all the way to the center ridge to make sure the repair is secure.

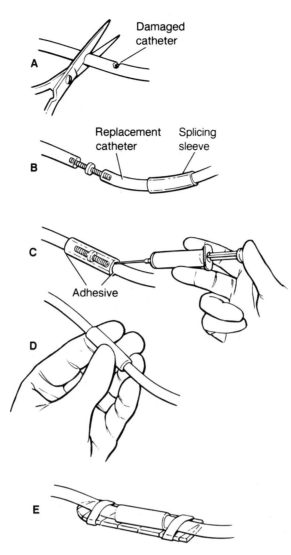

Damaged catheter

Replacement catheter   Splicing sleeve

Adhesive

Fig. 18–4 Repairing Hickman or Broviac right atrial catheter. (*A*) Cut catheter just proximal to damaged section. (*B*) Use connector to link damaged catheter and replacement tubing. (*C*) Apply adhesive liberally over ends of catheters and slide splicing sleeve along replacement segment and over connector. Additional adhesive can be inserted between catheter and sleeve using syringe. (*D*) Roll sleeve in fingers to spread adhesive. (*E*) Splint joint with protected tongue blade and tape.

   i. Apply adhesive liberally over area of center ridge. Slide loose splicing sleeve on replacement segment over connector (Fig. 18–4*C*).

The center ridge should be in the center of the splicing sleeve.

   j. Inject adhesive under sleeve from both ends.

   k. Roll sleeve in your fingers to spread adhesive. Wipe excess with 4 × 4 (Fig. 18–4*D*).

   l. Replace sterile injection cap.

   m. Splint joint with protected tongue blade and tape for 48 hours (Fig. 18–4*E*).

This protects the joint until the adhesive achieves maximum strength. *Caution:* Do not use the catheter for infusion for 2 hours after the repair.

   n. Before using catheter, remove any air remaining in replacement segment with syringe until blood fills entire segment. Flush catheter with heparin solution.

13. Protect long-term RA catheters according to the following procedure:

   a. Wrap catheter with piece of tape that is 1-cm wide about 4 cm from connector or injection cap.

Alternative method: Use a rubber-shod clamp when clamping the catheter. This prevents the clamps from damaging the catheter.

b. When clamping catheter, place clamp over tape.

14. Change injection cap weekly on RA catheter ports that are used intermittently.	Changing of the injection cap prevents leakage from the injection port.

EVALUATION PHASE

ANTICIPATED OUTCOMES	NURSING ACTIONS
1. Prevention of complications of TPN	
a. Catheter insertion	After catheter insertion, evaluate for hydrothorax, pneumothorax, arterial puncture, air or catheter embolism, and myocardial perforation. Infuse isotonic IV fluids only, at a keep-open rate until the catheter position is verified by a chest film and there is no evidence of hematoma.
b. Catheter-related sepsis	Evaluate serial temperatures. Observe the catheter site for redness or discharge. Notify the physician for catheter removal if the catheter is septic.
c. Metabolic complications	Evaluate for hyperglycemia or hypoglycemia; hyperosmolar hyperglycemic nonketotic coma; hypocalcemia; and electrolyte, vitamin, or fatty acid deficiencies.
2. Weight gain within individual limits (average 1.1 kg [2.5 pounds] per week)	Comply with all TPN protocols. Monitor the client's weight daily.
3. Increase in lean muscle mass **4.** Improvement of wound healing	Monitor laboratory work as ordered (*e.g.,* complete blood count, serum albumin, serum electrolytes, nitrogen balance studies).

PRODUCT AVAILABILITY

LUER-LOK EXTENSION SET (FOR USE WITH CENTRACIL CATHETER)

Quest Medical, Inc.

STERIDRAPE

3M Company

TPN PRODUCTS

McGaw Laboratories
Travenol Laboratories, Inc.

HICKMAN CATHETER REPAIR KIT

Evermed

SELECTED REFERENCES

Anderson MA, Aker SN, Hickman RO: The double-lumen Hickman catheter. Am J Nurs 82:2:272–275, 1982
Guidelines for Isolation Precautions in Hospitals. Washington DC, US Department of Health and Human Services Publication No. (CDC) 83-8314, 1983

Holloway NM: Nursing the Critically Ill Adult. Menlo Park, CA, Addison–Wesley, 1979
Hudak CM, Lohn T, Gallo BM: Critical Care Nursing, 3rd ed. Philadelphia, JB Lippincott, 1982
Vogel TC, McKimming SA: Teaching parents to give indwelling C.V. catheter care. Nursing '83 13:1:55–56, 1983

Lipid therapy

Objectives

To provide a parenteral source of calories and essential fatty acids for clients requiring parenteral nutrition for extended periods

To provide a parenteral source of essential fatty acids when a deficiency occurs

ASSESSMENT PHASE

- Does the client have the following clinical signs of essential fatty acid deficiency (EFAD): poor wound healing; hemolytic anemia; poor immune response; ECG changes; dehydration; dry, scaly skin; or sparse hair growth?
- Does the client have a disturbance of normal fat metabolism (*e.g.*, pathologic hyperlipemia, acute pancreatitis with hyperlipidemia)? IV lipids may be contraindicated.
- Is the client prone to fat embolism (*e.g.*, multiple fractures)?
- Does the client have conditions that might be complicated by the administration of IV lipids (*e.g.*, liver damage, pulmonary disease, anemia, or blood coagulation disorders)?
- Is a suitable IV available? Lipids may be infused as a separate peripheral infusion; into a central vein as a "Y" type of infusion; concurrently with amino acid/dextrose solutions, using a double-lumen RA catheter; or using a three-in-one admixture system in which a single container provides a 24-hour supply of amino acids, dextrose, fats, minerals, and electrolytes.

PRECAUTIONS

- **The addition of medications directly into the bottle or as a piggyback may interfere with the emulsion.**
- **Using an IV filter with IV lipids will clog the filter and may interfere with the emulsion.**

PLANNING PHASE

EQUIPMENT

IV infusion of lipid solution (500 ml) or 24-hour supply of premixed three-in-one admixture of dextrose, lipids, and amino acids
Alcohol swab
IV tubing (supplied with product)
IV drip controller

CLIENT/FAMILY TEACHING

- Discuss the reason for lipid infusion with the client and family.
- Caution the client to notify the staff of possible side-effects of lipid infusion, particularly early in the infusion period.

IMPLEMENTATION PHASE

NURSING ACTIONS	RATIONALE/AMPLIFICATION
1. Inspect solution for cracking (oiling out) of emulsion or frothy appearance.	Discard the bottle if these conditions are present.
2. If infusion has been refrigerated, allow it to warm to room temperature.	Intralipid 10% requires refrigeration; Liposyn 10% does not. Infusion of cold IV solutions can decrease the client's body temperature and cause venospasm.
3. Swab face of bottle stopper with alcohol sponge and pierce stopper with IV tubing spike.	Conventional IV sets contain polyvinylchloride, which contains diethyl hexyl phthalate. If possible, infuse lipids through a non-diethyl hexyl phthalate tubing (this is supplied with infusion set).
4. Prime and clamp tubing. Connect to drip controller. **5.** Connect bottle to one side of "Y" infusion or directly to IV cannula.	*Alternative method:* Obtain premixed three-in-one admixture from pharmacy. Prime the IV tubing with solution and connect it directly to the RA catheter. Infuse the admixture using an IV controller. Set the rate according to the physician's orders. *Alternative method:* Prime the IV tubing with lipid emulsion and connect it to the smaller lumen of the double-lumen RA catheter. Infuse the lipid emulsion concurrently with TPN.
6. Release clamp and set drip controller to deliver 1 ml/minute for first 15 minutes to 30 minutes of infusion.	Observe for the following early adverse reactions and report them to the physician: dyspnea, allergic reactions, nausea, flushing, sleepiness, chest or back pain, or local irritation at the infusion site.

7. If no adverse reactions occur, increase rate of infusion to 500 ml/4 hours for Intralipid and 500 ml/4 hours to 6 hours for Liposyn.

8. When infusion is complete, disconnect lipid tubing and continue regular IV solution with fresh tubing.

The usual daily rate is 2.5 g/kg for Intralipid and 3 g/kg for Liposyn.

RELATED NURSING CARE

NURSING ACTIONS	RATIONALE/AMPLIFICATION
1. Begin infusion of fat emulsions immediately after early morning blood samples are drawn.	Laboratory tests that are performed on blood drawn within 4 hours to 6 hours of the infusion may be altered because lipids have not been removed from the blood.
2. Decrease infusion rate or infuse lipids at night if client complains of unpleasant taste in mouth.	Emulsions containing safflower oil appear to have a less unpleasant taste than do those containing soybean oil. Changing the type of solution may eliminate the problem.

EVALUATION PHASE

ANTICIPATED OUTCOMES	NURSING ACTIONS
1. Establishment of lipid therapy in which IV lipids provide no more than 60% of total caloric intake	Monitor the total nutritional program.
2. Prevention of complications related to lipid therapy or to contamination	Evaluate for the following side-effects:
	a. Early reactions, such as hyperlipemia and coagulation problems
	b. Delayed reactions, such as liver or spleen problems, blood dyscrasias, or overload syndrome (fever, focal seizures, leukocytosis, spleen enlargement, shock)
	Monitor laboratory work as ordered by the physician, including serum triglycerides, liver function tests, plasma-free fatty acids, and blood coagulation studies.
	Evaluate for temperature elevation, thrombophlebitis caused by concurrent infusion of hypertonic solutions, infection of IV site, and clearance of fat from the blood within 6 hours. (Serum samples will be cloudy if fat is not cleared.)

PRODUCT AVAILABILITY

LIPID SOLUTIONS (10% AND 20%)

Abbott Laboratories
Cutter Laboratories Inc.

ADMIXTURE SYSTEMS (THREE-IN-ONE)

Travenol Laboratories, Inc.

SELECTED REFERENCES

Hutchison M McG: Administration of fat emulsions. Am J Nurs 82:2:275–277, 1982
Metheny NM, Snively WD: Nurses' Handbook of Fluid Balance, 4th ed. Philadelphia, JB Lippincott, 1983

IV

Respiratory techniques

19 *Airway management*

A patent airway is a prerequisite for sustaining life, and it is necessary for all respiratory care procedures. In performing client care, the health-care provider must not only be able to recognize the signs of both partial and complete airway obstruction, but must also be prepared to choose the best techniques to obtain and maintain an open, unobstructed airway.

Partial airway obstruction can usually be identified by noisy respirations. A snoring sound indicates possible obstruction of the airway by the tongue and can be remedied quickly by hyperextending the neck, displacing the mandible forward, or by inserting an oropharyngeal airway. A crowing sound on inspiration can be caused by epiglottitis, laryngotracheobronchitis, or postextubation edema. Treatment of these signs should include a combination of oxygen with aerosol and the administration of an aerosol decongestant, such as racemic epinephrine. In cases of postextubation edema, reintubation of the trachea may be necessary. Excess secretions produce rales over the affected area and require removal by endotracheal suctioning. All instances of partial airway obstruction may also be accompanied by retractions.

Although partial airway obstruction is potentially fatal because of hypoxia and hypercapnia, death resulting from complete airway obstruction is certain and rapid. Complete airway obstruction is characterized by the lack of air movement and the presence of supraclavicular and intercostal retractions. It requires immediate action by the health-care provider. In these situations, a patent airway must be established and manual or mechanical ventilation initiated if the client is apneic. Endotracheal intubation with manual ventilation is the best course of action, because it provides a patent upper airway and gives an indication of the patency of the lower airways. If time does not permit endotracheal intubation, an esophageal obturator airway (EOA) may be used as a temporary means of providing manual ventilation. The EOA, when properly inserted into the esophagus, prevents air from entering the stomach and allows lung ventilation through a series of small holes in the portion of the tube that is located in the upper airway. Endotracheal intubation should be performed as soon as possible and before the EOA is removed. If the client's condition requires long-term artificial airway placement, a tracheostomy should be performed, placing the airway into the trachea through a surgical incision.

Once an artificial airway has been inserted, the task of airway management has just begun. Meticulous care must be provided to ensure that the airway remains patent. Because the intubated client is unable to generate an effective cough, it is necessary to remove secretions by endotracheal suctioning. This procedure must be carried out under aseptic conditions to prevent iatrogenic infections. Placing an artificial airway also bypasses the normal humidification and filtering processes of the upper airway. To prevent a humidity deficit, which can dry mucous membranes and make secretions difficult to remove, inspired gases should be warmed and humidified with aerosol. Frequent changes in the client's position are also necessary. This maneuver aids in the draining of pulmonary secretions and facilitates their removal.

Many intubated clients also require some degree of mechanical ventilation. This presents the health-care provider with a new, more complex set of parameters to be measured, recorded, and evaluated.

While the instrumentation of airway management is important and, at times, lifesaving, the role of the health-care provider as observer must be emphasized. Observing and assessing the client for early signs of airway obstruction and respiratory failure are the best forms of airway management.

Blind endotracheal (nasotracheal) suctioning

Objective
To clear secretions from the trachea by aspiration

ASSESSMENT PHASE
- Does the client need to be suctioned? Listen to the client's breath sounds with a stethoscope. Can gurgling or coarse expiratory rales be heard?
- Is the client attempting to cough up secretions? If so, are these attempts successful, or does the client appear to choke on the secretions?

PRECAUTIONS
- **Use sterile technique along with sterile gloves and a sterile catheter to reduce the risk of infection.**
- **Because suctioning removes not only secretions but also air, time the suctioning procedure to avoid hypoxia (maximum time is 10 seconds to 15 seconds).**
- **The suction catheter should be large enough to easily remove secretions, but should be small enough to be easily inserted into the naris.**
- **Continuous repeated suctioning may produce tracheal irritation and coughing. Uninterrupted suctioning may damage the tracheal mucosa and is indicated by blood-streaked aspirate.**
- **Observe the cardiac pattern, if possible, for arrhythmias. Prolonged suctioning or repeated insertion of the suction catheter may produce vagal stimulation, which can cause profound bradycardia.**

PLANNING PHASE

EQUIPMENT
Stethoscope
Oxygen administration equipment
Vacuum source and connecting tube
Sterile suction catheter
Sterile gloves
Sterile, water-soluble lubricating gel
Disposable open container filled with sterile water
Unit-dose container (3 ml) of normal saline or 6-ml syringe filled with normal saline (remove needle)

CLIENT/FAMILY TEACHING
- Describe the purpose of the procedure.
- Explain the procedure, including what the client must do.
- Describe the expected sensations (*e.g.*, gagging and feeling short of breath).

IMPLEMENTATION PHASE

NURSING ACTIONS	RATIONALE/AMPLIFICATION
1. Explain procedure to client.	Because the procedure will require the cooperation of conscious clients, it is necessary that they understand procedure.
2. Place bedside table or other suitable tray within easy reach of client's bed.	Supplies should be readily available and within easy reach when suctioning.

3. Place supplies listed for suctioning on bedside table.

4. Check operation of vacuum source, regulator, and suction trap (bottle) to ensure correct operation.

A 6-ml syringe filled with sterile normal saline may be used in place of the unit-dose vial of saline.

Readjustment of the suction source may not be possible without contaminating your gloves or the catheter. Suction should not be set lower than −120 cm water pressure (cm H_2O) for adult client and not lower than −60 cm H_2O for the pediatric client.

5. Wash your hands with disinfectant soap.

Handwashing reduces the risk of iatrogenic infections.

6. Preoxygenate client using oxygen mask to increase client's fractional concentration of inspired oxygen (F_IO_2).

Preoxygenation decreases the possibility of hypoxia during the suctioning procedure.

7. Place client in sitting position.

8. Glove both of your hands, keeping one hand and catheter sterile.

The use of sterile gloves prevents the transmission of infection to the nurse.

9. Lubricate catheter tip.

Lubrication of the tip facilitates passage of the catheter through the naris and nasal passages.

10. Insert catheter into naris with slightly downward slant.

Inserting the catheter straight back or with an upward slant may damage nasal mucosa.

11. Advance catheter slowly, stopping at any sign of obstruction.

Slow advancement of the catheter avoids damage to nasal mucosa and turbinate bones. It may be necessary to use the other naris.

12. With catheter in oropharynx (this will usually stimulate gag reflex), ask client to take slow deep breath.

A deep breath causes retraction of the epiglottis and allows the catheter to pass through the vocal cords and into the trachea.

13. Instruct client to continue to take slow deep breaths through mouth.

Slow deep mouth breathing reduces the gag reflex and the feeling of suffocation.

14. Slowly advance catheter as far as possible *without applying suction*. Withdraw $\frac{1}{2}$ inch to 1 inch (1 cm to 2 cm).

This should place catheter tip just above carina level.

15. Withdraw catheter slowly, rotating it between your thumb and forefinger. Apply *intermittent* suction.

Rotation of the catheter prevents the catheter tip from adhering to the tracheal wall, causing mucosal damage.

16. If secretions are particularly thick, instill 5 ml to 10 ml 0.9% saline through catheter.

Saline dilutes and thins the secretions, facilitating removal of the catheter.

17. Apply suction for *10 seconds to 15 seconds only.*

Suctioning for only short periods at a time reduces the possibility of hypoxia.

18. Reoxygenate and allow client to rest before repeating procedure.

This allows oxygenation to return to normal.

19. If procedure will not be repeated, return client's F_IO_2 to previous setting.

20. When procedure is completed, discard gloves, catheter, and other materials.

Discarding of used materials minimizes contamination of the client area.

RELATED NURSING CARE

NURSING ACTIONS	RATIONALE/AMPLIFICATION
1. Auscultate client's chest frequently.	Evaluate the need for endotracheal suctioning to avoid *unnecessary* suctioning and related complications.
2. Encourage client to take deep breaths and cough.	Deep breaths and coughing help to clear excess secretions.

3. Ensure adequate hydration.

Hydration may be accomplished by administering fluids by aerosol, IV infusion, or orally. Adequate fluid intake helps to thin secretions.

4. Encourage ambulation.

5. Assist client in making frequent position changes and incorporate chest physiotherapy (see Chest Drainage in Chap. 22).

Changes in the client's position and chest physiotherapy utilize gravity to drain excess secretions.

EVALUATION PHASE

ANTICIPATED OUTCOMES	NURSING ACTIONS
1. Maintenance of patent airway	A patent airway can be maintained by auscultating the client's chest. Observe the client for signs of an obstructed airway.
2. Prevention of atelectasis	Auscultation of the client's chest and suctioning as necessary prevent atelectasis.
3. Reduction of risk of secondary infections	Removal of excess secretions that promote bacterial growth and infection reduces the risk of secondary infection. If the secretions increase, a bacterial infection may have developed. Notify the physician and request a culture of secretions.

PRODUCT AVAILABILITY

SUCTION CATHETERS

Argyle Division, Sherwood Medical
Portex, Inc.
Travenol Laboratories, Inc.—Medical Products Division

SELECTED REFERENCES

Fuchs PL: Streamlining your suctioning techniques, Part 1, NT Suctioning. Nursing '84 14(5):55–61
Hamilton H: Procedures. Springhouse, PA, Intermed Communications, Inc., 1983
Millar S: Methods in Critical Care, The AACN Manual. Philadelphia, WB Saunders, 1980

Morrison M: Respiratory Intensive Care Nursing, 2nd ed. Boston, Little Brown, 1979
Young CS: A Review of the adverse effects of airway suctioning. Physiotherapy 70(3):104–106, 1984

Insertion of esophageal obturator airway or esophageal gastric tube airway

Objectives
To provide an emergency method of ventilation by personnel who lack training or experience in endotracheal intubation techniques
To prevent aspiration of stomach contents in an unconscious client

ASSESSMENT PHASE

• Is the client apneic?
• Is the client unresponsive?
• Can orotracheal intubation be performed within a reasonable amount of time?
• Does the client require mechanical ventilation?

PRECAUTIONS

• **Use of EOAs is recommended only in the apneic and unresponsive adult (over age 16).**
• **EOAs should be used only as a means of providing emergency airway maintenance. If the client needs mechanical ventilation, tracheal intubation should be performed as soon as possible.**

- **Reduce the risk of esophageal trauma or rupture by avoiding the use of EOAs in clients who have preexisting esophageal pathology.**
- **Do not force the EOA during insertion. If the EOA does not pass easily into the esophagus, stop the procedure and ventilate the client with a manual resuscitator and face mask.**

PLANNING PHASE

EQUIPMENT

EOA or esophageal gastric tube airway (EGTA, Fig. 19–1)
50-ml syringe
Gastric tube (if using EGTA)
Manual resuscitator with 100% oxygen source
Stethoscope

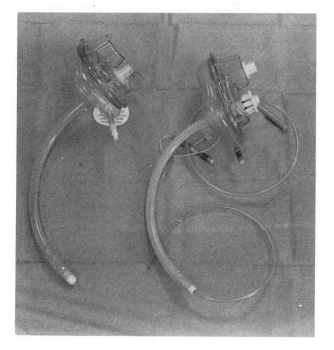

Fig. 19–1 Esophageal obturator airway *(left)* and esophageal (gastric tube) airway *(right)* with masks attached.

CLIENT/FAMILY TEACHING

- Provide emotional support for the family if an emergency situation exists. Provide realistic reports of the client's progress.
- Explain to the family the purpose of the EOA/EGTA.
- Inform the family of the possibility that mechanical ventilation will be required.

IMPLEMENTATION PHASE

NURSING ACTIONS	RATIONALE/AMPLIFICATION
1. Ventilate client with manual resuscitator and oxygen until EOA is ready for insertion.	The use of a manual resuscitator and oxygen maintains adequate ventilation and allows for assessment of the patency of the upper airway.
2. Check equipment.	
a. Inflate cuff on EOA, checking for even inflation and leaks.	
b. If EOA mask has inflatable seal, inflate seal and check for leaks.	
3. Place client's neck in neutral position. Remove dentures if applicable.	Hyperextension of the client's neck may cause the EOA tube to enter the trachea.

Fig. 19–2 Crossed-finger technique for opening mouth.

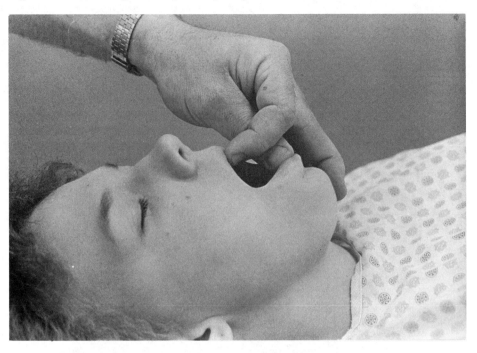

4. Open client's mouth using crossed-finger technique (Fig. 19–2).

5. Lift client's tongue and jaw by inserting thumb at base of tongue and placing two fingers on jaw and lifting straight upward.

6. Insert EOA into client's mouth. Slide over tongue into posterior pharynx.

7. Advance tube into proper position in esophagus.

If resistance is encountered, withdraw the tube slightly and readvance it. *Caution:* Do not use excessive force.

8. Advance tube until mask is tightly sealed on client's face.

A tight seal is necessary to perform ventilation with the manual resuscitator.

9. Holding mask firmly in place, ventilate client with manual resuscitator. Check for chest excursion and auscultate chest sounds.

A lack of chest excursion and breath sounds across the lung fields, along with gastric distention, indicates that the EOA has been placed in the trachea. If this occurs, remove the EOA and ventilate the client for several breaths with the manual resuscitator and face mask before attempting to reinsert the EOA.

10. Once EOA is properly positioned, inflate cuff just until seal is created.

Sealing of the esophagus allows ventilation and protects the trachea.

11. Ventilate client with manual resuscitator and oxygen at rate of approximately 12 breaths per minute.

RELATED NURSING CARE

NURSING ACTIONS	RATIONALE/AMPLIFICATION
1. Monitor chest sounds and excursion for length of ventilation.	Monitoring chest sounds and excursion ensures that proper tube position is maintained.

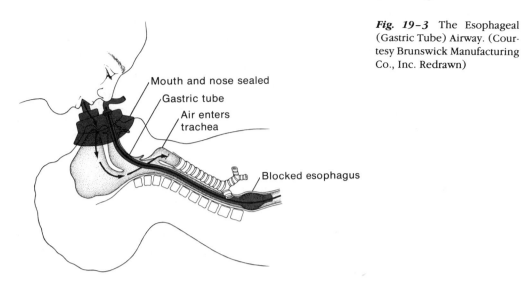

Fig. 19-3 The Esophageal (Gastric Tube) Airway. (Courtesy Brunswick Manufacturing Co., Inc. Redrawn)

Mouth and nose sealed
Gastric tube
Air enters trachea
Blocked esophagus

2. If EGTA is used, insert gastric tube into proper port on face mask (Fig. 19–3).

The gastric tube permits stomach contents to be removed, decreasing the chance of aspiration, and allows for the removal of any air that may have been introduced into the stomach during ventilation with the manual resuscitator.

EVALUATION PHASE

ANTICIPATED OUTCOMES	NURSING ACTIONS
1. Maintenance of temporary emergency airway	Maintain a temporary airway until the EOA can be safely removed or replaced with an endotracheal or tracheostomy tube.
2. Prevention of complications of EOA	Observe chest excursion and listen for bilateral breath sounds to determine correct placement of the EOA.

PRODUCT AVAILABILITY

ESOPHAGEAL OBTURATOR AIRWAYS

Argyle Division, Sherwood Medical
Armstrong Industries, Inc.

SELECTED REFERENCES

Hamilton H: Procedures. Springhouse PA, Intermed Communications, Inc., 1983
McPherson SP: Respiratory Therapy Equipment, 3rd ed. St. Louis, CV Mosby 1985

Millar S: Methods in Critical Care, the AACN Manual. Philadelphia, WB Saunders, 1980

Removal of esophageal obturator airway or esophageal gastric tube airway

Objectives
To remove the EOA when an artificial airway is no longer needed, or to provide a permanent method of airway management by endotracheal intubation

ASSESSMENT PHASE

• Is the client breathing spontaneously, or will the client need endotracheal intubation to maintain a patent airway after EOA removal? If the client is not breathing spontaneously, or if respirations are labored, endotracheal intubation is indicated.

- Will the client require supplemental oxygen/aerosol therapy after EOA removal? If the client will be intubated, aerosol is necessary to provide for adequate airway humidification. If the client will not be intubated, supplemental oxygen therapy may be provided by means of a nasal cannula or a medium-concentration mask and a proper humidification device.
- Will the client require mechanical ventilation after EOA removal and endotracheal intubation? Mechanical ventilation is indicated if the client is apneic or if normal arterial blood gas (ABG) values cannot be maintained with spontaneous ventilation.

PRECAUTIONS

- **Have suction equipment ready in the event of regurgitation when the EOA is removed.**
- **If indicated, intubate the client before removing the EOA.**
- **EOA removal should never be performed by a care-giver who does not possess the skills needed to perform endotracheal intubation.**

PLANNING PHASE

EQUIPMENT

Suction equipment
Intubation equipment
Oxygen administration equipment with a nasal cannula or a medium-concentration mask (use if the client will not be intubated)
Oxygen/aerosol equipment with Brigg's adapter (T tube) (use if the client will be intubated but will not require mechanical ventilation)
Ventilator (use if the client requires mechanical ventilation)

CLIENT/FAMILY TEACHING

- Discuss plans for future airway management with the client, if appropriate, and family.

IMPLEMENTATION PHASE

NURSING ACTIONS	RATIONALE/AMPLIFICATION
1. Wash your hands with appropriate antimicrobial solution.	Handwashing decreases the possibility of contamination.
2. If EOA has gastric tube, use gastric tube to suction stomach contents.	Suctioning of the stomach contents decreases the possibility of regurgitation after EOA removal.
3. Remove EOA mask.	
4. Suction client's mouth and oropharynx with EOA in place.	Suctioning of the client's mouth and oropharynx prevents obstruction of the airway by secretions.
If endotracheal intubation *is* indicated, complete steps 5, 6, and 7. If endotracheal intubation is *NOT* indicated, go to step 8.	
5. Prepare oral endotracheal intubation equipment.	
6. Perform endotracheal intubation with EOA in place (Fig. 19–4).	Placement of the endotracheal tube before EOA removal ensures airway maintenance.
7. Inflate cuff of endotracheal tube with EOA in place.	Inflation of the cuff seals the airway to prevent aspiration in the event of regurgitation.
8. Deflate EOA cuff.	
9. Remove EOA.	
10. Place client on oxygen or ventilator as appropriate.	
11. If appropriate, check endotracheal tube placement by auscultating client's chest.	

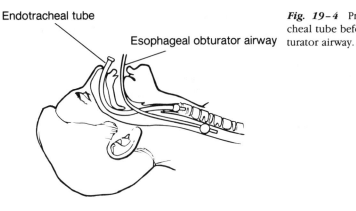

Endotracheal tube

Esophageal obturator airway

Fig. 19-4 Proper positioning of endotracheal tube before removal of esophageal obturator airway.

RELATED NURSING CARE

NURSING ACTION	RATIONALE/AMPLIFICATION
Observe client for signs of respiratory distress	Complete the following procedures if indicated: **a.** Administration of supplemental oxygen **b.** Nasotracheal suctioning **c.** Endotracheal intubation **d.** Mechanical ventilation

EVALUATION PHASE

ANTICIPATED OUTCOME	NURSING ACTIONS
Successful removal of EOA/EGTA	Prevent regurgitation and aspiration of the stomach contents by preparing the gastric tube and testing the vacuum source before removal of the EOA/EGTA. Prepare the intubation equipment.

SELECTED REFERENCES   Hamilton H: Procedures. Springhouse, PA, Intermed Communications, Inc., 1983   Millar S: Methods in Critical Care, The AACN Manual. Philadelphia, WB Saunders, 1980

Oropharyngeal airway insertion

Objectives
To provide short-term maintenance of a patent airway by inserting an oropharyngeal airway, which will prevent the tongue from blocking the upper airway
To prevent damage to the tongue and soft tissue of the mouth by utilizing an oropharyngeal airway as a bite-block

ASSESSMENT PHASE
- Are signs of upper airway obstruction by the tongue present (*i.e.*, does the client's breathing produce snoring sounds)?
- Can the client be maintained in a side-lying position or with neck hyperextension for general nursing care?
- Is the client having seizures and in danger of biting the tongue?

PRECAUTIONS
- **Select an oropharyngeal airway that is the proper size for the client. If the oropharyngeal airway is too large, it may actually cause airway obstruc-**

tion. If the oropharyngeal airway is too small, it will not hold the tongue in the proper position.
- Once the airway is in position, tape it in place. An airway that becomes dislodged could cause airway obstruction.
- Maintain neck hyperextension or place the client in a side-lying position.

PLANNING PHASE

EQUIPMENT

Oropharyngeal airway (use proper size for client)
Tongue depressor

IMPLEMENTATION PHASE

NURSING ACTIONS	RATIONALE/AMPLIFICATION
1. Place client supine with head tilted backward.	Tilt the client's head to displace the tongue anteriorly and to allow for passage and proper placement of the airway.
2. Wash your hands with appropriate antimicrobial solution.	Handwashing decreases the possibility of contamination.
3. Open client's mouth using crossed-finger technique or tongue depressor and insert airway into side of mouth.	This ensures that the tip of the airway is in proper position on the posterior portion of the tongue.
4. Rotate airway into place.	Rotation of the airway allows for proper insertion and placement with minimum trauma.
5. Check for correct placement of airway.	When it is correctly placed, an oropharyngeal airway displaces the tongue anteriorly and allows the client to breathe around the airway.
6. Tape airway in place.	Taping the airway in place prevents it from becoming dislodged.

RELATED NURSING CARE

NURSING ACTIONS	RATIONALE/AMPLIFICATION
1. Place client in side-lying position.	A side-lying position eliminates the possibility of the tongue blocking the airway.
2. Rotate client to opposite side every hour.	Changing the client's position prevents pooling of secretions and pressure necrosis.
3. Replace oropharyngeal airway every 24 hours.	Replace the airway to prevent the buildup of secretions on the airway and to reduce the risk of iatrogenic infection.

EVALUATION PHASE

ANTICIPATED OUTCOME	NURSING ACTION
Maintenance of patent airway	Reposition the oropharyngeal airway if the client shows signs of dyspnea or develops snoring or inspiratory crowing sounds.

PRODUCT AVAILABILITY

OROPHARYNGEAL AIRWAYS

Hudson Oxygen
Ohmeda
Puritan – Bennett Corporation

SELECTED REFERENCES   McPherson SP: Respiratory Therapy Equipment,   Morrison M: Respiratory Intensive Care Nursing,
3rd ed. St. Louis, CV Mosby, 1985   2nd ed. Boston, Little, Brown, 1979

Endotracheal intubation

Objective

To insert an endotracheal tube into the trachea to provide a patent airway for ventilatory support or to manage secretions

ASSESSMENT PHASE

- Does the client require intubation? Why is intubation being considered?
- Based on time considerations and on the condition of the client, should nasal or oral intubation be attempted?
- Will the client need mechanical ventilation after intubation?

PRECAUTIONS

- **Avoid damage to the client's teeth and soft tissue, which can be caused by improper use of the laryngoscope and tubes or by unnecessary force during the procedure.**
- **Ensure the availability of an oxygen source. Ventilate the client with a manual resuscitator using 100% oxygen if intubation cannot be accomplished within a reasonable period.**
- **Have suction equipment set up and operable at the client's bedside before performing the procedure.**
- **Avoid bronchial intubation (which most often occurs when the tube is inserted into the right main stem bronchus) by correctly positioning the endotracheal tube above the level of the carina.**
- **Be alert for signs of esophageal intubation. These signs include abdominal distention, belching, and lack of breath sounds in the lung fields after intubation.**

PLANNING PHASE

EQUIPMENT (FIG. 19–5)

Endotracheal tubes with low-pressure cuffs in various sizes (most common sizes for adult client range from 5 mm to 9 mm, inside diameter)
Laryngoscope handle and several sizes of both curved and straight blades
Topical anesthetic spray and sedative (if ordered)
Water-soluble anesthetic lubricating jelly
Flexible stylet
Forceps (for nasal intubation)
10-ml syringe
Oral airway or bite-block
Tape, benzoin tincture, and alcohol swabs
Suction equipment
Manual resuscitator with oxygen source

CLIENT/FAMILY TEACHING

- If the client is conscious, explain the need for endotracheal intubation and explain the procedure.
- Explain sensations that may be experienced during the procedure (*e.g.,* gagging and a feeling of suffocation).
- Explain the need for endotracheal intubation and explain the procedure to the family.

IMPLEMENTATION PHASE

NURSING ACTIONS	RATIONALE/AMPLIFICATION
1. Ensure that client is properly oxygenated using manual resuscitator with 100% oxygen.	Proper oxygenation prevents hypoxia before the intubation procedure.

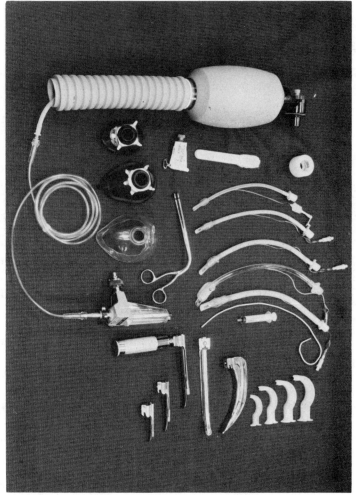

Fig. 19–5 Equipment used for endotracheal intubation.

2. Administer medications as ordered.

3. Check equipment.

Checking the equipment reduces the risk of equipment malfunction.

    a. Use syringe to inflate tube cuff. Check for uniform inflation and leaks before use.

    b. Check laryngoscope batteries and light by attaching proper-sized blade.

4. If using stylet, lubricate entire length and insert into endotracheal tube. Make sure tip of stylet does not extend beyond tip of endotracheal tube.

Lubrication of the tube facilitates removal of the stylet after intubation. Keep the tip of the stylet within the endotracheal tube to prevent trauma to the vocal cords and mucosal tissue.

5. Remove client's dentures or partial plates if applicable.

Removal of dentures prevents damage to dental prostheses and prevents them from obstructing the airway.

6. Hyperextend client's neck or place client's head in brandy-sniffing position (Fig. 19–6).

This places pharynx, larynx, and trachea in a straight line.

7. Open client's mouth using crossed-finger technique if necessary. Spray posterior pharynx with topical anesthetic. Suction mouth and pharynx if necessary.

A topical anesthetic prevents the gag reflex and reduces discomfort during the procedure. Suctioning clears the upper airway of secretions.

8. Hold laryngoscope in left hand. Insert blade into right side of client's mouth, moving to center of mouth to displace tongue.

Insert the blade into the right side of the client's mouth to facilitate visualization of the epiglottis. (Right-handed larynogoscopes are available.) Whenever possi-

Fig. 19–6 Positions used for endotracheal intubation. (*A*) Neck hyperextension position. (*B*) "Brandy-sniffing" position.

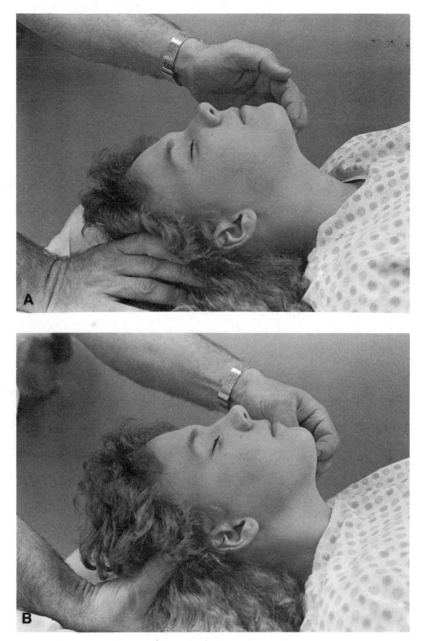

ble, the laryngoscope should be held in the nondominant hand.

9. Advance blade until epiglottis is visualized. If straight blade is used, advance blade past epiglottis. If curved blade is used, position tip of blade anterior to epiglottis in the vallecula (Fig. 19–7*A*).

10. Lift laryngoscope to a 45-degree angle. *Caution:* Do not use teeth as pivot.

Lifting the laryngoscope exposes the vocal cords and the larynx. Pressure on the client's teeth may cause tooth loss or damage.

11. If oral intubation will be used, insert endotracheal tube through mouth into larynx between vocal cords. Advance tube until cuff disappears behind vocal cords

Do not use the stylet if nasal intubation is being used.

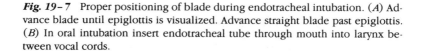

Fig. 19-7 Proper positioning of blade during endotracheal intubation. (*A*) Advance blade until epiglottis is visualized. Advance straight blade past epiglottis. (*B*) In oral intubation insert endotracheal tube through mouth into larynx between vocal cords.

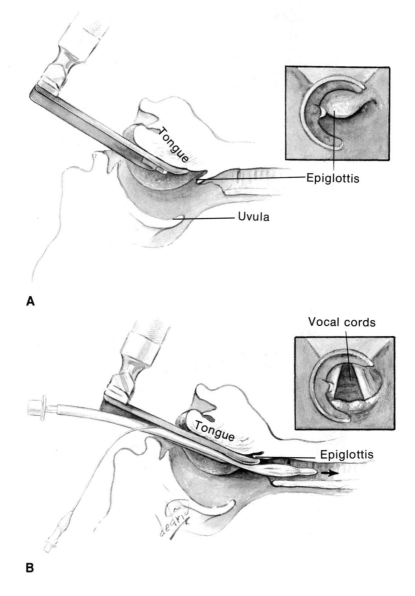

(Fig. 19-7*B*). If nasal intubation will be used, insert endotracheal tube through naris into pharynx. Forceps may now be used to guide tube between vocal cords and into larynx. Advance tube until cuff disappears behind vocal cords.

12. Holding tube in place, remove stylet, if used, and inflate cuff.

13. Ventilate client with manual resuscitator and 100% oxygen. Auscultate chest during ventilation. Suction endotracheal tube if necessary.

Ventilation of the client allows you to check the placement of the endotracheal tube. Bilateral breath sounds indicate proper placement. If bilateral breath sounds are not present, deflate the cuff, withdraw the tube 2 cm to 3 cm (approximately 1 inch), and auscultate again.

14. Secure tube with adhesive tape. Before applying tape, wipe client's cheeks with alcohol and benzoin.

15. Obtain chest film.	A chest film shows the actual position of the tube. The tip of the endotracheal tube should be 2 cm to 4 cm (1 inch to 1½ inches) above the carina.
16. Connect client to oxygen/aerosol using Brigg's adapter (T tube) or to mechanical ventilator.	
17. Check cuff inflation using pneumometer (see Fig. 19–14). Pressure should not exceed 25 cm H_2O. Record pressure and volume of air required to maintain seal.	Monitoring the pressure of the cuff minimizes damage to tracheal mucosa caused by excessive pressures.

RELATED NURSING CARE   See following section on Cuffed Tube Management.

EVALUATION PHASE   See following section on Cuffed Tube Management.

PRODUCT AVAILABILITY   ENDOTRACHEAL TUBES

Ohmeda
Portex, Inc.
Shiley, Inc.

LARYNGOSCOPES AND ACCESSORIES

AO Scientific Instruments
Fraser Harlake Inc.
Ohmeda
Puritan–Bennett Corporation
Welch Allyn

SELECTED REFERENCES   Burton GG, Hodgkin JE: Respiratory Care, 2nd ed. Philadelphia, JB Lippincott, 1984
McPherson SP: Respiratory Therapy Equipment, 3rd ed. St. Louis, CV Mosby, 1985
Millar S: Methods in Critical Care, Then AACN Manual. Philadelphia, WB Saunders, 1980

Shapiro BA, Harrison RA, Trout CA: Clinical Application of Respiratory Care, 2nd ed. Chicago, Year Book Medical Publishers, Inc., 1979

Endotracheal suction with airway in situ

Objective
To provide suction with an artificial airway, using sterile technique to clear secretions from the trachea and the airway

ASSESSMENT PHASE
• Is the client receiving supplemental oxygen, or are the client's respirations being supported by mechanical ventilation?
• Does the client need suctioning? Listen to the client's breath sounds with a stethoscope. Can gurgling or coarse expiratory rales be heard?
• Does the client appear to choke because of secretions? Are respirations labored, with episodes of forced expiratory maneuvers used for coughing? (Remember that a client cannot cough effectively with an artificial airway in place.)

PRECAUTIONS
• **Suctioning not only removes secretions but also removes air from the lower airways. Never suction continuously for more than 15 seconds because severe hypoxemia may occur.**
• **Prolonged suctioning or repeated insertion of the suction catheter may produce vagal simulation, which can cause profound bradycardia.**
• **Continuous repeated suctioning may produce tracheal irritation and coughing. Uninterrupted suctioning may produce damage to the tracheal mucosa and is indicated by blood-streaked aspirate.**

- The suction catheter should be of adequate size to remove secretions, but it should not so large that it obstructs the airway to be suctioned.
- Sterile technique should be used along with sterile gloves and a sterile suction catheter. Sterile technique is necessary to reduce the risk of iatrogenic infection of the airway.

PLANNING PHASE

EQUIPMENT

Sterile suction catheter
Sterile glove(s)
Water-soluble lubricant
Vacuum source and connecting tube
Disposable open container filled with sterile water
Unit-dose container (3 ml) of normal saline or 6-ml syringe filled with normal saline
Stethoscope
Oxygen source and equipment to raise client's inspired oxygen (if needed)

CLIENT/FAMILY TEACHING

- In some instances the client may not be alert when suctioning is required. In such cases, suction the client as needed. If the client appears alert or conscious, explain the procedure to reduce anxiety or fear. If there is a question about the client's level of consciousness, explain the procedure.
- Discuss the reason for suctioning through an artificial airway (to remove secretions accumulating in the trachea and bronchi).
- Describe the procedure and possible sensations, such as choking when the suction catheter is passed through the artificial airway into the trachea.
- Encourage the client to take deep breaths during the suctioning procedure to reduce the effects of the removal of air from the respiratory airways.

IMPLEMENTATION PHASE

NURSING ACTIONS	RATIONALE/AMPLIFICATION
1. Place bedside table or other suitable tray within easy reach of client's bed.	Supplies should be readily available and within easy reach when suctioning.
2. Place supplies listed for suctioning on bedside table.	A 6-ml syringe filled with sterile normal saline may be used in place of the unit-dose vials of saline.
3. Check vacuum source, regulator, and suction trap (bottle) to ensure correct operation.	Readjustment of the suction source may not be possible without contaminating your gloves or the catheter. Suction should not be set lower than -120 cm H_2O for an adult (-60 cm H_2O to -80 cm H_2O for pediatric clients).
4. Wash your hands with disinfectant soap to reduce risk of iatrogenic infections.	
5. If client is receiving supplemental oxygen, F_1O_2 should be increased. Clients on ventilators should receive sigh ventilations before suctioning. Clients who are able to take deep breaths should be instructed to do so. Clients unable to take deep breaths can be ventilated with bag and mask resuscitator to increase alveolar oxygen levels.	Suctioning removes gas from the respiratory airways, producing hypoxia.
6. Using sterile technique, open suction package, put on sterile gloves, and attach catheter to suction connection tube.	
7. Disconnect client from ventilator or oxygen delivery device and introduce suction catheter (Fig. 19–8).	Do *not* suction while inserting a catheter into an airway. Suction *only* intermittently while removing the catheter. When catheters do not slide easily through an arti-

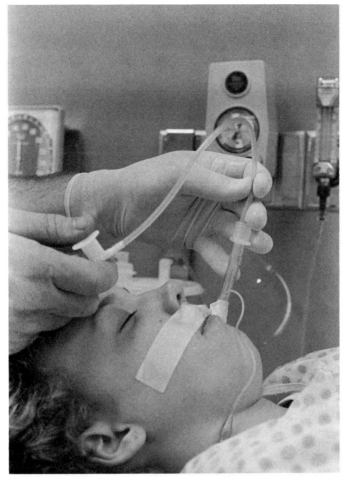

Fig. 19-8 Suctioning client with an endotracheal tube in place.

8. Obstruct suction port intermittently while rotating catheter between your thumb and forefinger as it is removed.

9. Client should be reoxygenated before suctioning is repeated. Suctioning should be repeated until secretions are clear or client shows signs of tiring.

10. If secretions are thick and tenacious, normal saline should be instilled into airway (Fig. 19-9). Hyperventilate and oxygenate client before suctioning. Repeat suctioning procedure.

11. After airway is suctioned, catheter can be rinsed with tap water and then reused to suction oropharynx.

12. Once suctioning is completed, reoxygenate client and return F_IO_2 to previous setting (Fig. 19-10).

13. Correctly dispose of catheter by wrapping it around fingers of gloved hand and pulling glove over catheter. Discard glove in proper waste container. Wash connecting tube with tap water until tube is clear.

14. Note all changes in heart rate, breath sounds, and characteristics of sputum on client's chart.

ficial airway, a sterile water-soluble lubricant can be applied to the lower portion of the catheter.

Because of the construction of some catheters, prolonged suctioning may result in injury to the respiratory mucosa. Suctioning should be intermittent and, in most cases, should last no longer than 15 seconds.

The client should not become hypoxic. Tachycardia is a sign of hypoxia.

Instilling normal saline helps to thin secretions and makes them easy to remove.

High level of oxygen can cause toxic changes to the lung parenchyma.

Proper disposal of contaminated catheters and setups reduces nosocomial infections.

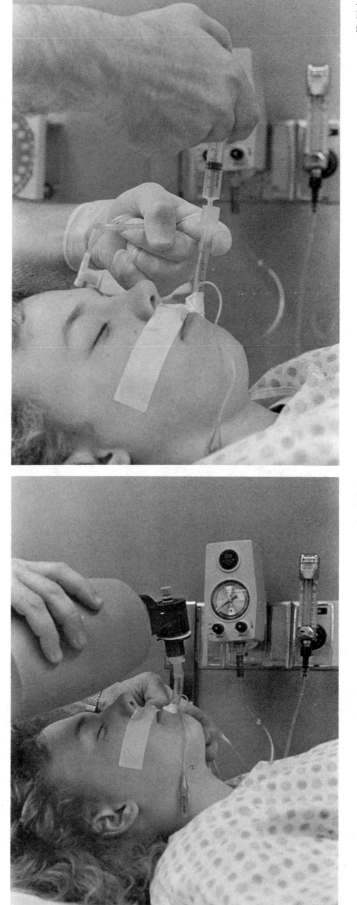

Fig. 19-9 Normal saline may loosen thick secretions for easy removal by suctioning.

Fig. 19-10 Reoxygenating client after suctioning using a manual resuscitator connected to oxygen outlet.

RELATED NURSING CARE

NURSING ACTIONS	RATIONALE/AMPLIFICATION
1. Determine that endotracheal tube is positioned correctly.	Suctioning may dislodge the endotracheal tube from the proper position.
2. See previous section on Blind Endotracheal (Nasotracheal) Suctioning.	

EVALUATION PHASE

ANTICIPATED OUTCOMES	NURSING ACTIONS
See previous section on Blind Endotracheal (Nasotracheal) Suctioning.	

PRODUCT AVAILABILITY

SUCTION CATHETERS

Argyle Division, Sherwood Medical
Ohmeda
Portex, Inc
Travenol Laboratories, Inc.

SELECTED REFERENCES   See previous section on Blind Endotracheal (Nasotracheal) Suctioning.

Assisting with emergency tracheostomy

Objective
To assist the physician in performing a tracheostomy to establish an artificial airway in the client in respiratory distress

ASSESSMENT PHASE

Note: The decision to perform a tracheostomy is made by the physician. Depending on the preferences of the physician, some assessments may have limited applicability.
- Is an endotracheal tube in place, and are the client's respirations being supported by mechanical ventilation?
- Is the client alert or aware of the seriousness of the situation?
- Does the client have spontaneous respirations, or is mechanical ventilation required?
- Is the client's condition stable or rapidly deteriorating?

PRECAUTIONS

- **A tracheostomy is a surgical procedure and must be performed under sterile conditions in all except extreme emergencies. Proper gowns, masks, and sterile equipment will be required to reduce the risk of iatrogenic infections.**
- **Support equipment must be available and in operable condition.**
- **Critical clients must be continuously monitored to detect any change in their condition.**

PLANNING PHASE

EQUIPMENT

Only equipment used in supporting an Emergency tracheostomy is included in this list.
Sterile gloves
Mask and gown
Stethoscope
6-ml syringe

Tracheostomy tubes (different sizes)
Vacuum source, trap, and connecting tube
Suctions kits
Sterile 4 × 4
Tracheostomy-tube ties
Manual resuscitator
Oxygen source and equipment (to raise client's inspired oxygen concentration)
Ventilator (if needed)

CLIENT/FAMILY TEACHING
- Discuss the reason for the tracheostomy with the client and family if possible. In most situations the physician will talk to the client and family. Reinforce the physician's explanation and answer any questions.
- Explain to the client that medications will be used to anesthetize the area around the incision but that some discomfort may be experienced.
- Explain to the client that talking will not be possible when the tracheostomy is in place. (A fenestrated tube is an exception.)
- Describe the need for suctioning of the artificial airway because of the accumulation of secretions.
- Describe the need for humidifying the inspired air whether the client is on a ventilator or ambient oxygen.

IMPLEMENTATION PHASE

NURSING ACTIONS	RATIONALE/AMPLIFICATION
1. Position client supine with neck hyperextended.	
2. Move aerosol tubes, oxygen tubes, or ventilator tubes to position that allows easy access when client's neck is draped.	
3. Place suction equipment within easy access. Check equipment before starting tracheostomy procedure.	Two suction sources will be required: one for airway suction and one for the surgical procedure.
4. Check cuff of tracheostomy tube before insertion.	Inflate the cuff and immerse it in sterile water to check for leaks.
5. Assist physician by suctioning, holding retractors, and providing necessary equipment and tubes while monitoring client's condition and ventilatory status.	
6. Once tracheostomy tube is in place, check ties and dressings around stoma. Assess breath sounds.	
7. If client requires mechanical ventilation, inflate cuff using pneumometer.	The cuff pressure should not exceed 25 cm H_2O.
8. Suction as necessary to remove excess secretions.	

RELATED NURSING CARE   See following section on Cuffed Tube Management.

EVALUATION PHASE

ANTICIPATED OUTCOMES	NURSING ACTIONS
1. See following section on Cuffed Tube Management.	
2. Prevention of complications of emergency tracheostomy	

a. Hemorrhage	Monitor the tracheostomy stoma for bleeding. Notify the physician *immediately* if excessive hemorrhaging is observed. (The tube may have eroded a blood vessel.) Suction the client to maintain a patent airway and prepare suture equipment while waiting for the physician.
b. Infection	Observe sterile technique. Assess the tracheal secretions for signs of infection (*e.g.*, changes in color, amount, and consistency of secretions). Monitor the client's vital signs.

PRODUCT AVAILABILITY

TRACHEOSTOMY TUBES

Argyle Divison, Sherwood Medical
Bivona Surgical Inc.
Olympic Medical
Shiley, Inc.

TRACHEOTOMY KITS

Argyle Division, Sherwood Medical
Oxequip Health Industries

SELECTED REFERENCES

Burton GG, Hodgkin JE: Respiratory Care, 2nd ed. Philadelphia, JB Lippincott, 1984

McPherson SP: Respiratory Therapy Equipment, 3rd ed. St. Louis, CV Mosby, 1985

Tracheostomy care

Objectives

To maintain the patency of a tracheostomy tube by routine cleaning
To reduce the risk of stomal irritation and infection by keeping the wound dry and free of exudate
To correctly secure the tube to prevent trauma and accidental decannulation

ASSESSMENT PHASE

- Is the client alert and able to assist with the care of the tracheostomy tube?
- Are supplemental, ambient oxygen and humidity being provided? Does the client need mechanical ventilation?

PRECAUTIONS

- **Cleaning the tracheostomy tube and stoma requires removal of the ties. Once the ties have been removed, the tracheostomy tube may be easily coughed out. Always support the tracheostomy tube by gently applying pressure to the flange to prevent accidental decannulation when the ties are removed.**
- **Although a sterile field cannot be maintained around a tracheostomy site because of exudate and bronchial secretions, sterile gloves should be used when giving tracheostomy care.**
- **Avoid moving the tracheostomy tube as much as possible to reduce tracheal irritation. Secure all ventilator and aerosol tubes to prevent unnecessary movement of the tracheostomy tube.**
- **If the client requires mechanical ventilation to support respirations, a clean inner cannula should be available to replace the one being cleaned. Avoid prolonged interruption of ventilation, particularly if the client's condition is unstable.**

PLANNING PHASE

EQUIPMENT

Tracheostomy cleaning kit
  Disposable sterile container (for cleaning inner cannula)
  Tracheostomy ties
  Sterile pipe cleaners or small tube brush

Sterile drape
Sterile tracheostomy dressing precut to fit around tube
Hydrogen peroxide
Sterile water
Sterile 4 × 4
Equipment for suctioning
Sterile tracheostomy tube (tape to head of bed for emergency use)

CLIENT/FAMILY TEACHING

- Discuss the reason for keeping the stoma site and tracheostomy tube clean.
- Describe the procedure and possible sensations, such as the feeling of choking when the inner cannula is removed, when the tracheostomy tube is suddenly moved, or when the tracheostomy tube is suctioned.
- If mechanical ventilation is required, reassure the client that disconnection from the ventilator will be minimal.

IMPLEMENTATION PHASE

NURSING ACTIONS	RATIONALE/AMPLIFICATION
1. Place client in semi-Fowler's position.	
2. Assemble tracheostomy kit on bedside table next to client.	
3. Assemble and test suction setup before cleaning tracheostomy site.	
4. Oxygenate client and suction airway and trachea.	
5. Reoxygenate client and remove inner cannula for cleaning (Fig. 19–11).	If the client requires continuous ventilation, insert a second, clean inner cannula into the tracheostomy tube and reconnect the client to the ventilator.

Fig. 19–11   Inner cannula of tracheostomy tube can be removed for cleaning.

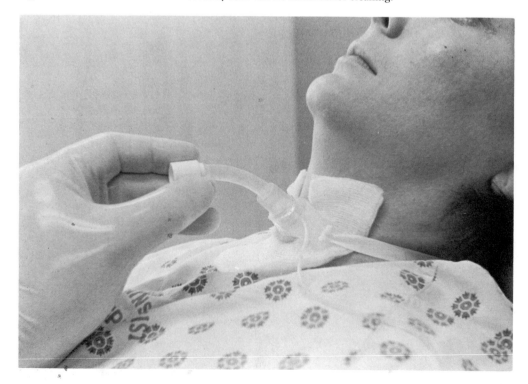

Fig. 19–12 Secretions can be removed from inside inner cannula using small brush supplied in tracheostomy cleaning kit.

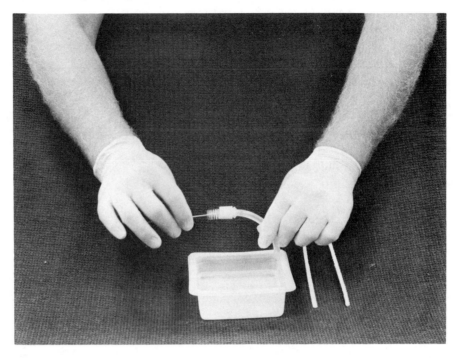

6. Clean inner cannula with 3% hydrogen peroxide using tube brush or pipe cleaners. Inner cannula should be rinsed with sterile water (Fig. 19–12).

7. If second inner cannula was not used, reposition inner cannula in tracheostomy tube. Be sure to lock cannula into correct position.

Rinse the inner cannula with sterile water to remove the hydrogen peroxide. Hydrogen peroxide may irritate the skin if it is not removed.

Fig. 19–13 A sterile dressing is placed around tracheostomy tube to absorb drainage.

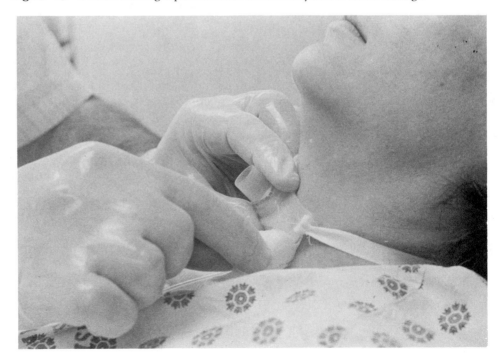

8. Using 4 × 4 soaked in hydrogen peroxide, gently remove dried exudate from stoma. Rinse area with sterile water, and with another dry 4 × 4 gently pat area around stoma until it is dry.

When cleaning around the stoma, note the condition of the skin and signs of inflammation or infection.

9. Unless excessive amounts of exudate are noted around stoma, area should be kept dry and uncovered. If drainage presents problem, place tracheostomy dressing around tracheostomy tube (Fig. 19–13).

The area around the stoma should be dry and open to air. Wet dressings seem to promote infections and the breakdown of tissue.

10. Remove tracheostomy ties and replace them with clean ones. Secure tracheostomy tube by gently applying pressure to flange of tube while ties are being changed. Ties should be knotted to prevent accidental cannulation.

Avoid tying the ties too tight and restricting circulation in the client's neck.

Fig. 19–14   A cuff pneumometer is used to inflate tracheostomy cuff to proper level.

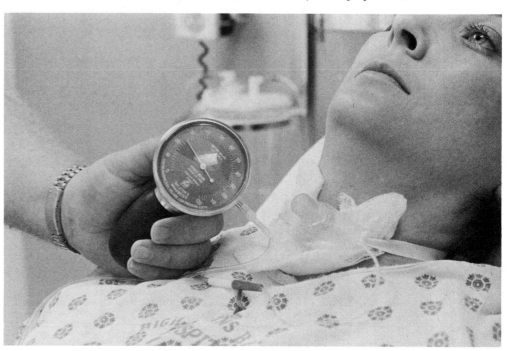

11. If secretions are present in airways after cleaning tube, change gloves and resuction airway with new sterile suction catheter. If cuff is inflated, suction airway, deflate cuff, and resuction airway before reinflating cuff.

Remember to reoxygenate the client before suctioning. If the cuff is deflated, be sure to check the cuff pressure using a cuff pneumometer to avoid over inflating the cuff and possibly causing necrosis of the epithelium of the trachea. Cuff pressure should not exceed 20 cm H_2O to avoid the risk of epithelial necrosis (Fig. 19–14).

RELATED NURSING CARE

NURSING ACTIONS	RATIONALE/AMPLIFICATION
1. Frequently recheck ties to avoid loss of circulation.	There should be enough slack in the ties to allow a finger to be inserted between the tie and the client's neck without discomfort.
2. Routinely check cuff pressure if it is inflated.	Failure to hold pressure may indicate a leaking cuff. Excessive pressure may cause tissue necrosis.

3. Suction as needed.	Suction only when needed, because unnecessary suctioning increases the risk of trauma and iatrogenic infections.

EVALUATION PHASE

ANTICIPATED OUTCOMES	NURSING ACTIONS
1. Prevention of respiratory tract infection	Monitor the amount of secretions. If the secretions become more abundant or if changes are noted, notify the physician. Request a culture of secretions. Monitor the client's vital signs.
2. Prevention of infection at stoma site	Keep the stoma site clean and dry. Note the production of purulent secretions at the stoma sight and notify the physician.
3. Prevention of tube obstruction by secretions	Remove and clean the inner cannula and ensure adequate humidification of inspired gases.

PRODUCT AVAILABILITY   TRACHEOSTOMY CARE KITS

American Hospital Supply Corp.
Argyle Division, Sherwood Medical
Inspiron Corporation
NCC Division, Malinkrodt, Inc.
Superior Plastic Products Co.

SELECTED REFERENCES   Burton GG, Hodgkin JE: Respiratory Care, 2nd ed. Philadelphia, JB Lippincott, 1984
Hamilton H: Procedures. Springhouse, PA, Intermed Communications, Inc. 1983
Millar S: Methods in Critical Care, The AACN Manual. Philadelphia, WB Saunders, 1980

Nelson EJ: Critical Care Respiratory Therapy, A Laboratory and Clinical Manual. Boston, Little, Brown, 1983
Shapiro BA, Harrison RA, Trout CA: Clinical Application of Respiratory Care, 2nd ed. Chicago, Year Book Medical Publishers, Inc., 1979

Accidental tracheostomy decannulation

Objective
To maintain a patent airway when accidental decannulation occurs

ASSESSMENT PHASE   *Note:* This is an emergency procedure and allows only limited assessment.
• Can the client breathe without assistance once the tracheostomy has been displaced?
• Is the airway obstructed, or are secretions causing a problem with gas exchange in the lungs?

PRECAUTIONS
• **Never leave a client unattended if the ties to the tracheostomy tube are removed.**
• **Periodically check the ties to be ensure that the tracheostomy tube is secure.**
• **Have a second sterile tracheostomy tube of equal size or smaller in the client's room.**
• **Keep the obturator to the tracheostomy tube in an accessible area near the bed or in the room.**

PLANNING PHASE
EQUIPMENT
Sterile tracheostomy tube (same size or smaller)
Manual resuscitator and mask with oxygen source
Obturator that will fit existing tracheostomy tube (Fig. 19–15)

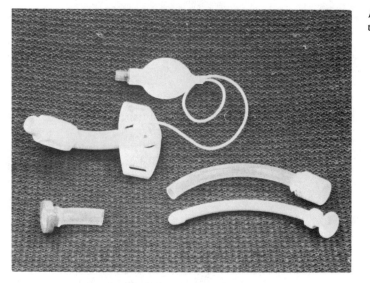

Fig. 19-15 Tracheostomy tube and obturator.

Tracheostomy cleaning kit with suction catheter
Suction equipment

CLIENT/FAMILY TEACHING

- Describe the procedure for reinserting the tracheostomy tube to the client if time permits.
- Instruct the client, if able, to hold the tracheostomy tube in place when coughing to avoid displacing the tube.

IMPLEMENTATION PHASE

NURSING ACTIONS	RATIONALE/AMPLIFICATION
1. Place client flat and hyperextend neck if possible.	A towel may be rolled and placed under the client's neck.
2. If tracheostomy tube has not been grossly contaminated, remove inner cannula, insert obturator into tracheostomy tube, and attempt to reinsert tracheostomy tube into stoma.	If the cuff was inflated, remove the air before continuing. Sometimes a tube can be reinserted without the obturator, but the chances that forcing the tube into the stoma will obstruct the airway and further complicate the client's condition are increased.
3. If tracheostomy tube is grossly contaminated, there are three possible options:	
a. Rinse tracheostomy tube with sterile water and attempt to replace tube.	In an emergency, the reestablishment of a patent airway must take precedence over the possibility of introducing a bacterial infection. This option should be used only if a second tracheostomy tube is unavailable.
b. Use new tracheostomy tube to reestablish patent airway.	Healing of the stoma may prevent the reinsertion of a tube of the same size. A smaller tube should be available.
c. Cover tracheal stoma with sterile pressure dressing and reestablish ventilation by using bag and mask resuscitator.	In most instances ventilation may be reestablished with the use of a manual resuscitator if the stoma is sealed. This technique is not an option if the client has had the upper airways removed.
4. If repeated attempts to reinsert tracheostomy tube	Ventilation must be reestablished as soon as possible to

are unsuccessful, seal stoma and ventilate client with manual resuscitator.

5. If tracheostomy tube is reinserted, assess ventilation by listening for breath sounds; suction if secretions are present in airways.

6. Secure tracheostomy tube by replacing ties.

reduce the risk of neural damage from hypoxia. Supplemental oxygen may be increased temporarily to offset the effects of hypoxia.

Reinflate the cuff if the client requires ventilation or if secretions are a problem. If the tube has not been in place long enough to establish a tract, it can be accidentally inserted into the soft tissues of the neck rather than into the trachea.

RELATED NURSING CARE

NURSING ACTIONS	RATIONALE/AMPLIFICATION
1. Check client's vital signs.	Look for signs of system(s) failure.
2. Notify client's physician.	
3. Initiate emergency procedures if patent airway cannot be maintained.	

EVALUATION PHASE

ANTICIPATED OUTCOME	NURSING ACTIONS
Reestablishment of ventilation	Evaluate the client for signs of respiratory distress. Auscultate the client's chest frequently.

SELECTED REFERENCES   Hamilton H: Procedures. Springhouse, PA. Intermed Communications, Inc., 1983
McIntyre KM, Lewis AJ (eds): Textbook of Advanced Cardiac Life Support, Dallas, American Heart Association, 1981

Cuffed tube management

Objectives
To provide proper care and maintenance of artificial airways
To decrease the risk of iatrogenic infections
To decrease the chance of tracheal damage
To decrease the risk of accidental extubation
To provide a patent airway for ventilation and removal of secretions

ASSESSMENT PHASE

- Does the client have a tracheostomy or oral endotracheal or nasal endotracheal tube in place?
- Does the client require mechanical ventilation?
- Does the client tolerate the artificial airway well?

PRECAUTIONS

- **Ensure adequate humidification of inspired gases.**
- **Ensure that the artificial airway is properly secured to prevent accidental extubation.**
- **Auscultate chest sounds frequently to ensure proper tube placement.**
- **Use a cuff pneumometer or minimal-leak technique to maintain cuff pressures at an acceptable level to reduce tracheal damage.**

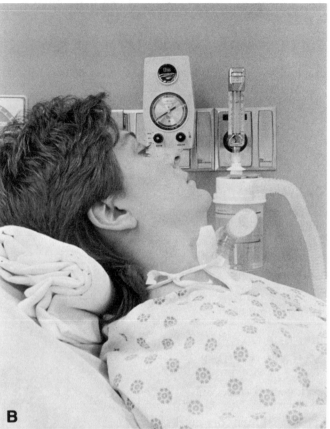

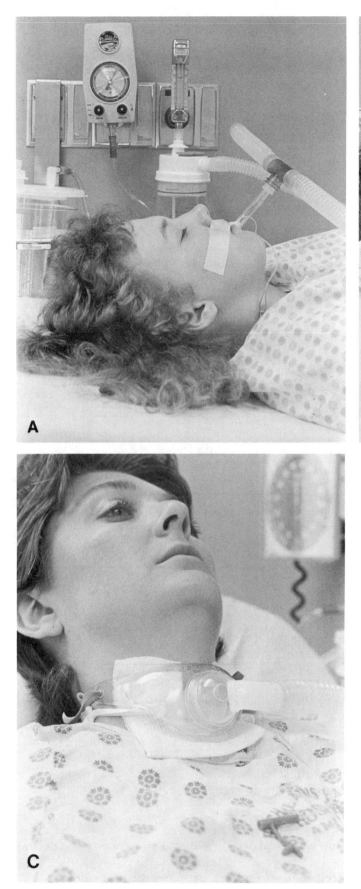

Fig. 19–16 Methods of delivering aerosol by artificial airways. (*A*) Brigg's adapter (T tube) attached to endotracheal tube. (*B*) Brigg's adapter (T tube) attached to endotracheal tube. (*C*) Tracheostomy collar used with tracheostomy tube.

PLANNING PHASE

EQUIPMENT

Cuff pneumometer (or pressure manometer with three-way stopcock and syringe)
Stethoscope
Oxygen/aerosol source with tubing and Brigg's adapter (T tube) or tracheostomy collar
Tape (to secure endotracheal tubes)
Suction equipment (at bedside)

CLIENT/FAMILY TEACHING

- Explain to the client the reason for the insertion of the airway.
- Discuss the need for airway care.
- Discuss the procedure for airway care.
- Describe ways in which the client or family can assist in airway care.

IMPLEMENTATION PHASE

NURSING ACTIONS	RATIONALE/AMPLIFICATION
1. Ensure adequate humidification of inspired gases by attaching oxygen/aerosol source to airway. Use Brigg's adapter (T tube) with oral and nasal endotracheal tubes. If tracheostomy tube has been inserted, use either Brigg's adapter or tracheostomy collar (Fig. 19–16).	The use of an artificial airway bypasses the natural humidification processes of the upper airway. The use of an aerosol restores humidification to proper levels. The use of a heated aerosol may also be indicated for clients with thick secretions.
2. Ensure that tube is properly secured.	Proper securing of the tube prevents dislodging and accidental extubation.
3. Auscultate chest sounds at least hourly.	The auscultation of chest sounds ensures that the tube has not been dislodged from the proper position. If breath sounds are heard on only one side, the tube has probably slipped into either the right or left main stem bronchus. Withdraw the tube 1 cm to 2 cm ($\frac{1}{2}$ inch to 1 inch) and recheck breath sounds. If breath sounds are still unilateral, obtain a chest film to determine the position of the tube.
4. Reposition or retape tube as necessary (Fig. 19–17).	The tube should be retaped whenever it is repositioned or when the tape becomes soiled. *Caution:* Obtain assistance when you are retaping the tube. This procedure is much easier and safer when the tube is held in place while retaping is performed.

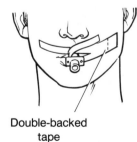

Double-backed tape

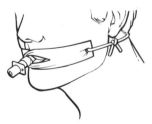

Fig. 19–17 Methods of taping endotracheal tubes in place.

5. Check cuff pressure at least every 8 hours. **a.** Attach manometer to pilot balloon port using stopcock with attached syringe. To measure cuff pressure, close stopcock to syringe. **b.** Record measured pressure. To adjust pressure	Monitoring of the cuff pressure prevents tracheal damage and ensures that the cuff is not leaking. A cuff that takes more air each time it is checked may indicate tracheomalacia. A cuff that will not hold pressure has a leak, and the tube must be replaced.

close stopcock to manometer. Now it is possible to inflate or deflate cuff.

c.   Close stopcock to syringe and measure pressure again. Cuff pressure should not exceed 20 cm H_2O. Record pressure and amount of air added or removed.

d.   Remove stopcock from pilot balloon port quickly to prevent air from leaking from cuff. Using one of the new models of cuff pneumometers will alleviate need for stopcock and syringe (see Fig. 19–14).

If manometer or pneumometer is unavailable, use minimal leak technique.

a.   Make sure cuff is deflated. Have client inhale and slowly inflate cuff with 10-ml syringe attached to pilot balloon port.

b.   As cuff is inflated, place stethoscope on client's neck. Once air leakage around cuff is no longer heard, stop inflating cuff.

c.   With stethoscope in place, remove air from cuff just until slight leak is heard. This should be minimum volume needed to seal airway. If client is on mechanical ventilation, perform this maneuver during inspiratory phase. Note amount of air required to achieve minimal leak.

6.   Aspirate secretions from airways as chest sounds indicate (see previous section on Endotracheal Suction with Airway *In Situ*).

RELATED NURSING CARE

NURSING ACTIONS	RATIONALE/AMPLIFICATION
1. Restrain client if necessary.	Restraining the client helps to prevent accidental extubation.
2. Prevent ventilator or aerosol tubing from pulling on tube. This can be accomplished by pinning or taping tubing to bedsheet (Fig. 19–17).	Securing the tube allows for lateral movement of the client's head. It also helps to prevent dislodging of the tube or accidental extubation.
3. Maintain ready access to manual resuscitator with mask and oxygen and intubation equipment. Know who is responsible for intubation in your institution.	If accidental extubation occurs, quickly assess the client's condition and provide manual ventilation, if necessary, until the client can be reintubated.
4. Monitor placement of tube.	If the tube becomes displaced, deflate the cuff, reposition the tube, and assess breath sounds. Retape the tube securely.

EVALUATION PHASE

ANTICIPATED OUTCOME	NURSING ACTIONS
Maintenance of patent airway	Evaluate the patency of the tube cuff. Notify the physician if the cuff will not hold the pressure. This situation may require replacement of the tube. Initiate emergency procedures if the client is accidentally extubated.

PRODUCT AVAILABILITY

CUFF PNEUMOMETERS

Portex, Inc.
Posey Co.

SELECTED REFERENCES

Burton GG, Hodgkin JE: Respiratory Care, 2nd ed. Philadelphia, JB Lippincott, 1984
Hamilton H: Procedures. Springhouse, PA, Intermed Communications, Inc., 1983
Millar S: Methods in Critical Care, The AACN Manual. Philadelphia, WB Saunders, 1980

Nelson EJ: Critical Care Respiratory Therapy, A Laboratory and Clinical Manual. Boston, Little, Brown, 1983

Extubation

Objective

To remove either an oral or nasal endotracheal tube after it has been determined that the client can breathe without assistance and that secretions can be removed without an airway in place

ASSESSMENT PHASE

- Can the client's ABG values be maintained without assisted ventilation?
- Has the client's underlying condition (the reason the client was intubated) improved to the point at which an artificial airway is no longer required?
- Does the client have spontaneous respirations without the assistance of a ventilator?
- Will the client require supplemental oxygen after extubation?
- Are secretions a problem? Will the client be able to cough and clear secretions after the endotracheal tube is removed?

PRECAUTIONS

- **Extubations should only be attempted after the client is well rested, especially in clients who have been intubated for long periods. Extubation may be more successful in the morning than in the late afternoon or evening.**
- **Never remove an endotracheal tube unless the personnel who are trained to reintubate are present. If respiratory failure follows extubation, a patent airway must be reestablished.**
- **A suction setup with sterile catheters and gloves must be present during the extubation process to remove secretions in the client's airway.**

PLANNING PHASE

EQUIPMENT

Sterile suction catheter
Sterile gloves
Scissors
Water-soluble lubricant
Vacuum source, regulator, and trap
Unit-dose container of sterile normal saline or 6-ml syringe filled with normal saline
Stethoscope
Aerosol setup with supplemental oxygen
Emergency airway box
 Manual resuscitator with mask
 Laryngoscope and blades
 Endotracheal tubes

CLIENT/FAMILY TEACHING

- Discuss the procedure for removing the endotracheal tube.
- Describe the suctioning process that will be used concurrently with the extubation procedure.
- Encourage the client to cough and breathe deeply, after the endotracheal tube is removed. Describe the benefits of coughing and deep breathing and explain why these procedures will reduce the risk of reintubation.

IMPLEMENTATION PHASE

NURSING ACTIONS	RATIONALE/AMPLIFICATION
1. Elevate head of bed to semi-Fowler's position or as high as client can tolerate.	Respiratory muscles function more effectively in an upright than in a prone position.
2. Assemble equipment for suctioning as described in previous section on Blind (Nasotracheal) Endotracheal Suctioning.	
3. Assemble equipment to give supplemental oxygen after endotracheal tube is removed.	
4. Remove tape or other means of securing tube in place.	Do not remove the air from the cuff at this time. Scissors may be required to remove the ties, especially if secretions have dried on them.
5. Using sterile technique, suction secretions from endotracheal tube.	
6. Increase client's F_IO_2.	This avoids the complications of hypoxia.
7. Insert syringe into one-way valve in pilot balloon and be prepared to deflate cuff.	Be prepared to deflate the cuff, but do not do so at this time.
8. Instruct client to breathe deeply. Reinsert suction catheter 1 inch to 2 inches below end of endotracheal tube, deflate cuff, and apply suction while endotracheal tube is removed.	If the client is not able to take a deep breath, a manual resuscitator may be used to hyperinflate the client's lung. The bag is quickly removed, the suction catheter is inserted, the cuff is deflated, and suction is applied while the endotracheal tube is removed.
9. Supplemental oxygen and aerosol should be administered to client as needed.	
10. Tracheostomy tubes are removed in approximately same way as endotracheal tubes are. More attention is given to stoma after tracheostomy tube is removed. Sterile dressing should be applied to stoma after tube is removed. Permanent closure of stoma usually occurs within few days of extubation.	Often the tracheal stoma will decrease in size to that of the tracheostomy tube. Even with the cuff deflated, the tube may not pass easily through the stoma. A sterile water-soluble lubricant may be applied to the stoma to make extubation easier.
11. After reoxygenation, encourage client to cough and breathe deeply. Suction oropharynx.	
12. Correctly dispose of tubes, catheters, and gloves.	Correct disposal of used material reduces the risk of nosocomial infection.

RELATED NURSING CARE

NURSING ACTIONS	RATIONALE/AMPLIFICATION
1. Encourage client to cough and breathe deeply.	Coughing and breathing deeply prevents atelectasis and the accumulation of tracheal secretions.
2. Suction as needed to remove secretions from oropharynx and trachea.	
3. *Caution:* Do not leave client unattended! Observe for any signs of respiratory failure and airway obstruction.	

EVALUATION PHASE

ANTICIPATED OUTCOME	NURSING ACTIONS
Prevention of complications of extubation	Evaluate the client's breath sounds. Snoring or crowing sounds from the upper airway may indicate edema. Hoarseness is not uncommon, but it is usually not persistent unless there are underlying complications. Monitor ABG values as ordered. Blood gases should be drawn 30 minutes to 1 hour after extubation to evaluate the client's condition. Observe for fatigue and respiratory failure. If failure occurs, be prepared to ventilate the client with a manual resuscitator. Call the physician if failure occurs.

SELECTED REFERENCES   Burton GG, Hodgkin, JE: Respiratory Care, 2nd ed. Philadelphia, JB Lippincott, 1984

Nelson EJ: Critical Care Respiratory Therapy, A Laboratory and Clinical Manual. Boston, Little, Brown, 1983

Shapiro BA, Harrison RA, Trout CA: Clinical Application of Respiratory Care, 2nd ed. Chicago, Year Book Medical Publishers, Inc., 1979

20

Ventilatory support

For help in understanding abbreviations and symbols used in this chapter, refer to Table 20–1.

BACKGROUND

Ventilatory support is indicated for the client whose own ventilation is inadequate. Signs of inadequate ventilation include dyspnea, tachypnea, somnolence, cyanosis, decreasing arterial oxygen partial pressure (PaO_2), increasing arterial carbon dioxide partial pressure ($PaCO_2$), decreasing pH, and unconsciousness. Ventilatory support may take several forms, including ambient oxygen administration, incentive spirometry, intermittent positive pressure breathing (IPPB), and mechanical ventilation.

Ambient oxygen administration is most effective for clients showing signs of hypoxia. The primary indication for oxygen therapy is a decreasing PaO_2. In the absence of arterial blood gases (ABGs), the health-care provider should watch for tachycardia, dyspnea, tachypnea, cyanosis, restlessness, confusion, and unconsciousness. Ambient oxygen can be delivered by several different methods. Regardless of the method chosen, all oxygen, whether from a cylinder or from a bulk system wall outlet, must be humidified before delivery. This humidification is accomplished by bubbling the oxygen through a humidifier that is filled with water. The humidifier is attached to the oxygen source by a flowmeter. The flowmeter regulates the flow of oxygen to the client and is calibrated in liters per minute (lpm). The oxygen administration device is connected to the humidifier by tubing.

OXYGEN ADMINISTRATION DEVICES

The most common oxygen administration device is the nasal cannula. It consists of two small prongs that fit into the nares. Depending on the rate at which the liter flow is set (usually 1 lpm to 6 lpm) and the client's breathing pattern, the nasal cannula is capable of delivering a fractional inspired oxygen concentration (F_IO_2) of 24% to 44% (approximate). To deliver higher or more precise concentrations of oxygen, a mask should be used instead of a nasal cannula. One type of oxygen mask, the Venturi mask, mixes oxygen and room air to deliver a precise F_IO_2. Most Venturi masks come with a variety of adapters to deliver between 24% and 60% oxygen. Liter flows for Venturi masks vary with desired F_IO_2 and manufacturer. To use a Venturi mask properly, the care-giver should follow the manufacturer's instructions. The simple mask or medium-concentration mask delivers between 35% and 55% oxygen (approximate) and is the most commonly used mask. Actual delivered F_IO_2 depends on the liter flow of oxygen (this type of mask should not be set at less than 5 lpm) and on the client's breathing pattern and respiratory rate. Two other types of oxygen masks use reservoir bags and deliver relatively high F_IO_2 levels. The partial rebreathing mask has an unobstructed opening between the mask and the reservoir bag. As the client exhales, some of the exhaled gases enter this bag and are rebreathed on the next inspiration. Because the first air to be exhaled has not taken part in gas exchange in the lungs, this air contains a relatively high oxygen concentration. The partial rebreathing mask delivers oxygen concentrations in the 60% to 80% range. The highest F_IO_2 that can be achieved without intubating the client comes from the non-rebreathing mask. The non-rebreathing mask is similar to the partial rebreathing mask, except that it has a

Table 20–1
Symbols and abbreviations used in ventilatory support

Primary symbols (capital letters; indicate physical quantities)	Secondary symbols (qualifying symbols; denote location of quantity)	Measurements of oxygenation and ventilation		Lung volumes and capacities and tests of ventilatory mechanics		
F fractional concentration of	A alveolar gas	P_IO_2	inspired oxygen partial pressure	VC	vital capacity	maximum volume that can be exhaled from the point of maximum inspiration
P partial pressure, tension	D dead space gas	P_AO_2	alveolar oxygen partial pressure	V_T	tidal volume	same as V_T. Used to indicate lung volume
V volume of a gas	E expired gas	P_ACO_2	alveolar carbon dioxide partial pressure	TV	tidal volume	maximum volume of gas that can be inspired from end-tidal inspiration
	I inspired gas	PaO_2	arterial oxygen partial pressure	IRV	inspiratory reserve volume	maximum volume of gas that can be expired from end-tidal expiration
	T tidal gas	$PaCO_2$	arterial carbon dioxide partial pressure	ERV	expiratory reserve volume	maximum amount of gas that can be inspired from end-tidal expiration
	a arterial	V_T	tidal volume. Amount of inspired or expired gas per breath.	IC	inspiratory capacity	volume of gas remaining in the lungs at the end of a maximum expiration
	v venous	$\dot{Q}$	cardiac output	RV	residual volume	amount of gas remaining in the lungs at end-tidal expiration
	v̄ mixed venous	$\dot{V}/\dot{Q}$	ventilation/perfusion ratio	FRC	functional residual capacity	amount of gas contained in the lungs at the end of a maximum inspiration
	c capillary	F_IO_2	fractional inspired oxygen concentration	TLC	total lung capacity	VC made at maximum effort
		F_EO_2	fractional expired oxygen concentration	FVC	forced vital capacity	

Note: Slash (¯) over a letter indicates mixed or mean volume (v̄ = mixed venous).
Dot (˙) over a letter indicates time ($\dot{V}$ = volume of ventilation per minute).
(After Harper RW: A Guide to Respiratory Care. Philadelphia, JB Lippincott, 1981)

271

one-way valve between the mask and the reservoir bag. This valve allows gas to exit from the bag on inspiration, but it does not allow exhaled gases to enter. Because the only gas in the reservoir bag when the client inhales is oxygen, the delivered F_1O_2 is between 80% and 95%. Both of the reservoir-type masks depend on the gas in the reservoir to deliver a high F_1O_2, so it is important to set the oxygen flow high enough to prevent the reservoir bag from completely deflating during inspiration (this may require flows of 10 lpm to 15 lpm for some clients).

The wide range of ambient-oxygen administration devices available makes it possible to choose a device that will deliver the required ranges of F_1O_2. Regardless of the type of oxygen administration device chosen, it is important that it be properly fitted. A device that fits poorly and is uncomfortable will not be tolerated by the client.

INCENTIVE SPIROMETRY

Incentive spirometry is a procedure that has gained popularity over the last several years as a replacement for IPPB. While it cannot and should not replace IPPB in all situations, incentive spirometry is useful as a method of increasing ventilation for short periods of time. Incentive spirometry should be the treatment of choice when the client can produce an increase in tidal volume without assistance. Incentive spirometry usually includes a volume-measuring device on which previous attempts can be recorded. These previous attempts provide an inspired volume level that the client should try to improve with each subsequent attempt.

There are many different types and styles of incentive spirometry devices available. The health-care provider should become thoroughly familiar with the device to be used before attempting to instruct the client on its use. Incentive spirometry can be effective in preventing or counteracting atelectasis in the postoperative client. It can also be effective in improving the client's cough and the ability to expectorate secretions. It should be remembered, however, that the effectiveness of incentive spirometry depends entirely on the client's ability and cooperation.

INTERMITTENT POSITIVE PRESSURE BREATHING

IPPB is indicated when a short-term increase in ventilation is necessary and the client is either unable or unwilling to voluntarily provide the necessary increase. After the client has initiated inspiration, IPPB provides positive pressure that increases the inspired volume. Because IPPB requires only that the client be able to initiate an inspiration, it can be useful even in clients who cannot voluntarily increase tidal volume because of pain or muscle weakness. Like incentive spirometry, IPPB aids in preventing or counteracting atelectasis and in improving the client's ability to expectorate secretions. IPPB is also indicated for the delivery of aerosolized medications to the lungs. IPPB should only be considered for this purpose if the client is unable to voluntarily increase tidal volume. If the client can increase tidal volume without assistance, a hand-held or small-volume nebulizer should be considered.

HAND-HELD NEBULIZERS

Hand-held nebulizers are a relatively new form of therapy but have proven to be effective in delivering aerosolized medications. The necessary equipment consists of a small hand-held nebulizer, a mouthpiece, connecting tubing, and a flowmeter. Most of these devices may be combined with an incentive spirometer. This allows for documentation of inspired volumes, as well as delivery of medication. Hand-held nebulization has the advantage of being less complicated for both the client and the health-care provider.

MECHANICAL VENTILATORY SUPPORT

Mechanical ventilatory support is indicated for the apneic client or for the hypoventilating client who would not benefit from the short-term increase in ventilation provided by IPPB. ABGs, when available, are the best indicator of the need for mechanical ventilatory support. In general, ABGs for the client in ventilatory failure will indicate acute acidemia (pH < 7.35), hypoxia ($PaO_2 < 50$ mm Hg), and hypercapnia ($PaCO_2 > 60$ mm Hg). In the absence of ABGs, the health-care provider should watch for the signs of inadequate ventilation and hypoxia previously discussed. In addition, be alert for signs of fatigue in the dyspneic or tachypneic client. Mechanical ventilation is always more effective when it is initiated before the client has to be resuscitated than after.

Because mechanical ventilation requires a patent, sealed airway, tracheal intubation of the client is the first step in the procedure. Once this has been accomplished, the next step involves choosing a ventilator and ventilatory parameters. In general, a volume ventilator provides a wide range of capabilities. Before attempting to initiate mechanical ventilation, the health-care provider should become thoroughly familiar with the equipment by reading the operator's manuals, by attending manufacturer's seminars, and by practicing with lung simulators. Initial ventilator settings should be based on the client's condition and on baseline ABG results. ABG analysis should be repeated 20 minutes to 30 minutes after the start of mechanical ventilation. Thereafter, requests for ABG analysis should be based on observations of the client's condition. However, because ABG analysis is the only adequate means of evaluating mechanical ventilation, it should be performed often enough so that sufficient documentation of the client's condition is available.

Frequent chest auscultation is essential during mechanical ventilation. Not only will it reveal the need for tracheobronchial suctioning, but it will also confirm the proper positioning of the endotracheal tube. Close attention should also be paid to the client's cardiac rate and rhythm and blood pressure. Assessment of these parameters will indicate the cardiovascular effects, if any, of mechanical ventilation.

Positive end-expiratory pressure (PEEP), intermittent mandatory ventilation (IMV), and pressure support are adjuncts that may be used in conjunction with mechanical ventilation. PEEP provides a positive pressure at the end of exhalation, when airway pressures normally fall to zero. PEEP increases functional residual capacity, which increases gas exchange in the alveoli and permits F_1O_2 to be kept as low as possible. Used primarily as techniques to wean clients from mechanical ventilatory support, IMV and pressure support may also be used as the primary mode of ventilation. IMV allows the client to take spontaneous breaths while continuing to deliver a reduced number of mandatory positive pressure ventilator-initiated breaths. As the client's condition improves, the number of ventilator breaths is reduced until the client is again breathing independently. Pressure support is very much like IPPB in that it supplies a preset inspiratory pressure, but it does not deliver a preset volume. As the client's condition improves, the present inspiratory pressure is reduced until the pressure support is no longer needed.

The decision to commit a client to mechanical ventilation should not be taken lightly. Mechanical ventilation is, in most instances, a supportive rather than a curative treatment. It will provide life support until the underlying disease process can be arrested. Therefore, before the decision to initiate mechanical ventilation is made, it should be evident that the client has a reasonable chance for survival. Once the decision is made, everything must be done to make the ventilatory course as short and uneventful as possible.

The advent of life-prolonging treatments such as mechanical ventilation has presented health-care personnel with moral, religious, and ethical problems that probably will not be answered in the near future. This, however, does not relieve us of our committment to provide the best care possible for each of our clients.

Oxygen administration

Objective
To administer ambient oxygen by nasal catheter, cannula, or mask to prevent or counteract hypoxia

ASSESSMENT PHASE
- Is the client hypoxic? Do the client's ABGs indicate decreased PaO_2?
- Is the client dyspneic? Are respirations labored or is the client using accessory respiratory muscles?

• Is the client cyanotic? Do nailbeds, skin, or buccal membranes show signs of cyanotic discoloration?
• Does the client have symptoms of cardiovascular impairment?

PRECAUTIONS

• **Humidify all oxygen delivered from either a cylinder or a wall outlet.**
• **Check the flowmeter frequently to ensure that proper flow is maintained.**
• **Do not administer oxygen at flows that are greater than 2 lpm (approximately 28%) to clients with known or suspected chronic obstructive pulmonary disease until ABGs are obtained and interpreted.**
• **When using oxygen masks (except Venturi masks), do not use oxygen flows that are less than 5 lpm.**
• **Instruct the client, family, and visitors about oxygen precautions (*e.g.,* no smoking) and place the precaution sign on the door.**

PLANNING PHASE

EQUIPMENT (FIG. 20–1)

Oxygen source
Oxygen flowmeter
Humidifier
Sterile distilled water
Administration device (*e.g.,* cannula, mask; as ordered)
Oxygen precaution (no smoking) sign for door

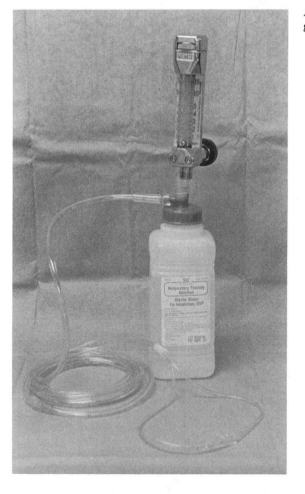

Fig. 20–1 Equipment used to deliver oxygen by nasal cannula.

CLIENT/FAMILY TEACHING

• Explain procedure to client, including the reason for oxygen therapy, how the administration device should be worn, and when oxygen will be used.
• Explain the oxygen precautions to the client, family, roommates, and visitors. Oxygen precautions include no smoking and using only hospital-approved electric appliances.

**IMPLEMENTATION
PHASE**

NURSING ACTIONS	RATIONALE/AMPLIFICATION
1. Assess client's condition.	Verify the need for oxygen therapy.
2. Review client's chart.	Verify the physician's order and the method of oxygen administration.
3. Collect necessary equipment, choosing appropriate administration device (see Fig. 20–2 for descriptions and recommendations for use).	

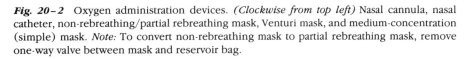

Fig. 20–2 Oxygen administration devices. *(Clockwise from top left)* Nasal cannula, nasal catheter, non-rebreathing/partial rebreathing mask, Venturi mask, and medium-concentration (simple) mask. *Note:* To convert non-rebreathing mask to partial rebreathing mask, remove one-way valve between mask and reservoir bag.

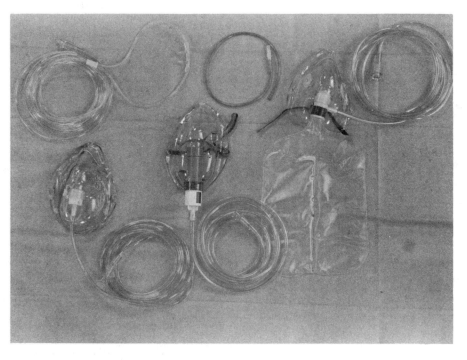

NURSING ACTIONS	RATIONALE/AMPLIFICATION
4. Explain procedure to client.	
5. Assemble and test equipment.	
a. Fill humidifier with sterile distilled water. Attach humidifier to flowmeter and attach setup to oxygen source. Turn on oxygen flow to check patency of humidifier. Attach administration device to humidifier and check patency.	This first step may not be necessary if prefilled humidifiers are available.
6. Place administration device on client.	
a. If nasal catheter is used, first check patency of nares. To insert catheter, lubricate tip with water or water-soluble lubricant and advance it into naris. Using tongue depressor, observe positioning of catheter tip in nasopharynx. Advance catheter until tip is visible below uvula. Withdraw catheter until tip disappears behind uvula. Tape catheter in place.	

b. If nasal cannula is used, insert prongs so that curve is downward, following natural curve of nasal passages. Loop tubing behind client's ears and under chin, securing cannula in place. Avoid securing cannula too tightly to decrease risk of pressure-related irritation.

c. If using oxygen mask, place mask over client's nose, mouth, and chin. Adjust metal band to fit bridge of nose. To secure mask, place elastic band behind head (or loop tubing behind ears) and adjust for snug but comfortable fit. If using partial rebreathing or non-rebreathing mask, check for proper functioning of one-way valves and reservoir bag.

7. Set flowmeter to prescribed flow.

Set the flow as ordered by the physician. If a specific flow was not ordered, set the flow according to the client's condition and the device used (see Fig. 20–2 for recommendations).

8. Explain precautions to client.

9. Put oxygen precaution sign on door.

RELATED NURSING CARE

NURSING ACTIONS	RATIONALE/AMPLIFICATION
1. Observe client for signs of hypoxia.	Watch for dyspnea, tachycardia, cyanosis, decreased level of consciousness, and restlessness.
2. Observe client for signs of oxygen toxicity.	Oxygen toxicity may produce signs of hypoxia (see step 1). ABGs will indicate respiratory failure.
3. Replace or refill humidifier as necessary.	The administration of unhumidified oxygen causes mucous membranes to dry.
4. Change nasal catheters every 8 hours. Use other naris if possible.	Alternate nares to decrease the risk of pressure necrosis and irritation to mucosa.
5. Replace nasal cannulas and masks as necessary.	
6. Periodically check skin under straps.	Periodic inspection of the client's skin decreases the risk of pressure necrosis and irritation.

EVALUATION PHASE

ANTICIPATED OUTCOME	NURSING ACTION
Reversal of hypoxia	Observe the client for signs of hypoxia.

PRODUCT AVAILABILITY

OXYGEN FLOWMETERS

Hudson Oxygen
OEM Medical
Ohmeda
Puritan–Bennett Corporation

OXYGEN HUMIDIFIERS

Airlife, Inc.
Inspiron Corporation

Respiratory Care, Inc.
Travenol Laboratories, Inc. — Medical Products Division

OXYGEN ADMINISTRATION DEVICES

Airlife, Inc.
Hudson Oxygen
Inspiron Corporation
Puritan – Bennett Corporation

SELECTED REFERENCES

Burton GG, Hodgkin JE: Respiratory Care, 2nd ed. Philadelphia, JB Lippincott, 1984
Hamilton H: Procedures. Springhouse, PA. Intermed Communications, Inc., 1983

McPherson SP: Respiratory Therapy Equipment, 3rd ed. St. Louis, CV Mosby, 1985

Intermittent positive pressure breathing therapy

Objectives
To decrease $PaCO_2$ and increase PaO_2
To improve expectoration
To prevent or counteract atelectasis
To relieve bronchospasm and decrease mucosal edema
To treat pulmonary edema through the use of positive pressure inspirations

ASSESSMENT PHASE

- Is the client hypoxic or hypercapnic? Is the client dyspneic? Do the client's ABGs indicate decreased PaO_2 or increased $PaCO_2$?
- Is the client unable to cough up secretions? Do the client's breath sounds indicate the retention of secretions?
- Do the client's breath sounds or chest films indicate the presence of atelectasis? Are breath sounds absent? Do chest films show areas of consolidation or atelectasis?
- Is the client experiencing bronchospasm? Does auscultation reveal wheezing or rhonchi? Are wheezes audible without a stethoscope? Does the client have a history of bronchospastic disorders?
- Is the client experiencing mucosal congestion? Does auscultation reveal stridor? Is stridor audible without a stethoscope?
- Is the client developing pulmonary edema? Are the client's secretions frothy? Can fine rales be heard on auscultation? Do the client's ABGs indicate decreased PaO_2?

PRECAUTIONS

- **Check the client's pulse rate and blood pressure before, during, and after treatment to gauge cardiovascular effects. If the pulse rate increases more than 20 beats per minute (bpm) or if blood pressure readings show a rapid change, stop treatment and consult the physician.**
- **Avoid administering IPPB therapy immediately before or after meals.**
- **Observe the client for signs of gastric distention caused by swallowing air.**
- **Coach the client in proper breathing patterns to prevent hyperventilation. Observe the client for signs of dizziness.**
- **Make sure that the medication cup contains enough solution for the duration of the treatment.**
- **Start the treatment (especially the first treatment) with the flow and pressure set at comfortable levels until the client becomes accustomed to the procedure. Adjust the flow and pressure to prescribed levels as tolerated.**
- **If possible, administer IPPB treatments with compressed air to clients with chronic obstructive pulmonary disease.**

PLANNING PHASE

EQUIPMENT (FIG. 20 – 3)

Stethoscope, sphygmomanometer
IPPB machine
Breathing circuit

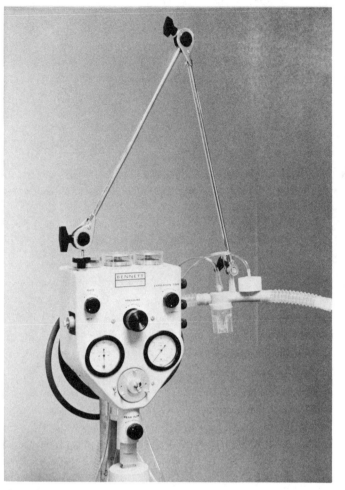

Fig. 20-3 Equipment used to administer IPPB therapy.

Mouthpiece, mouthseal, mask, and noseclips (as needed)
Medications (as ordered)
Tissues, emesis basin, and specimen cup
Suction equipment (if necessary)

CLIENT/FAMILY TEACHING

• Explain the treatment to the client, including need for the treatment, the treatment procedure, how often the treatment will be administered, proper breathing patterns, and proper coughing techniques (see Client/Family Teaching under Postural Drainage in Chap. 22).

IMPLEMENTATION PHASE

NURSING ACTIONS	RATIONALE/AMPLIFICATION
1. Review client's chart for medication orders and other pertinent information.	
2. Assess client before treatment.	Record the client's pulse rate, blood pressure, and breath sounds.
3. Explain procedure to client. Allow time for client to ask questions and answer questions as completely as possible.	Effective administration of IPPB therapy requires the client's cooperation, and client cooperation depends entirely on client understanding.
4. Assemble equipment. Attach breathing circuit to machine, and attach mouthpiece or mask to tubing.	

5. Administer treatment.

   a. If possible, place client in sitting position. Unless client must remain supine, raise head of bed to at least 45-degree angle (Fig. 20–4).

   b. Choose correct delivery mode.

Depending on the client's condition, use a mouthpiece, a mouthseal, or a mask. If a mouthseal or mask is used, leave the client's dentures, if present, in place to help ensure adequate sealing. Use noseclips if the client has trouble breathing through the mouth.

Fig. 20–4 Positioning of client during administration of IPPB therapy. Head of bed should be elevated to at least a 45-degree angle.

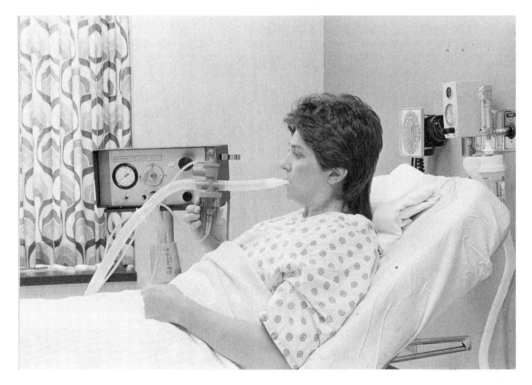

   c. Add medication to medication cup on breathing circuit. Adjust nebulizer control if necessary.

Ensure proper humidification during the treatment.

   d. Adust flow and pressure settings.

Start with flow and pressure set at comfortable levels and gradually adjust them to prescribed levels.

   e. Instruct client in proper breathing patterns.

The client should breathe at a normal rate, with a slight pause at the end of inspiration.

   f. Observe client for proper breathing patterns and for any unfavorable reactions to treatment.

Hyperventilation may cause dizziness.

   g. Assess client during treatment.

Record the client's pulse rate, blood pressure, and breath sounds.

   h. Instruct client on proper coughing techniques during and after treatment. Suction client to remove secretions if necessary.

   i. After treatment, assess client's condition.

Record the client's pulse rate, blood pressure, and breath sounds. Assessments made before, during, and after the treatment should be used for comparison and to gauge the effectiveness of the treatment.

j. Rinse medication cup and mouthpiece and store equipment.

All residual medication should be removed from the medication cup.

RELATED NURSING CARE

NURSING ACTIONS	RATIONALE/AMPLIFICATION
1. Observe client for signs of dyspnea and hypoxia.	Watch for shortness of breath, use of accessory respiratory muscles, and cyanosis.
2. Encourage client to breathe deeply and to cough between treatments.	Breathing deeply maintains patent airways and removes secretions.
3. Perform chest auscultation frequently.	Chest auscultation helps to assesses the client's ability to expectorate secretions.
4. Change client's position every hour if tolerated.	Changes in the client's position help to prevent the pooling and retention of secretions.

EVALUATION PHASE

ANTICIPATED OUTCOMES	NURSING ACTIONS
1. Relief of hypoxia	Persistent hypoxia is relieved by ambient-oxygen therapy, which requires a physician's order.
2. Mobilization of secretions	Assess the client's breath sounds.
3. Reduction of atelectasis	If atelectasis persists, encourage the client to breathe deeply and cough. Consult with the physician about the effectiveness of therapy.

PRODUCT AVAILABILITY

IPPB MACHINES

Bird Products/3M
Puritan – Bennett Corporation

IPPB BREATHING CIRCUITS

Airlife, Inc.
Hudson Oxygen
Inspiron Corporation
Puritan – Bennett Corporation

SELECTED REFERENCES

Burton GG, Hodgkin JE: Respiratory Care, 2nd ed. Philadelphia, JB Lippincott, 1984
McPherson SP: Respiratory Therapy Equipment, 3rd ed. St. Louis, CV Mosby, 1985

Spearman CB et al: Egan's Fundamentals of Respiratory Therapy, 4th ed. St. Louis, CV Mosby, 1982

Hand-held (small-volume) nebulizer therapy

Objective

To deliver aerosolized medications to increase airway humidification, to improve expectoration, to relieve bronchospasm, and to reduce bronchial mucosal congestion

ASSESSMENT PHASE

• Is the client unable to expectorate secretions? Do the client's breath sounds indicate the retention of secretions?
• Is the client experiencing bronchospasm? Does auscultation reveal wheezing? Are wheezes audible without a stethoscope? Does the client have a history of bronchospastic disorders?

• Is the client experiencing mucosal congestion? Does auscultation reveal rhonchi? Is stridor audible without a stethoscope?

PRECAUTIONS

• **If a bronchodilator is being administered, check the client's pulse rate and blood pressure before, during, and after treatment to gauge cardiovascular effects. If the pulse rate increases more than 20 bpm or if blood pressure readings show a rapid change, stop the treatment and consult the physician.**
• **Teach the client proper breathing patterns to prevent hyperventilation. Observe the client for signs of dizziness.**
• **If possible, administer nebulizer therapy with compressed air to clients with chronic obstructive pulmonary disease.**

PLANNING PHASE

EQUIPMENT

Stethoscope, sphygmomanometer
Hand-held nebulizer with mouthpiece and connecting tubing
6-inch section of corrugated tubing
Flowmeter
Medications (as ordered)
Tissues, emesis basin, and specimen cup
Suction equipment (if necessary)

CLIENT/FAMILY TEACHING

• Explain the treatment to the client, including the need for the treatment, the treatment procedure, how often the treatment will be administered, proper breathing patterns, and proper coughing techniques (see Client/Family Teaching under Postural Drainage in Chap. 22).

IMPLEMENTATION PHASE

NURSING ACTIONS	RATIONALE/AMPLIFICATION
1. Review client's chart for medication orders and other pertinent information.	Note all drug allergies.
2. Assess client before treatment.	Record the client's pulse rate, blood pressure, and breath sounds.
3. Explain procedure to client. Allow time for client to ask questions and answer questions as completely as possible.	Effective administration of hand-held nebulizer therapy requires the client's cooperation, and client cooperation depends entirely on client understanding.
4. Assemble equipment.	
a. Attach flowmeter to gas source.	
b. Attach connecting tubing to flowmeter and nebulizer. Attach mouthpiece to one side of nebulizer "T." Attach six-inch piece of tubing to opposite side of "T."	A 6-inch piece of tubing will serve as a reservoir for medication that is nebulized during exhalation.
5. Administer treatment.	
a. If possible, place client in sitting position. Unless client must remain flat, raise head of bead to at least 45-degree angle (Fig. 20–5).	The sitting position allows for more complete expansion of the lungs.
b. Add medication to reservoir in nebulizer.	
c. Adjust flowmeter to approximately 4 lpm to 5 lpm. Instruct client on proper breathing patterns.	The rate ensures the proper nebulization of medication. The client should breathe deeply at a slower than normal rate, with a 1-second to 2-second pause at the end of inspiration.

Fig. 20–5 Positioning of client during therapy with hand-held nebulizer. Head of bed should be elevated to at least a 45-degree angle.

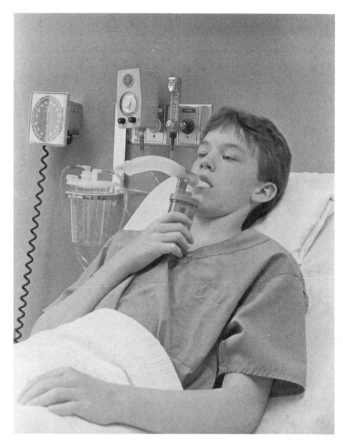

d. Observe client for proper breathing patterns and for any unfavorable reactions to treatment. Assess client's condition during treatment.

Hyperventilation may cause dizziness. Record the client's pulse rate, blood pressure, and breath sounds.

e. Instruct client in proper coughing techniques during and after treatment. Suction client to remove secretions if necessary. After treatment, assess client's condition.

Record the client's pulse rate, blood pressure, and breath sounds. Assessments made before, during and after the treatment should be used for comparison and to gauge the effectiveness of the treatment.

f. Rinse medication cup and mouthpiece and store equipment.

All residual medication should be removed from the medication cup.

RELATED NURSING CARE

NURSING ACTIONS	RATIONALE/AMPLIFICATION
1. Observe client for signs of dyspnea and hypoxia.	Watch for shortness of breath, use of accessory respiratory muscles, and cyanosis.
2. Encourage client to breathe deeply and to cough between treatments.	Breathing deeply maintains patent airways and removes secretions.
3. Perform chest auscultation frequently.	Chest auscultation helps to assess the client's ability to expectorate secretions. Compare breath sounds before and after treatment.

4. Change client's position every hour if tolerated.

Changing the client's position helps to prevent the pooling and retention of secretions.

EVALUATION PHASE

ANTICIPATED OUTCOMES	NURSING ACTIONS
1. Relief of bronchospasm	If wheezing persists, consult with the physician about increasing the frequency of hand-held nebulizer treatments or the administration of parenteral bronchodilators.
2. Increase in expectoration	Auscultate the client's chest frequently. Obtain an order to suction the client's airways if necessary.

PRODUCT AVAILABILITY HAND-HELD (SMALL-VOLUME) NEBULIZERS

Airlife, Inc.
Hudson Oxygen
Inspiron Corporation
Puritan – Bennett

SELECTED REFERENCES Burton G, Hodgkin J: Respiratory Care, A Guide to Clinical Practice, 2nd ed. Philadelphia, JB Lippincott, 1984

McPherson SP: Respiratory Therapy Equipment 3rd ed. St. Louis, CV Mosby, 1985

Incentive spirometry

Objectives
To prevent or counteract atelectasis
To return lung volumes to normal
To provide the client with a method of observing progress

ASSESSMENT PHASE

• Has the client complained of pain when breathing deeply? If so, the client may be splinting because of the pain. This can result in alveolar hypoventilation and can lead to atelectasis.
• Does the client have an effective cough? If not, secretions can accumulate in the airways, decreasing ventilation and causing atelectasis. The deep breathing associated with incentive spirometry may help to increase the effectiveness of the cough mechanism.
• Can the client follow instructions? The success of incentive spirometry depends entirely on the client's ability to spontaneously perform a series of deep-breathing maneuvers.

PRECAUTIONS

• **If the client cannot follow instructions and perform deep-breathing maneuvers, the ordering physician should be contacted. It may be necessary to change therapy modalities.**
• **Set realistic volume goals for the client, but increase these goals as tolerated.**

PLANNING PHASE

Incentive spirometer (Fig. 20–6)

EQUIPMENT

CLIENT/FAMILY TEACHING

• Explain the procedure to the client.
• Demonstrate the desired technique.

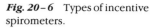

Fig. 20–6 Types of incentive spirometers.

IMPLEMENTATION PHASE

NURSING ACTIONS	RATIONALE/AMPLIFICATION
1. Assemble incentive spirometer.	
2. Place client in sitting position.	
3. Instruct client to insert mouthpiece, to breathe in as deeply as possible and to sustain maximum inspiration for 2 seconds to 5 seconds (Fig. 20–7).	The sustained maximum inspiration increases not only lung volume but also transpulmonary pressure, which reverses atelectasis.
4. Tell client that exhalation should be passive maneuver. Instruct client to exhale through pursed lips.	Exhaling through pursed lips will maintain a positive airway pressure during exhalation.

Fig. 20–7 Positioning of client during administration of incentive spirometry. Head of bed should be elevated to at least a 45-degree angle.

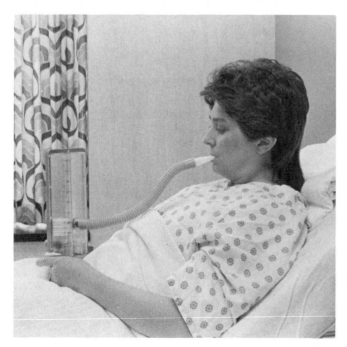

5. Record total number of breaths and number of times client reaches this goal.

RELATED NURSING CARE

NURSING ACTION	RATIONALE/AMPLIFICATION
Auscultate chest frequently.	Decreased or absent breath sounds indicate the need for more frequent incentive spirometry exercises or a change in therapy modalities.

EVALUATION PHASE

ANTICIPATED OUTCOMES	NURSING ACTIONS
1. Reduction of atelectasis	Auscultate the client's chest for increased breath sounds. Evaluate chest films for reduced areas of consolidation.
2. Improvement in lung volumes	The client should be able to achieve progressively higher volume goals during treatments.

PRODUCT AVAILABILITY

INCENTIVE BREATHING EXERCISES

Chesebrough–Ponds, Inc. (Voldyne Volumetric Exerciser)
Dart Respiratory—Division of Dart Industries, Inc. (Volume Plus)
Inspiron Corporation (Inspirx)

SELECTED REFERENCES

Burton GG, Hodgkin JE: Respiratory Care, 2nd ed. Philadelphia, JB Lippincott, 1984
Indihar F, Forsberg D, Adams A: A prospective comparison of three procedures used in attempts to prevent postoperative pulmonary complications. Respir Care 27(5):564–568, 1982

Shapiro BA, Peterson J, Cane RD: complications of mechanical aids to intermittent lung inflation. Respir Care 27(4):467–470, 1982

Initiating mechanical ventilation

Objective
To provide mechanical ventilatory support to the apneic or hypoventilating client

ASSESSMENT PHASE
- Is the client apneic?
- Is the client hypoventilating? Do the client's ABGs indicate acidemia ($pH < 7.35$), hypoxia ($PaO_2 < 50$ mm Hg) or hypercapnia ($PaCO_2 > 60$ mm Hg)?

PRECAUTIONS
- **Obtain baseline ABGs. These values will be the guide for future changes in mechanical ventilation parameters. Try to determine the client's normal ABGs and set these as the goal of mechanical ventilation.**
- **Obtain a baseline blood pressure reading. Blood pressure may fall rapidly after the initiation of mechanical ventilation in the hypoxic client. In addition, an excessive tidal volume during mechanical ventilation may decrease cardiac output, causing blood pressure to fall.**
- **Request a chest film after endotracheal intubation to confirm endotracheal tube positioning.**
- **Auscultate the client's chest frequently. Listen closely for bilateral breath sounds. Chest auscultation will also indicate the need for endotracheal suctioning.**

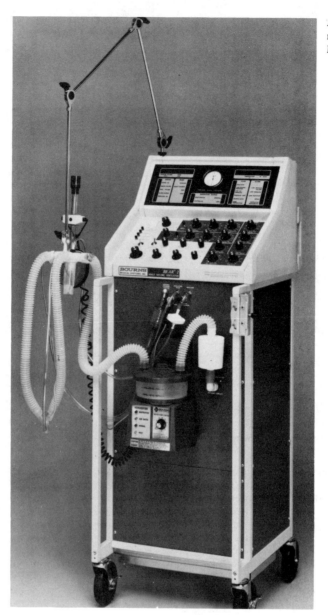

Fig. 20-8 Volume ventilator with humidifier and circuit. (Courtesy Bear Medical Systems)

PLANNING PHASE

EQUIPMENT (FIG. 20-8)

Mechanical ventilator with breathing circuit
Heated humidifier and sterile distilled water
O_2 and air sources (50 pounds per square inch [psi])
O_2 analyzer
Manual resuscitator
Stethoscope
Sphygmomanometer
Suction equipment

CLIENT/FAMILY TEACHING

• Explain the treatment to the client, including the need for mechanical ventilation, a step-by-step account of the procedure, and sensations the client can expect to feel.
• Explain the procedure to the client's family to alleviate their anxiety.

IMPLEMENTATION PHASE

NURSING ACTIONS	RATIONALE/AMPLIFICATION
1. Assess need for mechanical ventilation by measuring vital capacity (this should be less than 10 ml/kg), respiratory rate (normal = 12 bpm to 15 bpm; rates above and below this may indicate need for mechanical ventilation) and ABGs.	This ensures that the client cannot be maintained by less complicated methods.
2. Intubate client if endotracheal tube is not already in place.	Because ventilation is achieved by positive pressure, a cuffed endotracheal tube is required.
3. Set ventilator controls. **a.** Tidal volume = 10 ml to 12 ml/kg **b.** Respiratory rate = 12 bpm to 15 bpm **c.** F_IO_2 = 40% to 60%, depending on client's condition	These settings provide a starting point for mechanical ventilation. Changes in these settings can be made according to ABG results.
4. Ensure that all alarms are activated and functioning properly. Refer to operating manual for use of ventilator.	Alarms provide audible or visual warning of changes in the client's condition or problems with equipment or connections.
5. Connect client to ventilator. Maintain secure connection.	Try to maintain the aseptic condition of tubing connector and the client's endotracheal tube.
6. Auscultate chest, checking for bilateral breath sounds.	Chest auscultation confirms the location of endotracheal tube at a level that is high enough to allow ventilation of both lungs.
7. Monitor pulse rate and blood pressure.	Watch for signs of adverse cardiovascular effects.
8. Place O_2 analyzer in line on inspiratory side of ventilator breathing circuit.	This step confirms that delivered F_IO_2 is the same as the preset F_IO_2.
9. Check ABGs after client has been on ventilator for 20 minutes to 30 minutes. Adjust settings as indicated by results.	ABGs indicate the effectiveness of ventilation ($PaCO_2$) and oxygenation (PaO_2).

RELATED NURSING CARE

NURSING ACTIONS	RATIONALE/AMPLIFICATION
1. Auscultate client's chest frequently.	Chest auscultation indicates proper positioning of the endotracheal tube if bilateral breath sounds are heard. It also indicates the need for endotracheal suctioning (see Endotracheal Suction with Airway *In Situ* in Chap. 19).
2. Perform ABG analysis as ordered or as indicated by client's condition.	ABGs are the only reliable way to monitor the need for ventilator changes.
3. Talk with client and make sure emergency call signals are within easy reach.	Talking with the client helps to alleviate the client's fears and anxiety.
4. Restrain client if necessary.	Restraint prevents accidental or self-extubation or disconnection.

(See also Related Nursing Care under Ventilator Management in previous section.)

EVALUATION PHASE

ANTICIPATED OUTCOME	NURSING ACTIONS
Adequate ventilation	Auscultate the client's chest for bilateral breath sounds. Assess the client's ABGs.

PRODUCT AVAILABILITY

VENTILATORS

Bear Medical Systems, Inc.
J.H. Emerson Company
Engstrom Division of Gambro, Inc.
Ohmeda
Puritan – Bennett Corporation
Sechrist Industries, Inc.
Siemens – Elema Ventilator Systems

VENTILATOR BREATHING CIRCUITS

Airlife, Inc.
Bear Medical Systems, Inc.
J.H. Emerson Company
Hudson Oxygen
Inspiron Corporation
Ohmeda
Puritan – Bennett Corporation
Siemens – Elema Ventilator Systems

SELECTED REFERENCES

Burton GG, Hodgkin JE: Respiratory Care, 2nd ed. Philadelphia, JB Lippincott, 1984
McPherson SP: Respiratory Therapy Equipment, 3rd ed. St. Louis, CV Mosby, 1985

Shapiro BA, Harrison RA, Trout CA: Clinical Application of Respiratory Care, 2nd ed. Chicago, Year Book Medical Publishers, Inc., 1979

Ventilator management

Objectives

To maintain adequate ventilatory support for a client who needs mechanical assistance with breathing

To establish routine ventilator checks and maintenance and to alter ventilator functions to match the client's respiratory needs

ASSESSMENT PHASE

- Is the ventilator, at the current settings, keeping the client's ABGs within acceptable ranges?
- Can the client tolerate short periods of disconnection from the ventilator, or does the client become apneic when disconnected?
- Are breath sounds adequate and heard bilaterally?
- Does the client have single-system failure or multisystem failure?
- Does the ventilator require special maintenance when used for an extended period?
- Does the ventilator have adequate alarms to monitor client/ventilator failure, and are the alarms operational?
- Is the ventilator humidification system adequate to keep the client's tracheal and bronchial secretions thin and mobile?
- Is a manual resuscitator available in the event of ventilator or power failure? An oxygen source is usually needed with a manual resuscitator when the client's inspired oxygen must be above 21%.

PRECAUTIONS

- **Never leave a client who is attached to a ventilator unattended if there is a question about the reliability of the ventilator or if the client's condition is unstable.**
- **If a ventilator's operation is questionable, remove the client from the ventilator and ventilate with a manual resuscitator. If a question about the ventilator's reliability remains, change the ventilator if possible.**

PLANNING PHASE

EQUIPMENT (FIG. 20–9)

The ventilator and support equipment are the same as that described in the previous section on Initiating Mechanical Ventilation.
Stethoscope
Oxygen analyzer
Respirometer (used to measure exhaled volumes)
Pressure manometer (used to measure negative inspiratory pressure [NIP])
Pressure manometer (used to measure cuff pressures)
Manual resuscitator with oxygen source

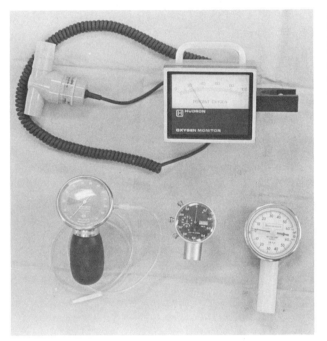

Fig. 20–9 Equipment used to assess client's condition and ventilator performance. *(Clockwise from top)* Oxygen analyzer, negative inspiratory pneumatometer, respirometer, and pneumatometer for assessing cuff pressures on airways.

CLIENT/FAMILY TEACHING

- Explain any changes in ventilator settings, modes of ventilation, or new procedures to the client.
- Explain the procedure that will be followed in daily checking of ventilator function.
- Demonstrate the alarms to the client and reassure the client that the staff will give prompt attention to determining the cause of the alarm.
- Provide the family with realistic reports of the client's progress.

IMPLEMENTATION PHASE

NURSING ACTIONS	RATIONALE/AMPLIFICATION
1. Perform routine client assessment.	Client assessment should be completed when ventilator checks are made.
a. Assess client's breath sounds for adequate ventilation.	
b. Note rate of respiration.	

c. Measure client's tidal volume and minute volume while client is using ventilator.

d. Measure client's forced vital capacity while client is not using ventilator.

e. Measure client's negative inspiratory pressure.

f. Measure effective or static compliance as required.

g. Make sure that endotracheal or tracheostomy tube is secured to prevent accidental extubation.

h. Ask whether client is comfortable or needs anything.

2. Assess the ventilator for correct functioning.

a. Drain condensed water from all tubes.

Water should be drained from the tubes and should never flow back into the humidifier reservoir.

b. Ensure that all tubes are securely connected.

c. Check all ventilator settings routinely.

Note any undocumented changes.

d. Check and fill humidifier as needed.

e. Check temperatures and adjust them as needed to maintain client's comfort and mobilization of secretions.

The ideal temperature is 30°C to 35°C.

f. Analyze oxygen concentration of ventilator and adjust if needed.

Compare the analyzed concentration with the oxygen setting.

g. Measure delivered tidal volume and adjust if needed. Check all alarms to ensure proper function.

Compare the measured volume with the ventilator setting.

h. Change ventilator setup and humidifier every 24 hours.

Changing of equipment reduces the risk of iatrogenic infections.

3. Perform additional assessments as needed.

a. Request ABGs when significant changes in client's condition are noted and when significant changes have been made to ventilator.

b. Request chest films when significant changes in breath sounds are noted, placement of endotracheal tube is in question, and client's condition appears to deteriorate suddenly.

RELATED NURSING CARE

NURSING ACTIONS	RATIONALE/AMPLIFICATION
1. Suction airways as needed.	Suctioning reduces the risk of atelectasis and infection.
2. Assist client to make frequent position changes.	Frequent changes in the client's position prevent pooling of secretions and pressure necrosis.
3. Provide client with means of communication.	Provide the client with a pad and pencil or picture board to use for communication.
4. Perform routine mouth care.	
5. Restrain client if necessary.	Restraint reduces the risk of accidental extubation.

EVALUATION PHASE

ANTICIPATED OUTCOMES	NURSING ACTIONS
1. Maintain acceptable ABG values through mechanical ventilatory support, regardless of changes in client's condition	Monitor ABGs and the client's condition.
2. Provide mechanical ventilation until such support is no longer necessary	Assess respiratory parameters as described previously under Routine Client Assessment.

PRODUCT AVAILABILITY

CUFF PRESSURE MANOMETER

Posey Co.
Portex, Inc.

RESPIROMETERS

Boehringer Laboratories, Inc.
Fraser Harlake, Inc.
Ohmeda

NEGATIVE INSPIRATORY PRESSURE MANOMETERS

Boehringer Laboratories, Inc.

SELECTED REFERENCES

Burton GG, Hodgkin JE: Respiratory Care, 2nd ed. Philadelphia, JB Lippincott, 1984
McPherson SP: Respiratory Therapy Equipment, 3rd ed. St. Louis, CV Mosby, 1985
Shapiro BA, Harrison RA, Trout CA: Clinical Application of Respiratory Care, 2nd ed. Chicago, Year Book Medical Publishers, Inc., 1979
Spearman B et al: Egan's Fundamentals of Respiratory Therapy, 4th ed. St. Louis, CV Mosby, 1982

Continuous positive airway pressure and positive end-expiratory pressure

BACKGROUND

Continuous positive airway pressure (CPAP) is a procedure that produces positive airway pressure throughout the respiratory cycle. *Positive end-expiratory pressure* (PEEP) is a procedure that produces positive airway pressure with mechanical ventilation. PEEP is also used in describing spontaneous ventilation in which positive pressure is only maintained during exhalation.

Objectives

To increase the client's functional residual capacity (FRC) by elevating the mean airway pressure above atmospheric pressure
To allow for normal breathing without mechanical assistance
To decrease physiologic shunting
To maintain acceptable PO_2 with a low inspired oxygen concentration (F_IO_2).

ASSESSMENT PHASE

• Is the client unable to maintain acceptable ABG values because of a decrease in FRC?
• Are the client's respiratory muscles and thoracic cage intact and capable of moving air if positive pressure is applied?
• Is the client intubated?

PRECAUTIONS

• **Since respiratory failure may occur even with CPAP or PEEP, be prepared to ventilate the client if needed.**
• **High levels of CPAP or PEEP can reduce cardiac return and cause circulatory failure.**
• **High levels of CPAP and PEEP can cause barotrauma to the lungs.**

- **If CPAP or PEEP is administered through a face mask, be aware of possible injury to the client's face and necrosis of tissue. Masks that are strapped on must be released every 15 minutes to 30 minutes to allow circulation to return to pressure areas.**
- **Levels of CPAP or PEEP should be monitored carefully with an in-line pressure manometer.**
- **Note changes in breath sounds and breathing patterns. Be aware of the risks and signs of respiratory failure and pneumothorax.**
- **Overall, an endotracheal tube may have an advantage over a face mask because of the ease with which CPAP and PEEP can be applied. If a face mask is used, a clear mask is preferred because it allows an observer to note any signs of vomitus, thereby reducing the risk of aspiration.**

PLANNING PHASE

EQUIPMENT

Due to the variety of CPAP and PEEP devices used, a representative diagram of each is shown, but specific equipment will not be described (Figs. 20–10 and 20–11).

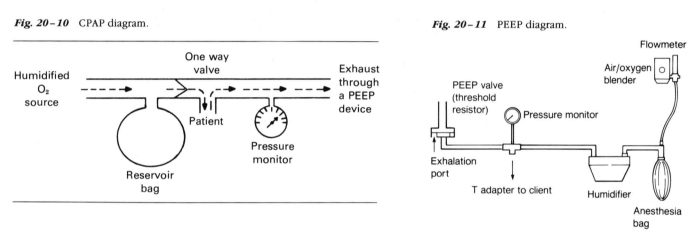

Fig. 20–10   CPAP diagram.

Fig. 20–11   PEEP diagram.

CLIENT/FAMILY TEACHING

- Explain to the client the reason for using CPAP or PEEP.
- If the client will be intubated, explain that talking will not be possible because of the tube. Explain to the client that breathing may actually be easier once CPAP or PEEP is initiated than before.
- Provide the family with realistic reports of the client's progress.

IMPLEMENTATION PHASE

NURSING ACTIONS	RATIONALE/AMPLIFICATION
1. Client assessment should include ABG determinations, vital signs, breath sounds, and central venous pressure (CVP) and pulmonary artery (PA) pressure if available.	Because of the effects of pressure on the lungs, baseline studies are needed as references that help to monitor the client's progress.
2. Set up equipment.	
a. Check connectors and oxygen delivery lines.	
b. Add water to humidifier and set temperature.	
c. Begin flow through device.	
3. Connect device to client.	
4. Adjust level of CPAP or PEEP.	
5. After 10 minutes to 15 minutes, reassess client's vital signs.	Excessive airway pressures and failure to tolerate the procedure may be indicated by failing vital signs.
6. *Caution:* Do not leave client unattended.	

7. After 30 minutes, ABGs can be drawn to assess effectiveness of treatment.	If ABGs have not improved, mechanical ventilation may be necessary.

RELATED NURSING CARE

NURSING ACTIONS	RATIONALE/AMPLIFICATION
1. Suction as needed.	Suctioning prevents atelectasis and infection.
2. Assess vital signs and breath sounds as needed.	The client's condition can deteriorate rapidly.
3. Assess CVP, ABGs, and PA pressure as needed and if available.	

EVALUATION PHASE

ANTICIPATED OUTCOME	NURSING ACTIONS
Improvement of ventilatory status	Observe whether the client's breathing is labored; assess sensorium, and evaluate ABGs. Failure to improve will require mechanical ventilation in most cases.

PRODUCT AVAILABILITY

CPAP DEVICES

Argyle Division, Sherwood Medical
Healthdyne, Inc.
Siemens–Elema Ventilator Systems
Novametrix Medical Systems, Inc.
Respironics, Inc.

PEEP DEVICES

Armstrong Industries, Inc.
J.H. Emerson Company
Laerdal Medical Corp.
Puritan–Bennett
Siemens–Elema Ventilator Systems

SELECTED REFERENCES

Burton GG, Hodgkin JE: Respiratory Care, 2nd ed. Philadelphia, JB Lippincott, 1984
Gregory GA, Kitterman JA, Phibbs RH et al: Treatment of idiopathic respiratory distress syndrome with continuous positive airway pressure. N Engl J Med 284:1333, 1971

Millar S: Methods in Critical Care, The AACN Manual. Philadelphia, WB Saunders, 1980
Morrison M: Respiratory Intensive Care Nursing, 2nd ed. Boston, Little, Brown, 1979

Discontinuance of mechanical ventilation

Objective
To terminate mechanical ventilation in a manner that will allow the client to resume normal breathing without undue stress

ASSESSMENT PHASE

- Has the client's underlying disease improved such that mechanical ventilation is no longer needed?
- Have breath sounds improved, and is the client able to clear secretions effectively?
- Does the client have a forced vital capacity greater than 20 ml to 25 ml/kg?
- Can the client generate an NIP that is less than −25 cm H_2O?
- Is tidal volume 5 ml to 7 ml/kg of ideal body weight, and are respirations less than 25 breaths per minute?

• How long has the client required a ventilator?
• Can the client support acceptable ABGs after removal from a ventilator?

PRECAUTIONS

• **Begin to discontinue mechanical ventilation in the morning, when the client is rested. The procedure should not be attempted in the evening or if the client appears fatigued.**
• **Discontinuance of the ventilator should be the only major procedure that is attempted during the day. Avoid any activities that will tire the client.**
• **Any sign of cardiovascular instability may require returning the client to the ventilator.**
• **Discontinuance of the ventilator may not be accomplished in 1 day, especially with clients who have been using mechanical ventilation for long periods.**
• **Do not leave the client unattended until it has been determined that the client is not in immediate danger.**
• **Do not remove the ventilator from the immediate area until it has been determined that it will no longer be needed by the client.**

PLANNING PHASE

EQUIPMENT

To assess the adequacy of ventilation, use the following:
Stethoscope
Respirometer
NIP manometer
For the traditional method of ventilator discontinuance, use the following:
Heated aerosol with capability of delivering different oxygen concentrations
Large-bore tubing with thermometer and proper endotracheal tube adapter (Fig. 20–12)

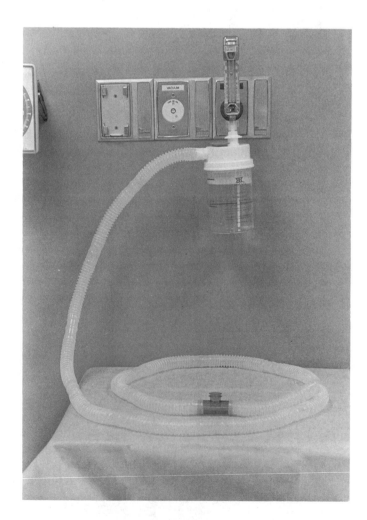

Fig. 20–12 Aerosol setup with Brigg's adapter (T tube).

For the IMV method of ventilator discontinuance, use the following:
Ventilator with IMV mode or rate controls down to 2 breaths per minute
IMV circuit that can be added to ventilator

CLIENT/FAMILY TEACHING

- Explain the procedure that will be used to discontinue ventilatory support.
- Reassure the client that someone will be nearby during the discontinuation process and that if complications arise, mechanical ventilation will be restarted. Place the emergency call button within the client's reach.
- Describe the feelings that the client may experience when breathing is no longer supported by mechanical means. Be realistic in setting goals for the client.

IMPLEMENTATION PHASE

NURSING ACTIONS	RATIONALE/AMPLIFICATION

1. Assess client's condition.
  a. Determine level of sensorium.
  b. Listen to breath sounds.
  c. Measure tidal volume while client is not using ventilator (Fig. 20–13).
  d. Measure vital capacity.
  e. Measure NIP.
	Ventilator discontinuance may be attempted with clients whose assessments are lower than those described previously under Assessment Phase. However, clients with low assessments will have a lower success rate than those with high assessments.

Fig. 20–13 Measuring exhaled tidal volume using respirometer.

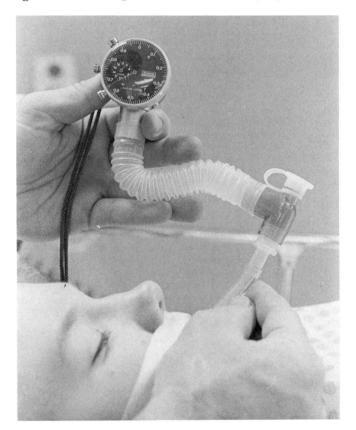

2. Traditional method of ventilator discontinuance proceeds as follows:

  a. Set up heated aerosol.

b. Describe procedure to client and suction airways.

Obstructed airways make breathing difficult; suction the airways as needed.

c. Disconnect client from ventilator and place on heated aerosol for 5 minutes to 10 minutes.

Stay nearby and reassure the client.

d. After 5 minutes to 10 minutes, return client to ventilator for remainder of hour. Increase time that client breathes without ventilator assistance each hour.

Observe for signs of fatigue.

e. If client cannot maintain respirations, return to ventilator. If progress is good, client may be extubated. If there is any doubt about client's ability to breathe without assistance by evening, return client to ventilator and start again next morning.

If any major changes in the client's condition occur, return the client to the ventilator and call the physician. Positive indications that the client will be able to breathe without assistance include good assessments of ventilatory parameters, respirations that do not become labored, and the continued good outlook of the client.

3. Alternative method of ventilator discontinuance using IMV proceeds as follows:

This method is helpful in weaning the client from the respirator gradually.

a. Set ventilator to give client specified number of breaths per minute at specified tidal volume.

If the client needs to breathe more often than the rate set on the ventilator, an additional circuit or demand valve will make air available to the client. The amount of air inspired through the IMV circuit is determined by the client's strength. Air used in the IMV circuit is usually humidified and is available at the same F_IO_2 that is set on the ventilator.

b. Slowly decrease ventilator rate while client assumes work of breathing.

The client cannot trigger the ventilator rate because it is set at a predetermined rate.

c. If client has setback during weaning process, increase rate of ventilation.

d. Gradually decrease ventilator rate until client is doing all work of breathing.

IMV can be used at night. Most changes are made during the day when the client is stronger, more alert, and better able to tolerate the changes.

e. Extubate when client is able to breathe without mechanical assistance.

RELATED NURSING CARE

NURSING ACTIONS	RATIONALE/AMPLIFICATION
1. Suction as needed.	Suctioning prevents atelectasis and infection.
2. Assess vital signs and breath sounds as needed.	The client's condition can deteriorate rapidly.
3. Assess ABGs as needed.	Observe for signs of pulmonary instability.

EVALUATION PHASE

ANTICIPATED OUTCOMES	NURSING ACTIONS
1. Improvement of ventilatory status	Observe whether the client's breathing is labored, assess sensorium, and evaluate ABGs. Failure to improve will require a return to mechanical ventilation.
2. Discontinuance of mechanical ventilation	Assess the client's ability to maintain normal ventilatory status without the use of the ventilator.

PRODUCT AVAILABILITY

AEROSOL NEBULIZERS

Disposable
Airlife
Inspiron Corporation
Respiratory Care Inc.
Travenol Laboratories, Inc. — Medical Products Division

Nondisposable
Airlife
Ohmeda
Puritan – Bennett
Respiratory Care Inc.

MECHANICAL VENTILATORS

Bear Medical Systems Inc.
Puritan – Bennett
Siemens – Elema Ventilator Systems

SELECTED REFERENCES

Burton GG, Hodgkin JE: Respiratory Care, 2nd ed. Philadelphia, JB Lippincott, 1984
Hamilton H: Procedures. Springhouse, PA. Intermed Communications, Inc., 1983
McPherson SP: Respiratory Therapy Equipment, 3rd ed. St. Louis, CV Mosby Co., 1985
Millar S: Methods in Critical Care, The AACN Manual. Philadelphia, WB Saunders, 1980

Pressure support

BACKGROUND

Pressure support closely parallels IPPB in function. A level of inspiratory pressure support is preset on the ventilator control panel. When the client initiates an inspiration, the ventilator provides the flow needed to raise the inspiratory pressure to the preset level. Throughout the inspiration, the preset pressure is constant while the flow rate is variable. Expiration begins when the inspiratory flow falls below 25% of the peak flow.

On the Siemens Servo Ventilator 900C, there are two built-in safety systems for this mode of ventilation. Both ensure that inspiratory flow does not fall below 25% of the peak flow. The first system ensures that expiration will begin if the inspiratory pressure rises to +3 cm H_2O above that set on the "Inspiratory pressure level above peep" control. The second system ensures that expiration will begin after 80% of the preset time that is allowed for one respiratory cycle has elapsed. For this reason the "Breaths/minute" control should be set at a reasonably normal setting.

Objective

To provide pressure-supported inspiration for the client whose own breathing is insufficient or for the client who is being weaned from mechanical ventilatory support (This mode is currently available only on the Siemens Servo Ventilator 900C. Directions are given under Implementation Phase in this section.)

ASSESSMENT PHASE

• Is the client hypoventilating? Do the client's ABGs indicate hypoxia or hypercapnia? The client must be intubated for this procedure.
• Is the client ready to be weaned from mechanical ventilatory support?

PRECAUTIONS

• **If the client will be weaned from mechanical ventilatory support, assess the client's condition to ensure that weaning is appropriate.**
• **Set the "Breaths/minute" control on the ventilator to a reasonable rate. This preset rate determines how long inspiration will be allowed to continue in the event of equipment malfunction.**
• **If there is any question about the client's ability to tolerate weaning from mechanical ventilatory support, the client should not be left unattended.**

PLANNING PHASE

EQUIPMENT (FIG. 20-14)

Siemens Servo Ventilator 900C
Intubation equipment (if necessary, see Endotracheal Intubation in Chap. 19)

Fig. 20-14 Siemens–Elema Servo Ventilator 900C. (Courtesy Siemens–Elema Corp.)

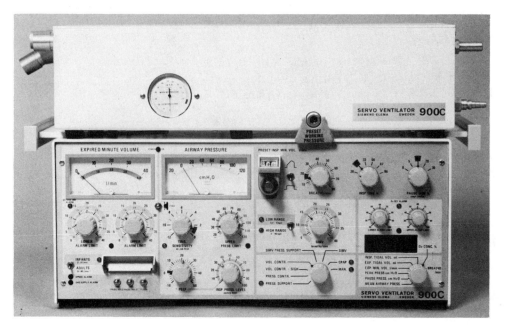

CLIENT/FAMILY TEACHING

• If pressure support will be used with a hypoventilating client, explain the need for the procedure, including the technique of endotracheal intubation (see Endotracheal Intubation in Chap. 19).
• If pressure support will be used as a weaning procedure, prepare the client for its use. Explain what pressure support is and that the client must initiate inspiration.

IMPLEMENTATION PHASE

NURSING ACTIONS	RATIONALE/AMPLIFICATION
1. Assess client's condition.	If pressure support will be used with a hypoventilating client, this assessment will ensure that treatment goals cannot be achieved by less complicated methods (see Assessment Phase under Intermittent Positive Pressure Therapy in previous section). If pressure support will be used as a weaning procedure, this assessment will ensure that the client is ready to be weaned from mechanical ventilatory support (see Ventilator Management in previous section).
2. Explain procedure to client.	
3. Set "Breaths/minute" control on the ventilator at reasonable rate (12 bpm to 15 bpm).	This is one of two built-in safety systems for this mode of ventilation on the Siemens Servo Ventilator 900C.
4. Set "Inspiratory pressure level above peep" control on ventilator to desired level.	This control sets the maximum inspiratory pressure for each spontaneous breath. Remember that this pressure setting will be *added* to any existing PEEP.
5. Select "Press support" control on mode selector on ventilator.	

RELATED NURSING CARE

NURSING ACTIONS	RATIONALE/AMPLIFICATION
1. Monitor ventilator indicators for airway pressure and expired minute volume.	Be sure that the maximum pressure setting is not exceeded and that tidal volume is sufficient for the client.
2. Observe client closely, especially during early phase of procedure. Perform ABG analysis after 20 minutes or as indicated by client's condition.	Watch for signs of hypoxia and respiratory distress (*e.g.*, tachycardia, restlessness, tachypnea and cyanosis).

EVALUATION PHASE

ANTICIPATED OUTCOME	NURSING ACTIONS
Improvement of ventilation or discontinuance of mechanical ventilatory support	Observe whether breathing is labored and monitor signs, sensorium, and ABGs. Check the client's ventilatory parameters to determine whether discontinuance of mechanical ventilatory support is appropriate.

PRODUCT AVAILABILITY
PRESSURE SUPPORT EQUIPMENT

Siemens–Elema Ventilator Systems (Siemens Servo Ventilator 900C)

SELECTED REFERENCES
McPherson SP: Respiratory Therapy Equipment, 3rd ed. St. Louis, CV Mosby, 1985

Arterial blood gases

Objective
To obtain an anaerobic sample of arterial blood to determine a client's level of oxygenation, ventilation, and acid–base status

ASSESSMENT PHASE
- Does the client have an arterial line?
- If the client does not have an arterial line, can the blood sample be obtained from the radial, brachial, or femoral artery?
- Does the client have an abnormally low or high blood pressure reading?

PRECAUTIONS
- **Sterile technique should be used when drawing a sample of blood from an arterial line to prevent the possibility of bacteremia.**
- **Clean the client's skin with an alcohol-soaked swab to prevent infection when performing arterial sticks.**
- **Observe for signs of rupture of an artery near the puncture site in clients with elevated blood pressure.**
- **Avoid sticking arteries with poor collateral circulation unless other sites are unavailable.**
- **Do not allow air to enter the syringe, because ABG values may change dramatically when exposed to room air. Remove any bubbles from the syringe as quickly as possible after obtaining the sample.**
- **Blood samples that cannot be analyzed within 20 minutes should be placed in an ice slurry to prevent changes in measured values because of the metabolism of the red blood cells.**
- **If possible, avoid using the same sample site on consecutive sticks.**
- **Note the client's allergies if a local anesthetic is used.**
- **Note whether a client is on anticoagulant therapy.**

• **Avoid sites that are covered with scar tissue or surgical incisions (*i.e.*, sticks in areas of synthetic arterial grafts).**

PLANNING PHASE	Blood gas kit*
EQUIPMENT	Ampule of sodium heparin (use if syringe is not preheparinized)
	22-gauge, 1-inch needle, "B" bevel (radial, brachial, and some femoral sticks)
	22-gauge, 1½-inch needle, "B" bevel (deep femoral sticks)
	Sterile 4 × 4s
	Alcohol preparation pads
	Adhesive bandage or adhesive tape
	Container for transporting syringe in ice-slurry pack
	Label for syringe

CLIENT/FAMILY TEACHING

• Explain the procedure to the client and emphasize the importance of remaining calm to prevent hyperventilation.
• Tell the client that although some discomfort may be experienced, sudden movements should be avoided.
• Explain the reasons for obtaining an arterial blood sample and how the procedure differs from a venous sampling procedure.

IMPLEMENTATION PHASE

NURSING ACTIONS	RATIONALE/AMPLIFICATION
1. Wash your hands before preparing equipment.	Handwashing prevents iatrogenic infections.
2. Prepare syringe.	
a. If syringe is not heparinized, draw 1 ml of sodium heparin into syringe. Lubricate walls of syringe by drawing plunger in and out. Change needles on syringe. Hold needle up and eject heparin. Cap needle.	The heparin will prevent the blood from clotting and will allow the plunger to move with less resistance. Air should not be in the syringe or in the needle. *Only* heparin should be in the syringe and needle, and the plunger should be fully pushed in. This is adequate to prevent coagulation. Excessive amounts of heparin will alter ABG values.
b. If syringe is heparinized, place needle on syringe.	Preheparinized syringes may contain liquid heparin (sodium heparin) or dry lithium heparin. Some syringes with lithium heparin can be preset to the desired sample size (up to 3 ml).
3. Set up equipment within easy reach.	A bedside table can be used.
4. Wash your hands before starting procedure.	
5. Select arterial sampling site (Fig. 20–15).	
a. Radial arteries are small but close to surface and are easily stabilized. Collateral circulation is easily checked by Allen's test.	The three most common sites, listed in order of preferred selection, are the radial artery, the brachial artery, and the femoral artery. The Allen's test is done by having the client make a fist and applying pressure over the radial and ulnar arteries. The client then opens the hand and pressure is released from the ulnar artery. Return of color to the palm indicates collateral circulation by way of the ulnar artery.
b. Brachial arteries may be used as second choice when radial sites are unavailable. These arteries are larger and deeper than radial arteries.	It is more difficult to stop bleeding from brachial arteries. They are also more difficult to stabilize and may "roll" when puncture is attempted.

* A 3- to 5-ml syringe designed for arterial blood sampling may be used instead of a blood gas kit. Syringes that are preheparinized are available, or heparin can be added before the sample is drawn.

Fig. 20–15 Arteries used for puncture. (*A*) Brachial. (*B*) Femoral.

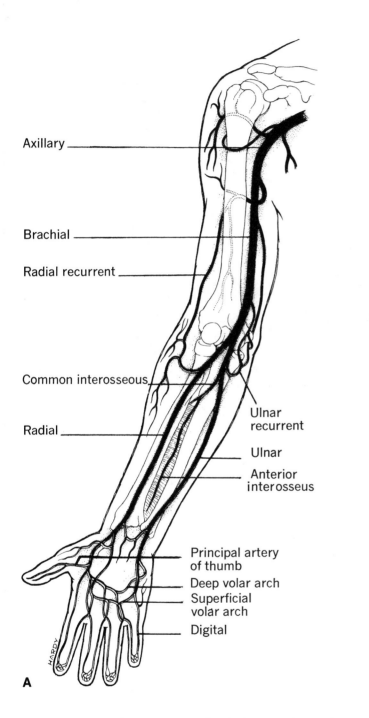

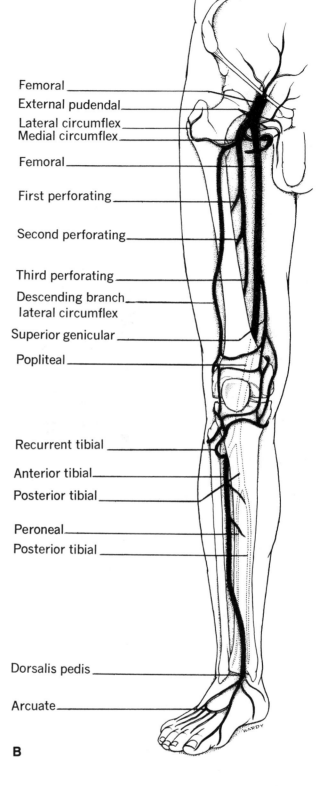

c. Femoral arteries are third choice when other sites are unavailable or client's blood pressure is very low. Some hospitals require physician approval before this site can be used.

Femoral arteries are the largest and deepest of the arteries listed. There is no collateral circulation, and the artery lies in close proximity to the femoral vein. Venous samples are sometimes mistaken for arterial samples, especially in critical clients with low blood pressures. It is difficult to apply adequate pressure to control bleeding.

6. Technique for radial artery sampling is as follows:

a. Place client supine, with arm at side and palm facing upward.

A small towel may be rolled and placed under the wrist to hyperextend the wrist.

b. Clean puncture site and your fingertips with alcohol pad (Fig. 20–16).

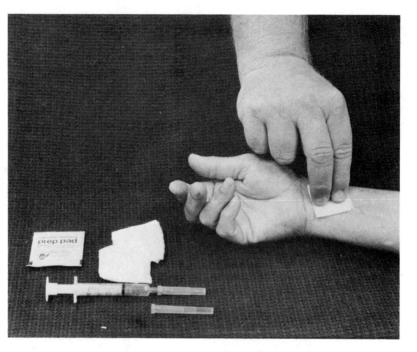

Fig. 20–16   Preparing site for radial artery puncture.

c. Palpate radial artery.

d. After locating puncture site, clean area again with alcohol pad. Remove cap from needle and hold syringe as you would hold a pen.

The needle should enter the puncture site at a 30-degree to 40-degree angle to wrist, and it should be pointed toward the elbow.

e. Smoothly puncture surface of skin. Advance needle into artery (Fig. 20–17).

The client may be warned just before the insertion of the needle that there will be a "stick." A flash of blood into the hub of the needle will indicate that the needle is in the vessel.

f. Aspirate or allow blood to fill to proper level.

Stabilize the needle to prevent any unnecessary tissue damage.

g. Place 4 × 4 over needle and puncture site and immediately apply pressure once needle is removed. Remove air bubbles from syringe.

Pressure must be applied to the puncture site for 3 minutes to 5 minutes after the needle is removed.

h. Cap syringe, label it to identify client, place syringe in ice slurry if more than 20 minutes will elapse before sample is measured. Transport sample to blood gas laboratory.

Be sure to indicate the client's name, the time the sample was drawn, and the oxygen concentration that the client is breathing, if known.

7. Technique for brachial artery sampling is as follows:

a. Client should be placed supine with arm at side and palm facing upward. (Fig. 20–18). Arm may be hyperextended.

There is not an effective test to demonstrate collateral circulation.

b. Skin should be prepared with alcohol pad and artery should be palpated.

Fig. 20-17 Radial artery puncture.

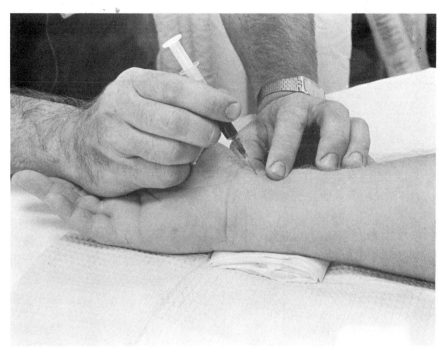

Fig. 20-18 Palpation of brachial artery.

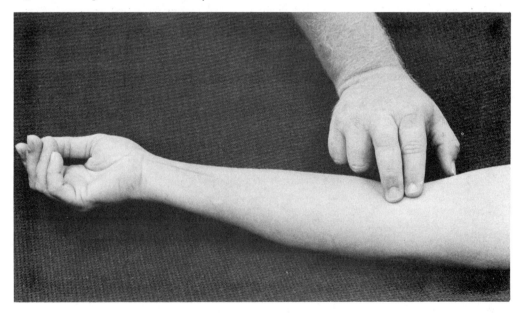

c. Same procedure should be followed for puncturing brachial artery as that used for radial artery puncture (Fig. 20-19).

d. Once sample of blood is obtained, pressure should be applied to area for 3 minutes to 5 minutes.

e. Handling of syringe is same as that used for radial artery.

Fig. 20-19 Brachial artery puncture.

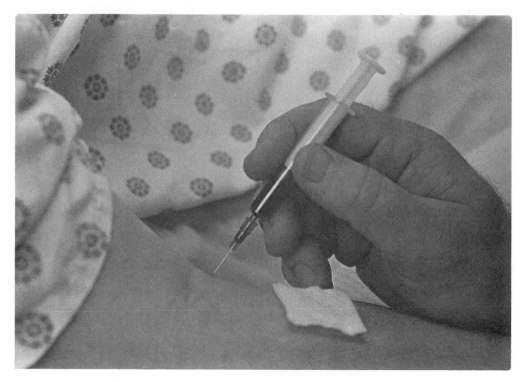

8. Technique for femoral artery sampling is as follows:

   a. Place client supine.

   b. Palpate femoral artery.

   c. Prepare puncture site with alcohol pad.

   d. Insert needle at 90-degree angle to surface of skin.

   A 1½-inch needle may be required for large clients.

   e. Once sample is obtained and needle is removed, apply pressure to site for 3 minutes to 5 minutes.

   f. Handling of syringe is same as for radial artery.

9. Technique for obtaining sample from arterial line is as follows (Fig. 20-20):

   See Obtaining Blood Sample from Arterial Line in Chap. 5 for description of technique.

   a. Two syringes will be needed. One syringe should be heparinized.

   b. Remove cap from sampling port and place on sterile gauze.

   c. Clean port with alcohol pad, insert syringe without heparin, turn stopcock so that indwelling catheter is open to port, and aspirate 2 ml to 3 ml of blood.

   d. Quickly remove syringe and replace with heparinized syringe.

   A 4 × 4 can be placed under the stopcock to absorb any blood that may be lost during the exchange.

   e. Handle syringe as described above in procedure for radial artery sampling.

   f. Flush arterial line. Replace cap on sampling port.

Fig. 20–20 Removing sample from arterial line.

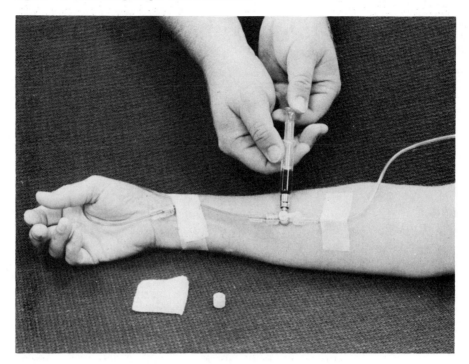

RELATED NURSING CARE

NURSING ACTIONS	RATIONALE/AMPLIFICATION
Recheck sampling site if needle is used. Look for signs of hematoma; note any changes in strength of pulse. Notify physician if there are any significant changes.	

EVALUATION PHASE

ANTICIPATED OUTCOMES	NURSING ACTIONS
1. Obtaining arterial blood	Note whether blood is pulsating in the syringe when drawing the sample.
2. Prevention of bleeding or hematoma at puncture site	Monitor the condition of the puncture site. Apply a pressure dressing if necessary.

PRODUCT AVAILABILITY　　BLOOD GAS KITS

Airlife, Inc.
American Scientific Products
Bard–Parker
Chesebrough–Ponds, Inc.
Corning Medical
Marquest Medical Products, Inc.

SELECTED REFERENCES　　Burton GG, Hodgkin JE: Respiratory Care, 2nd ed. Philadelphia, JB Lippincott, 1984
Millar S: Methods in Critical Care, The AACN Manual. Philadelphia, WB Saunders, 1980

Shapiro BA, Harrison RA, Walton JR: Clinical Application of Blood Gases, 3rd ed. Chicago, Year Book Medical Publishers, Inc., 1984

21 *Infection control for respiratory techniques*

BACKGROUND

Clients in critical care units frequently require assistance with respiratory problems ranging from help with coughing and breathing deeply to mechanical ventilation. Pneumonia is a major infection-control problem because it accounts for 10% to 20% of all nosocomial (hospital-associated) infections, and it is the infection that is most likely to occur in the critical care unit.

Conditions that increase the risk of respiratory infection are recent surgery, artificial airways or other conditions that increase the possibility of aspiration, colonization with gram-negative aerobic bacilli, and impaired immunologic function. In addition, clients who are exposed to contaminated respiratory therapy equipment or who receive respiratory care without appropriate infection-control precautions are vulnerable to respiratory infection.

To protect vulnerable clients from respiratory infection, perform vigorous pulmonary toilet and ambulate the client as soon as his condition permits. Use precautions to prevent aspiration, for example, not overfeeding tube-fed clients and keeping the head of the bed elevated. Use aseptic techniques if suctioning is required and avoid traumatizing the delicate tissue of the respiratory tract. Use adequate handwashing techniques between contacts with different clients.

Herpes whitlow, a painful infection of the pulp space of the finger, can be acquired from clients who have active herpes lesions of the mouth. Wear gloves for all contact with oral secretions.

The Centers for Disease Control (CDC) publish guidelines for two categories of respiratory isolation, which may be used to effectively protect personnel against diseases spread by airborne contamination. They are acid-fast bacillus (AFB) isolation and respiratory isolation. AFB isolation is used to protect clients against tuberculosis; respiratory isolation is used to prevent the spread of airborne diseases.

Acid-fast bacilli (AFB) isolation

Objective
To prevent cross-infection of tuberculosis to personnel or other clients

ASSESSMENT PHASE

- Is a private room available? A private room is indicated for isolation of this infection.
- Is the client cooperative? Will the client use a tissue to cover his mouth when coughing?

PRECAUTIONS

- **Early identification of a client who has tuberculosis is the most effective method of prevention of cross-infection.**
- **Use a mask when you are caring for an uncooperative client or when you are giving mechanical ventilation.**

PLANNING PHASE	Isolation cart
EQUIPMENT	AFB isolation sign (gray)
	Gowns (as needed)
	Masks
	Tissues (for client's use)

CLIENT/FAMILY TEACHING	• Share the information on the CDC sign with the client and family. This is an excellent way of informing the client of the precautions that will need to be observed.
	• Teach the client to use tissues to cover his mouth when coughing and to dispose of them appropriately. Emphasize that it is the tuberculosis bacilli — not the client — that is being isolated. Reassure the client that the quality of nursing care will not be affected.
	• Does the client have tuberculosis at a stage that requires isolation? (See list of diseases requiring AFB isolation.)

Diseases requiring AFB isolation*

This isolation category is for patients with current pulmonary TB who have a positive sputum smear or a chest x-ray appearance that strongly suggests current (active) TB. Laryngeal TB is also included in this category. In general, infants and young children with pulmonary TB do not require isolation precautions because they rarely cough and their bronchial secretions contain few AFB compared with adults with pulmonary TB. To protect the patient's privacy, this instruction card is labeled AFB (acid-fast bacilli) Isolation rather than Tuberculosis Isolation.

* A private room with special ventilation is indicated for AFB isolation. In general, patients infected with the same organism may share a room.

IMPLEMENTATION PHASE

NURSING ACTIONS	RATIONALE/AMPLIFICATION
1. Place CDC "AFB Isolation" sign on client's door.	This is a guide for the client, family, and personnel.
2. Label outside of client's record "AFB Isolation." Label all interdepartmental requisitions (*e.g.*, x-ray film requests) "AFB Precautions."	Labeling provides interdepartmental communication about AFB precautions.
3. Follow specifications on front of CDC card (see list of AFB isolation protocols).	

AFB isolation

VISITORS — REPORT TO NURSES' STATION BEFORE ENTERING ROOM

1. Masks are indicated only when patient is coughing and does not reliably cover mouth.
2. Gowns are indicated only if needed to prevent gross contamination of clothing.
3. Gloves are not indicated.
4. HANDS MUST BE WASHED AFTER TOUCHING THE PATIENT OR POTENTIALLY CONTAMINATED ARTICLES AND BEFORE TAKING CARE OF ANOTHER PATIENT.
5. Articles should be discarded, cleaned, or sent for decontamination and reprocessing.

EVALUATION PHASE

ANTICIPATED OUTCOME	NURSING ACTION
Prevention of cross-infection of tuberculosis	Monitor compliance with CDC AFB guidelines until the client has been on medication long enough to show clinical improvement and it is determined that the client is no longer infectious.

Respiratory isolation

Objective
To prevent cross-infection of airborne diseases

ASSESSMENT PHASE
- Is a private room available? A private room is necessary; however, clients who have the same infection may share a room.
- Does the client have a respiratory disease that requires isolation? (See list of diseases requiring respiratory isolation.)

Diseases requiring respiratory isolation*

Epiglottitis, *Haemophilus influenzae*
Erythema infectiosum
Measles
Meningitis
　Haemophilus influenzae, known or
　　suspected
　Meningococcal, known or suspected
Meningococcal pneumonia

Meningococcemia
Mumps
Pertussis (whooping cough)
Pneumonia. *Haemophilus influenzae,* in
　children (any age)

* A private room is indicated for Respiratory
Isolation; in general, however, patients infected
with the same organism may share a room.

PRECAUTIONS
- **Early implementation of isolation precautions is essential because respiratory diseases may be infectious before and immediately at the onset of symptoms.**
- **Wear gloves and use good handwashing practices when you are in contact with oral secretions to prevent herpetic whitlow.**

PLANNING PHASE

EQUIPMENT
Isolation cart
　Respiratory isolation sign (blue)
　Masks
　Tissues (for client's use)
　Gowns (if contact with respiratory secretions is possible)

CLIENT/FAMILY TEACHING
See previous section on Acid-Fast Bacilli (AFB) Isolation.

IMPLEMENTATION PHASE

NURSING ACTIONS	RATIONALE/AMPLIFICATION
1. Place CDC "Respiratory Isolation" sign on door of client's room.	This is a guide for the client, family, and personnel.

2. Label outside of client's record "Respiratory Isolation." Label all interdepartmental communication (*e.g.,* x-ray film requests) "Respiratory Isolation."

Labeling provides interdepartmental communication.

Respiratory isolation

VISITORS—REPORT TO NURSES' STATION BEFORE ENTERING ROOM

1. Masks are indicated for those who come close to patient.
2. Gowns are not indicated.
3. Gloves are not indicated.
4. HANDS MUST BE WASHED AFTER TOUCHING THE PATIENT OR POTEN- TIALLY CONTAMINATED ARTICLES AND BEFORE TAKING CARE OF ANOTHER PATIENT.
5. Articles contaminated with infective material should be discarded or bagged and labeled before being sent for decontamination and reprocessing.

3. Follow specifications on front of CDC Respiratory Isolation sign (see list of respiratory isolation protocols).

EVALUATION PHASE

ANTICIPATED OUTCOME	NURSING ACTION
Prevention of cross-infection of airborne infections	Monitor compliance with CDC guidelines for respiratory infections.

SELECTED REFERENCES

Craig CP, Connelly S: Effect of intensive care unit nosocomial pneumonia on duration of stay and mortality. Infect Control 12:233–238, 1984

Garner JS, Simmons BP: CDC Guidelines for the prevention and control of nosocomial infections: Guideline for isolation precautions in hospitals. Am J Infect Control 12(2):103–166, April 1984

Guidelines for Isolation Precautions in Hospitals. Washington, D.C., Department of Health and Human Services (HHS Publication No. [CDC] 83-8314), 1983

Guidelines for Prevention of TB Transmission in Hospitals. Washington, D.C., Department of Health and Human Services (HHS Publication [CDC] 82-8371), 1982

Stanford JP, Pierce AK: Lower respiratory tract infections. In Bennett JV, Brachman PS (eds): Hospital Infections, p 255–286. Boston, Little, Brown, 1979

22 *Chest drainage*

Postural drainage, chest percussion, and chest vibration are techniques that are used to facilitate the removal of secretions from the airways. The purpose of these three techniques is to allow secretions to drain from smaller peripheral airways into larger central airways, where their removal can be easily accomplished by coughing and expectoration or by tracheobronchial suctioning.

Postural drainage consists of positioning the client such that the lobe or segment of the lung that requires draining is in the uppermost location. This positioning uses gravity to help drain the secretions. To achieve optimal effectiveness, each position should be maintained for a minimum of 15 minutes to 20 minutes, if the positions are tolerated by the client. Because many of the postural drainage positions are based on Trendelenburg's position, extreme caution should be exercised with clients who show signs of unstable heart rate and rhythm or who have a history of dyspneic episodes. Trendelenburg's position should not be used with clients who are experiencing fluid imbalance or increased intracranial pressure. If there is any question about the client's ability to tolerate a specific position, do not leave the client unattended during the treatment. When used properly and cautiously, postural drainage can be an effective part of airway-clearance therapy.

The objective of both chest percussion and chest vibration is to loosen thick, tenacious secretions. Chest percussion is accomplished by clapping the chest wall with cupped hands. Cupping your hands traps air in the resulting pocket, producing sufficient force to be effective without directly striking the skin. Chest vibration is performed during expiration only. Vibration is accomplished by placing one hand over the other and gently vibrating the chest wall. It is believed that vibration is effective because it increases the velocity of exhaled air, thus increasing the movement of secretions. When used in conjunction with postural drainage, chest percussion and chest vibration can enhance secretion clearance.

Postural drainage

Objective

To position the client such that gravity helps to drain secretions from small into large airways that may then be cleared by coughing and expectoration

ASSESSMENT PHASE

- Has the client been unable to remove secretions by coughing and expectoration?
- Can the client tolerate the required positions?
- Does the client experience episodes of dyspnea?
- Are the client's cardiac rate and rhythm stable?

PRECAUTIONS

- **Stay with clients who are placed in Trendelenburg's position.**
- **Avoid Trendelenburg's position in clients who have dyspnea, arrhythmias, increased intracranial pressure, or fluid imbalances.**
- **Avoid treatment immediately before or after meals.**

· **When more than one lung segment will be drained, start with the uppermost segment and work downward.**

PLANNING PHASE	Stethoscope
EQUIPMENT	Bed or postural drainage platform capable of elevating client's head and feet
	Pillows
	Emesis basin and tissues
CLIENT/FAMILY TEACHING	· Explain the procedure to the client.
	· Tell the client to be alert for conditions that warrant stopping the procedure (*e.g.,* dyspnea, chest pain, nausea).
	· Instruct the client in the proper techniques for producing an effective cough.

IMPLEMENTATION PHASE

NURSING ACTIONS	RATIONALE/AMPLIFICATION
1. Use chest films and chest auscultation to determine which lung segments require drainage.	Chest films and auscultation will determine the proper client positioning.
2. Place client in proper position to drain specific lobe or segment (Fig. 22–1).	Proper positioning is essential to the efficient use of gravity.
3. Ensure client's comfort by using pillows for support.	Since the positions will be maintained for 15 minutes to 20 minutes, client support and comfort are important.
4. Monitor cardiac rate and rhythm, breathing pattern, and skin color during procedure.	Arrhythmias, dyspnea, or cyanosis are contraindications for postural drainage.
5. Maintain postural drainage position for 15 minutes to 20 minutes if tolerated.	Maintain the position for 15 minutes to 20 minutes to allow adequate time for drainage.
6. Reposition client for drainage of next segment and repeat steps 2 to 5 as necessary.	
7. Place client in sitting position.	Because an effective cough requires a deep breath, the sitting position is more effective than the supine one.
8. Instruct client in proper coughing techniques.	
a. Ask client to take several deep breaths and to hold each for three counts.	
b. Ask client to take several deep breaths and hold while performing Valsalva's maneuver. To perform this maneuver, client should be instructed to "close" throat and contract or tighten abdominal muscles. After tightening abdominal muscles, client should be instructed to "open" throat and forcibly expel air from lungs.	
9. Assist client in coughing and expectoration by coaching and by supporting any incisions.	Coaching will reinforce the use of proper coughing techniques. Supporting incisions will decrease the pain associated with coughing.
10. If client is unable to generate effective cough, perform nasotracheal suctioning (see Blind Endotracheal [Nasotracheal] Suctioning in Chap. 19).	

RELATED NURSING CARE

NURSING ACTIONS	RATIONALE/AMPLIFICATION
1. Aerosol therapy, bronchodilator therapy, and pain medication should precede postural drainage.	The delivery of these adjunct procedures will enhance the efficiency of postural drainage.

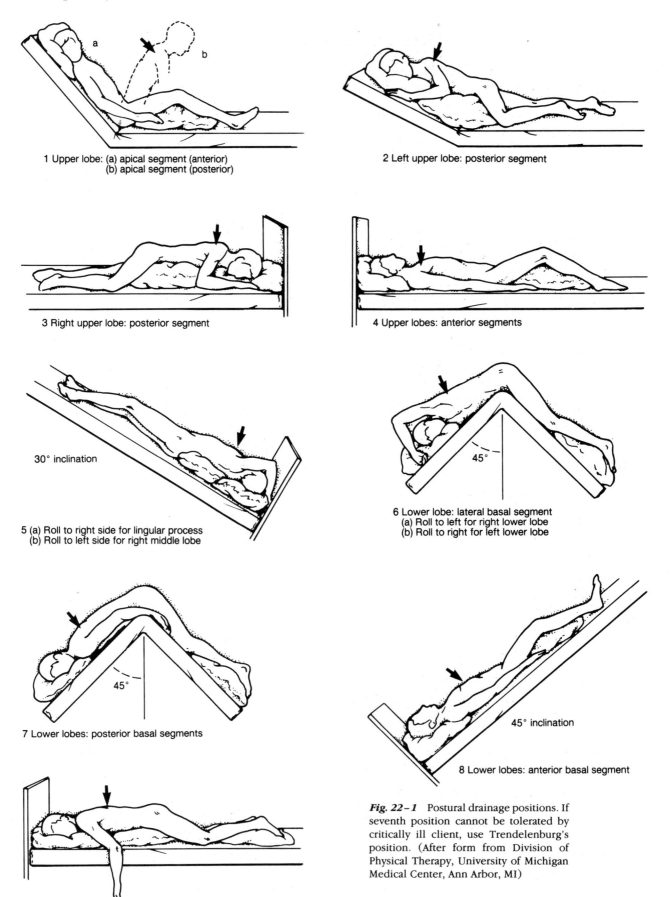

1 Upper lobe: (a) apical segment (anterior)
(b) apical segment (posterior)

2 Left upper lobe: posterior segment

3 Right upper lobe: posterior segment

4 Upper lobes: anterior segments

30° inclination

5 (a) Roll to right side for lingular process
(b) Roll to left side for right middle lobe

6 Lower lobe: lateral basal segment
(a) Roll to left for right lower lobe
(b) Roll to right for left lower lobe

45°

7 Lower lobes: posterior basal segments

45° inclination

8 Lower lobes: anterior basal segment

9 Lower lobes: apical segments

Fig. 22-1 Postural drainage positions. If seventh position cannot be tolerated by critically ill client, use Trendelenburg's position. (After form from Division of Physical Therapy, University of Michigan Medical Center, Ann Arbor, MI)

2. Encourage client to breathe deeply and to cough between postural drainage treatments.

Breathing deeply and coughing help to keep secretions mobile and airways clear.

EVALUATION PHASE

ANTICIPATED OUTCOME	NURSING ACTIONS
Effective mobilization of secretions	If expectoration does not improve, ensure that adequate humidification is being provided to facilitate the removal of secretions. Coach the client in breathing deeply and in proper coughing techniques between treatments. If respiratory problems suddenly develop because of excess secretions, raise the client's head and suction if possible.

PRODUCT AVAILABILITY

POSTURAL DRAINAGE TABLES

The John Bunn Company
Strom Corp.

SELECTED REFERENCES

Burton GG, Hodgkin JE: Respiratory Care, 2nd ed. Philadelphia, JB Lippincott, 1984
Gaskell DV, Webber BA: The Brompton Hospital Guide to Chest Physiotherapy, 4th ed. Oxford, Blackwell Scientific Publications, 1980
Morrison M: Respiratory Intensive Care Nursing, 2nd ed. Boston, Little, Brown, 1979
Tyler ML: Complications of Positioning and Chest Physiotherapy. Respir Care 27(4):458–466, 1982

Chest percussion and vibration

Objectives

To position the client such that gravity will help to drain secretions from small to large airways

To perform chest percussion or vibration to loosen secretions in the airways

ASSESSMENT PHASE

- Has the client been unable to remove secretions by coughing and expectoration?
- Can the client tolerate the required positions?
- Does the client experience episodes of dyspnea?
- Are the client's cardiac rate and rhythm stable?

PRECAUTIONS

- **Stay with clients who are placed in Trendelenburg's position.**
- **Avoid Trendelenburg's position in clients who have dyspnea, arrhythmias, increased intracranial pressure, or fluid imbalances.**
- **Avoid treatment immediately before or after meals.**
- **When more than one lung segment will be drained, start with the uppermost segment and work downward.**
- **Avoid percussion and vibration over the spine and the bony protrusions of the thorax.**
- **Avoid percussion and vibration over incisions and chest tubes.**
- **Avoid percussion and vibration over the kidneys, the liver, and the spleen.**
- **Avoid percussion and vibration on bare skin and on female clients' breasts.**

PLANNING PHASE

EQUIPMENT

Stethoscope
Bed or postural drainage platform capable of elevating client's head and feet
Pillows
Towel
Emesis basin and tissues

Suction equipment (as needed)
Mechanical percussor (if applicable)

CLIENT/FAMILY TEACHING
- Explain the procedure to the client.
- Tell the client to be alert for conditions that warrant stopping the procedure (*e.g.,* dyspnea, chest pain, nausea).
- Instruct the client in the proper techniques for producing an effective cough.

IMPLEMENTATION PHASE

NURSING ACTIONS	RATIONALE/AMPLIFICATION
1. Use chest films and chest auscultation to determine which lung segments require percussion or vibration.	Chest films and auscultation will determine the proper client positioning.
2. Place client in proper position to drain specific lobe or segment (see Fig. 22–1).	Proper positioning is essential to the efficient use of gravity.
3. Ensure client's comfort by using pillows for support.	Because the position will be maintained for 15 minutes to 20 minutes, client support and comfort are important.
4. Monitor cardiac rate and rhythm, breathing pattern, and skin color during procedure.	Arrhythmias, dyspnea, or cyanosis are contraindications for postural drainage.
5. Use towel to cover area to be percussed.	Percussion performed on bare skin or through thin clothing can be painful.
6. Perform percussion:	
a. Stand opposite of side to be percussed.	This allows your arms to be held in a comfortable position.
b. Cup hands with fingers flexed and thumbs held tightly against forefingers (Fig. 22–2).	Cupping your hands allows air to be trapped beneath, which cushions the blow to the chest wall.

Fig. 22–2 Proper hand positioning for performing percussion.

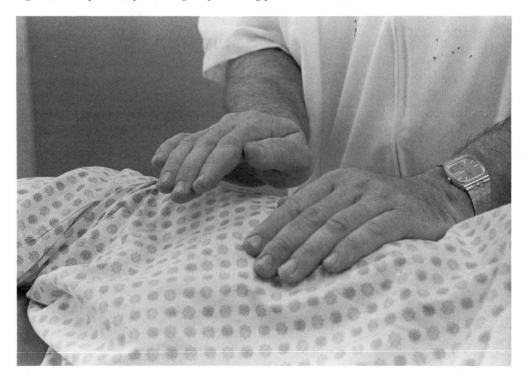

c. Clap chest wall, alternating hands, in rhythmic manner. Movement of the hands should be from the wrists only; your arms and shoulders should remain relaxed.

When performed properly, clapping should produce a characteristic popping sound.

d. Percuss each segment for 2 minutes to 3 minutes.

7. Perform vibration.

a. Instruct client to inhale deeply and exhale slowly through pursed lips.

Exhaling through pursed lips prolongs the expiratory phase.

Caution: Perform vibration during exhalation only.

Performing vibration during the inspiratory phase may produce effects that are opposite of those desired.

b. Place one hand on top of the other and gently vibrate the chest wall.

Vibration increases the velocity of the exhaled gas, facilitating the removal of secretions.

c. Vibrate over each segment during approximately five exhalations.

8. Maintain postural drainage position for 5 minutes to 10 minutes if tolerated.

Maintain the position for 5 minutes to 10 minutes to allow adequate time for drainage.

9. Reposition client for drainage of next segment and repeat steps 2 to 8 as necessary.

10. Place client in sitting position.

Because an effective cough requires a deep breath, a sitting position is more effective than a supine one.

11. Instruct client in proper coughing techniques.

a. Ask client to take several deep breaths and to hold each for three counts.

b. Ask client to take several deep breaths and hold while performing Valsalva's maneuver. (See previous section on Postural Drainage for a description of Valsalva's maneuver.)

12. Assist client in coughing and expectoration by coaching and supporting any incisions.

Coaching will reinforce the use of proper coughing techniques. Supporting incisions will decrease the pain associated with coughing.

13. If client is unable to generate effective cough, perform nasotracheal suctioning (see Blind Endotracheal [Nasotracheal] Suctioning in Chap. 19).

RELATED NURSING CARE

NURSING ACTIONS	RATIONALE/AMPLIFICATION
1. Aerosol therapy, bronchodilator therapy, and pain medication should precede postural drainage and percussion treatments.	Delivery of these adjunct procedures will enhance the efficiency of postural drainage and percussion.
2. Encourage client to breathe deeply and to cough between postural drainage and percussion treatments.	Breathing deeply and coughing help to keep secretions mobile and airways clear.

EVALUATION PHASE   See previous section on Postural Drainage.

SELECTED REFERENCES   Burton GG, Hodgkin JE: Respiratory Care, 2nd ed. Philadelphia, JB Lippincott, 1984
Gaskell DV, Webber BA: The Brompton Hospital Guide to Chest Physiotherapy, 4th ed. Oxford, Blackwell Scientific Publications, 1980

Morrison M: Respiratory Intensive Care Nursing, 2nd ed. Boston, Little, Brown, 1979
Tyler ML: Complications of positioning and chest physiotherapy. Respir Care 27(4):458–466, 1982

Thoracentesis

Objectives
To remove fluid, blood, or air from the pleural space
To relieve pulmonary compression and restore respiratory integrity
To obtain pleural fluid specimens for laboratory analysis
To obtain pleural tissue samples for biopsy
To instill medication directly into the pleural space

ASSESSMENT PHASE

- Are chest films available for documentation of fluid location?
- Is the client coughing enough to interrupt the procedure? If the needle punctures the lung, pneumothorax will result. Administer a cough suppressant before the procedure begins.
- Does the client have a clotting disorder? Is the client taking anticoagulants? Bleeding may be a problem after thoracentesis.

PRECAUTIONS

- **If the lung is punctured during the procedure, pneumothorax will result.**

PLANNING PHASE

EQUIPMENT

Sterile thoracentesis tray
    Sterile drapes
    Sterile gloves
    Antiseptic solution
    5-ml syringe with 21- or 25-gauge needle
    17-gauge thoracentesis needle
    50-ml Luer-Lok syringe
    Three-way stopcock
    Sterile tubing
    Sterile hemostat
    Sterile gauze 4×4s
Local anesthetic (1% or 2% lidocaine)
Band-Aid
Optional items
    Underwater-seal drainage setup
    Sterile specimen containers and labels
    Sterile Teflon catheter
    Biopsy needle
    Sterile specimen containers with 70% alcohol solution

CLIENT/FAMILY TEACHING

- Explain the procedure and its purpose to the client and family. Assist the physician as necessary in obtaining an informed consent from the client.
- Explain that pressure will be felt when the needle is inserted. Reassure the client that a local anesthetic will be administered.
- Advise the client to remain still during the thoracentesis to prevent injury.

IMPLEMENTATION PHASE

NURSING ACTIONS	RATIONALE/AMPLIFICATION
1. Obtain baseline vital signs.	These serve as a basis for evaluating client status during and after the procedure.
2. Assess client's respiratory status, including auscultation of lung fields.	Pre- and post-thoracentesis comparisons are made to determine the therapeutic value of the procedure to the client.
3. Position client in one of the following ways:	

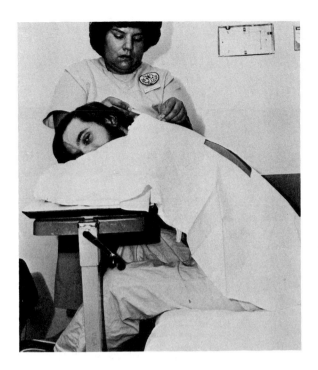

Fig. 22–3 Client rests over bedside table for thoracentesis. Secure sterile drape with adhesive strips so that it will not slip over work area.

a. Sitting on edge of bed with legs supported and head and arms placed on pillow on overbed table (Fig. 22–3)

The upright position causes fluid to pool at the base of the lungs. Arching of the back or stretching of the thorax provides easier palpation of the intercostal spaces than the upright position does.

b. Straddling chair with head and arms on back of chair

c. Lying on unaffected side in bed with opposite arm stretched overhead, and head of bed raised 30° to 40°.

4. Expose client's back.

5. Wash your hands. Open thoracentesis tray on bedside table to provide sterile field. Open sterile supplies on field.

6. Assist physician in preparing skin with antiseptic solution and administering local anesthetic.

If an iodophor solution is used, do not clean the puncture site after the procedure.

7. Monitor client's tolerance and vital signs during procedure.

The physician will assemble the thoracentesis needle, stopcock, and 50-ml syringe. The stopcock prevents air from entering the pleural space while the space is being penetrated. The needle is inserted into the pleural space through the appropriate interspace. Suction is applied to the syringe when the pleural space is entered. The needle is anchored with a hemostat during fluid drainage to prevent perforation of the lung or tearing of the pleura by the needle (Fig. 22–4).

8. If Teflon catheter is inserted through catheter, connect second catheter to sterile tubing and water-seal drainage or a Heimlich valve (see following section on Chest Tube and Water-Seal Drainage).

If the catheter is indwelling, underwater-seal drainage will be required to prevent air from entering the pleural space.

9. After needle or catheter is removed, apply manual pressure with sterile 4 × 4 until bleeding or leaking of pleural fluid stops.

Manual pressure at the puncture site keeps air from entering the pleural space.

Fig. 22-4 Needle is inserted into pleural space. Stopcock prevents air from entering pleural space during penetration. Needle is anchored with a hemostat to prevent perforation of lung.

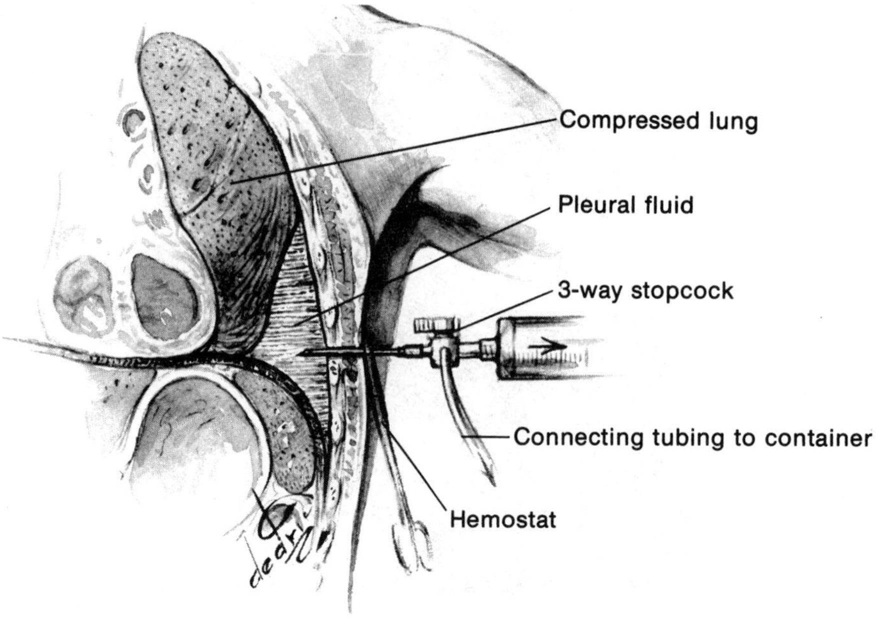

Labels on figure:
- Compressed lung
- Pleural fluid
- 3-way stopcock
- Connecting tubing to container
- Hemostat

10. Dress site with Band-Aid.

11. Label and send pleural specimens to laboratory.

Tests that are frequently ordered include bacteriology, specific gravity, cell count and differential, protein, glucose, lactate dehydrogenase (LDH), and cytology.

RELATED NURSING CARE

NURSING ACTIONS	RATIONALE/AMPLIFICATION
1. Assess client's vital signs and respiratory function every 15 minutes until stable. Decrease frequency of monitoring as client's condition allows.	Tachycardia, tachypnea, faintness, hypotension, respiratory stridor, diaphoresis, chest pain, and uncontrollable coughing may indicate pneumothorax or hypovolemic shock.
2. Obtain chest film after procedure is completed.	This will rule out pneumothorax.
3. Note and record color, consistency, odor, and amount of pleural fluid drained.	An accurate description aids in diagnosis and future treatment. Hypovolemic shock may result from a rapid shift of fluid from the circulating volume to the pleural space as fluid from the circulating volume replaces the aspirated pleural fluid.

EVALUATION PHASE

ANTICIPATED OUTCOMES	NURSING ACTIONS
1. Removal of pleural fluid	Evaluate physical assessment findings to determine whether reaccumulation of the pleural effusion has occurred.
2. Prevention of complications of thoracentesis	
a. Pneumothorax	Monitor for pleuritic or shoulder pain, which indicates pleural irritation by the needle. Monitor the client's respiratory status and vital signs.

b. Hypovolemic shock

Usually no more than 1000 ml of fluid is removed during each thoracentesis. Monitor the client's hemodynamic parameters.

c. Infection

Monitor the client's vital signs and temperature. Evaluate the use of aseptic technique during the procedure.

3. Restoration of respiratory function

Evaluate lung sounds after the procedure and compare them with the baseline assessment. Observe the rate, depth, symmetry, and ease of respiratory movements. Monitor the client for improvement in sensorium.

PRODUCT AVAILABILITY

DISPOSABLE THORACENTESIS TRAY

Travenol Laboratories, Inc.
Abbott Laboratories
Pharmaseal Inc.

SELECTED REFERENCES

Kaye W: Invasive therapeutic techniques. Heart and Lung 12(3):300–319, May 1983

Rhodes M: Update on chest trauma. Crit Care Quart 6(2):59–66, September 1983

Chest tube and water-seal drainage

BACKGROUND

The insertion of a chest tube connected to a water-seal drainage system restores normal respiratory function when the integrity of the pleural space is interrupted. This can occur as a result of a collection of air (pneumothorax), of blood (hemothorax), of blood and air (hemopneumothorax), or of serous fluid (pleural effusion) in the pleural space. Causes include trauma, surgery, and spontaneous pneumothorax. All of these interfere with normal respiration.

Air that enters the pleural space interferes with normal intrathoracic pressure and thus prevents expansion of the lung. If air continues to enter the pleural space after the lung is totally collapsed, enough pressure can develop to push the mediastinal structures toward the unaffected side, causing tension pneumothorax (Fig. 22–5). This is an emergency condition that requires immediate insertion of a chest tube to correct impaired venous return and severe respiratory distress.

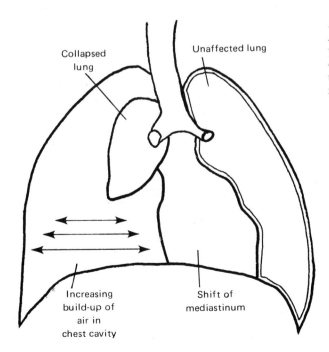

Collapsed lung

Unaffected lung

Increasing build-up of air in chest cavity

Shift of mediastinum

Fig. 22–5 Tension pneumothorax. As air enters lung on inspiration and is unable to escape, each inspiration causes further lung collapse, mediastinal shift, and encroachment on unaffected lung.

WATER-SEAL DRAINAGE

A chest tube is inserted into the pleural space to drain air or fluid. However, another mechanism is used to prevent air from entering the pleural space through the chest tube while the client inhales. Water-seal drainage accomplishes this by acting as a one-way, low-resistance valve that prevents the return of air or fluid through the tube.

A single-bottle system is used in cases in which gravity alone provides drainage. An air vent is always used to prevent a buildup of pressure in the bottle, which would prevent more air or fluid from draining into the bottle (Fig. 22–6). Occasionally, suction may be applied to the air vent tube at 20 cm of water pressure (cm H_2O) to facilitate drainage. If suction is required, a two- or three-bottle system is used to regulate the amount of suction that is applied to the pleural space.

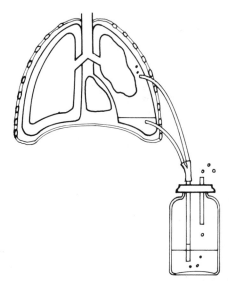

Fig. 22–6 One-bottle underwater-seal drainage system.

The three-bottle drainage system includes a collection bottle, an underwater-seal bottle, and a bottle that regulates suction pressure (Fig. 22–7). If only one bottle is used as both an underwater seal and as a trap for drainage, the level of fluid can rise enough to cause resistance to expulsion of air or fluid from the lung. Using the three-bottle system, lung secretions are removed before they reach the water-seal drainage bottle. Air is removed from the system by the vacuum source. The second bottle serves as the water seal, preventing air from entering the pleural space by

Fig. 22–7 Three-bottle drainage system. (*1*) Drainage-collection bottle. (*2*) Water-seal bottle. (*3*) Suction-control bottle.

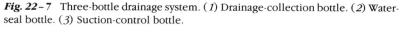

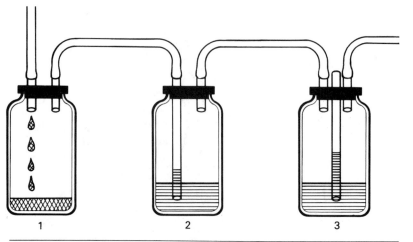

1   2   3

creating a seal that is equal to the subatmospheric thoracic pressure in the pleural space during inspiration.

The third bottle is a suction regulator. It is a sealed bottle with an atmospheric vent, or manometer tube, and is used to measure and control applied suction. For every centimeter of water pressure applied to the system, the water column in the atmospheric vent is pulled 1 cm beneath the surface. The upper limit of suction is achieved when the water level is at the bottom of the tube. In a two-bottle system, the water-seal and collection bottles are combined. In a system that is functioning correctly, gentle bubbling will be observed in the suction-control bottle. Fluid in the water-seal bottle will rise and fall with normal respiration. This pattern will be reversed if the client is on a positive-pressure ventilator.

ALTERNATIVES TO TRADITIONAL WATER-SEAL DRAINAGE

Disposable plastic chest drainage systems are similar to the three-bottle drainage system (Fig. 22–8). Chest drainage can also be accomplished using an Emerson chest-suction system. This is a three-bottle system that can remove large amounts of air or fluid from the pleural space while maintaining a low controlled negative pressure from 9 cm H_2O to 60 cm H_2O.

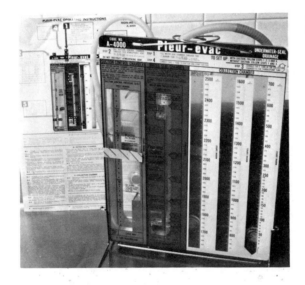

Fig. 22–8 Pleur-evac disposable chest drainage system. (Courtesy Deknatel Corp.)

When decreased drainage from the chest tube is observed, the underwater drainage system may be replaced with a Heimlich valve to increase the client's mobility. The Heimlich valve is a one-way valve that is attached directly to the chest tube to allow air or fluid to escape, and to prevent the entry of air into the pleural space. Attach a plastic bag loosely to the valve to prevent drainage fluid from staining the linen.

Objectives

To remove air, blood, or serous fluid from the pleural space and to facilitate reexpansion of the lung

To prevent the entry of air into the pleural space using an underwater drainage system

ASSESSMENT PHASE

- Is the client exhibiting signs or symptoms of pneumothorax or hemothorax? Check for shortness of breath, subcutaneous crepitus, altered breath sounds, and restlessness.
- Is the pneumothorax or hemothorax serious enough to warrant the insertion of chest tubes? Will a thoracentesis be sufficient?
- Has the client had chest trauma, lung surgery, or open-heart surgery? Chest tubes may be required to reexpand the lung. Chest tubes may also be inserted into the mediastinal cavity for drainage after open-heart surgery.
- Are signs or symptoms of tension pneumothorax present? Check for respiratory

distress, mediastinal shift, and shock. Reexpansion of the lung is an emergency procedure that prevents cardiovascular collapse. Keep advanced cardiac life support equipment on standby.

- Does the client have respiratory support? Provide supplemental oxygen if necessary and make sure that ventilator equipment and personnel are available.

PRECAUTIONS

- **Do not clamp the chest tubes. If the chest tubes are clamped, the risk of a tension pneumothorax increases. The effects of tension pneumothorax are far more damaging than those caused by a simple pneumothorax from an unclamped tube.**
- **Keep the water seal intact to prevent the entry of air into the pleural space.**

PLANNING PHASE

EQUIPMENT

4×4s
Antiseptic solution (povidone–iodine)
Sterile gloves
Xylocaine 1% (without epinephrine)
10-ml non–Luer-Lok syringes — 2
30-ml non–Luer-Lok syringes — 2
25-gauge needle ($\frac{1}{2}$ inch)
22-gauge needle ($1\frac{1}{2}$ inch)
Scalpel handle
Blades — Nos. 11 and 15
2-0 silk suture with cutting needle
Kelly clamp
Mosquito forceps
Scissors
Sterile five-in-one barrel connector — 2
Sterile "Y" connector (if two chest tubes are inserted)
Sterile dressing materials
Chest tube assortment with obturators
Water-seal drainage equipment
Sterile connecting tube (two will be needed if suction is required)
Sterile normal saline
Suction source (wall suction or Emerson suction)
Razor

CLIENT/FAMILY TEACHING

- If the client's condition permits, reinforce the physician's explanation of the purpose of chest tubes and the expected results.
- Explain the function of the water-seal drainage system.
- Reassure the client that a local anesthetic will help to alleviate discomfort during the procedure.

IMPLEMENTATION PHASE

NURSING ACTIONS	RATIONALE/AMPLIFICATION
1. Open sterile drape on bedside table to provide sterile field. Open sterile supplies on sterile field.	
2. Fill water-seal bottle with sterile saline to water-level marking.	Saline is unlikely to cause cell hemolysis when it comes into contact with lung tissue.
3. Place water-seal tube bottle so that tip of tube is 2 cm to 3 cm below fluid level. Prepare suction-control bottle.	For every centimeter that the end of the tube is underwater, 1 cm of positive pressure will be required to force air out of the pleural space.
4. Position client upright or semi-upright for procedure to ensure that lung will fall away from chest wall.	When it is used to remove intrapleural air, a chest tube is usually inserted anteriorly in the region of the second or

third intercostal space at the midclavicular line. It is inserted in the eighth or ninth intercostal space posteriorly when it is used to remove blood or fluid. Chest tubes may be placed at both sites if the pleural space contains both air and fluid.

5. Shave operative site if necessary. Assist physician with skin preparation, draping, and drawing up local anesthetic as necessary.

6. Monitor client's condition while physician inserts chest tube. Connect chest tube to underwater seal using sterile connector and connecting tube. Connect drainage system to wall suction using sterile connecting tube if appropriate.

Air bubbles in the water-seal drainage compartment indicate that air is escaping from the pleural space. A decrease in the leak indicates healing. The tube is sutured in place with a skin suture.
Alternative method: Connect the chest tube to an Emerson pump.

7. If two chest tubes are inserted, connect both to same drainage bottle using "Y" connector.

Using two separate drainage systems can cause fluid from one system to be suctioned through the chest and into the second system.

8. Secure all connections with tape strips or Parham band (Fig. 22–9*A* and *B*).

Obscuring the connections can prevent the identification of a possible air leak by hiding a loose connection (Fig. 22–9*C*).

Five-in-one connector

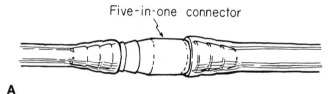

A

Fig. 22–9 Connections are secured with tape strips or Parham band. (*A*) Connector. (*B*) Correct method using tape strips or Parham band. (*C*) Wrong method of taping. (Reproduced with permission from Fishman NH: Thoracic Drainge: A Manual of Procedures. Copyright © 1983 by Year Book Medical Publishers, Inc., Chicago)

CORRECT:

Tape strips

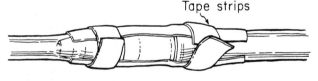

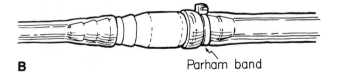

B

Parham band

WRONG: Complete wrapping

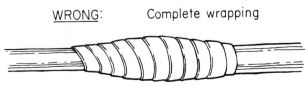

C

9.   Cover chest tube insertion site with dry, sterile occlusive dressing.

RELATED NURSING CARE

NURSING ACTIONS	RATIONALE/AMPLIFICATION
1. Keep excess tubing coiled and flat on bed instead of allowing it to hang over side of bed.	A dependent loop of tubing that has fluid in it can obstruct flow and increase pressure.
2. "Milk" vinyl chest tube as necessary by rolling tubing over hemostat.	Milking a chest tube serves to break up clots and to facilitate drainage by forcing air and fluid through the tube.
3. If drainage has decreased sufficiently and suction is no longer required, apply Heimlich valve to chest tube (Fig. 22–10).	
a. Disconnect tubing from chest tube.	
b. Attach Heimlich valve while client performs Valsalva's maneuver.	Using a Heimlich valve prevents air from entering the pleural space. Clamping the chest tubes is inadvisable because of the problems that occur if the clamps are not removed.
c. Attach plastic bag to Heimlich valve to collect drainage.	Make a loose connection between the valve and the bag so that air can continue to escape from the pleural space.

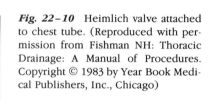

Fig. 22–10   Heimlich valve attached to chest tube. (Reproduced with permission from Fishman NH: Thoracic Drainage: A Manual of Procedures. Copyright © 1983 by Year Book Medical Publishers, Inc., Chicago)

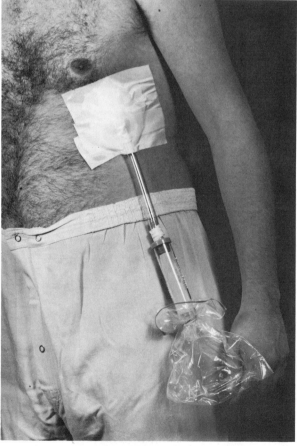

4. Place chest drainage bottles on stand, if available, to prevent accidental breakage. If system is disturbed, re-establish water seal as quickly as possible.

Plastic drainage systems are suspended from the bed frame.
Bottles may also be taped to the floor to prevent breakage.

5. If chest tube is removed accidentally, apply pressure to insertion site with combine dressing during inhalation. Release pressure during exhalation to allow air to escape from pleural space. Notify physician for immediate reinsertion of chest tube.

6. Label drainage collection bottle with time. Observe and record amount of drainage in collection bottle or chamber every hour. Notify physician if more than 100 ml collects every hour or if frank bleeding from chest tube is observed.

The presence of either of these conditions indicates the need for further intervention.

7. If drainage bottle becomes full, replace it with new sterile bottle while client performs Valsalva's maneuver.

Alternative method: Empty the bottle into a receptacle at the client's bedside and reconnect the chest tube. Use aseptic technique.

8. Remove chest tube when lung has reexpanded and accumulation of air or drainage has ceased.

a. Prepare occlusive dressing of sterile petroleum jelly on 4 × 4 or use commercially prepared occlusive dressing.

An occlusive dressing prevents the recurrence of pneumothorax because it forms a seal over the opening created by the chest tube.

b. Use sterile scalpel blade to cut skin suture that holds chest tube in place.

c. Place linen protector on client's bed. Clamp tube between fingers and remove steadily with one motion. Place tube on linen protector.

d. Have client perform Valsalva's maneuver by bearing down as tube is removed.

Valsalva's maneuver increases the intrathoracic pressure and serves to force any remaining fluid or air from the pleural space while preventing air from reentering.

e. Quickly cover chest tube insertion site with sterile occlusive dressing before client inhales.

Cover the insertion site to prevent the entry of air into the chest. The dressing should remain in place 48 hours to 72 hours.

EVALUATION PHASE

ANTICIPATED OUTCOMES	NURSING ACTIONS
1. Correct functioning of chest tube and water-seal drainage	An air leak may require surgical intervention. Evaluate the whole system for secure connections. Make sure that the point at which the chest tube exits the chest is airtight. Reinforce the occlusive dressing and notify the physician if it is not airtight. If necessary, determine the source of the air leak by clamping the chest tube briefly with a rubber-shod clamp. If bubbling in the water-seal bottle continues, there may be a problem with the integrity of the drainage system. If the system is functioning properly, the problem is with the chest tube insertion site. Evaluate for the following complications: pleural erosion, hemorrhage, hematomas of the lung or chest wall, or infection.

2. Reexpansion of affected lung   Auscultate breath sounds over affected and unaffected lung fields during at least every shift. Evaluate for respiratory function.

PRODUCT AVAILABILITY

TROCAR CATHETER AND CHEST DRAINS

Argyle
Sherwood Medical
Chesebrough Ponds

DISPOSABLE DRAINAGE UNITS

Anderson
Deknatal Inc.

HEIMLICH VALVE

Bard Parker

EMERSON PUMP

Emerson Co.

BOTTLE DRAINAGE SYSTEMS

Chesebrough Ponds

SELECTED REFERENCES

Fishman NH: Thoracic Drainage: A Manual of Procedures. Chicago, Year Book Medical Publishers, Inc., 1983

Morgan CV, Orcutt TW: The care and feeding of chest tubes. Am J Nurs 72(2):305–308, February 1972

V

Neurologic techniques

23 *Neurologic assessment*

BACKGROUND

The influence of the brain and its related structures is diverse and can affect, both directly and indirectly, the function of other body systems. Consequently, neurologic assessment is a valuable tool to use with persons who have diseases of other body systems, as well with the client who has a specific neurologic dysfunction. The client with septic shock, cardiac dysrhythmias, or chronic lung disease may develop neurologic deficits just as the client with an acute subdural hematoma or a brain tumor may.

The acutely ill client whose condition is changing or the client whose condition has the potential to change rapidly may require more frequent neurologic assessments than the client whose condition has stabilized. The baseline information provided by the initial neurologic assessment will dictate future actions.

Why is it imperative that the nurse be familiar with and comfortable in assessing the nervous system? First, the complete neurologic assessment provides initial baseline information that the nurse can use to evaluate all other neurologic checks as well as plan appropriate nursing care. Additionally, it can assist in evaluating care by determining deterioration or improvement in the client's condition.

The foundation of the neurologic assessment is skilled observation; that is, looking for the subtle as well as the obvious changes. Along with observational skill, the nurse must be able to interpret the observations so that appropriate interventions may be determined.

The neurologic assessment can be approached on two levels. The first includes the complete neurologic physical examination, which is performed by the physician or neuroscience clinical specialist. The purpose of this examination is to determine the presence or absence of disease of the nervous system. In fact it is possible to pinpoint specific lesions of the central nervous system (CNS) based on a careful, thorough examination.

The second type of neurologic examination is an abbreviated form of the complete physical examination. It focuses on those specific parameters that allow the nurse to quickly evaluate client behaviors in terms of trends that indicate neurologic improvement or deterioration. It is important to remember that changes in neurologic status may occur as a result of other disease processes as well as increased intracranial pressure (ICP). However, most often the target of the emergency neurologic assessment is the evaluation of the ominous presence of increased ICP. Increased ICP initiates a vicious cycle of pathophysiologic changes that, if not interrupted, can result in distortion and shifting of cerebral contents. This cerebral distortion can produce irreversible brain damage or result in the client's death.

This abbreviated neurologic assessment focuses on specific neurologic parameters, including level of consciousness (LOC), pupillary size and reactivity, motor and sensory function, and vital signs. The abbreviated format is used to assess a client's changing neurologic status on a more frequent, perhaps hourly, basis. It also causes much consternation among nurses in both its performance and interpretation.

Most hospitals have developed their own neurologic assessment flow sheet to assist the nursing staff in making an organized, comprehensive assessment (see example of neurologic assessment form). Others may use the Glasgow Coma Scale (GCS)

329

University of Maryland NEURO ASSESSMENT

Stimulus

Voice	4
Shake or Shout	3
Peripheral Pain	2
Deep Pain	1

Orientation

Time, Place, Person	3
2 of 3	2
1 of 3	1
None	0
Untestable	U

Strength (R/L)

Strong	5
Mild Weakness	4
Moderate Weakness	3
Severe Weakness	2
Trace	1
None	0
Untestable	U

Eye Opening

Spontaneously	4
To Speech	3
To Pain	2
None	1
Untestable	U

Pupil Equality

= L > R; R > L

Best Motor Response

Obeys	6
Localizes	5
Withdraws	4
Flexes	3
Extends	2
None	1
Untestable	U

Verbal Response

Oriented	5
Confused	4
Inappropriate (words)	3
Incomprehensible (sounds)	2
None	1
Untestable	U

Medications

Sedation	S
Paralytic	PL
Tranquilizer	T
Pain	P

Pupil Reaction, Corneal Reflex, Facial Grimace

Normal	3
Decreased or Abnormal	2
Absent	1
Untestable	U

Date													
Time													
Initials													
Medications													
Stimulus													
Eye Opening													
Verbal Response													
Orientation													
Pupil Equality													
Pupil Reaction R/L													
Corneals R/L													
Facial Grimace R/L													
Best Motor Response													
* Strength Arms R/L													
* Strength Legs R/L													
Signature/Status													
* Record Strength if Motor Response 4 or Greater													

Table 23–1
*Glasgow coma scale**

Response	Level of response	Score
Eye opening response	Spontaneous	4
	To verbal command	3
	To pain	2
	No response	1
Best motor response	Obeys verbal commands	6
	Localizes to pain	5
	Normal flexion (withdrawal)	4
	Abnormal flexion	3
	Extension	2
	No response	1
Best verbal response	Oriented	5
	Confused conversation	4
	Inappropriate words	3
	Incomprehensible sounds	2
	No response	1

* The Glasgow Coma Scale is based on eye-opening, verbal, and motor response. A total score is given to the client. Scores of less than seven are defined as coma. The total possible score is 15.

(see Table 23–1). The GCS was developed in 1974 at the University of Glasgow by Drs. Jennett and Teasdale as an objective tool to quantitatively designate the severity of head injury. It provides a baseline assessment relating consciousness to motor responses, verbal responses, and eye opening. The GCS has gained increasing use and acceptance as both an accurate and effective means of evaluating a client's level of consciousness, because it is behavioral in nature and has been repeatedly demonstrated to have high interrater reliability. It can be found in a variety of clinical settings. The parameters measured on the GCS are included in most neurologic assessment tools.

INTRACRANIAL PRESSURE MONITORING

Neurologic status, specifically ICP, can also be evaluated through the use of invasive ICP monitoring techniques. These techniques include the intraventricular catheter (IVC), subarachnoid bolt, epidural sensors, and solid-state transducers.

The pressure exerted by the increasing bulk in the cranium produces mechanical impulses, which are converted to electric energy by a transducer system and then to waveforms that are visible on an oscilloscope. These waveforms are of a lower amplitude than those produced by arterial pressure monitoring. A chart recorder may be used to provide a readout strip for documentation. The nurse must interpret the waveforms and the ICP values generated by the system to plan and evaluate appropriate nursing interventions. Additionally, the nurse must be able to troubleshoot the monitoring system for the appearance of abnormal waveforms, identifying and solving any problem areas.

The principles governing the setup and maintenance of ICP monitoring systems are similar to those of any pressure-monitoring system. Ideally, the ICP device should be inserted by the physician under the sterile conditions of the operating room. However, the labile neurologic status of the client may necessitate that the device be inserted in the critical care unit. If so, the insertion and assembly of the entire system must be done using strict aseptic technique.

Neurologic vital signs

Objectives

To establish an objective baseline of neurologic function to identify significant changes in neurologic status

To determine the need for, or evaluate the effectiveness of, therapeutic interventions

ASSESSMENT PHASE

- Has the client had previous experience with the neurologic assessment?
- Is the client at risk of deterioration in neurologic status?
- Is the client receiving any medications that will depress the CNS (*e.g.,* narcotics, analgesics, barbiturates, antihistamines, benzodiazepines, hypnotics)?
- Is the client receiving any medications that affect the ability to move? Note the use of paralytic agents such as curare or pancuronium bromide.
- Is the patient receiving any medications that affect pupillary size? Note the use of topical miotics that produce pupillary constriction (*e.g.,* pilocarpine hydrochloride). Remember that certain systemic drugs (cholinergics) also may produce pupillary constriction. Note the use of topical mydriatics that produce pupillary dilation, such as anticholinergics (atropine, scopolamine, homatropine) and adrenergics (epinephrine). Systematic anticholinergics and adrenergics may also dilate pupils.

PRECAUTIONS

- **Neurologic status can change rapidly and dramatically.**
- **Avoid causing unnecessary trauma such as bruising of the skin during the assessment.**

PLANNING PHASE

EQUIPMENT

Penlight
Neurologic assessment flow sheet
Blood pressure cuff
Stethoscope

CLIENT/FAMILY TEACHING

- Explain to the client and family the need for frequent neurologic assessments.
- Explain the need to use painful or noxious stimuli in eliciting a response from the client.

IMPLEMENTATION PHASE

NURSING ACTIONS	RATIONALE/AMPLIFICATION
1. If possible, place client supine with head of bed elevated 30°.	This position allows for observation of the client as a whole, as well as comparison of the client's right and left sides. Clients with vertebral column instability or an unstable hemodynamic status must be evaluated in the supine position.
2. Assess level of consciousness, including arousability and content of consciousness.	Level of consciousness reflects the functional integrity of the brain and is the most sensitive indicator of neurologic function.
3. Arousability is tested as follows.

 a. Begin with verbal stimuli and progress to application of painful stimuli only if client does not respond. | Arousability refers to the stimuli needed to wake the client. The degree of arousability depends on the functional integrity of the reticular activating system (RAS) and the cerebral hemispheres, as well as the feedback mechanism that operates between them. Both structural (trauma, brain tumors) and metabolic processes (ischemia, electrolyte imbalance) may interfere with the normal arousability process. |
b. Call client by name.	Use the name the client is used to being called. Ask the family about preferred nicknames.
c. If client does not answer to name, shake client vigorously by grabbing his shoulders.	
d. If shaking client fails to elicit response, apply painful stimuli, including compression of nail beds with pen, pinching of the trapezius muscle, application of pressure to supraorbital ridge, or application of pressure to sternum (Fig. 23–1).	Noxious stimuli should not cause the client further injury. Be careful not to gouge or scratch the client. Twisting or pinching of nipples is inappropriate and can result in injury.

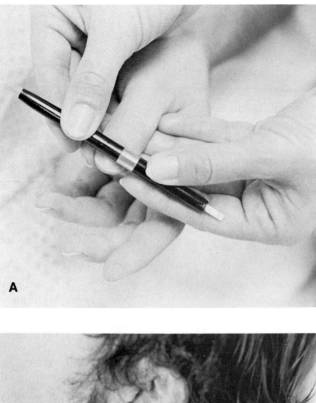

A

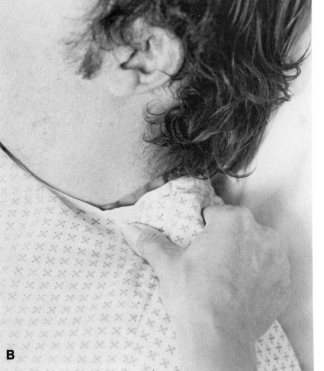

B

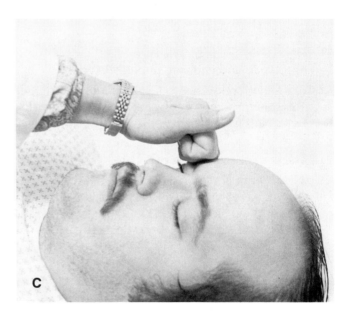

C

Fig. 23-1 Application of painful stimuli in neurologic assessment. (*A*) Compressing nail beds with pen. (*B*) Pinching trapezius muscle. (*C*) Applying pressure to supraorbital ridge.

4. Arouse client to maximum level of wakefulness and assess content of consciousness by ascertaining client's orientation to environment.

a. Ask alert, verbal client, "Tell me where you are."

b. Ask client who is intubated questions that require yes/no answers: "Is this place your house?" "Is this place a hospital?" "Is this place a store?" "Is your name Jim?"

The client may appear oriented and give you correct answers. If the same questions have been asked repeatedly, the client may have memorized the answers. Vary the questions or the order in which the questions are asked.

c. Ask client what date is and what events preceded hospitalization.

d. Assess client's ability to follow commands such as "Hold up one finger," or "Open your eyes."

5. Does client demonstrate any behavioral changes, such as restlessness, irritability, or combativeness?

6. Determine whether client is able to speak. If so, is speech clear? Garbled? Slurred? Does client make incomprehensible sounds? Does client understand what is said? Do answers to questions make sense?

7. Assess pupillary action.

a. Observe size, shape, and equality of pupils, as well as pupils reaction to light.

b. Assess and compare pupils bilaterally.

c. Record pupil size as small, medium, or large, unless transparent ruler is available to measure exact pupil size (Fig. 23–2).

8. Assess motor movement (Fig. 23–3).

a. If client is alert and cooperative, test strength of all muscle groups against resistance, comparing right and left sides (Fig. 23–3*A*).

Early indications of a decreased LOC include recent memory loss, disorientation, or uncooperative behavior.

Be careful about asking the client to squeeze your hand. Clients with diffuse cerebral injury, particularly frontal lobe injury, have a strong grasp reflex, much like that of an infant. If you tell the client, "Squeeze my hand," also request that the client let go.

Assess for other physiological causes for the behavior (*e.g.,* hypoxia, hypoglycemia, or pain)?

The left cerebral hemisphere is responsible for the interpretation and production of speech in all right-handed and most left-handed persons. Cranial nerves (CN) V, VII, IX, X, and XII are responsible for phonation and articulation of speech.

Pupils should be round and should react briskly to light. The oculomotor nerve (CN III) (parasympathetic fibers) and the brain stem (sympathetic fibers) control pupil size and reactivity. Sluggish pupils indicate that pressure is beginning to be exerted on CN III. Often a lesion can be identified by the pupil size. Pinpoint pupils indicate pontine involvement; ipsilateral dilation indicates a lesion of one hemisphere. Abnormal pupil size may be the result of iridectomy, cataract surgery, inflammatory processes, or traumatic injury. The structures that control pupil reaction are relatively resistant to toxic insults. Approximately 17% of the population has anisocoria, a benign pupillary asymmetry.

Note any medication taken by the client that may affect pupillary reaction and size. Pupil size may be altered by eye trauma, eye surgery, or blindness as a result of diseases of the retina or optic nerve.

Injuries at certain levels of the neurologic axis produce characteristic patterns of motor activity. Voluntary movement is controlled by the fibers of the lateral corticospinal or pyramidal tracts originating in the frontal lobe of the cerebral cortex. Motor fibers descend

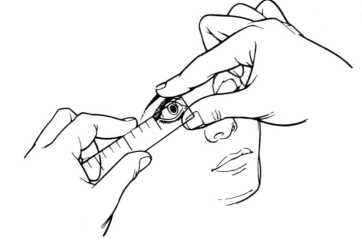

Fig. 23–2 Measuring pupil size with transparent ruler.

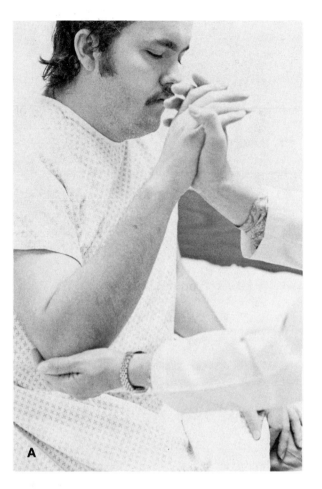

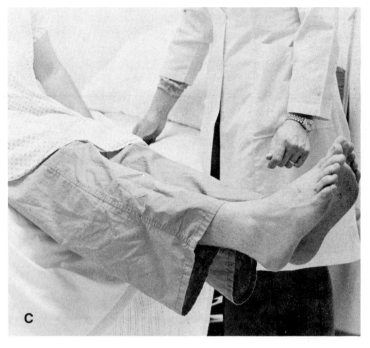

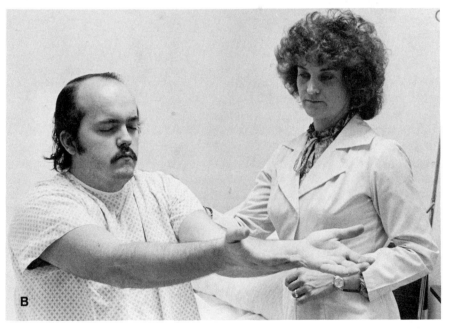

Fig. 23–3 (*A*) Testing muscle strength of upper extremity against resistance. (*B*) Testing muscle strength of upper extremities using palmar drift method. (*C*) Testing muscle strength of lower extremities in alert client.

b. *Alternative method:* Test motor strength of upper extremities using palmar drift method. Ask client to extend arms in front, palms upward, with eyes closed (Fig. 23–3*B*).

through the brain stem, where most cross over (decussate) and continue down the spinal cord.

If the client has a weakness in one arm, the palm will turn over and the arm will slowly drift downward.

c. To test for leg strength, have client sit on edge of bed, holding legs out in front for 10 seconds (Fig. 23–3*C*).

The weaker leg will start to drop. *Alternative method:* Ask client to "push on the gas" against your hand. With the stuporous or comatose client, apply light pressure to the legs. If the client does not respond, apply deep pressure to the Achilles tendon.

d. If client cannot follow commands, apply painful stimuli and evaluate client's response.

(1) Observe for purposeful movement, which indicates intact neurologic axis.

Purposeful movement occurs when the client grimaces, pushes the assessor away, or withdraws the affected area from the stimulus.

(2) Observe for localization, which indicates cortical dysfunction.

Localization occurs when the client can grossly locate the general area of the painful stimulus, purposefully moving toward the stimulus.

(3) Evaluate for nonpurposeful responses, which indicate dysfunction deeper in cerebral hemispheres and midbrain. Nonpurposeful responses result in incomplete removal of the painful stimulus. The client may try to withdraw only that part being stimulated or may move only slightly without trying to move away from the pain.

(4) Assess for decorticate posturing (flexion), which follows interruption of corticospinal pathways by lesions of cerebral hemispheres or internal capsule (Fig. 23–4).

Flexion results from the loss of cerebral cortex influence over movement.

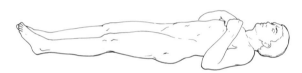

Fig. 23–4 Decorticate posturing. Note flexion of arms, wrists, and legs; adduction of upper extremities; plantar flexion; and grasping of thumb in hand.

(5) Assess for decerebrate posturing (extension), which results from deep cerebral hemisphere lesions that extend into upper brain stem (Fig. 23–5). Extension indicates more severe brain dysfunction and has a poorer prognosis than flexion.

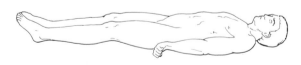

Fig. 23–5 Decerebrate posturing. Note rigid extension of all extremities with adduction and internal rotation of arms.

e. Assess for lack of response to painful stimuli.

Lack of response indicates severe brain injury with poor prognosis.

9. Report changes in motor movement to physician at once.

10. Document client's behavior in response to stimuli and quality of verbal responses.

Avoid using labels (*e.g.,* decorticate, decerebrate) to describe the client's condition. Avoid using vague ter-

11. Measure vital signs.

a. Evaluate blood pressure for increasing systolic pressure, widening pulse pressure, followed by sharp drop in blood pressure.

b. Evaluate pulse for bradycardia followed by sharp rise in rate.

c. Evaluate respirations for changes in rate, rhythm, ratio of inspiration and expiration, and periods of apnea.

d. Assess for Cushing's triad (increased systolic blood pressure, decreased diastolic blood pressure, decreased pulse rate), and changes in respiratory patterns.

12. Assess oculocephalic reflex (doll's eye response) (Fig. 23–6).

minology such as stupor, lethargic, or semicomatose because such terms are easily misinterpreted.

The vasomotor center, located in the lower third of the pons and the upper two thirds of the medulla, regulates vascular tone by inhibiting or exciting sympathetic vasoconstrictor fibers, which allows vessels to constrict or dilate. Cardiac activity is regulated by stimulation of sympathetic nerve fibers and vagus nerve (CN X) parasympathetic fibers.

The respiratory center is located in the medulla and lower pons. It is influenced by higher cerebral structures and by metabolic conditions.

Changes in vital signs as a result of neurologic deterioration occur late in the clinical course. They are considered to be a consequence of rather than a prelude to deterioration.

Caution: Do not test oculocephalic response if cervical injury is suspected.

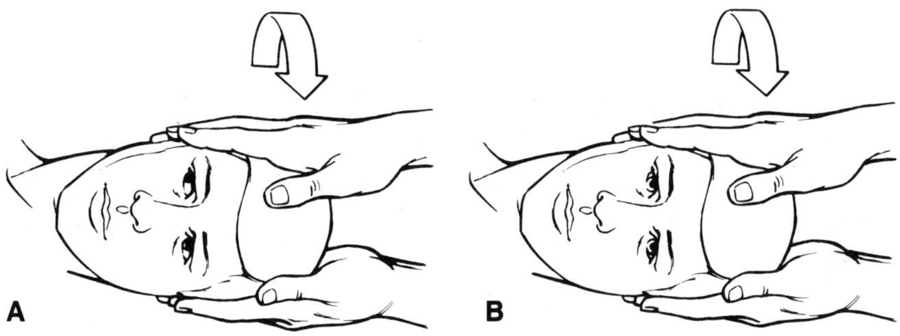

Fig. 23–6 Testing oculocephalic reflex (doll's eye response). (*A*) Normal finding. Note eye deviation away from direction head is turned. (*B*) Abnormal finding. Note eye movement in same direction in which head is turned.

a. Hold client's eyes open.

b. Briskly turn client's head from side to side, pausing to assess eyes on each side.

The oculocephalic response can only be elicited in clients with depressed LOC, because alert clients override the reflex by looking at objects as the head is turned.

If the reflex is normal (doll's eye response present), conjugate eye deviation to the direction opposite to that in which the head is turned (Fig. 23–6*A*) will occur (*i.e.,* the eyes remain fixed in space as the head is turned). It may occur in a comatose client whose brain stem is intact between CN III and CN VIII, or in a client in any altered state of consciousness whose brain stem is intact.

If the reflex is abnormal (doll's eye response absent), the eyes may move with the head or dysconjugate eye movements may occur (Fig. 23–6*B*). This occurs in comatose clients with brain stem injury. (Oculovestibular reflex [calorics] is usually tested by the physician.)

EVALUATION PHASE

NURSING ACTIONS	RATIONALE/AMPLIFICATION
1. Provide frequent eye care with artificial tears if client is unable to blink.	Blinking is a protective reflex that is often absent in comatose clients. Its absence predisposes comatose clients to inadequate lubrication and corneal abrasions.
2. Coordinate nursing care with neurologic assessments.	Promote rest for the client. The need for frequent assessments that require the client to be fully aroused predisposes the client to sensory overload.

EVALUATION PHASE

ANTICIPATED OUTCOMES	NURSING ACTIONS
1. Observation of early signs of neurologic deterioration	Monitor and evaluate trends presented by the client's condition rather than isolated responses to a specific parameter of the assessment.
2. Prevention of inadvertent trauma	Evaluate the structural integrity of the eyes and skin. Use the correct techniques to determine LOC.

SELECTED REFERENCES

Anderson MS: Assessment under pressure: When your patient says, "My head hurts." Nursing, September 1984, pp 34–41

Core Curriculum for Neuroscience Nursing. Chicago, American Association of Neuroscience Nurses, 1984

Hickey J: The Clinical Practice of Neurological and Neurosurgical Nursing. Philadelphia, JB Lippincott, 1981

Shpritz DW: Craniocerebral trauma. Critical Care Nurse, March–April 1983, pp 49–61

Walleck C: A neurologic assessment procedure that won't make you nervous. Nursing, December 1982, pp 50–57

Young MD: Understanding the signs of intracranial pressure. Nursing, February 1981, pp 59–63

Intracranial pressure monitoring

Objectives
To provide continuous measurement of ICP
To detect trends of increasing ICP
To identify ICP waveforms
To determine the need for appropriate therapeutic interventions
To evaluate the effectiveness of therapeutic interventions
To measure cerebral perfusion pressure
To evaluate the amount of compliance in the cranial vault

ASSESSMENT PHASE
• Is the client at risk of developing increased ICP?
• Is the client's neurologic status unstable or deteriorating?
• Do the results of the neurologic assessment indicate an increase in ICP?

PRECAUTIONS
• **Use of ICP monitoring devices is not a substitute for skilled observation.**
• **Neurologic status can change rapidly and dramatically.**
• **Strict aseptic technique is mandatory.**

PLANNING PHASE

EQUIPMENT
Razor
Local anesthesia
Sterile operating room ventriculostomy tray with twist drill
ICP monitoring device
Sutures
Transducer setup with high-pressure tubing

Sterile normal saline solution without preservative
Three-way stopcocks
Povidone–iodine solution
Occulsive dressing supplies
Transfer pack (optional)

CLIENT/FAMILY TEACHING
- Explain to the client and family the need for the insertion of an ICP monitoring device.
- Explain to the family what the client's physical appearance will be after the insertion of the ICP monitoring device.

IMPLEMENTATION PHASE

NURSING ACTIONS	RATIONALE/AMPLIFICATION
1. Assemble necessary equipment at bedside.	Strict aseptic technique is mandatory.
2. Assemble transducer system (Fig. 23–7).	Use normal saline without preservative to fill the transducer dome or to flush the system. Never use heparin.

Fig. 23–7 (*A* and *B*) Intraventricular catheter. (*C*) Basic components of continuous pressure monitoring system.

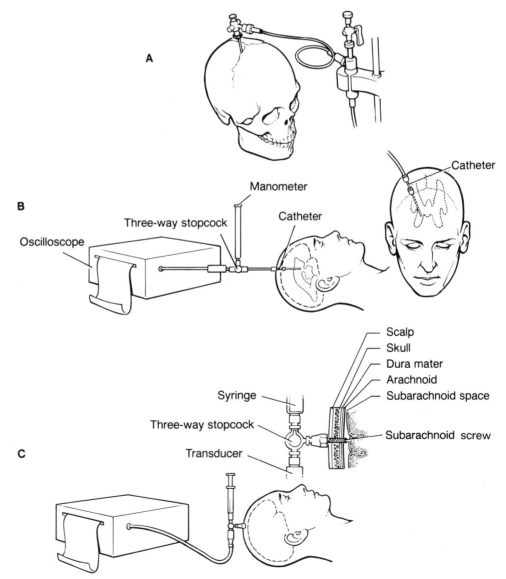

A

B
Oscilloscope
Three-way stopcock
Manometer
Catheter
Catheter

C
Syringe
Three-way stopcock
Transducer
Scalp
Skull
Dura mater
Arachnoid
Subarachnoid space
Subarachnoid screw

3. Position transducer level with client's foramen of Monro (tragus of ear).

Adjust the level of the transducer if the bed height is changed. For every 1 inch that the transducer is below the pressure source, there is an error rate of approximately 2 mm Hg.

4. Position client supine with head of bed elevated 30° to 45°.

Hold the client's head during insertion.

5. After device is inserted, clean area with povidone–iodine solution.

The device is inserted into the anterior horn of the lateral ventricle on the nondominant side (IVC) or into the subarachnoid or epidural space (bolt).

6. Apply occlusive dressing.

A two-layer dressing system is used in some protocols. The inner layer covers the insertion site and is changed only by the physician. A second layer covers the device–tubing–transducer connection and is changed by the nurse.

7. Calibrate at least every 4 hours.

Calibrate after dressing changes, flushing, and removal of CSF, and when a dampened waveform occurs or a waveform is lost.

8. Change transfer pack as needed.

An alternative method of measuring ICP is the external ventriculostomy. The IVC is connected to an external pressure reservoir (transfer pack). CSF drains continuously against positive pressure to maintain the desired ICP. To maintain an ICP of 10 cm water pressure (cm H_2O), the transfer pack is positioned 10 cm above the zero ICP reference point (the external auditory meatus —the foramen magnum). When the ICP reaches or exceeds the desired ICP, CSF drains into the bag. ICP can be regulated by raising or lowering the bag. A manometer can be used with the system for intermittent ICP measurements. However, these measurements are only indicative of ICP.

RELATED NURSING CARE

NURSING ACTIONS	RATIONALE/AMPLIFICATION
1. Record ICP hourly or more often as client's condition indicates.	A normal ICP is 0 to 15 mm Hg, or 50 cm H_2O to 150 cm H_2O.
2. Use nursing interventions to prevent increased ICP during and after insertion.	Nursing research has shown that many routine nursing activities precipitate increases in ICP.
a. Preoxygenate before suctioning.	
b. Elevate head of bed 30° to 45°.	
c. Maintain client's head in proper alignment.	Use sandbags, padded IV bags, or a Philadelphia collar.
d. Avoid clustering of nursing activities.	
e. Avoid use of Valsalva's maneuver.	
3. Monitor ICP waveforms (Fig. 23–8).	
a. A or plateau waves indicate sustained rises in ICP to 50 mm Hg to 100 mm Hg for 5 minutes to 20 minutes.	These waves indicate decompensation and loss of autoregulation. Report them to the physician immediately.
b. B waves are sharp, rhythmic oscillations that occur every 30 seconds to 2 minutes and are not associated with sustained rises in ICP; they rapidly return to baseline.	These waves occur with sneezing, coughing, or rigorous movement.

Fig. 23-8 A or plateau waves.

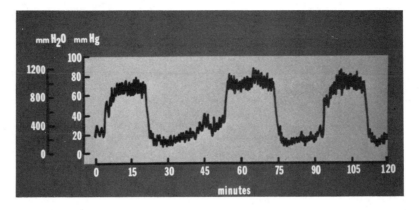

c. C waves are rhythmic oscillations that occur 4 times to 8 times per minute. They may reach abnormal levels, but they are not sustained rises in ICP.

These waves are not clinically significant and correlate with changes in blood pressure or respirations.

d. Monitor for loss of waveform or dampened waveform.

A waveform may be lost or dampened if brain tissue or clots occlude the device, if air is present in the system, if there is a loose connection in the system, or with changes in the client's position in relation to the position of the transducer.

4. Anticipate interventions for increased ICP.

Interventions for increased ICP include hyperventilation, drug therapy (steroids, osmotic diuretics, barbiturates), fluid restriction, hypothermia, CSF venting, and operative decompression.

5. Calculate cerebral perfusion pressure (CPP):*

$$CPP = MABP - ICP$$

$$MABP = \frac{(diastolic\ blood\ pressure \times 2) + systolic\ blood\ pressure}{3}$$

Cerebral autoregulation is used to maintain constant blood flow and pressure needed to provide oxygen and nutrients to brain tissue. Optimal CPP is 60 mm Hg. With CPP that is less than 50 mm Hg, autoregulation begins to fail. A CPP that is less than 30 mm Hg is associated with hypoxia and irreversible brain death.

6. Measure intracranial compliance.

Intracranial compliance is measured by the physician only.

7. Change dressing every 24 hours.

Use strict aseptic technique.

8. Daily laboratory analysis of CSF may be ordered.

9. Provide continual support of family and client.

10. Never irrigate system.

Irrigation of the system is done by the physician only.

EVALUATION PHASE

ANTICIPATED OUTCOMES	NURSING ACTIONS
1. Prevention of increased ICP	Monitor and evaluate the trends of increasing ICP values and waveforms. Use nursing interventions to avoid increasing ICP. Evaluate client response to therapeutic interventions.
2. Prevention of infection	Use strict aseptic technique.

*When calculating CPP, both values (ICP, mean arterial blood pressure [MABP]) must be the same unit of measurement (mm Hg) (1.36 cm H_2O = 1 mm Hg).

SELECTED REFERENCES

Gardner D: Intracranial pressure monitoring. In Millar S, Sampson LK, Soukup M, Sr., Weinberg SL (eds): Methods in Critical Care, p 291–295. Philadelphia, WB Saunders, 1980

Hanlon K: Description and uses of ICP monitoring. Heart and Lung, March–April 1976, pp 277–282

Hickey J: The Clinical Practice of Neurological and Neurosurgical Nursing. Philadelphia, JB Lippincott, 1981

Jones CC, Cayard CH: Care of ICP monitoring devices: A nursing responsibility. J Neurosurg Nurs, October 1982, pp 255–261

Kinney MR, Dear CB, Packa DR, Voorman DMN (eds): AACN's Clinical Reference for Critical Care Nursing. St. Louis, CV Mosby, 1981

Shpritz D: Craniocerebral trauma. Critical Care Nurse, March–April 1983, pp 49–61

Smith SL: Continuous intracranial pressure monitoring: Implications and applications for critical care. Critical Care Nurse, July–August 1983, pp 42–51

24

Fixed skeletal traction

BACKGROUND

Trauma to the spinal cord is one of the most devastating injuries a person can experience. Approximately 10,000 spinal cord injuries (SCI) occur annually, the majority of which are males between the ages of 18 years and 30 years. The rate of SCI among females is increasing. While the cause of SCI is variable, the majority of injuries are the result of car or sports accidents.

Injury to the cervical spine (C2, C4–6) is the most common site of injury, followed by the lower thoracic and lumbar areas (T11–L2). Despite the variety of causes, injury in these areas occurs when a relatively mobile part of the spinal column meets a relatively fixed point. Injuries in the cervical area are considered to be the most unstable, because this is an area of free mobility that permits neck movement.

The permanency of neurologic deficits and loss of function depends on the degree and type of injury. Edema usually occurs in the spinal cord after injury and can temporarily inhibit function. Once the edema subsides, function may return in clients with incomplete lesions, provided the injury is stabilized and immobilized with skull tongs or halo traction. The highest priority is to prevent further neurologic damage. The client in skull tongs or a halo apparatus may be placed on a Stryker frame or Roto Rest kinetic treatment table to facilitate turning without risk of disturbing vertebral alignment (see Chap. 32, Pressure Control Devices).

SKULL TONGS

A variety of skull tongs are available, including Crutchfield, Vinke, Barton, Garnder–Wells, and Trippe–Wells tongs. The type of tongs used depends on availability within the institution and physician preference. Gardner–Wells tongs are the most commonly used, although Crutchfield tongs are still used in some areas (Figs. 24–1 and

Fig. 24–1 Placement of Crutchfield tongs.

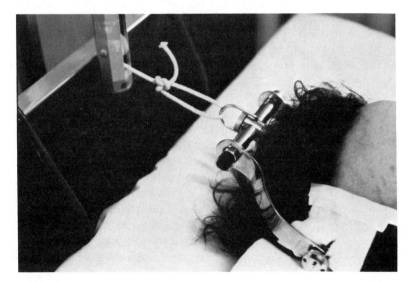

Fig. 24–2 Placement of Gardner–Wells tongs. (Source: Dr. W. J. Gardner)

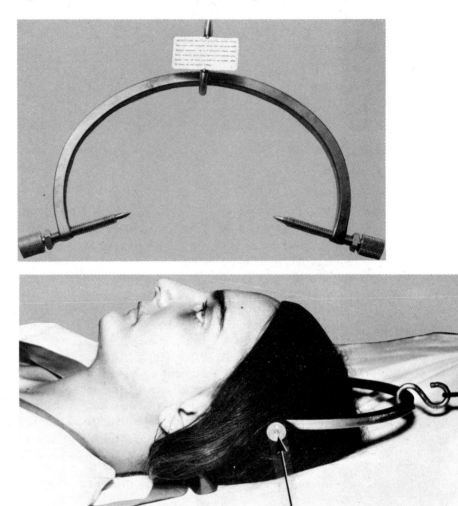

24–2). Although both tongs use two pins, the Gardner–Wells tongs do not require an incision or drill holes to seat the tongs. The skull area may or may not require shaving. The Trippe–Wells Dual-Purpose Cranial Tongs were developed for the purpose of placing the client directly from traction into a halo vest. These tongs have four pins, two occipital and two frontal, instead of the usual two temporal pins. The halo vest can be directly attached to the tongs after stabilization and satisfactory alignment have been accomplished with skeletal traction.

HALO VEST APPARATUS   The halo vest apparatus (Fig. 24–3) is an alternative to skull tongs. It consists of an adjustable metal ring that fits over the client's head and metal bars or struts that connect the ring to a rigid, plastic, sheepskin-lined vest. With the halo vest, there is a complete inability to flex, extend, or rotate the neck. The site of injury or fusion is completely immobilized, thus allowing callus formation and healing.

The halo vest allows the client greater mobility than skull tongs do, and the risk of disturbing spinal alignment is minimal. The paralyzed client can be turned from side to side, placed in a sitting position, or helped out of bed. The client with voluntary muscle control may be able to ambulate and resume many of his usual activities. However, the client may have difficulty maintaining balance because the halo appa-

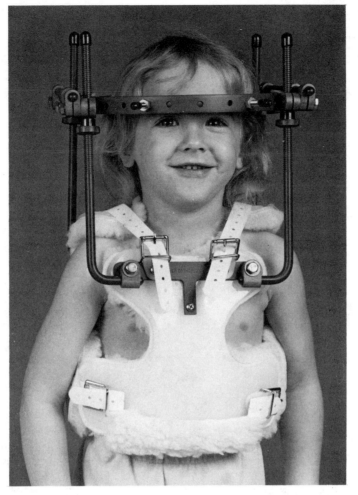

Fig. 24–3 Halo vest. (Courtesy Bremer Orthopedics, Jacksonville, FL)

ratus weighs approximately 10 pounds (2.2 kg). There are some mobility restrictions because the client cannot see his feet or turn his head without turning his whole body. The halo vest can be expected to remain in place for 10 weeks to 12 weeks.

Skull tongs

Objectives
To reduce vertebral fractures or dislocation through the use of traction
To immobilize the site of injury or fusion
To maintain spinal alignment
To prevent infection of pin sites

ASSESSMENT PHASE
- Does the client have a preexisting scalp infection?
- Has the client or family had previous experience with any type of traction?
- What is the client's functional and physiological level of injury?
- Has the injury site been surgically stabilized?
- Is the SCI a complete or an incomplete injury?

PRECAUTIONS
- **Never add weights to or subtract weights from the traction apparatus without a physician's order.**
- **Weights must hang freely.**

PLANNING PHASE

EQUIPMENT

For tong placement use the following items:

    Skull tongs
    Lidocaine without adrenaline
    3-ml syringe with 25-gauge needle
    Sterile gloves
    Povidone–iodine solution

For routine skull tong care use the following items:

    Hydrogen peroxide
    Normal saline solution
    Sterile 4 × 4s
    Cotton-tip applicators
    Antibiotic ointment

CLIENT/FAMILY TEACHING

- Explain the procedure thoroughly to the client and family.
- Reiterate the physician's explanation of the need for the procedure.
- Explain the need for and the use of a turning frame in conjunction with the tongs.
- Answer questions.

IMPLEMENTATION PHASE

NURSING ACTIONS	RATIONALE/AMPLIFICATION
1. Assist physician with tong placement.	Provide emotional support to the client during the procedure.
2. Give routine pin site care.	Pin site care should be done at least every 8 hours or more often if infection is present. Care of the pin site helps to prevent infection and removes exudate that could block drainage, leading to abscess formation.
a. Assemble equipment.	
b. Wash your hands.	
c. Observe pin sites carefully for signs of infection or loose pins.	Swelling, redness, purulent drainage, pain, or loose pins indicate a possible infectious process. Some serosanguineous drainage normally occurs 2 days to 3 days after tong insertion.
d. Cleanse around each pin site with cotton-tip applicator soaked in 1:1 solution of hydrogen peroxide and normal saline, using gentle scrubbing motion. Separate applicators should be used for each pin site.	Do not penetrate the pin sites. Exceptionally encrusted sites may require wrapping the pin with hydrogen peroxide-soaked gauze and moving the gauze in a firm but gentle scrubbing motion. Discard the solution after use because peroxide loses strength quickly.
e. Apply antibiotic or iodophor ointment around insertion sites, if ordered.	The use of dressings around pin sites is controversial. Some feel that it promotes infection by holding moisture and bacteria next to open skin; others feel that it protects the area from contamination.

3. Give care of infected pin sites.
    a. Culture exudate.
    b. Increase pin site care to at least four times daily.
	Infected pin sites usually result in loose pins. If a loose pin is suspected, do not turn the client. Call the physician to examine the site. The physician may order that the pin site be wrapped with iodoform gauze.

RELATED NURSING CARE

NURSING ACTIONS	RATIONALE/AMPLIFICATION
1. Provide emotional support to client and family.	
2. Maintain client safety.	Pay specific attention to intravenous infusion lines, catheters, and monitoring lines while turning the client.
3. Know principles and use of turning frame.	Nurse knowledge and confidence help to decrease client anxiety. Clients become very familiar with the equipment and will often remind nurses of areas to check when using the turning device.
4. Assess neurologic status and spinal cord integrity at least every 4 hours to 8 hours until stable, pre- and post-operatively, and when client's activity level or medical treatment changes.	Some units use flow sheets specifically designed for the SCI client. If these are not available, be sure to check movement and sensation bilaterally.
5. Check weights every 2 hours and each time client is turned.	Maintain effective traction by ensuring that the knot on the rope that connects the weights to the tongs is always clear of the pulley. Weights should be hanging freely.

EVALUATION PHASE

ANTICIPATED OUTCOMES	NURSING ACTIONS
1. Prevention of infected pin sites	Care at the pin site should be given as described above at least during every shift.
2. Prevention of dislodged pins	Check the pins every 2 hours. If the pins become dislodged, remove the weights, maintain the client's neck in a neutral position with small sandbags, alleviate client anxiety, do not leave the client unattended, and notify the physician.
3. Maintenance of traction	Weights must hang freely, and the knot on the rope should always be clear of the pulley. Maintain proper body alignment. Never add or subtract weights without a physician's order, because this can cause further neurologic impairment. Obtain a cervical spine film after weights have been added or subtracted.

Halo vest apparatus

	Objectives See previous section on Skull Tongs.
ASSESSMENT PHASE	• See previous section on Skull Tongs. • Will the client be discharged with a halo vest? • Will the client be able to walk?
PRECAUTIONS	• **A wrench should be kept at the bedside at all times for emergency removal of the vest front.** • **Do not unbuckle the shoulder straps.** • **Do not use the vest or the superstructure to turn, lift, or reposition the client.** • **Know the procedure for removal of the front of the halo apparatus in case cardiopulmonary resuscitation (CPR) is required.**

PLANNING PHASE

EQUIPMENT

Halo vest apparatus*
  Halo ring (sterile)
  Plastic vest
  Halo ring conversion chart
  Allen wrench
  Conventional wrenches—2
  Sterile skull pins and locking plates—5
  Sterile positioning pins—4
  Torque screwdriver
  Sheepskin liner for vest
  Vest superstructure
Positioning board covered with sterile towel
Razor and scissors
Sterile gloves
4 × 4s
Hydrogen peroxide
Povidone–iodine solution
Lidocaine in multidose vial
3-ml syringe with 25-gauge needle
Cotton-tip applicators
Sterile normal saline solution

CLIENT/FAMILY TEACHING

- Explain the procedure used for applying the halo vest apparatus to the client and family.
- Reiterate the physician's explanation of the purpose of the halo vest apparatus.
- Answer questions thoroughly.
- Begin preparation for discharge teaching about the halo vest apparatus with the client and family.

IMPLEMENTATION PHASE

NURSING ACTIONS	RATIONALE/AMPLIFICATION
1. Assemble and prepare equipment, ensuring sterility throughout procedure.	Application is done in two stages: application of the halo ring, then application of the vest and superstructure.
2. Assist physician with application of halo ring.	
a. Place client supine with head extending beyond edge of bed.	
b. Measure client's head for appropriate ring size.	The ring should clear the client's head by 1.5 cm and should fit 1 cm above the bridge of the nose.
c. Support head with padded board placed under client's back and head.	Support the client's head to maintain spinal alignment.
d. Hold head in neutral position until halo vest is applied.	
e. Shave and trim hair about 5 cm around each pin site.	Shaving facilitates pin care and helps to prevent infection.
f. Cleanse scalp with povidone–iodine solution	
g. Remove halo from package.	
h. Position halo ring around head with raised portion in back.	

*The halo vest apparatus can be obtained as a unit containing software (jacket, liner), hardware (halo, pins, bars, screws), and tools (wrenches, screwdriver, screws).

i. Physician will select four pin sites.

The two frontal sites are 1 cm above the lateral one third of each eyebrow. The two occipital sites are 1 cm above the top of each ear.

j. Positioning pins are placed in holes next to those to be used for skull pins.

Positioning pins holds the halo ring in place for placement of the skull pins. This helps to ensure symmetrical placement around the skull.

k. Assist physician in preparing anesthetic that will be used to infiltrate four pin sites.

Tell the client to close his eyes because this relaxes the skin around the pin sites and prevents puckering of the skin around the site.

l. Physician will insert the four skull pins into holes, tightening by hand and alternating front with back pin.

m. When physician determines that position of pins is correct and that skin is not under tension, opposing skull pins are simultaneouly tightened with torque screwdriver to desired tightness.

The desired tightness for skull pins is 5 inches to 5.5 inches/lb for adults; 4 inches/lb for children or adults with osteoporosis. Simultaneous torquing helps to ensure the balance of the halo ring. Torque skull pins again 24 hours to 36 hours after application, allowing tissue necrosis to occur at pin site.

n. Tighten locking plate on each screw.

o. Remove positioning pins.

3. Assist physician applying halo vest and superstructure.

a. Measure client's chest and abdomen.

b. Select vest of appropriate size.

c. Place sheepskin liners inside front and back of vest.

Sheepskin liners provide comfort and help to prevent decubitus ulcers.

d. Attach two angled uprights to posterior vest.

e. Attach two straight uprights to anterior vest.

f. Logroll client to one side.

You may also raise the client to a partial sitting position while maintaining alignment.

g. Slide posterior vest under client's back.

Shoulder pieces should touch the client's shoulders.

h. Return client to supine position.

i. Place anterior vest on client.

Straps that attach the anterior and posterior sides of the vest may have buckles or Velcro attachments.

j. Fasten anterior vest to posterior vest.

k. Attach metal support bars to halo ring and vest.

Alternative method: The application of the halo ring to the suprastructure depends on the manufacturer. Use the manufacturer's directions as guidelines.

l. Tighten each bolt.

m. Obtain cervical spine films.

Cervical spine films verify cervical alignment.

RELATED NURSING CARE

NURSING ACTIONS	RATIONALE/AMPLIFICATION
1. Check routine and neurologic vital signs and spinal cord integrity every 2 hours for 24 hours, then every 4 hours until stable.	Notify the physician of any decrease in motor movement or any sensation that could indicate further spinal cord trauma.
2. Give pin site care every 4 hours to 8 hours. Cleanse around each pin site with cotton-tip applicator soaked in 1 : 1 solution of hydrogen peroxide and normal saline,	Care at the pin site helps to prevent infection. Remove exudate that could block drainage and potentially lead to abscess formation.

using gentle scrubbing motion. Separate applicators should be used for each pin site.

3. Assess pin sites for loose pins, swelling, redness, purulent drainage, or pain.

These may indicate infection.

4. Examine halo apparatus every shift for loose bolts or screws.

Call the physician if bolts are loose. Do not tighten or adjust the shoulder straps. If the client can nod or shake his head, the bolts are loose.

5. Provide skin care daily by loosening side buckles/Velcro attachments individually and reaching under vest to wash and dry skin.

Inspect the client's skin for pressure sores. Check for areas in which greatest pressure is exerted by the vest by running your hand under the vest. Do not put stress on the halo vest structure; this could disturb the alignment. If sheepskin is wet, use a hairdryer to thoroughly dry it, because moisture will predispose the skin to breakdown.

6. Lightly apply medicated powder or cornstarch to skin.

Powder or cornstarch prevents itching.

EVALUATION PHASE

ANTICIPATED OUTCOMES	NURSING ACTIONS
1. Protection of client from extraneous environmental stimulation	Do not let anything touch the metal superstructure of halo ring. Bone is an excellent conductor of sound and the client will be sensitive to any noise that is made by striking the metal.
a. Protection of pin sites from infection	Care at the pin site should be given as described above.
b. Ensure that skin remains intact	Inspect the client's skin daily and give daily skin care
c. Maintenance of good hygiene	Change the sheepskin lining after prolonged use or when it becomes soiled. Remove the lining from top to bottom. The lining can be machine washed; it should be laid flat to dry.
2. Maintenance of safe environment	Walk with ambulatory clients. The client will have difficulty maintaining balance and will notice decreased peripheral vision. The client will not be able to see his feet or be able to turn his head without turning his whole body.

SELECTED REFERENCES

Altier T: Care of skull tongs. In Procedures (Nurse's Reference Library), pp 647–649. Springhouse, PA, Springhouse Corporation, 1983

Hickey J: The Clinical Practice of Neurological and Neurosurgical Nursing. Philadelphia, JB Lippincott, 1981

Hummelgard A, Martin E: Management of the patient in a Halo brace. J Neurosurg Nurs, June 1982, pp 113–119

Kindel K: Halo-vest traction. In Procedures (Nurse's Reference Library), pp 644–647. Springhouse, PA, Springhouse Corporation, 1983

Maryland Institute for Emergency Medical Services Systems. Master Care Plan for Spinal Cord Injury. Baltimore, MD, 1981

Pires M: Spinal cord injury—Coping with devastating damage. In Coping with Neurological Problems Proficiently, pp 99–123. Springhouse, PA, Springhouse Corporation, 1984

Rudy EB: Advanced Neurological and Neurosurgical Nursing. St. Louis, CV Mosby, 1984

Rutecki B, Seligson D: Caring for the patient in a Halo apparatus. Nursing, October 1980, pp 73–77

University of Maryland Hospital. Procedure manual. Baltimore, MD, 1983

25

Neurologic diagnostic techniques

Lumbar and cisternal puncture

BACKGROUND

The lumbar puncture (LP) and cisternal puncture (CP) involve the introduction of a hollow needle with a stylet into the subarachnoid space of the spinal canal, for the purpose of removing cerebrospinal fluid (CSF). Both punctures may be done for diagnostic or therapeutic purposes, and both are done under strict aseptic technique.

The LP, the most common method of obtaining CSF, is contraindicated if sepsis is present near the puncture site, because the site could become contaminated and meningitis could result; when there is evidence that the intracranial pressure (ICP) is elevated, because the sudden relief of the increased pressure could lead to herniation through the foramen magnum; or when a myelogram is planned, because CSF can be obtained at that time.

The CP involves inserting a needle 5 cm to 6 cm above the spinous process of the second cervical vertebrae, into the space between the cerebellum and the medulla (cisterna magna) (Fig. 25–1). The CP is indicated when it is vital to obtain CSF and an LP has been unsuccessful because of technical difficulties or local sepsis. Additionally, it may be used to inject radiopaque dye above a blocked spinal canal for a myelogram or when lumbar myelography has been unsuccessful. The CP is more difficult to perform. Contraindications are the same as those for the LP. It should also be avoided if a lesion in the cisterna magna or a congenital anomaly at the level of the foramen magnum is suspected.

Objectives
To remove CSF for laboratory analysis
To measure CSF pressure
To inject dyes or air for radiologic examination
To administer drugs or anesthetic agents
To remove CSF to alleviate increased ICP

ASSESSMENT PHASE

• Has the client had previous experience with lumbar or cisternal punctures?
• Is a developmental anomaly at the foramen magnum level suspected?
• Does the client have a lumbar deformity?
• Does the client exhibit behaviors indicative of increased ICP?
• Is the client receiving anticoagulant therapy?
• Does the client have osseous or cutaneous infection at the potential puncture site?

PRECAUTION

• **LP or CP is contraindicated for clients with increased ICP.**

PLANNING PHASE

EQUIPMENT

Overbed table
Disposable LP tray
Local anesthetic

Fig. 25–1 Cisternal puncture. Imaginary line is drawn between external auditory meatus and nasion. Needle enters above spinous process of first cervical vertebra, parallels this line, and enters cisterna magna. Medulla is approximately 2.5 cm anterior to posterior occipitoatloid ligament. (After Thorek P: Surgical Diagnosis, 3rd ed. Philadelphia, JB Lippincott, 1977)

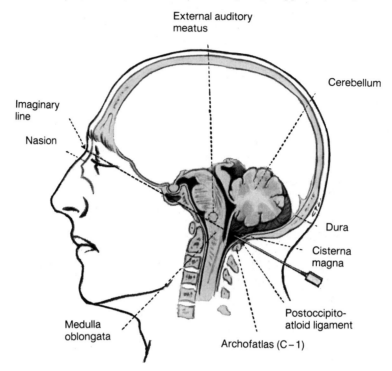

Test tubes for laboratory analysis
Band-Aid
Razor (for CP)
Good light source
Emergency equipment for intubation and respiratory and circulatory support

CLIENT/FAMILY TEACHING

- Explain the procedure thoroughly to the client and family.
- Tell the client to breathe slowly and deeply through the mouth during the procedure.
- Explain the necessity for the client to avoid sudden movements, coughing, or sneezing during the procedure.
- Explain to the client that a burning sensation and local discomfort will occur with the injection of local anesthesia.
- Tell the client to inform you of the type and location of pain or sensations (*e.g.,* pain shooting down leg). Irritation of a nerve root may be occurring, and the needle must be repositioned.
- Tell the client that pressure will be felt as the needle is inserted and the dura is penetrated.
- Explain postprocedure activity restrictions to the client and family.
- Answer questions.
- Inform the client that a headache may be experienced after the procedure.

IMPLEMENTATION PHASE

NURSING ACTIONS	RATIONALE/AMPLIFICATION

1. Have client void before procedure.

2. Provide privacy.

3. Open LP tray on overbed table.

4. Provide adequate lighting.

5. Adjust height of bed to allow physician to be comfortable during procedure.

6. Administer preprocedure medication if ordered by physician.

7. Shave area, if needed.

8. Position client appropriately. For LP, lateral recumbent position, with back to the edge of bed, back arched, neck flexed forward onto chest, and knees drawn up to abdomen is used (Fig. 25–2).

The needle is inserted between the L4–5 interspace to avoid injuring the spinal cord, which ends at the L1 interspace. The lateral recumbent position widens the space between the vertebrae to facilitate needle insertion.

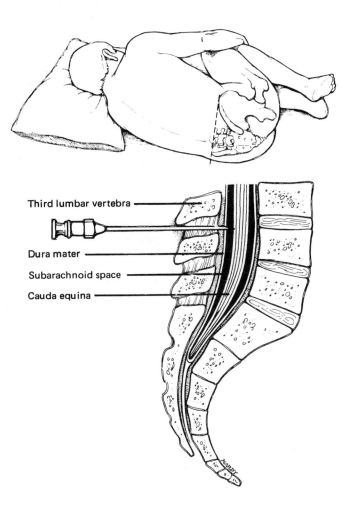

Fig. 25–2 Technique of lumbar puncture. Interspaces between spines of L3 and L5 are just below line joining anterosuperior iliac spines.

Third lumbar vertebra

Dura mater

Subarachnoid space

Cauda equina

9. Help client to maintain position by placing one hand behind client's neck, the other behind his knees, and pulling forward gently.

This prevents accidental displacement of the needle or disconnection of the system. It also helps to minimize discomfort.

10. For CP, sitting position with head flexed forward onto chest is used.

Alternative position: A lateral position at the edge of the bed with the chin flexed onto the chest can also be used.

11. Instruct client to breathe normally.

12. Stand facing client.

13. Assist client to maintain position throughout procedure.

This support will help to prevent the client from making sudden movements.

14. Physician will perform procedure.

    a. Prepare site with povidone–iodine solution.

Povidone–iodine solution prevents contamination of the site by normal skin flora. If povidone–iodine sponges rather than swabs are used, provide a second pair of gloves to prevent the introduction of povidone–iodine into the subarachnoid space with the LP needle.

    b. Drape client with fenestrated drape to provide sterile field.

    c. Anesthetize skin.

    d. Insert needle; remove stylet.

Instruct the client to breathe normally and to stay still.

    e. Attach stopcock and manometer to needle to measure CSF pressure.

Help the client to slowly straighten his legs to provide an accurate pressure reading. A false increase in CSF pressure may occur because of abdominal compression and muscle tension.

    f. Remove manometer. CSF is removed for analysis, dye is injected, or CSF is drained.

Between 1 ml and 3 ml are required for laboratory analysis; a total of only 5 ml to 8 ml should be removed unless CSF is being therapeutically removed. CSF should not be removed with a syringe; it should drip out on its own because a syringe could precipitate herniation or make an incomplete spinal blockage complete.

15. Label specimen tubes in order of sequence.

The sequence in which tubes were collected can differentiate a traumatic tap from a subarachnoid hemorrhage. Local trauma to the tissue can result in bleeding, which is evident in the first tube and progressively clears in subsequent tubes. Send the tubes to the laboratory *immediately.*

16. Physician may check for Queckenstedt's sign.

This is done if spinal subarachnoid obstruction is suspected.

    a. Initial CSF pressure reading should be taken.

    b. Compress jugular vein for 10 seconds, one side at a time and then simultaneously.

Compression of the jugular vein temporarily obstructs blood flow from the cranium and increases ICP. In the absence of subarachnoid blockage, CSF pressure increases also, indicating that the pathways between the skull and the LP needle are open. With a complete blockage, there is no rise in pressure; with a partial blockage, CSF may fluctuate, rise slowly, and remain at a new level.

    c. Repeat pressures every 5 seconds to 10 seconds.

Use of a blood pressure cuff is believed to create a more consistent pressure.

17. Monitor client's condition during procedure.

18. Monitor neurologic status and vital signs during procedure, notifying physician of any significant changes.

Observe for adverse reactions that could indicate sudden release of increased ICP, resulting in herniation of cerebellar tonsils or medullary collapse (decreased level of consciousness and respiratory distress). Document the details of the procedure, opening and closing pressures, and laboratory tests to be performed.

EVALUATION PHASE

ANTICIPATED OUTCOMES	NURSING ACTIONS
1. Prevention of CNS infection	Monitor the client's body temperature, white blood cell count, the presence of nuchal rigidity, and redness at the puncture site.
2. Prevention of postprocedure headache caused by irritation of meninges or CSF leak at puncture site	Instruct the client to lie flat for the amount of time specified by the physician (4 hours to 24 hours) to allow the dura to seal, to prevent CSF leakage, and to decrease the severity of headache. Headache is not a usual occurrence with CP.
3. Prevention of post-LP complications, such as nuchal rigidity, chills, and fever, which may result from meningeal irritation	Administer analgesics and antiemetics as needed.
4. Prevention of transient voiding problems, lower backache, spasms of lower back or thighs, which may result from nerve root irritation	Monitor the presence and duration of problems, and notify the physician if problems persist. Provide emotional support to the client.
5. Prevention of post-CP complications, such as increased ICP, herniation syndromes, or shock, which results from penetration of brain tissue or distortion of cerebral contents	Monitor the client's vital signals and give special attention to the respiratory pattern. Notify the physician if complications persist. Have emergency equipment for intubation available.
6. Alleviation of increased ICP, if used as therapeutic modality	Monitor the client's neurologic vital signs.

SELECTED REFERENCES

Core Curriculum for Neuroscience Nursing. Chicago, American Association of Neuroscience Nurses, 1984

Hickey J: The Clinical Practice of Neurological and Neurosurgical Nursing. Philadelphia, JB Lippincott, 1981

Rose MB (ed): Procedures (Nurse's Reference Library). Springhouse, PA, Intermed Communications, Inc., 1983

Rudy EB: Advanced Neurological and Neurosurgical Nursing. St. Louis, CV Mosby, 1984

Ricci M: Assisting with lumbar and cisternal punctures. In Millar S, Sampson LK, Soukup M Sr., Weinberg SL: Methods in Critical Care, pp 296–300. WB Saunders, 1980

26

Controlling body temperature: hypothermia and hyperthermia

BACKGROUND

Hypothermia and hyperthermia, disorders in thermoregulation, are common clinical syndromes. Thermoregulation is controlled by the hypothalamus, which is found in the deep structures of the brain. It lies above the pituitary gland and below the thalamus, and it is responsible for integration and regulation of autonomic–somatic responses, one of which is the regulation of body temperature.

As the blood flows through the hypothalamus, receptors sense the temperature of the blood and stimulate afferent impulses to return the body to a normothermic state. When the core body temperature rises, the hypothalamus sends out somatic signals to increase heat loss and inhibit heat production. Perspiration enables the body to loose heat by evaporative action—the sweat evaporates and cools the skin. The tachypnea that accompanies an increase in temperature also produces heat loss by evaporation. Peripheral vasodilation allows heat to be lost though the skin (radiation).

With a decrease in body temperature, the hypothalamus signals vasoconstriction, and piloerection ("goose bumps") reduces heat loss and inhibits sweat production. The shivering that accompanies a decrease in body temperature increases cell metabolism, thus producing body heat and increasing core temperature.

Thermoregulation can be disrupted by infection or irritation of the hypothalamus, which can be caused by head trauma, surgery in or around the third or fourth ventricle, or strokes of the hypothalamus or brain stem. Metabolic diseases may result in increased heat production (thyrotoxicosis) or decreased heat production (myxedema). Obesity and the absense of sweat glands may also result in disorders of heat loss.

It is imperative to control elevated body temperature because it may precipitate increased intracranial pressure (ICP). With an increase in body temperature, a series of catabolic events begins. Increases in arterial and venous blood pressure bring about an increase in cerebral blood flow and an increase in cerebral metabolic rate. With the increase in cerebral metabolic rate, there is an increase in oxygen consumption and glucose metabolism by the brain. This is followed by a consequent increase in the production of carbon dioxide and lactic acid, both of which are potent vasodilators that contribute to increased ICP.

Increased body temperature should be lowered gradually to prevent shivering, which can increase both cell metabolism and body temperature, thus defeating the therapeutic intervention. Chlorpromazine and diazepam may be ordered by the physician to control shivering and to help return the body to a normothermic state.

Objective

To maintain the client's body temperature at a predetermined level

Hypothermia

To lower an elevated temperature

To decrease metabolic oxygen demands during intracranial surgery, cardiac surgery, or with cerebral edema

To control bleeding or intractable pain in clients with amputations, burns, or cancer

Hyperthermia

To maintain normothermia in clients with spinal cord injury

To return a client to a normothermic state after severe hypothermia

To maintain normothermia before the diagnosis of brain death

ASSESSMENT PHASE

- Has the client had previous experience with hypothermia or hyperthermia?
- Does the client have impaired circulation, which could predispose the client to severe tissue damage?
- Is other electric equipment being used in conjunction with the blanket unit, which could increase the risk of electric shock?
- Is the client receiving oxygen?
- Is a consent form necessary?

PRECAUTIONS

- **Avoid the use of pins because accidental puncture of the blanket can result in fluid leakage and burns.**
- **Place the control unit at least 3 feet from the client and the oxygen source.**
- **Avoid the use of hospital gowns with metal snaps/closure because they could potentially cause injury.**
- **Avoid a sharp rise or fall in temperature.**

PLANNING PHASE

EQUIPMENT

Hypo/hyperthermia control unit with operations manual

Fluid for the control unit (use distilled water or solution suggested by manufacturer)

Thermistor probe (rectal, skin, esophageal)

Thermometer

Hypothermia–hyperthermia coiled blankets—2 (disposable blankets are available for single client use)

Bath blankets

Lanolin, cold cream, or mineral oil

ECG monitor

Sphygmomanometer

Stethoscope

CLIENT/FAMILY TEACHING

- Explain to the client and family the need for the hypo/hyperthermia blanket.
- Explain the procedure that will be used to place the client on the blanket.
- Explain the need for frequent assessment of vital signs, neurologic status, and skin condition.

IMPLEMENTATION PHASE

NURSING ACTIONS	RATIONALE/AMPLIFICATION
1. Obtain physician's order for parameters to follow in initiating therapy.	
2. Prepare equipment.	
a. Read operations manual.	Types of units and operating instructions may vary.
b. Inspect unit and blanket for leaks, kinks, and frayed or broken wires.	Return defective equipment to central supply for repair.
c. Connect blanket to control unit.	The tubing must not be allowed to kink because this interrupts the flow of the fluid.
d. Place control unit at foot of bed.	Be sure the unit is properly grounded.
e. Set control for manual or automatic operation.	
f. Set desired body/blanket temperature.	

g. Add liquid to unit if needed.

h. Place single sheet on mattress.

i. Place one coiled blanket on top of sheet.

A second blanket may be placed on top of the client to increase the contact area if needed.

j. Cool or warm blanket before use with client.

This allows you to test the blanket for proper operation and allows the client to receive immediate benefit from the unit.

k. Place bath blanket on top of coiled blanket.

A bath blanket absorbs perspiration and condensation.

3. Prepare client.

a. Help client to put on hospital gown.

b. Do baseline assessment, including vital signs, temperature, neurologic status, and skin condition.

4. Place client on blanket; position client supine with arms and legs extended.

The top edge of the blanket should be aligned with the client's neck. A pillow may be placed under the client's head.

5. Cover client with sheet or, if ordered, another coiled blanket.

The sheet insulates the client against the environmental temperature and increases the benefit of the unit by trapping cooled or heated air.

6. Select automatic or manual mode.

a. Automatic operation proceeds as follows:

The automatic mode allows the client's body temperature to control the heating or cooling process by a thermistor probe.

(1) Insert thermistor probe into client's rectum and tape in place.

Tape prevents accidental dislodgement. If the use of a rectal probe is contraindicated, a skin probe inserted deep into the axilla or an esophageal probe may be used. The esophageal probe is most often used with comatose or anesthetized clients.

(2) Connect probe to control unit.

(3) Obtain client temperature through probe.

Check the correlation to the probe temperature.

(4) Follow manufacturer's directions to set hypo/hyperthermia coiled blanket temperature.

(5) Set desired temperature.

b. Manual operation proceeds as follows:

Manual operation allows the nurse to set the unit's temperature. The blanket will maintain this temperature regardless of the client's temperature.

(1) Obtain client temperature.

(2) Set desired hypo/hyperthermia blanket setting.

(a) For hypothermia, place temperature dial at 4°C (40°F) for 5 minutes, then reset to 10°C to 16°C (50°F to 60°F).

(b) For hyperthermia, place temperature dial at 100°F for 5 minutes, then reset to 27°C to 32°C (80°F to 90°F).

(3) Adjust temperature setting of coiled blanket gradually to attain desired temperature.

Cooling that occurs too rapidly can cause frostbite or fat necrosis; warming that occurs too rapidly can cause burns

(4) Adjust temperature setting to maintain desired client temperature.	A $-7°C$ to $-4°C$ ($20°F$ to $25°F$) difference between the blanket temperature and the client's temperature will maintain the desired temperature.

RELATED NURSING CARE

NURSING ACTIONS	RATIONALE/AMPLIFICATION
1. Apply lanolin, cold cream, or mineral oil to client's skin where it touches blanket. Reapply as needed.	These substances help to protect skin integrity, because excessive heat or cold may lead to tissue breakdown.
2. Wrap client's hands and feet with Kerlix.	Wrapping promotes comfort and decreases shivering and chilling. It preserves skin integrity by protecting bony prominences from frostbite.
3. Place pillow under client's head.	The rigid surface of the coiled blanket is uncomfortable.
4. Provide frequent eye care with artificial tears if client is unable to blink.	Lack of the protective blinking reflex predisposes the client to corneal abrasions.
5. Perform range of motion (ROM) exercises every 2 hours to 4 hours.	ROM exercises reduce circulatory stasis and help to maintain the functional position of the extremities.
6. Reposition every 1 hour to 2 hours, unless contraindicated, and give back care with lotion.	Repositioning help to prevent skin breakdown, stimulates circulation, and promotes comfort. Report any skin discoloration, edema, or breakdown.
7. Change bath blanket, gown, or sheet when it becomes wet.	Freezing can occur if moisture accumulates on the blanket.
8. Monitor vital signs, neurologic status, lip color, and capillary refill every 15 minutes until desired body temperature is reached and stabilized. Repeat every hour.	Hypothermia produces depression of vital functions, such as renal output, cardiac output, respirations, and sensorium.

EVALUATION PHASE

ANTICIPATED OUTCOMES	NURSING ACTIONS
1. Maintenance and stabilization of predetermined temperature	Monitor the client's body temperature every hour.
2. Avoidance of excessive shivering during hypothermia, because this will increase metabolism, temperature, ICP, and oxygen usage as well as cause hyperventilation	The physician may order chlorpromazine (Thorazine) or diazepam (Valium) to control shivering.
3. Note that temperature may drift as much as $-15°C$ ($5°F$) after desired temperature has been reached and after discontinuation of procedure	Stop the procedure when the temperature is within $1°F$ to $3°F$ of the desired temperature.
4. Avoidance of complications of hypothermia or hyperthermia, such as respiratory distress or arrest, cardiac arrest, and oliguria	Have emergency equipment available. Assess the client's condition frequently.
5. Anticipation of secondary defense reaction (vasodilation or vasoconstriction) with either procedure, which may cause rebounding of temperature and defeat purpose of procedure	Carefully monitor vital signs and neurologic status for several days after the procedure.

6.   Discontinuation of procedure

Remove equipment.

Make sure that the client is comfortable.

Monitor vital signs, intake and output, specific gravity, and neurologic status every 30 minutes until the client is stable for 2 hours; then monitor every hour.

Monitor the client's temperature until it stabilizes.

SELECTED READINGS

Conway–Rutkowski BL: Carini and Owens' Neurological and Neurosurgical Nursing. St. Louis, CV Mosby, 1982

Coping with Neurologic Problems Proficiently. Springhouse, PA, Springhouse Corporation, 1984

Hickey, J: The Clinical Practice of Neurological and Neurosurgical Nursing. Philadelphia, JB Lippincott, 1981

Procedures (Nurse's Reference Library). Springhouse, PA, Springhouse Corporation, 1984

Ricci M: Hypothermia and hyperthermia. In Millar S, Sampson LK, Soukup M Sr., Weinberg SK (eds): Methods in Critical Care. Philadelphia, WB Saunders, 1980

Rudy EP: Advanced Neurological and Neurosurgical Nursing. St. Louis, CV Mosby, 1984

University of Maryland Medical Systems Nursing Procedure Manual. Baltimore, MD, 1981

VI *Renal/genitourinary techniques*

27 *Hemodialysis techniques*

BACKGROUND

The use of hemodialysis as a technique for maintaining life in the client with kidney failure became a technologic reality in the early 1960s. It was in 1970 and thereafter that diverse population groups were able to undergo hemodialysis regardless of economic or geographic circumstances. Hemodialysis of the critically ill client is a common procedure, but utilization of this complex technology requires that nursing staff be trained in the techniques, the equipment, and the care of the client who is undergoing the procedure.

CAUSES OF ACUTE RENAL FAILURE

The causes of acute renal failure are generally classified into the following categories: prerenal, postrenal, and renal parenchymal (intrinsic). Prerenal causes of acute renal failure include those that result from lack of adequate renal perfusion, causing the development of azotemia and oliguria. Hypoperfusion of the kidneys may result from a significant myocardial infarction, congestive heart failure, or cardiogenic shock, or it may result from severe hemorrhage or other intravascular volume-depletion causes. Prerenal causes of acute renal failure are often reversible if adequate perfusion is restored, either through fluid/blood volume replacement or support of the cardiac pump. If perfusion is not restored, acute renal failure usually results.

Postrenal acute renal failure occurs if there is bilateral obstruction to the outflow of formed urine, or if the sole functioning kidney is obstructed. Postrenal failure is often caused by obstructive processes within the genitourinary tract, but it may develop from extrinsic causes as well. Obstruction may result from prostatic hypertrophy, bladder tumors, or ureteral compression from pelvic or abdominal tumors. Renal or ureteral calculi in the client who has only one kidney may also result in obstruction and postrenal acute renal failure. Reversal of the renal destruction is possible, in fact probable, if the cause of the obstruction is identified and removed. Failure to identify and remove the obstruction may result in acute renal failure and could even lead to chronic renal failure.

Renal parenchymal damage involves injury to the glomeruli, the tubules, or the interstitium of the kidney. Causes of renal parenchymal, or intrinsic, acute renal failure may be related to prolonged unresolved hypoperfusion (ischemia) and to exposure to nephrotoxins such as aminoglycoside antibiotics, radiographic contrast material, or a variety of other medications that may be nephrotoxic or related to prostaglandin inhibition.

In the critical care setting, the development of sepsis may be a common cause of acute renal failure. Similarly, crush injuries or trauma may result in severe muscle damage and the release of myoglobin. Myoglobin is a large protein molecule, similar to hemoglobin, that is present only if muscle damage has occurred. The myoglobin molecule is believed to clog the renal tubules and thus to cause damage to the renal parenchyma. *Rhabdomyolysis* is the name given to any process that results in the destruction of skeletal muscle. Viral infections, prolonged seizures, and extensive exercise are other causes of rhabdomyolysis.

CLINICAL MANIFESTATIONS

The clinical manifestations of acute renal failure depend on the type of acute renal failure and the severity of the response. The age of the client and the presence of any preexisting renal insufficiency are also important factors in the development of acute renal failure. Acute renal failure may be either oliguric or nonoliguric. *Oliguria* is defined as a urine output of less than 400 ml/24 hours. Nonoliguric renal failure means that urine output is normal or slightly increased.

PRERENAL AZOTEMIA

Clients with prerenal acute renal failure have a decrease in urine output and are usually oliguric. The urine is concentrated and has a sodium content that is less than 10 mEq/liter. In prerenal states there is a decrease in renal perfusion. This results in extensive tubular reabsorption of sodium and water because the kidney tries to restore intravascular volume and thus restore perfusion. If a lack of circulating blood volume has caused the hypoperfusion, this renal resorptive response is beneficial. The volume-depleted client will be hypotensive, cold, and clammy.

If impaired cardiac pumping ability is the cause of the hypoperfusion, the sodium and water retention may be disastrous. In this situation the client will be hypertensive, edematous, or both. Pulmonary edema and symptoms of fluid-volume overload from heart failure, with secondary and continued hypoperfusion of the kidneys will result.

When renal perfusion is decreased, urea nitrogen is reabsorbed, but creatinine is not. Therefore, the blood urea nitrogen (BUN) : creatinine ratio is increased.

POSTRENAL ACUTE RENAL FAILURE

The client with postrenal acute renal failure will usually manifest a profound drop in urinary output. Frequently, the client is anuric. *Anuria* is defined as urine output of less than 100 ml/24 hours. Occasionally, the client will have intermittent periods of anuria and polyuria; thus early recognition of obstruction is more difficult. The urine is initially low in sodium content, but after 24 hours to 48 hours, the urine sodium content is increased.* BUN and serum creatinine levels will also rise, and azotemia will be present. If the obstruction is at or below the bladder neck, there will be abdominal distention and perhaps overflow incontinence. Flank pain, lower abdominal pain, or colic suggest intraureteral or renal pelvic processes.

ACUTE RENAL FAILURE — RENAL PARENCHYMAL

Clinically, the client with acute renal failure resulting from renal parenchymal, or intrinsic renal, causes may exhibit a variety of symptoms and laboratory manifestations. If the acute renal failure is nonoliguric, normal or slightly increased urine output will be maintained. However, BUN and serum creatinine levels will gradually rise. The specific gravity of the urine, which reflects the ability of the kidneys to concentrate urine, is low and is similar to the plasma osmolality.

In the client with oliguric acute renal failure, there is a decrease in urinary output in the range of 100 ml to 400 ml/24 hours. BUN and creatinine levels rise in the serum. The specific gravity and the urine osmolality are fixed, reflecting the inability of the nephrons to concentrate urine. The sodium content of the urine is elevated to greater than 40 mEq/liter. Other laboratory manifestations seen in the client with oliguric acute renal failure include hyperkalemia, metabolic acidosis (decreased bicarbonate reserve), hyperphosphatemia, and hypocalcemia.

Clinically, the symptoms experienced by the client with acute renal failure vary. If awake and alert, the client will have anorexia, nausea and vomiting, hiccups, muscle cramps, and generalized fatigue and lethargy. Fine tremors, myoclonus, asterixis, or alterations in sensorium or attention span indicate an increase in metabolic imbalances. Although these symptoms may be present in nonoliguric states, the presentation is generally milder than in oliguria.

Evidence of fluid imbalance is generally related to volume overload. A continuing decrease in output in relation to intake, increasing weights as measured on a daily basis, and elevation of blood pressure, especially the diastolic pressure, are all manifestations of fluid retention. Hemodynamic measurements, such as the central venous pressure (CVP) and the pulmonary capillary wedge (PCW) pressure may be helpful is assessing fluid status (see Chap. 5, "Hemodynamic Pressure Monitoring"). The CVP

* Bastle CP, Rudnick MR, Norris RG: Diagnostic approaches to acute renal failure. In Brenner BM, Stein JH (eds): *Acute Renal Failure.* New York, Churchill Livingstone, 1980

and PWC pressure will be elevated in clients with volume expansion. Edema may be detected in the pedal, pretibial, periorbital, or presacral areas, or in the pulmonary fields. The presence of rales on pulmonary auscultation, shortness of breath, or difficulty in breathing are commonly observed manifestations.

Sixty percent of the causes of acute renal failure are related to surgery or severe trauma, 30% result from general medical causes, and 10% are related to pregnancy. An important distinction of acute renal failure, in terms of prognosis, is whether the client is oliguric or nonoliguric. In clients with oliguric acute renal failure, the mortality is 50% or greater. Mortality in nonoliguric acute renal failure is approximately 30%. Mortality is highest among those with extensive disease, severe trauma, or sepsis.*

INDICATIONS FOR DIALYSIS

Indications for dialysis for the client with acute renal failure include situations in which the fluid or electrolyte imbalances threaten the homeostasis or stability of the client. Fluid overload, hyperkalemia, metabolic acidosis, and the systemic effects of uremia are the prime indications for dialysis. Fluid overload may result in pulmonary edema and a decreased ability to maintain adequate oxygenation. Hyperkalemia, if uncorrected, will cause arrhythmias (*e.g.,* idioventricular rhythm), which may be fatal, when the serum level exceed 7 mEq/liter. Metabolic acidosis, in which the bicarbonate base reserve is decreased, may be temporarily compensated for by respiratory mechanisms. However, as the bicarbonate level diminishes and bicarbonate is no longer available as a blood buffer and as the breathing muscles become fatigued, acidemia will result. This must be corrected by dialysis.

Other manifestations of uremia, such as increasing lethargy or uremic encephalopathy, generally indicate the need to initiate dialysis to prevent grand mal seizures. Uremia also enhances bleeding, because the ability of the platelets to aggregate blood is impaired. Gastrointestinal bleeding occurs more readily in a uremic environment than in a nonuremic one. Because blood is a protein that the liver will convert to urea, reabsorption of blood will increase BUN and worsen other symptoms.

MODALITY SELECTION

The modality of dialysis selected will depend on several variables (see Chap. 28, "Peritoneal Dialysis"). The clinical status of the client, especially that of the cardiovascular system, is an important consideration. For hemodialysis to be considered, adequate systolic blood pressure must be present to allow the extracorporeal pathway of blood to flow through the dialysis machine. Hemodialysis is quickly initiated, and chemical and fluid imbalances may be stablized rapidly. Rapid correction of hyperkalemia or severe metabolic acidosis may be necessary to prevent the occurrence of other life-threatening sequelae. Hemodialysis offers these options. Rapid reduction of BUN and creatinine levels should be avoided, however, to prevent dialysis disequilibrium from developing. Headaches and seizures occur in the dialysis disequilibrium syndrome. Delayed removal of BUN from the cerebrospinal fluid, with the movement of water into the cerebrum is believed to be the cause of this syndrome.

VASCULAR ACCESS/ PERITONEAL ACCESS

Regardless of the modality selected, some form of access is required for the initiation of dialysis. If hemodialysis is selected, vascular access must be established. Short-term vascular access options include the external arteriovenous (AV) shunt and the subclavian or femoral catheter. The AV fistula, or graft, requires several weeks to months to mature before it can be used. Thus in the critical care setting a newly created fistula is not an option.

ANTICOAGULANT REGIMEN

Anticoagulation is required for clients receiving hemodialysis. In general the two options for administering anticoagulants are systemic heparinization and regional heparinization.

Systemic heparinization involves the administration of low-dose heparin at the initiation of hemodialysis and at the midpoint of the treatment. The dosage of heparin

---

* Anderson RJ, Schrier RW: Clinical spectrum of oliguric and non-oliguric acute renal failure. In Brenner BM, Stein JH (eds): *Acute Renal Failure.* New York, Churchill Livingstone, 1980

is small and is given to prevent clotting of blood in the blood lines and in the artificial kidney unit (dialyzer). However, because the client receives heparin systemically, there is a risk of bleeding.

Regional heparinization involves the administration of heparin to the blood as it begins the extracorporeal circulation. As the blood is returned to the client, protamine sulfate is infused. Consequently, the blood is only heparinized while it is in the extracorporeal circuit. The risk of client bleeding is minimized, and the blood does not clot in the blood lines or in the dialyzer.

Hemodialysis

Objectives

To control fluid balance

To normalize serum potassium levels

To reverse metabolic acidosis

To control uremic manifestations

ASSESSMENT PHASE

- Is there evidence of fluid-volume excess (hypervolemia)? Check for the following:
    Tachycardia, third heart sound (S_3), or gallop rhythm
    Systolic and diastolic hypertension
    Increase in body weight
    Intake in excess of output, oliguria, or anuria
    Neck-vein distention; or pedal, pretibial, periorbital, or presacral edema
    Presence of rales
    Elevated PCW pressure or CVP
- Is there evidence of hyperkalemia? Check for the following:
    Profound skeletal muscle weakness
    Complaints of intestinal colic
    Changes in voice quality, such as increased hoarseness
    ECG changes such as peaked T waves, widened QRS complex (beginning of Q wave to end of S wave), prolonged P-R interval, and flattened or absent P waves
    Premature ventricular contractions
    Increased serum potassium levels
- Is there evidence of metabolic acidosis? Check for the following:
    Decrease in serum bicarbonate (serum CO_2 or CO_2 combining power)
    Changes in level of consciousness (LOC), such as drowsiness or disorientation
    Decrease in arterial pH of blood
    Asterixis, myoclonus, or seizures
- Is there evidence of the ability to compensate for metabolic acidosis? Check for tachypnea; decreased pCO_2; and normal arterial pH.
- Is there evidence of uremia? Check for the following:
    Nausea, vomiting, hiccups, muscle cramps, and pruritis
    Anorexia with possible weight loss
    Fatigue, lethargy, changes in behavior, slurred speech, or changes in LOC
    Occult blood in stool or emesis
    Ecchymoses or easy bruising
    Asterixis, tremors, myoclonus, or seizures
    BUN elevation (usually > 100 mg/dl)
    Serum creatinine elevation
- Do the physician orders for each treatment specify the following?
    Dialyzer. The choice of dialyzer is based on the clearance characteristics, the ultrafiltration rate, and the blood volume required to fill the dialyzer. Impaired cardiac function may worsen if a large blood volume is required.
    Frequency of treatment. For the critically ill client, daily dialysis treatments may be required. Stable chronic dialysis clients usually dialyze two times or three times per week.

Length of treatment. The length of treatment for the client in the critical care unit varies from 2½ hours to 4½ hours. Stable chronic dialysis clients usually dialyze from 3½ hours to 4½ hours.

Blood flow. Blood flow through the dialyzer during the treatment is generally 200 ml to 300 ml/minute. Blood flow is increased gradually. Ideally, optimum blood flow is obtained within 30 minutes after the initiation of the hemodialysis treatment.

Anticoagulant regimen. Heparin administration may be given either systemically or regionally.

Dialysate bath concentration. The dialysate bath is composed of sodium, potassium, chloride, magnesium, and calcium electrolytes. Acetate or bicarbonate and glucose are also present. The concentration of one or more of these substances may be altered to meet the individual needs of the client's changing electrolyte status.

Weight/fluid loss. Fluid loss during hemodialysis is based on the principle of filtration. The amount of positive or negative pressure applied to the membrane of the dialyzer may be altered to remove more or less fluid.

Blood pressure maintenance. Hypotension is associated with the fluid removal of a hemodialysis treatment. The method of maintaining blood pressure should be specified in case hypotension occurs. Methods that are available to maintain blood pressure include bolus fluid administration, continuous fluid administration, vasopressors, and blood product administration.

Laboratory work. Pretreatment laboratory work is generally done to determine BUN, serum creatinine and electrolyte levels. Client needs will vary. Post-treatment laboratory work should be delayed for 4 hours to 6 hours after the treatment to permit equilibration of the electrolytes in the intracellular, interstitial, and intravascular fluid spaces.

Physician phone number or pager availability. It is essential that the nurse performing the hemodialysis treatment know how to reach the attending nephrologist.

PRECAUTIONS

- **Extracorporeal blood flow increases the risk of hypotension, angina, and arrhythmias.**
- **Improper dialysate temperature could cause hemolysis.**
- **Improper dialysate conductivity can result in an undesirable electrolyte exchange between the client and the dialysate.**
- **The presence of air in the blood circuit and failure to activate the air/foam detector could result in an air embolus.**
- **An acetate dialysate will increase vasodilatation and may precipitate hypotension.**
- **Contact of the client's blood with the synthetic materials of the dialyzer may result in signs and symptoms of hypersensitivity.**
- **Procedures involving frequent contact with blood or blood products increase the possibility of developing hepatitis**
- **The presence of vascular access devices increases the risk of local infection or systemic bacteremia.**

PLANNING PHASE

EQUIPMENT

Water source
Electric source
Dialyzer
Dialysate
Blood lines
Blood pump
Dialysis machine
Conductivity-standardizing solution and meter-line clamps
Vascular access supplies (used to initiate and discontinue treatment)
Vascular access dressing-change supplies

Blood pressure maintenance supplies (*e.g.,* saline, intravenous [IV] tubing, medications, or blood products)
Laboratory supplies for blood work to be drawn
Stethoscope and sphygmomanometer
Cardiac monitor
Physician orders
Nursing notes

CLIENT/FAMILY TEACHING

- Discuss the reason for the hemodialysis treatment.
- Describe the procedure and possible sensations of hypotension, chest pain, headache, nausea, vomiting, or muscle cramps.
- Reassure the client that you, or another dialysis nurse, will always be present.

IMPLEMENTATION PHASE

NURSING ACTIONS	RATIONALE/AMPLIFICATION
1. Attach dialysis machine to water and electric source.	
2. Rinse machine with high-level disinfectant.	Use of disinfectant prevents unwanted client contact and exposure.
3. Place concentrate line in dialysate.	A concentrate line achieves the proper dialysate concentration.
4. Prime blood lines and dialyzer.	Priming maintains a sterile and air-free circuit.
5. Establish dialysate conductivity.	The establishment of dialysate conductivity ensures proper electrolyte exchange between the client and the dialysate.
a. Confirm proper dialysate selection.	
b. Note conductivity monitor reading.	
6. Begin client teaching.	Client teaching improves the client's response and cooperation.
7. Obtain client's pretreatment weight.	The pretreatment weight establishes the fluid removal goal.
8. Obtain vital signs and temperature; assess LOC, breath sounds, and evidence of peripheral edema.	These vital signs provide baseline data for the client's status.
9. Draw pretreatment laboratory work as ordered.	Pretreatment laboratory work establishes baseline data, and laboratory work drawn during or within 4 hours to 6 hours after the treatment is invalid.
10. Prepare vascular access (see following section on Vascular Access for Hemodialysis).	Utilize sterile technique to prevent infection.
11. Attach blood lines to client access.	Secure the lines to prevent hemorrhage.
12. Initiate gradual blood flow.	A gradual blood flow prevents hypotension and leukopenia.
13. Set and activate machine alarms, pressure parameters, and detectors. Perform line-accuracy checks.	These checks on machine function minimize the risk of access infiltration, air embolus, and line separations.
a. Air/foam detector should be in operating position.	
b. Blood detector should be in operating position.	
c. Set venous pressure upper and lower limits (-50 mm Hg).	

d. Securely attach lines to client, dialyzer, and transducer.

e. Dialysate flow should be present as ordered.

14. Monitor and assess client's condition during treatment, including assessments of vital signs; cardiac monitor; medication, fluid, and blood administration; anticoagulant administration; arterial and venous line pressures; fluid removal calculations; blood flow; access performance; and client tolerance of treatment.	Monitoring and assessing the client's condition detect and prevent complications.
15. Return client's blood at termination of treatment.	Returning the client's blood minimizes the blood loss.
16. Note presence of clotted blood in dialyzer.	Assess the anticoagulant regimen.
17. Terminate medication and fluid administration as indicated.	Avoid the administration of excess fluid, vasopressor, or anticoagulant.
18. Disconnect blood lines from vascular access.	Maintain the sterility of the vascular access.
19. Complete vascular access care (see following section on Vascular Access for Hemodialysis).	Vascular access care improves the access survival rate.
20. Obtain client's post-treatment weight.	Assess the amount of fluid removed and compare it with the goal.
21. Complete post-treatment assessment; including vital signs and temperature, LOC and patency of vascular access.	Complete documentation of client's condition.
22. Report to critical care nurse and physician.	Communication among staff enhances the continuity of client care.
23. Discard disposable equipment.	Discarding of disposable equipment minimizes accidental exposure among personnel.
24. Disinfect machine and reusable equipment.	Disinfect reusable equipment to improve machine performance and to prevent cross-contamination.

EVALUATION PHASE

ANTICIPATED OUTCOMES	NURSING ACTIONS
1. Normalization of serum potassium, sodium, and bicarbonate level	Obtain blood specimens 4 hours to 6 hours after the completion of the dialysis treatment.
2. Correction of fluid-volume excess or deficit	Assess the client's blood pressure, peripheral edema, post-treatment weight, and breath sounds.
3. Prevention of complications of hemodialysis	Assess the client's blood pressure every 15 minutes and administer fluid, medication, or blood as prescribed.
a. Hypotension	
b. Hemorrhage	Assess blood line connections and access insertion sites.
c. Arrhythmias	Increase the oxygen flow during treatment and observe the cardiac monitor.
d. Air emboli	Set the air/foam detector and monitor.
e. Disequilibrium syndrome	Initiate dialysis at a low blood flow and increase it gradually.
f. Discomfort such as nausea, vomiting, and muscle cramps	Monitor the client's blood pressure, fluid removal, and dialysate conductivity.
4. Establishment of patent vascular access	Assess for desired venous pressure and good blood flow; palpate thrill and auscultate bruit in shunt or fistula.

PRODUCT AVAILABILITY

DIALYSIS MACHINES

C. D. Medical
Drake Willock
Hospal Ltd.
Travenol Laboratories, Inc.
Organon Teknika

CONCENTRATE

Renal Dynamics
Travenol Laboratories, Inc.
3-C Medical

BLOOD TUBING

C. D. Medical
Travenol Laboratories, Inc.
Drake Willock
Hospal Ltd.
Terumo Corporation, USA

PUMPS

Drake Willock
Hospal Ltd.
C. D. Medical
Travenol Laboratories, Inc.

DIALYZERS

Travenol Laboratories, Inc.
Hospital Ltd.
C. D. Medical
Drake Willock
3-C Medical

CONDUCTIVITY EQUIPMENT

American Medical Equipment
C. D. Medical
Drake Willock
Travenol Laboratories, Inc.

HEPARIN INFUSION PUMPS

American Medical Equipment
C. D. Medical

Vascular access for hemodialysis

BACKGROUND

A variety of vascular access devices have been developed for hemodialysis. The two major requirements for vascular access are a route for blood outflow and one for blood inflow. The outflow route must supply an adequate volume of blood. The inflow route must be of adequate diameter to accept the blood flow at a rapid rate of return. The desired rate of extracorporeal blood flow is 200 ml to 300 ml/minute. Therefore small blood vessels will not be adequate for hemodialysis treatments. Blood flow does not have to originate from an arterial source. In the critical care setting, blood outflow and inflow are usually obtained from specially designed catheters that have been placed in the subclavian or femoral veins. In addition, shunt tubing may be placed in forearm blood vessels for temporary use.

SELECTION OF VASCULAR
ACCESS

Initially, the selection of the type of vascular access depends on the severity of the client's condition and the presence of life-threatening circumstances that require immediate dialytic intervention. Subclavian and femoral catheters permit relatively immediate initiation of hemodialysis. Either the subclavian or femoral catheter may be inserted at the client's bedside. The AV shunt and the AV fistula require a surgical procedure, and thus time is a factor to be considered.

TYPES OF VASCULAR ACCESS

AV fistula. The AV fistula is the internal surgical anastomosis of an artery to a vein. The side-to-side or end-to-side anastomosis of the artery to the vein results in the direct flow of arterial blood into the vein (Fig. 27–1). Over a period, usually 4 weeks to 8 weeks, the vein distends under the pressure of the arterial blood flow. In addition, the wall of the vein toughens and thickens, becoming more like the wall of an artery. The distention and toughening of the normally thin wall of the vein allows for frequent needle insertions into the fistula. Fistula needles are usually 15 gauge and thus provide a sufficient blood outflow and inflow diameter (Fig. 27–2). Generally, two needles are placed for each dialysis treatment and are removed at the termination of the treatment.

Fig. 27–1 Arteriovenous fistula. (*A*) Side-to-side anastomosis. (*B*) End-to-end anastomosis.

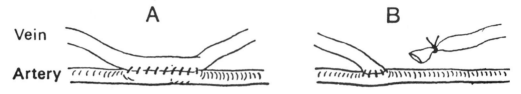

Fig. 27–2 Needle placement in fistula.

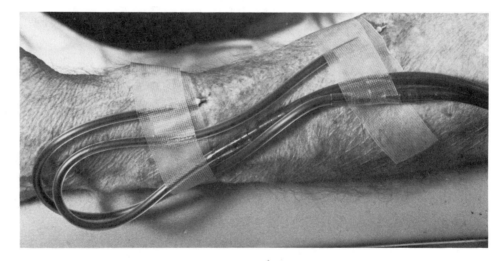

The major advantages of the AV fistula include the potential for access longevity, minimal client restriction, and lack of foreign material. Regular rotation of the cannula insertion sites will promote the longevity of the fistula. The lack of any external tubing allows the client greater freedom of activity, such as bathing and dressing, and is less traumatic to body-image considerations. Because no synthetic materials are in place, there is a decreased risk of infection or clotting of the fistula.

The major disadvantages of the AV fistula include the length of time needed for fistula development and the risks of improper or repeated cannulations. Up to 8 weeks are required for the fistula's development for cannulation (maturing period). For some clients the fistula is never adequate and another vascular access procedure may be needed. Improper cannulation may result in infiltration and subsequent hematoma formation. Repeated venipunctures with fistula needles may result in strictures or the development of aneurysms in the fistula. Phlebitis, infection, and clotting are also potential problems with the AV fistula.

AV shunt (external cannula). The AV shunt is the external connection of an artery to a vein by specially treated synthetic tubing. The internal diameter of the tubing is generally about 2.7 mm. One piece of tubing, sometimes referred to as a "limb" of tubing, is inserted into an artery by a stab wound through the skin; the second limb of tubing is inserted into a nearby vein by a stab wound the skin. Each limb of shunt tubing is sutured in place. The two external ends are joined by a connecting device, resulting in a loop of tubing that lies on the outside of the skin (Fig. 27–3). The connecting device may be a straight connector or a T connector (Fig. 27–4). The presence of a T connector allows for blood access between dialysis treatments. Dialysis is readily initiated by simple disconnection of the two limbs of the shunt.

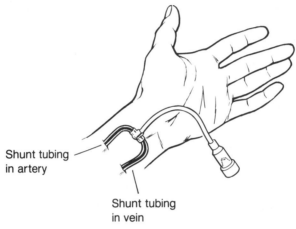

Fig. 27–3 Shunt tubing placed in forearm vessels.

Shunt tubing
in artery

Shunt tubing
in vein

Fig. 27–4 Shunt with straight connector.

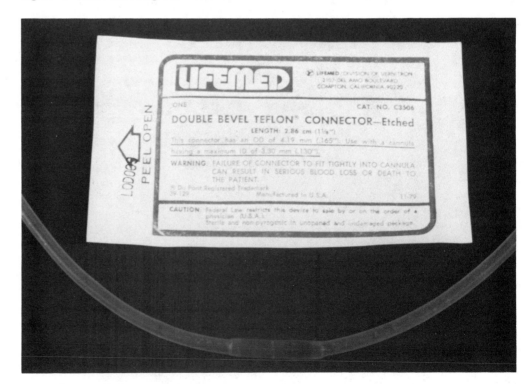

The major advantages of the AV shunt include ease of surgical placement, lack of patient discomfort, and efficiency of dialysis treatments. Generally, less than 1 hour is needed for the surgical placement of the AV shunt. The discomfort associated with the shunt insertion is mild and of short duration. The constant outflow and inflow of blood during dialysis permits good clearance of fluids, electrolytes, and nitrogenous wastes from the blood. When a T connector is in place, frequent venipunctures may be minimized, thus increasing client comfort and preventing other peripheral vein trauma.

The major disadvantages of the AV shunt result from the synthetic quality of the tubing, external placement, and the care required for maintenance. The presence of synthetic or artificial tubing increases the risk of local infection. Local infections may become systemic blood infections or may result in localized skin erosion. Blood viscosity is increased within the external shunt tubing as a result of lower external body temperature. Sluggish or slowed blood flow increases the potential for clotting of the AV shunt. Considerable care is needed to prevent the accidental dislodgement of the shunt tubing, the development of infection, and clotting of the access. Impaired collateral circulation may result because reconstruction of the vessels used for the shunt placement is generally not possible. Vessel spasm may occur in the first several hours after surgical placement and may result in discomfort or may impair the efficiency of the hemodialysis treatment. Fortunately, impaired collateral circulation and vessel spasm are not common occurrences. Another disadvantage of the AV shunt is the visibility of the shunt tubing. Even when covered with an Ace wrap, many clients experience concerns about altered body image.

Subclavian catheter. Subclavian catheters for hemodialysis are specially designed, 15F catheters that are approximately 37.5 cm (15 inches) long. The subclavian catheter is inserted percutaneously into the subclavian vein below the clavicle. The catheter is advanced into the subclavian vein and terminates in the right atrium of the heart (Fig. 27–5). The catheter has small openings along the lower 3 inches to 4 inches and at the tip, through which blood flow is obtained for extracorporeal circulation (Fig. 27–6). The catheter's external ports designate the source of blood outflow and inflow.

Subclavian catheters may be single lumen or double lumen. Double-lumen catheters allow for continuous outflow and inflow of blood during the hemodialysis treat-

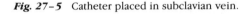

Fig. 27–5 Catheter placed in subclavian vein.

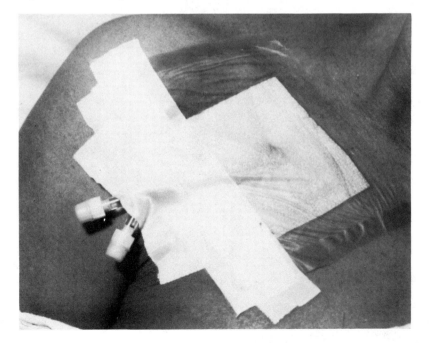

Fig. 27–6 Subclavian catheter with "Y" ports.

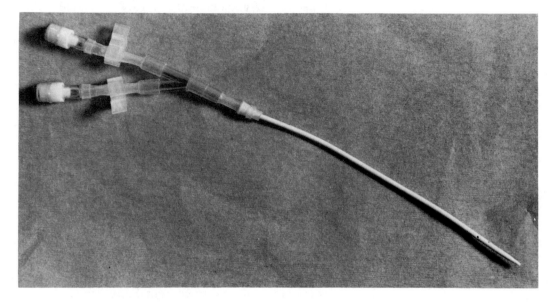

ment. The blood outflow and inflow in single-lumen catheters is temporarily inter-rupted by the blood pump so that major recirculation of the blood does not occur. The subclavian catheter is sutured to the skin at the site of insertion, and a sterile occlusive dressing is applied.

The primary advantage of the subclavian catheter is its ease of insertion. After insertion a chest film is obtained to ensure proper placement and lack of hemothorax or pneumothorax before the subclavian catheter may be used for hemodialysis. Care of the catheter is relatively simple because no irrigations or dressing changes are needed

Fig. 27–7 Subclavian catheter connected to machine.

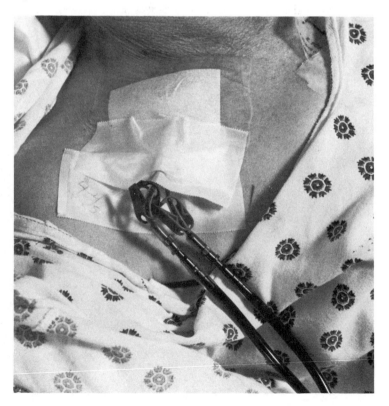

between dialysis treatments. Although it is generally preferred for inpatient care, the stable, alert client may go home with the subclavian catheter in place. The use of the subclavian catheter for outpatient dialysis treatment prevents the client from unnecessary or prolonged hospitalizations, which are costly and inconvenient. The double-lumen catheter provides a better clearance of waste products, electrolytes, and fluid than does the single-lumen catheter (Fig. 27–7).

The major disadvantage of the subclavian catheter is the risk of local or systemic infection. Clients have some activity restrictions because maintenance of a dry occlusive dressing is essential to decrease the risk of infections. Showers are not permitted. The potential for pneumothorax or hemothorax when inserted by inexperienced care-givers is also present. Certain clothing, such as shoulder straps, may promote dislodgement of the catheter. The suture may also become loose and contribute to the dislodgement of the catheter. The single-lumen catheter has decreased clearance

Fig. 27–8 (*A*) Double-lumen double-port femoral catheter. (*B*) Single femoral catheter.

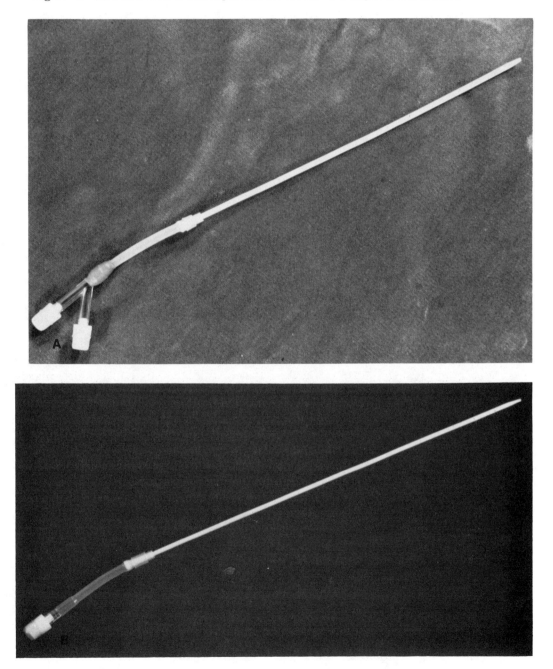

capacity for waste, electrolyte, and fluid removal, which results from the intermittent inflow and outflow of blood. The subclavian catheter is an externally visible piece of equipment that may result in negative body image.

Femoral catheter. Femoral catheters used for hemodialysis are specially designed to permit outflow and inflow of blood. A single-lumen double-port catheter or a double-lumen double-port catheter, or two single catheters may be placed (Fig. 27–8). Venous placement of the femoral catheter(s) is preferred. The catheter design is similar to that used for subclavian placement; however, some femoral catheters are several inches shorter than subclavian catheters. The concepts of blood flow for the single-lumen and double-lumen catheters that are placed in a femoral vein are similar to those discussed for the subclavian catheter. If two femoral catheters are placed, one catheter provides the outflow of blood and the second catheter is the means of inflow (Fig. 27–9). If a single-lumen double-port catheter is used, clearance rates are less efficient than those of the double-lumen double-port catheter.

Fig. 27–9 Two single femoral catheters in place.

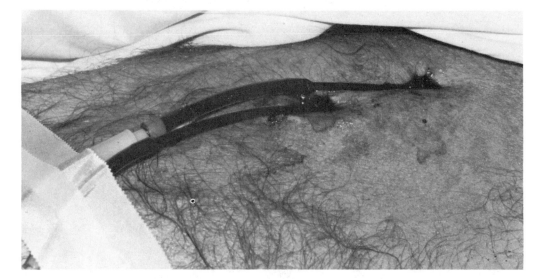

The primary advantage of a femoral catheter is that it may be easily and quickly inserted. Dialysis may be initiated immediately after placement.

A variety of disadvantages are involved in the use of femoral catheters. Client immobility, the risk of bleeding, and the potential for infection are factors that make the femoral catheter less desirable than the subclavian catheter. The client must be on bed rest with a less than 45-degree elevation of the head of the bed to prevent catheter dislodgement or vessel perforation. Thrombophlebitis and pulmonary emboli are potential problems associated with immobility and the presence of a foreign object in the blood vessel. Hematoma formation after insertion or resulting from accidental, vigorous movement of the client may also occur. Proximity to the genital area increases the risk of infection.

Arteriovenous fistula

BACKGROUND

Assessment of adequate arterial blood supply must be determined before the surgical creation of the AV fistula. Adequate collateral circulation must be ensured to prevent ischemia to tissue distal to the fistula.

After insertion, assess the fistula every hour for the first 24 hours to detect any bleeding or loss of patency. A thrill is a palpable rippling sensation that is felt over the venous route of blood flow. A bruit is the audible distention of the vein wall that is receiving the new arterial flow of blood. It is heard by placing the stethoscope over the same site where the thrill is palpated. Clotting is most common during this time period. Bleeding at the incision site is usually minimal.

Elevate the fistula arm slightly on a pillow to increase venous return and to prevent edema. Offer analgesics to ensure client comfort. Insertion of graft materials for blood access requires considerably more tissue dissection and thus client discomfort is substantially increased. Intramuscular injections of a narcotic analgesic are usually required after graft procedures.

Objectives
To prevent bleeding at the fistula site or throughout the body if a systemic anticoagulation regimen is used
To maintain patency of the fistula
To prevent infection at the fistula site
(See Objectives in previous section on Hemodialysis.)

ASSESSMENT PHASE

• Is there evidence of bleeding at the incision or fistula-needle insertion sites? Check for the following:
  Evidence of hematoma or infiltrate near needle insertion site(s)
  Presence of blood on surgical dressing
  Oozing or spurting of blood at needle insertion sites
• Is there evidence of clotting or decreased blood flow through the fistula? Check for the following:
  Absence of thrill or bruit in fistula
  Decrease in quality of thrill or bruit in fistula
  Altered access performance during hemodialysis treatment
• Is there evidence of inflammation at the site of the incision, the needle insertion sites, or the length of the fistula tract? Check for the following:
  Erythema, edema, tenderness, or drainage
  Increased white blood cell count
  Elevated temperature
  Chills

PRECAUTIONS

• **Accidental perforation of the wall of the fistula vein during needle insertion may result in hematoma formation and temporary loss of access function.**
• **The trauma associated with repeated attempts to insert the fistula needle may result in permanent loss of the vascular access.**
• **Dislodgement of fistula needles during the hemodialysis treatment could result in significant blood loss.**
• **Hypotensive episodes may result in clotting of the fistula because of decreased blood flow.**

PLANNING PHASE

EQUIPMENT

Clean gloves — 2 pairs
Tourniquet
Povidone – iodine swabs — 4
Xylocaine 1% without epinephrine
3-ml syringe for Xylocaine — 2
26-gauge needle — 2
Fistula needle — 2
Tape
Band-Aid — 2
Sterile gauze sponge — 2
Povidone — iodine ointment — 2 packets
Bactericidal cleansing agent

CLIENT/FAMILY TEACHING

- Discuss the fistula or graft as a permanent means of vascular access for hemodialysis treatments.
- Explain that the nondominant arm will be used so that the dominant arm will be free for use during the dialysis treatment.
- Advise the client that surgical placement usually takes about 1 hour and that a local anesthetic is generally given.
- Assure the client that medications will be given after the surgery to provide for comfort.
- Advise the client that elevation and extension of the arm will be requested after the surgery.
- Instruct the client not to permit blood pressure measurement or venipuncture in the fistula arm.
- Demonstrate palpation of the thrill and auscultation of the bruit after fistula establishment; initiate a return demonstration.
- Explain that a local anesthetic will be administered before the placement of the fistula needles.
- Explain that normal use of the fistula arm is permitted between dialysis treatments, but caution should be exercised to prevent compression or constriction of the fistula.
- Explain that normal bathing or showering is permitted.
- Emphasize the need to notify the physician or the dialysis unit staff if the thrill cannot be palpated or the bruit auscultated.
- Explain the need to apply pressure to the fistula-needle insertion sites after needle removal.

IMPLEMENTATION PHASE

NURSING ACTIONS	RATIONALE/AMPLIFICATION
1.–9. See steps 1 to 9 under Implementation Phase in previous section on Hemodialysis.	
10. Prepare vascular access.	
a. Check fistula for thrill and bruit.	Thrill and bruit ensure fistula patency.
b. Clense fistula with bactericidal agent for 3 minutes to 5 minutes.	Cleansing reduces the risk of infection.
c. Cleanse cannulation sites individually with povidone–iodine swabs.	
d. Inject Xylocaine epidermally at cannulation sites until wheal is formed.	Xylocaine minimizes client discomfort.
e. Apply tourniquet.	Use a tourniquet to identify the fistula tract and to facilitate needle insertion.
f. Insert fistula needle and tape securely in place.	
g. Allow blood flow to displace air from cannula.	This confirms proper needle placement.
h. Give heparin bolus, if ordered, after both needles are properly placed.	Heparin prevents bleeding.
11. Attach blood lines to client access.	
a. Apply povidone–iodine ointment at needle insertion sites.	Povidone–iodine ointment reduces the risk of infection.
b. Tape blood lines to reduce tension and trauma to the insertion sites.	Tape blood lines to extremity.

12.–17. See steps 12 to 17 under Implementation Phase in previous section on Hemodialysis.

18. Prepare to disconnect blood lines.

    a. Apply gauze pressure dressing over venous site and remove needle.

A pressure dressing prevents hemorrhage caused by the pressure of the artial blood flow and the remaining effects of anticoagulant administration.

    b. Repeat for arterial needle.

19. Complete vascular access care.

    a. Apply continuous pressure to each site for 5 minutes to 10 minutes or until bleeding has stopped.

    b. Apply povidone–iodine ointment and Band-Aid to each insertion site.

    c. Apply additional pressure dressings as indicated.

    d. Check for presence of thrill and bruit.

Thrill and bruit confirm patency of the fistula.

20.–24. See steps 20 to 24 under Implementation Phase in previous section on Hemodialysis.

RELATED NURSING CARE

NURSING ACTIONS	RATIONALE/AMPLIFICATION
1. Avoid blood pressure readings, phlebotomy, or IV therapy in fistula limb.	This increases the viability and longevity of the fistula. Constriction or compression of the fistula arm increases the potential for loss of fistula patency.
2. Rotate needle insertion sites for each dialysis.	Rotating the sites decreases the potential for the development of strictures, aneurysm, and infection.
3. Assess fistula for patency after hypotensive episodes.	Hypotensive episodes may result in clotting of the fistula because of the decreased blood flow.

EVALUATION PHASE

ANTICIPATED OUTCOMES	NURSING ACTIONS
1. See previous section on Hemodialysis.	
2. Prevention of complications of AV fistula dialysis	
a. Bleeding	Apply pressure at the needle insertion sites. The administration of systemic anticoagulants increases the potential for bleeding during and after dialysis.
b. Clotting	Avoid the application of tourniquets or other constrictive devices. Palpate thrill and auscultate bruit.
c. Infection	Scrub the fistula arm before cannulation. Cleanse and swab skin before needle insertion. Instruct the client on routine hygiene activities. Culture any drainage that may be present. Monitor for signs of infection and monitor the client's vital signs.

PRODUCT AVAILABILITY   FISTULA NEEDLES

C. D. Medical
Drake Willock
Terumo Corporation, USA

Arteriovenous shunt

BACKGROUND

Before surgical placement of the shunt, the surgeon will assess the blood flow and collateral circulation to the arm and to the hand of the arm selected for shunt placement. Adequate collateral circulation must be insured because the presence of the shunt may compromise distal blood flow.

The preferred site for shunt placement is the dominant forearm. However, the other arm or even an ankle may be a potential alternative. When an arm site has been selected, avoid the use of its peripheral blood vessels for IV infusions and venipunctures.

After insertion assess the shunt every hour for the first 24 hours to detect any bleeding or the loss of the thrill and bruit. Check circulation distal to the shunt insertion sites. Clamps should be available for application in case the tubing becomes disconnected. After the first 24 hours, make a shunt assessment every 4 hours. More frequently observation is indicated particularly if clotting becomes a problem.

Slightly elevate the arm in which the shunt is placed to promote blood flow and to decrease local edema in the area of the insertion sites. Mild discomfort is usually alleviated with the administration of oral non-narcotic analgesics or an agent such as acetaminophen with codeine.

Physician orders for use of the AV shunt for hemodialysis treatments should specify the use of a T connector or a straight connector. Interim care of the AV shunt, including the frequency of dressing change, irrigation procedures, and use of the shunt for blood drawing, IV medication, or fluid administration, should be carried out according to nursing policy or as prescribed by the physician.

Objectives
To prevent bleeding at the shunt site
To maintain patency at the shunt site
To prevent infection at the shunt site
See Objectives in previous section on Hemodialysis.

ASSESSMENT PHASE

- Is there evidence of bleeding at the shunt insertion sites or at the point of the shunt-tubing connection? Check for the following:
  Presence of blood on the dressing/Ace wrap that covers the shunt tubing
  Lack of tubing approximation over T connector or straight connector
  Any unusual tension on shunt tubing
  Decrease in blood pressure or increase in pulse rate
  Presence of alligator clamps on shunt dressing
- Is there evidence of clotting or decreased blood flow through the shunt tubing? Check for the following:
  Absence of thrill or bruit in shunt
  Evidence that blood is darkened or separated into serum and cells
  Decreased temperature of shunt tubing
  Kinking of shunt tubing
  Tightly applied dressing
  Altered access performance during treatment

• Is there evidence of inflammation at the shunt insertion sites? Check for the following:

    Erythema, edema, tenderness, or drainage
    Increased white blood cell count
    Elevated temperature
    Chills
    Skin erosion

PRECAUTIONS

- **The external tubing of the AV shunt increases the risk of dislodgement or disconnection.**
- **Excessive anticoagulant administration may result in hemorrhage or hematoma formation at the shunt insertion sites.**
- **External constriction of the shunt tubing or constriction of the shunt extremity increases the risk of loss of patency.**
- **Spasm of the artery or vein in which the shunt tubings are placed may compromise blood flow and result in loss of patency.**
- **Although arterial pulsation in the shunt tubing may be noted, it is not sufficient evidence that the shunt is patent.**
- **Wet shunt dressings or wraps increase the potential for local or systemic infection.**
- **Failure to use sterile techniques when initiating or discontinuing dialysis may increase the risk of local or systemic infection.**
- **Failure to use sterile technique when performing dressing changes increases the risk of local or systemic infection.**
- **The presence of artificial shunt tubing increases the potential for the direct entry of pathogens into the bloodstream.**

PLANNING PHASE

EQUIPMENT

Stethoscope
Doppler stethoscope (as required)
Alligator clamps — 2
Ace wrap
T connector or straight connector
Sterile drape — 2
Sterile gloves — 2 pairs
Sterile gauze sponges — 4
Tape
Iodine-soaked gauze pads — 4
3 ml heparinized saline (100 units/ml)
Dressing change supplies (see Related Nursing Care in this section)

CLIENT/FAMILY TEACHING

- Explain the reason for an AV shunt insertion and how it will be used for hemodialysis treatments.
- Advise the client that surgical placement of the shunt requires about 1 hour to complete and that the shunt may be used immediately after placement.
- Assure the client that medication will be given for the alleviation of the mild discomfort that is associated with insertion.
- Advise the client to elevate the shunt arm slightly and to avoid lying on the shunt arm.
- Instruct the client not to permit blood pressure measurements or venipuncture in the shunt arm.
- Demonstrate palpation of the thrill and auscultation of the bruit, and initiate a return demonstration by the client if possible.
- Discuss the potential sites of shunt bleeding and the appropriate corrective action.
- Instruct the client in methods that do not allow the dressing to become wet.
- Assure the client that the removal of the shunt will not require another surgical procedure and is often done at the bedside.

IMPLEMENTATION PHASE

NURSING ACTIONS	RATIONALE/AMPLIFICATION
1.–9. See steps 1 to 9 under Implementation Phase in previous section on Hemodialysis.	
10. Prepare vascular access.	
a. Check shunt for thrill and bruit.	Thrill and bruit ensure shunt patency.
b. Remove Ace wrap and external gauze dressing from shunt.	
c. Prepare alligator clamps in iodine-soaked gauze pad packet.	This reduces the potential for local or systemic infection.
d. Cleanse shunt tubing around connector with second iodine-soaked gauze pad.	
e. Place sterile drape under shunt tubing.	
f. Drop alligator clamps on drape; drop two sterile gauze sponges on drape.	
g. Prepare anticoagulant regimen.	
h. Identify arterial and venous blood lines and place them near drape.	
i. Put on sterile gloves.	
j. Clamp arterial and venous shunt tubing with alligator clamps.	
k. Separate shunt tubing and remove connector.	
11. Attach blood lines to client access.	
a. Grasp arterial blood line with sterile 4 × 3 and attach to arterial shunt limb, remove clamp, and note pulsation.	This ensures proper access performance, which is necessary for efficient nitrogenous waste and fluid removal.
b. Give heparin bolus, through venous shunt limb, if ordered.	A heparin bolus prevents clotting of the extracorporeal blood circuit.
c. Grasp venous blood line with another sterile 4 × 3 and attach to venous shunt limb; remove clamp.	
d. Securely anchor shunt tubing to extremity with tape.	Anchor the tubing to reduce tension and trauma to the insertion sites.
12.–17. See steps 12 to 17 under Implementation Phase in previous section on Hemodialysis.	
18. Prepare to disconnect blood lines.	
a. Prepare alligator clamps in iodine-soaked gauze pad packet.	This reduces the risk of local or systemic infection.
b. Cleanse connecting point of shunt tubing and blood line with second iodine-soaked gauze pad.	
c. Place sterile drape under shunt tubing, drop alligator clamps on drape, and drop two sterile gauze sponges on drape.	
d. Put on sterile gloves.	
e. Place alligator clamps on arterial and venous shunt tubing.	Clamps prevent blood loss.

f. Grasp each blood line with sterile gauze sponges and disconnect blood lines from shunt tubing.

19. Complete vascular access care.

a. Attach 3-ml heparinized saline syringe (without needle) to arterial limb of shunt; remove arterial clamp.

b. Inject heparinized saline into arterial limb of shunt until client detects slight burning sensation.

Heparinized saline minimizes the risk of clotting caused by temporary clamp placement.

c. Reclamp arterial limb and remove syringe.

d. Use sterile connector to join limbs of shunt tubing.

The sterile connectors reestablish shunt blood flow.

e. Remove clamps. Note blood flow through connector.

f. Complete dressing change if this was not done earlier during treatment.

g. Apply Ace wrap to extremity.

This protects the shunt site from trauma and accidental disconnection of tubing.

h. Attach alligator clamps to outside of Ace wrap.

i. Determine presence of thrill and bruit.

Thrill and bruit ensure patency.

20.–24. See steps 20 to 24 under Implementation Phase in previous section on Hemodialysis.

RELATED NURSING CARE

NURSING ACTIONS	RATIONALE/AMPLIFICATION
1. Change dressing.	Dressings for external AV shunts should be changed at least three times per week. Interim dressing changes should be done if the dressing becomes wet, soiled, or must be removed.
a. Assist client into comfortable position with arm extended.	
b. Wash hands and remove Ace wrap and inner dressing.	
c. Create sterile field and put on sterile gloves.	
d. Cleanse around insertion site(s) with separate acetone/alcohol swab.	Use of sterile technique minimizes the potential for development of infection at the insertion sites or systemically.
e. Cleanse around insertion site(s) with separate povidone–iodine swab.	
f. Apply povidone–iodine ointment to each insertion site with separate applicator.	
g. Place preslit sterile gauze 4 × 3 under shunt tubing next to skin.	Gauze placed under the tubing protects the skin from breakdown from pressure.
h. Cover with sterile gauze sponges; tape dressing lightly to keep it in place.	Avoid circular wrapping of the arm with the tape, which could impair circulation.
i. Cover dressing and all tubing with Ace wrap; place clamps on outside of wrap.	Covering the tubing decreases the risk of accidental dislodgement.
2. Remove clots from shunt.	Policies and procedures about the role of the nurse in removing clots from an external AV shunt vary among institutions. Identify the policy and procedure of your institution before initiating this intervention.

a. Assist client into comfortable position with arm extended.

b. Wash your hands and remove Ace wrap and inner dressing.

c. Create sterile field and put on sterile gloves.

d. Cleanse connection point of shunt tubing and adjacent tubing with povidone–iodine swabs.

Sterile technique is essential to prevent the development of systemic infection.

e. Place sterile alligator clamp on each limb of tubing.

An alligator clamp prevents loss of blood if one side of the shunt is patent.

f. Separate shunt tubing.

g. Attach empty sterile 10-ml syringe without needle to one limb of shunt tubing; hold it in one hand.

h. Remove alligator clamp with other hand.

i. Aspirate gently; reapply clamp.

Gentle aspiration may remove a newly formed clot and reestablish patency.

j. Repeat steps g through i with other limb of shunt tubing.

k. Rejoin limbs of shunt tubing with T connector or straight connector.

l. Check shunt for thrill and bruit.

Thrill and bruit indicate that patency has been restored.

m. Apply sterile dressing per procedure.

A sterile dressing prevents local or systemic infection.

n. Notify physician of need for Fogarty catheter embolectomy if patency is not restored.

EVALUATION PHASE

ANTICIPATED OUTCOMES	NURSING ACTIONS
1. See previous section on Hemodialysis.	
2. Prevention of complications of AV shunt dialysis	Ensure that the tubing is covered by the Ace wrap.
a. Bleeding	Ensure that two alligator clamps are placed on the outside of the Ace wrap.
	Determine that the limbs of the shunt tubing are approximated over the straight connector or over the T connector.
b. Clotting	Palpate thrill and auscultate bruit every 4 hours.
	Inspect shunt tubing to determine that blood is bright red and that no separation of cells and serum is present.
	Remove Ace wrap and look for kinks in the tubing if a decrease in the quality of the thrill or bruit is detected.
	Irrigate the T connector with 3 ml heparinized saline if clotting or sluggish blood flow is suspected.
	Notify the physician if the thrill and bruit are not restored.
c. Infection	Inspect the shunt insertion sites at each dialysis treatment.
	Change the dressing when it is wet, nonocclusive, or a minimum of three times per week.
	Obtain a culture of any drainage that may be present.

PRODUCT AVAILABILITY   SHUNT SUPPLIES

Lifemed
Quinton
3-C Medical

Subclavian catheter for hemodialysis

BACKGROUND

SITE SELECTION

The selection of a subclavian or femoral catheter access site is usually determined by the need for immediate hemodialysis and the lack of other vascular access. The subclavian catheter is considered to be a temporary form of access, but it can remain in place for several weeks. The femoral catheter is generally not left in place for longer than 48 hours. Options include the right or left subclavian vein or the right or left femoral or saphenous veins. Contraindications for site selection include previous vascular surgery or the presence of synthetic graft material, existing central lines, a history of difficult or multiple attempts at percutaneous line placement, known vascular anomalies, and temporary pacemaker wires.

ASSISTING WITH INSERTION

Assist the client into a comfortable supine position in bed. For a subclavian catheter, lower the head of the bed into a slight Trendelenberg's position. For a femoral catheter, elevate the head of the bed slightly, but not more than 15° to 30°.

During the insertion of the subclavian catheter, ask the client to turn the head away from the side of insertion. When the catheter is open to air, request that the client take a deep breath and hold it. Valsalva's maneuver creates positive pressure within the chest cavity and prevents the accidental intake of air through the open catheter.

For femoral catheter insertion, ask the client to refrain from moving the legs. A natural response is to flex the knees or to try to turn to the side. These movements make the insertion more difficult and increase the risk of hematoma formation.

CATHETER INSERTION

The subclavian and femoral catheters are placed by similar techniques. After skin preparation and a local injection of Xylocaine, a 3-inch to 4-inch cannula with a beveled needle introducer is inserted into the selected vein. Aspiration of blood confirms proper cannulation. The inner needle is withdrawn, and a guidewire is inserted through the outer cannula into the vein. After the removal of the outer cannula, the subclavian or femoral catheter is introduced into the selected vein over the guidewire. When the catheter is placed, the guidewire is removed. Flush each port and lumen (if double) with sterile saline. Apply Luer-Lok caps. To prevent clotting, instill a heparin/saline solution into each lumen. Apply clamp(s) to the external tubing of the catheter. The subclavian catheter is sutured in place. The femoral catheter is anchored securely with tape. Apply dry, sterile occlusive dressings.

POSTINSERTION CARE

After insertion of the subclavian catheter, obtain a chest film to ensure proper placement of the catheter and absence of pneumothorax or hemothorax. Instruct clients with a femoral catheter(s) in place to remain on bed rest and to avoid acute flexion of the hip. Assess the distal circulation. In addition, assess the vital signs and inspect the insertion site(s) for evidence of bleeding, hematoma formation, or dislodgement of the catheter.

Before the subclavian catheter is used for hemodialysis, a physician's order is needed to ensure that the proper location of the catheter has been confirmed. Nursing policy or a physician order should specify interim catheter care to prevent clotting.

One method used to prevent catheter occlusion is the instillation of a concentrated heparin/saline solution after insertion or at the termination of the hemodialysis treatment. The concentration recommended is generally 2500 units heparin/ml of saline. Because there is no blood flow through the catheter, the "dwell" solution fills the lumen of the catheter and prevents clot formation. This is effective in preventing clot formation for at least 48 hours. Aspirate the heparin/saline concentrate before using the catheter for any purpose.

Other methods of preventing catheter clotting involve routine irrigations of the catheter with a dilute heparin/saline solution, usually 100 units/ml saline. These irrigations need to be done every 4 hours to prevent clot formation.

The advantage of a concentrated heparin dwell procedure is that catheter manipulation and entry into the bloodstream are minimized. Ideally, catheters inserted for hemodialysis treatment should not be used for blood withdrawal or injection of IV medication, fluids, or blood. Infection is a major problem that is associated with these catheters.

Insertion of subclavian catheter

BACKGROUND

The presence of a synthetic catheter in the vasculature increases the potential for the direct entry of pathogens into the bloodstream. Systemic bacteremia necessiates temporary catheter removal. Complications of catheter insertion include hemorrhage, hematoma, internal jugular vein cannulation, pneumothorax, or hemothorax.

Objective
To obtain emergency vascular access

PRECAUTIONS

- **Excessive anticoagulation administration may result in hemorrhage or hematoma formation at the insertion site.**
- **Recirculation of the client's blood may occur if proper catheter performance is not assessed.**
- **Inadequate catheter irrigation at the completion of the treatment may result in a lack of catheter patency and a loss of function.**
- **Accidental removal or loss of Luer-Lok injection caps may result in air embolization or blood loss.**

PLANNING PHASE

EQUIPMENT

Clamp — 2
Sterile drape — 2
Sterile gloves — 2 pairs
Sterile gauze sponges — 4
Tape
Iodine-soaked gauze pads — 4
Luer-Lok injection cap — 2
5-ml syringe — 2
3-ml syringe with 3 ml sterile sodium chloride for injection — 2
Dressing change supplies (see Related Nursing Care in this section)
Heparin flush irrigation (as ordered by physician or according to nursing policy)
Single-needle pump device (if indicated)

CLIENT/FAMILY TEACHING

- Discuss the reason for the insertion of a subclavian catheter.
- Inform the client that the insertion will be done at the bedside.
- Describe the insertion procedure and possible sensations of pressure and discomfort.
- Discuss the need for a chest film after insertion and before the initiation of dialysis.
- Assure the client that medication will be given to alleviate the mild discomfort that is associated with the catheter insertion.
- Tell the client to notify the nurse if bleeding develops around the catheter or if the dressing feels wet.
- Provide information about general activity and precautions related to hygiene and clothing.

IMPLEMENTATION PHASE

NURSING ACTIONS	RATIONALE/AMPLIFICATION
1.–9. See steps 1 to 9 under Implementation Phase in previous section on Hemodialysis.	
10. Prepare vascular access.	
a. Clamp extension tubing if it is not already clamped.	Clamping prevents the entry of air into the catheter.
b. Cleanse each Luer-Lok injection cap, catheter extension tubing, and clamp with iodine-soaked gauze pad.	Cleansing reduces the risk of local or systemic infection.
c. Place sterile drape under extension tubing; place two 5-ml sterile syringes and two sterile gauze sponges on drape.	
d. Prepare anticoagulant regimen.	
e. Identify arterial and venous blood lines and place near drape.	
f. Put on sterile gloves.	
g. Remove catheter caps, attach sterile syringes, remove one clamp, and aspirate 3 ml to 5 ml of blood. Replace clamp and repeat with other port.	This step removes clots and ensures catheter patency.
11. Attach blood lines to client access.	
a. Remove syringe from arterial port; grasp blood line with sterile gauze sponges and attach it to arterial port.	This ensures proper access performance, which is necessary for the efficient removal of fluid and nitrogenous wates.
b. Attach heparin-bolus syringe to venous port, remove clamp, and administer heparin and reclamp.	This prevents clotting of blood in the extracorporeal circuit.
c. Remove bolus syringe; grasp venous blood line with another sterile gauze sponges and attach to venous port. Remove clamps on extension tubing.	
d. Securely anchor tubing to extremity with tape.	Secure the tubing to reduce tension and trauma to the insertion site.
12.–17. See steps 12 to 17 under Implementation Phase in previous section on Hemodialysis.	
18. Prepare to disconnect blood lines.	
a. Place clamps on extension tubing.	Clamps prevent the entry of air into the catheter.
b. Cleanse connecting points of catheter and blood lines; cleanse clamps.	Cleansing reduces the risk of local or systemic infection.
c. Place sterile drape under catheter; place two sterile 4 $\times$ 3s on drape.	
d. Prepare catheter flush solution (saline, or as ordered by physician).	
e. Put on sterile gloves.	
f. Grasp each blood line with sterile gauze sponges and disconnect blood lines from catheter.	

19.   Complete vascular access care.

    a.   Administer saline flush solution to each port.

Saline flush solution clears the extension tubing and the catheter of blood.

    b.   Administer additional heparin flush as ordered by physician.

A heparin flush ensures catheter patency.

    c.   Securely attach Luer-Lok injection caps.

Luer-Lok caps prevent the loss of blood or the entry of air.

    d.   Place clamps on extension tubing.

20.–24.   See steps 20 to 24 under Implementation Phase in previous section on Hemodialysis.

RELATED NURSING CARE

NURSING ACTIONS	RATIONALE/AMPLIFICATION

1.   Redress catheter after dialysis or when it is nonocclusive, soiled, or wet.

    a.   Place client in supine position with face turned away from insertion site.

This position prevents contamination from the client's breathing.

    b.   Wash your hands.

    c.   Remove outer occlusive dressing.

    d.   Put on sterile gloves and remove inner dressing; discard gloves and old dressing.

Sterile technique decreases the risk of infection.

    e.   Set up sterile field.

    f.   Observe site for drainage; note presence of suture.

Culture the drainage as required. Notify the physician if the suture is absent.

    g.   Put on sterile gloves.

    h.   Cleanse insertion site with acetone/alcohol swab.

Acetone/alcohol removes oils from the skin and enhances cleaning.

    i.   Cleanse insertion site with povidine–iodine swab; allow it to dry.

Povidone–iodine has bactericidal properties; skin irritation is likely to occur if drying does not precede the placement of the transparent film.

    j.   Apply povidone–iodine ointment at insertion site and at suture site.

    k.   Apply preslit gauze dressing over ointment and under catheter; apply another small gauze dressing over catheter.

    l.   Apply barrier skin preparation to skin that surrounds gauze, which will be covered by transparent film dressing.

This enhances adhesion and decreases skin irritation.

    m.   Apply transparent film dressing over gauze and catheter. Cut "V" wedge from lower side of transparent film dressing.

The transparent film dressing increases occlusion around the catheter.

    n.   Apply 4-inch to 5-inch piece of 2-inch tape over edge of transparent film where "V" was cut.

Tape reinforces the lower edge of the dressing.

2.   Irrigate subclavian catheter after blood withdrawal or medication administration.

    a.   Cleanse injection cap with povidone–iodine swab; allow it to dry.

Use of a bactericidal preparation decreases the risk of infection.

    b.   Flush catheter with 3 ml sterile saline.

Flushing clears blood or medication from the catheter.

c. Cleanse exit port with povidone–iodine sepp.

d. Instill 1 ml heparin/saline solution (usually 5000 units/ml mixed with 1 ml sterile saline).

The dwell solution will prevent clotting for 48 hours.

e. Reapply clamp.

Clamping prevents the accidental entry of air into the catheter.

3. Remove subclavian catheter as ordered.

a. Remove dressing.

b. Remove suture using sterile scalpel blade.

c. Cover catheter insertion site with sterile gauze sponges.

d. Instruct client to take deep breath and hold it; remove catheter.

This prevents the entry of air into the catheter.

e. Apply firm digital pressure over site.

Firm digital pressure prevents bleeding.

f. Apply povidone–iodine ointment and sterile dressing.

Povidone–iodine ointment decreases the risk of infection.

EVALUATION PHASE

ANTICIPATED OUTCOMES	NURSING ACTIONS
1. See previous section on Hemodialysis.	
2. Prevention of bleeding	Monitor the access site for frank bleeding. Monitor the client's vital signs. Ensure the closure of the clamps and caps. Avoid disconnection of the blood lines from the access site. Administer anticoagulant as ordered.
3. Prevention of clotting	Observe the catheter for clots. Administer anticoagulant if interim use is required. Assess the ease of blood aspiration from the catheter.
4. Prevention of infection	Inspect the catheter insertion and suture sites with each dressing change or with each dialysis treatment. Change the dressing if it is wet, nonocclusive, or at least three times per week, using strict sterile technique. Monitor for signs of infection. Culture any drainage that may be present.
5. Prevention of air in catheter	Utilize clamps when the catheter cap(s) are removed; encourage the client to perform Valsalva's maneuver when the catheter cap(s) are removed.

PRODUCT AVAILABILITY   SUBCLAVIAN CATHETERS

Shiley
Quinton
Vas-Cath

Femoral catheter for hemodialysis

Objectives
To obtain emergency vascular access for hemodialysis
To prevent bleeding at the insertion site

To maintain the patency of the catheter
To prevent infection at the insertion site

ASSESSMENT PHASE

See previous section on Insertion of Subclavian Catheter.

PRECAUTIONS

· **The presence of a synthetic catheter(s) in the vasculature increases the potential for the direct entry of pathogens into the bloodstream.**
· **Trauma during placement may result in hemorrhage or hematoma formation at the insertion site.**
· **Accidental placement of the catheter in the femoral artery instead of the femoral vein may occur.**
· **Pulmonary emboli may result from the presence of the femoral catheter(s).**
· **Excessive anticoagulation administration may result in hemorrhage or hematoma formation at the insertion site.**
· **Recirculation of the client's blood may occur if proper catheter performance is not assessed.**
· **The external tubing of the femoral catheter increases the risk of dislodgement or disconnection.**
· **Local access-site infection may result in systemic bacteremia and may necessitate temporary removal of the catheter.**
· **Inadequate catheter irrigation at the completion of the treatment may result in a lack of catheter patency and a loss of function.**
· **Accidental removal or loss of Luer-Lok injection caps may result in air embolization or blood loss.**
· **Groin trauma, catheter occlusion, or catheter breakage can occur if hip flexion is more than a 45°.**
· **A decrease in the circulation to the affected extremity may occur.**

EQUIPMENT

See previous section on Insertion of Subclavian Catheter.

CLIENT/FAMILY TEACHING

· Discuss the reason for the insertion of the femoral catheter.
· Inform the client that the insertion will be done at the bedside.
· Describe the insertion procedure and possible sensations of pressure and discomfort.
· Inform the client of the need to remain in bed with the head of the bed elevated no higher than 45°.
· Assure the client that medication will be given to alleviate the mild discomfort that is associated with the catheter insertion.
· Tell the client to notify the nurse if bleeding develops around the catheter or if the dressing feels wet.

IMPLEMENTATION PHASE

See previous section on Insertion of Subclavian Catheter.

RELATED NURSING CARE

NURSING ACTIONS	RATIONALE/AMPLIFICATION
1. Change dressing after dialysis and as required.	
a. Place client in supine position in bed.	
b. Wash your hands.	
c. Remove outer occlusive dressing.	
d. Put on sterile gloves and remove inner dressing; discard gloves and old dressing.	Sterile technique decreases the risk of infection.
e. Set up sterile field.	

f. Observe site for drainage; note presence of suture.

Culture drainage as indicated.

g. Put on sterile gloves.

h. Cleanse insertion site(s) with acetone/alcohol swab.

Acetone/alcohol removes oils from the skin and enhances cleaning.

i. Cleanse insertion site(s) with povidone–iodine swab; allow it to dry.

Povidone–iodine has bactericidal properties.

j. Apply povidone–iodine ointment at insertion site(s).

k. Apply preslit gauze dressing over ointment and under catheter; apply another small gauze dressing over catheter.

l. Cover insertion site(s) with sterile gauze sponges.

m. Tape dressing securely to skin.

The femoral catheter is not sutured; taping it securely helps to prevent dislodgement.

2. Irrigate femoral catheter after blood withdrawal or medication administration.

a. Cleanse injection cap with povidone–iodine swab; allow it to dry.

Use of a bactericidal preparation decreases the risk of infection.

b. Flush catheter with 3 ml sterile saline.

Flushing clears blood or medication from the catheter.

c. Cleanse exit port with povidone–iodine swab.

d. Instill 1 ml heparin/saline solution (usually 5000 units/ml mixed with 1 ml sterile saline).

The dwell solution will prevent clotting for 48 hours.

3. Remove femoral catheter as ordered.

a. Remove dressing.

b. Cover catheter insertion site with several sterile gauze sponges.

c. Apply pressure while catheter is removed.

Pressure prevents bleeding.

d. Apply firm pressure to site for 5 minutes to 10 minutes.

Pressure prevents hematoma formation.

e. Apply povidone–iodine ointment and pressure dressing.

Povidone–iodine prevents infection.

EVALUATION PHASE See previous section on Insertion of Subclavian Catheter.

PRODUCT AVAILABILITY See previous section on Insertion of Subclavian Catheter.

SELECTED REFERENCES Ash DM: Femoral catheterization: The nurse's role. Nephrology Nurse, September/October 1980, p 44

Connolly E et al: Complications of renal dialysis access procedures. Archives of Surgery 119:1325, November 1984

Parker SR, Lancaster LE: In Lancaster LE (ed): Access to the Circulation. The Patient with End Stage Renal Disease, 2nd ed. New York, John Wiley, 1984

Sims TW, Ulrich B: Successful utilization of catheters for hemodialysis and apheresis access. AANNT Journal, 10:6, December 1983

28 *Peritoneal dialysis*

Because of recent advancements in techniques, peritoneal dialysis is available to a growing number of clients and is considered to be an acceptable alternative to hemodialysis for both acute and chronic renal failure. Soft, pliable peritoneal catheters, which were developed in the early 1970s, have reduced the risk of peritonitis, making long-term peritoneal dialysis possible. The Tenckhoff Silastic catheter in use today has two bonded cuffs; one rests on the fascia covering the peritoneal membrane, the other in subcutaneous tissue. Tissue overgrowth prevents bacterial invasion along the catheter tunnel and provides an anchor for the catheter. The catheter is placed surgically with the client under local or general anesthesia or by endoscopy under peritoneoscopic visualization. The optimal position of the catheter is in the left lower quadrant between the bowel loops and the anterior abdominal wall.

CANDIDATES FOR PERITONEAL DIALYSIS

Peritoneal dialysis may be performed by the client with or without assistance, which is an advantage over hemodialysis. As economics play a greater part in medical care, peritoneal dialysis, which is considerably more inexpensive and more accessible than hemodialysis, will be an option for a greater number of people. Peritoneal dialysis can be performed in the critical care unit, or clients who dialyze at home may be admitted to the critical care unit for other health problems.

Because peritoneal dialysis is a slower process than hemodialysis, it is considered to be more physiologically normal, particularly for the client who has a cardiovascular disorder or for the pediatric client. Peritoneal dialysis is also considered to be an option for the client who does not have a vascular access or who does not have a shunt site. The technique may be contraindicated for clients with severe vascular disease (blood flow to the peritoneum may not be adequate to carry the dialysate and to remove metabolic end products) and for clients who have had extensive abdominal surgery (intact peritoneal surface is required for optimal dialysis).

DIALYSATE COMPOSITION

During dialysis, substances in the bloodstream and in the dialysate equilibrate across a semipermeable membrane, that is, the peritoneum. Peritoneal dialysis requires more time than hemodialysis because of the number of diffusion barriers that solutes must pass through to reach the dialysate. These include blood vessel walls, interstitial tissues, and capillaries of the peritoneum.

The thickness of the peritoneal membrane; the amount of surface area in contact with the dialysate; and the flow rate, temperature, pH, and osmolality of the dialysate are factors that affect peritoneal dialysis. Increasing flow rate increases water removal but does not remarkably increase the metabolic end product clearance. To improve the removal of wastes, the rate of exchanges should be increased rather than the amount of fluid infused with each cycle. Warming the dialysate to body temperature improves metabolic end product clearance and minimizes the loss of body heat. As a rule, pH generally does not affect clearance, but acid dialysate may cause pain on inflow.

Adding dextrose to the dialysate increases dialysate osmolality, thereby providing an increased solute clearance because of the osmotic pull of the dextrose. For dextrose to overcome the colloid osmotic and hydrostatic pressures of the vascular system, the dialysate solution generally should contain at least 1.5% dextrose. Fluid removal can be accelerated by increasing the dextrose concentration; however, the use of dextrose concentrations greater than 4.25% can result in hypernatremia, rapid fluid loss, and hypovolemic shock. Because dextrose that is absorbed from the dialysate can increase blood glucose levels, the diabetic client will probably need insulin-dosage adjustment. The nondiabetic client requires insulin therapy only if symptoms of hyperglycemia occur.

COMPLICATIONS

A common complication of peritoneal dialysis is peritonitis. Fever, rebound tenderness, tachycardia, nausea, malaise, and cloudy outflow (effluent) are symptoms manifested by peritonitis. Peritonitis may be treated by adding antibiotics to the dialysate. However, the best approach to peritonitis is prevention by strict aseptic technique. Timesaving shortcuts often lead to breaks in sterile technique.

Other complications encountered by the dialysis client include inflow pain, outflow difficulties, tunnel infection, and nutritional problems. Inflow pain results from intraperitoneal irritation, cold dialysate, acid dialysate, or stretching and irritation of the diaphragm (generally manifested as referred pain between the shoulder blades). Outflow failure is caused by a full colon, catheter obstruction, peritonitis, a dislodged catheter, or absorption of the initial small-volume exchanges. Tunnel infections, which occur around the subcutaneous segment of the implanted catheter, are difficult to manage, often requiring both local and systemic antibiotic therapy or replacement of the catheter.

Dietary restrictions for the client on peritoneal dialysis are much less rigid than those for hemodialysis. Protein is lost through the peritoneal membrane and is further depleted if peritonitis or local infection is present. Adequate protein intake becomes a problem if the client is a "picky" eater or has an aversion to meat, as do many clients with renal failure. Restriction of dietary potassium is seldom necessary. The dialysate is potassium free, encouraging potassium loss into the dialysate. Dietary restriction of sodium depends on blood pressure and fluid weight gains.

PERITONEAL DIALYSIS MODALITIES

Peritoneal dialysis using gravity flow. Dialysis may be accomplished by allowing dialysate to flow into the peritoneal cavity using gravity flow. The inflow of 2 liters of dialysate takes approximately 10 minutes to 20 minutes. "Dwell" time is determined by the client's needs and is ordered by the physician. Generally, a dwell time of approximately 10 minutes to 25 minutes is needed to achieve clearance. The collection bag is then placed below the level of the client's abdomen to facilitate outflow of the dialysate by gravity.

Continuous ambulatory peritoneal dialysis (CAPD). For CAPD the inflow and outflow of dialysate is controlled by gravity flow, using disposable solution bags and tubing. Upon completion of inflow, the bag and tubing are folded, secured to the client's torso in a pouch or pocket, and used later for the outflow, which takes about 20 minutes. Dwell time is between 4 hours and 6 hours. Four exchanges are completed each day, with the last exchange of the day allowed to dwell overnight. CAPD allows the client freedom from a dialysis center. This technique is also used for hospitalized clients.

Continuous cycled peritoneal dialysis (CCPD). Three to five exchanges are performed automatically at night using the cycler (Fig. 28–1). The abdomen is left full during the day. Exchanges are performed according to a preset schedule by the cycler, which uses gravity for inflow and outflow of fluid. A system of clamps attached to special tubing controls cycling time. An alarm system is activated by inflow or outflow problems.

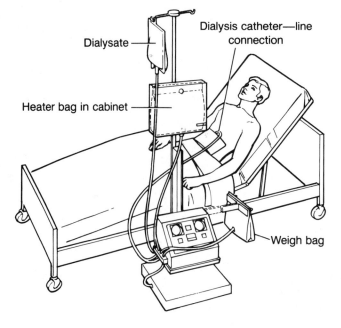

Fig. 28-1 The cycler.

Dialysate

Dialysis catheter—line connection

Heater bag in cabinet

Weigh bag

Peritoneal dialysis using gravity

Objective
To provide effect clearance of metabolic end products and excess fluid from the body in the presence of acute or chronic renal failure

ASSESSMENT PHASE

• Are the client and family familiar with the components of the disease process that require dialysis?
• Is this the client's first experience with peritoneal dialysis? If not, is the client willing to share helpful information about the previous experience?
• Does the client understand the principles of peritoneal dialysis?
• Is the client aware of the symptoms of a difficult dialysis? Is the client aware of symptoms that should be reported (*e.g.,* abdominal pain)?
• Is the client aware of fluid and dietary restrictions necessary to maintain equilibrium?
• Has the client been weighed before dialysis?
• Have baseline vital signs and an abdominal girth measurement been obtained? Fluid retention will be monitored using the abdominal girth measurement as well as a daily weight.

PRECAUTIONS

• **Adhere to strict aseptic technique throughout the procedure.**

PLANNING PHASE

EQUIPMENT

Face masks — 2
2-inch tape
4 × 4s — 8
Perforated sterile drape
Iodophor solution
Peroxide or alcohol solution
Sterile cups or basins — 2
Sterile gloves
Sterile inlet cap
Dialysate tubing
Dialysate solution (at room temperature)
Outflow bag or bottle (as indicated by dialysis mode) or disposable tray

CLIENT/FAMILY TEACHING
- Discuss the reasons for peritoneal dialysis.
- Discuss the significance of adhering to strict aseptic technique when initiating and discontinuing dialysis.
- Describe possible sensations (*e.g.,* abdominal fullness, inflow pain).
- Tell the client to report shortness of breath or abdominal pain after the procedure begins.
- Describe the symptoms of peritonitis and encourage the client to report any unpleasant symptoms.
- Discuss individual dietary and fluid restrictions.

IMPLEMENTATION PHASE

NURSING ACTIONS	RATIONALE/AMPLIFICATION
1. Remove dialysis tubing from protective package. Connect two flasks of dialysate to two tubing extensions. Prime and clamp tubing.	Allow the dialysate to warm to room temperature. Infusion of cold dialysate will cause abdominal discomfort and can lower the core body temperature. The dialysate may require additives, such as heparin to prevent clotting, potassium chloride to prevent a drop in serum potassium, antibiotics for the treatment of peritonitis, or lidocaine for the control of local discomfort.
2. Wear mask and put mask on client.	If the client is not able to wear a mask, turn the client's head away from the catheter site to prevent contamination.
3. Wash your hands.	
4. Pour iodophor solution into large sterile cup or basin.	*Alternative method:* Remove Ampak On–Off kit from the package. Use a clean, dry table for assembly. Open the package using sterile technique. Use forceps to separate the contents of the kit. Pour solution as described (Fig. 28–2).

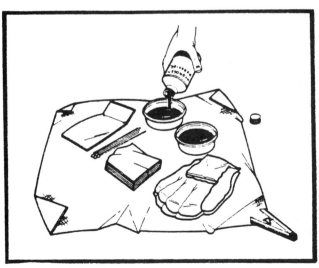

Fig. 28–2 Preparation of solutions using disposable peritoneal dressing change tray.

5. Soak four sterile 4 × 4s in iodophor solution.

6. Pour alcohol or peroxide into remaining sterile container.

7. Remove tape and outer dressings from catheter site, retaining 4 × 4s immediately covering catheter. This prevents contamination of the catheter site.

8.   Put on sterile gloves.

This prevents contamination of the sterile gloves.

9.   Using dry sterile 4 × 4, remove remaining 4 × 4 and expose catheter site.

10.   Grasp catheter tip and wrap iodophor-saturated 4 × 4 around exposed tip of catheter. Allow tip to soak for 5 minutes.

This will begin a 5-minute soak.

11.   Prepare insertion site with 4 × 4s that have been saturated with iodophor solution. Begin at insertion site and clean with circular motion using widening concentric circles. Discard 4 × 4 and repeat.

Using widening concentric circles without returning to the insertion site prevents contamination of the prepared area.

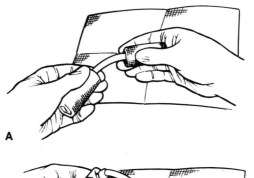

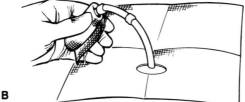

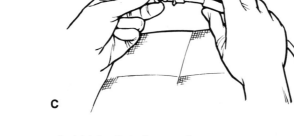

Fig. 28–3   Five-minute catheter soak. (*A*) Disinfecting catheter with 4 × 4 saturated with iodophor solution. Note that the iodophor soak is still intact around catheter tip. (*B*) Placement of sterile drape with iodophor soak still in place on catheter tip. (*C*) Connecting catheter to primed dialysis tubing.

12.   Using iodophor-saturated 4 × 4, disinfect catheter, moving from insertion site toward catheter tip. Discard 4 × 4 and repeat (Fig. 28–3*A*).

13.   Insert catheter tip (with iodophor-saturated 4 × 4 intact) through perforation in sterile drape (Fig. 28–3*B*).

14.   Remove 4 × 4 from catheter tip at end of 5-minute soak.

15.   Remove catheter cap and secure catheter to primed dialysis tubing (Fig. 28–3*C*).

16.   Dress catheter–client dialysis line connection with dry 4 × 4 and tape.

Dry dressings allow leaks to be easily detected and alleviate moisture, which is conducive to bacterial contamination.

17. Discard drape. Cleanse skin with iodophor solution.

If iodine sensitivity develops, cleanse the client's skin with an alcohol or a peroxide solution.

18. Apply dry occlusive dressing to insertion site.

Make certain that no part of the catheter is exposed.

19. Release clamp and begin infusion of dialysate.

Inflow is controlled by gravity.

20. On completion of inflow, clamp tubing.

Approximately 10 minutes to 20 minutes are allowed for inflow. Record the client's vital signs every 15 minutes during the first dialysis and every hour thereafter if the client's condition is stable.

21. Allow prescribed dwell time to elapse. Then begin outflow phase.

Dwell time is determined by the physician according to individual needs and the dialysis mode. The first exchange may be drained immediately to determine the patency of the catheter.

22. Position container below level of client's abdomen and allow dialysate to return by gravity flow (Fig. 28-4).

Facilitate the return of the dialysate by assisting the client to change position or by elevating the head of the bed.

23. On completion of outflow, clamp tubing. Record volume of dialysate infused and volume returned on dialysis flow sheet (see example of peritoneal dialysis flow sheet).

Notify the physician if the dialysate is not returned or if the volume returned is 500 ml more than the amount infused.

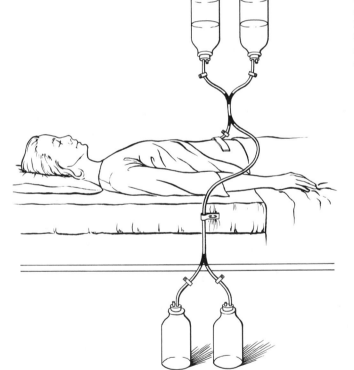

Fig. 28-4 Peritoneal dialysis. After solution flows into patient, it remains *in situ* for length of time ordered by physician. Then clamps on lower bottles are opened and solution is drained.

Peritoneal dialysis flow sheet.

DATE	WEIGHT		B.P.		PULSE		RESP.		TEMP.		NO. SOLUTION CONTAINERS			INFLOW VOLUME	OUTPUT VOLUME	VOLUME EXCESS/ DEFICIT	COMMENTS LAB RESULTS, MEDICATIONS
	PRE	POST	PRE	POST	PRE	POST	PRE	POST	PRE	POST	1.5%	2.5%	4.25%				
														1000 ml	1250 ml	−250 ml	1st exchange
														1000 ml	1100 ml	−350 ml	2nd exchange

24. If additional infusions of dialysate are not planned, prepare to disconnect dialysis tubing. Repeat steps 2 to 12. Place sterile drape under catheter.

It is not possible to insert the catheter through the perforation in the drape.

25. After 5 minute-soak is completed, disconnect dialysis line from catheter and apply sealing cap to end of catheter.

26. Discard drape. Cleanse skin with iodophor solution.

Use alcohol or peroxide if skin sensitivity develops.

27. Apply sterile, dry occlusive dressing to catheter site.

RELATED NURSING CARE

NURSING ACTIONS	RATIONALE/AMPLIFICATION
1. Provide catheter care between exchanges.	
a. If dressing remains dry and intact, do not disturb.	
b. If dressing becomes wet, redress.	Use the technique described above, including the 5-minute soak. Do not remove the catheter cap.
2. Assist client and family in managing dietary and fluid restrictions.	
3. Encourage client to use stool softeners or mild laxatives as prescribed by physician.	Colonic distention can interfere with optimal inflow, outflow, and effective clearance.

EVALUATION PHASE

ANTICIPATED OUTCOMES	NURSING ACTIONS
1. Effective clearance of waste products	Monitor the client's weight daily. Weigh the client at the same time daily on the same scales and make sure that the client wears similar clothing each time. Monitor laboratory studies, including electrolytes and blood chemistries. Alter the dialysate concentration as ordered to control sodium retention. Monitor the client's blood pressure and intake and output.
2. Prevention of complications of peritoneal dialysis.	
a. Infection	Maintain sterile technique during dressing changes and during the procedure. Monitor the client's vital signs. Evaluate the quality of outflow. Cloudy outflow indicates infection.
b. Nutritional problems	Evaluate the client's ability to select nutritional foods within the dietary restrictions. Monitor sodium and fluid intake. Encourage small and more frequent feedings if the client is anorexic.
c. Inflow pain	Evaluate for possible causes of inflow pain (*e.g.,* improper catheter position, infection, constipation).

	Determine that the client can implement a bowel-management program.
d. Improper catheter position	Report any complaints of pressure in the bladder, epigastrium, or rectum. Pressure in the bladder indicates that the catheter should be withdrawn slightly; epigastric pressure indicates that the catheter is entangled in the omentum. When a peritoneal catheter is first inserted, pressure in the rectal area indicates that the catheter is properly positioned. If the rectal pain continues, the catheter may need to be withdrawn slightly.
e. Fluid retention	Monitor the client's abdominal girth measurements to detect fluid retention. Respiratory distress and abdominal discomfort are also signs of retention.
f. Abnormal appearance of outflow fluid	Monitor the color of the outflow and report it to the physician if indicated. Brown outflow indicates bowel perforation; amber, bladder perforation; cloudy, infection; and bloody, abdominal bleeding, if blood continues to appear after the first few exchanges.

Continuous ambulatory peritoneal dialysis

Objective
To perform peritoneal dialysis while affording the client minimal interruption of activities of daily living

PLANNING PHASE

EQUIPMENT

See previous section on Peritoneal Dialysis Using Gravity.
Belt and pouch for attachment to abdomen

CLIENT/FAMILY TEACHING
- See previous section on Peritoneal Dialysis Using Gravity.
- If the client will perform the procedure at home, teach the client and family members the technical aspects of CAPD. Supervise return demonstrations until the client and partner are able to perform CAPD unassisted. It is necessary to train a partner as well as the client in case the client experiences complications during CAPD.
- Teach the client and partner how to recognize complications of peritoneal dialysis and to maintain an intake and output record.
- Refer the client to a home-health agency for nursing follow-up care.
- If the client using CAPD is hospitalized, assist with the procedure according to the client's condition. Encourage input from the client about tried and proven techniques.

IMPLEMENTATION PHASE

NURSING ACTIONS	RATIONALE/AMPLIFICATION
1. Check new container of dialysate for correct concentration, leaks, or particles in solution.	The solution is used at room temperature unless the client cannot tolerate it. If warming is required, use heating pads, place the tubing in a warm bath during inflow, or warm the solution in a microwave oven. *Caution:* Check the temperature carefully if you are using a microwave oven.

2. Wash your hands. Remove empty solution bag from pouch that secures it to client's body.

3. Position client comfortably. Place empty container below level of client's abdomen. Unclamp tubing and begin outflow (Fig. 28–5). Monitor client's vital signs every 15 minutes.

Dialysate remains in the peritoneal cavity for 4 hours to 6 hours. During this time, the bag used for inflow is rolled up and secured to the client's abdomen.

Allow approximately 15 minutes to 20 minutes for outflow.

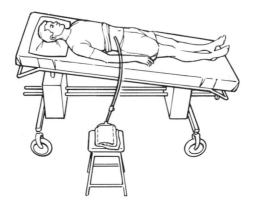

Fig. 28–5 Begin outflow by positioning dialysate container below level of client's abdomen and releasing clamp.

4. On completion of outflow, clamp tubing. Measure amount of outflow and record measurement on intake and output record or on dialysis flow sheet.

5. Remove tubing from outflow bag and spike new solution bag. Be careful not to contaminate ports.

6. Hang new solution bag and open clamp to begin inflow (Fig. 28–6).

Inspect the outflow solution for cloudiness or discoloration, which may indicate infection. Compare the amount of output with the amount of dialysate infused.

Allow 10 minutes to 20 minutes for inflow.

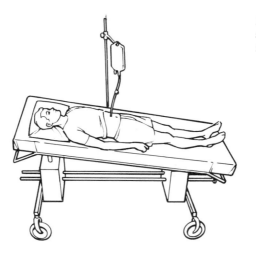

Fig. 28–6 Begin inflow phase by suspending dialysate container above level of client's abdomen and releasing clamp.

7. On completion of inflow phase, clamp tubing.

8. Fold empty bag so that entry port is folded toward inside. Secure bag to abdomen. Record amount of dialysate infused and client response to inflow phase.

Leave a small amount of fluid in the bag. This will prevent air from entering the system and will facilitate drainage.

RELATED NURSING CARE

NURSING ACTIONS	RATIONALE/AMPLIFICATION
Change inflow tubing every 24 hours. Change catheter dressing only when changing tubing set, unless it becomes soiled (see previous section on Peritoneal Dialysis Using Gravity).	

Continuous cycled peritoneal dialysis

Objective
To perform peritoneal dialysis more efficiently using automation
To provide freedom from the peritoneal dialysis procedure during the daytime

PLANNING PHASE

EQUIPMENT

See previous section on Peritoneal Dialysis Using Gravity.
Cycler

CLIENT/FAMILY TEACHING

• If the cycler will be used on an outpatient basis, instruct the client and a partner in the use of the machine. Familiarize the client and partner with the instruction manual that accompanies the cycler.
• A partner must be trained in addition to the client in case complications occur during nighttime dialysis. Continue the training sessions until both are comfortable with CCPD. Refer the client to a home-health agency for continued nursing consultation.
• If the client using CCPD is temporarily hospitalized, assist with CCPD as required. Allow the client to have maximal input into the procedure according to his condition. Encourage the client to give suggestions regarding proven techniques.

IMPLEMENTATION PHASE

NURSING ACTIONS	RATIONALE/AMPLIFICATION
1. Spike dialysate container with tubing. Prime tubing with dialysate and clamp tubing.	
2. Thread tubing through cycler.	Follow the specific instructions and precautions outlined in the manufacturer's instructions.
3. Connect primed tubing to peritoneal catheter using technique outlined in previous section on Peritoneal Dialysis Using Gravity.	
4. Connect remaining tubing to weigh bag, which is near base of machine.	
5. Set time controls for inflow, dwell, and outflow times.	Clamps open automatically according to preset times to allow for the exchange.
6. Activate cycler to begin exchange.	An alarm system will activate to alert the operator to inflow or outflow problems.
7. The final exchange is allowed to dwell during daytime. Record amount of inflow and number of exchanges on dialysis flow sheet.	
8. Remove bag and tubing from cycler and secure to client's abdomen in same manner as for CAPD.	

9. At end of day, thread tubing through cycler and allow for outflow. Record amount of outflow on dialysis flow sheet.

Observe the outflow solution for cloudiness or discoloration.

10. Secure new solution bags and initiate next exchange.

RELATED NURSING CARE   See previous section on Continuous Ambulatory Peritoneal Dialysis.

PRODUCT AVAILABILITY   TENCKHOFF PERITONEAL CATHETER
Cobe Laboratories

PERITONEAL CATHETER DRESSING TRAY
American Medical Products (Ampak tray)

DIALYSATE, TUBING, AND DIALYSIS PRODUCTS
Abbott Laboratories
American Medical Products
B–D Drake Willock
Cutter Laboratories
Gambro Inc.
Kormed Inc.
Lifemed
Medlon Inc.
Steward–Reiss Laboratories
Travenol Laboratories, Inc.
American Health Care Industries
American McGaw
Amicon Corporation

CYCLER
Travenol Laboratories, Inc.
Belmed, Inc.

SELECTED REFERENCES   County CM, Collins AJ: Dialysis therapy in the management of chronic renal failure. Med Clin North Am 68(2):399–421, March 1984
Denniston DJ, Burns KT: Home peritoneal dialysis, Am J Nurs 80(11):2022–2026, November 1980

Nursing Photobook Series. Implementing urologic procedures, pp 134–143. Springhouse, PA, Intermed Communications, Inc., 1981

29

Continuous bladder irrigation (Murphy drip)

BACKGROUND

Enlargement of the prostate gland caused by benign prostatic hypertrophy or cancer of the prostate compresses the urethra, narrowing the lumen and interfering with urine flow. Changes in urination patterns result. Narrowing of the urethra may be compensated for by a more forceful contraction of bladder muscles to achieve complete emptying. The muscle fibers form bands (trabeculae). The bladder wall may thin and slip between the trabeculate, forming pouches or diverticula. Incomplete bladder emptying allows urine to collect in the diverticula, become stagnant, and cause urinary tract infections. Frequently, gram-negative bacteria are implicated in these urinary tract infections.

Prostatectomy can be performed by an incision (suprapubic, perineal, or retropubic) or by a closed-technique, transurethral resection (TUR), in which tissue is removed with special instruments that are inserted into the bladder through a cystoscope. Continuous bladder irrigation (Murphy drip) is used to control hemorrhage after prostatectomy.

Objective

To provide continuous closed irrigation of the bladder, decreasing the probability of clot formation resulting in hemorrhage

To maintain patency of the catheter and to decrease the possibility of bladder distention and trauma

ASSESSMENT PHASE

- What type of anesthesia was used during surgery? Did the client have spinal or general anesthesia?
- What surgical technique was used (*i.e.,* open incision or TUR)?
- Is a triple-lumen bladder (Foley) catheter in place? The triple lumen is necessary to initiate continuous irrigation (Fig. 29–1).
- What is the color and consistency of the urine postoperatively? Immediately postoperatively the urine should be pink or light red.

PRECAUTION

- **Prevent hypothermia by avoiding the use of cool irrigating solutions.**

PLANNING PHASE

EQUIPMENT

Irrigating solution containers—2
Tandem irrigating tubing set
Urinary drainage bag
Large measuring container
IV pole
Asepto syringe catheter irrigation set or sterile bowl and Toomey syringe
Flask of sterile water
Iodophor solution
Sterile 4 × 4s
Sterile gloves
2.5-cm tape (1-inch)

Fig. 29–1 Three-way Foley catheter.

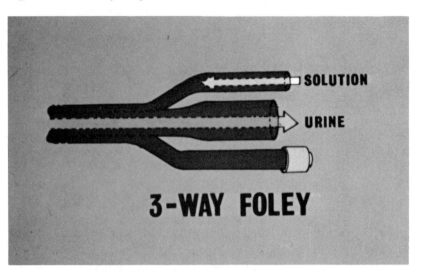

CLIENT/FAMILY TEACHING
- Tell the client that a catheter will remain in the bladder after surgery to drain and irrigate the bladder to control postoperative bleeding. The client should expect some discomfort from the catheter, although it should not be painful.
- Describe symptoms that should be reported to the nurse (*e.g.*, fullness, pressure, or bladder spasms).
- Tell the client and family that the urine will be blood stained after surgery.
- Teach the client that urgency and bladder irritation may be experienced postoperatively and will subside as healing continues. Dribbling of urine may be a temporary problem that will be alleviated as the client regains sphincter control.

IMPLEMENTATION PHASE

NURSING ACTIONS	RATIONALE/AMPLIFICATION
1. Inspect containers of irrigation solution for particles and clarity of solution.	The presence of particulate matter or cloudiness can indicate contaminated solution.
2. Remove tandem tubing from box and close clamps. Spike solution bags and open clamp above drip chamber to fill drip chamber.	
3. Open drip-rate control clamp to prime remainder of tubing.	
4. Connect urinary drainage bag to outflow lumen of triple-lumen catheter.	Have a large container available for frequent emptying and measuring of irrigant and urinary drainage. If existing drainage tubing must be removed to connect the urinary drainage bag, use sterile gloves to prevent contamination.
5. Pour iodophor solution into sterile basin. Wearing sterile gloves, saturate sterile 4×4 with solution. Cleanse solution port of catheter with iodophor.	
6. Connect primed tubing securely to inflow lumen (Fig. 29–2).	
7. Open drip control clamp to desired rate.	Titrate the drip rate according to the color and consistency of the urine. If increased bleeding is observed, increase the drip rate.

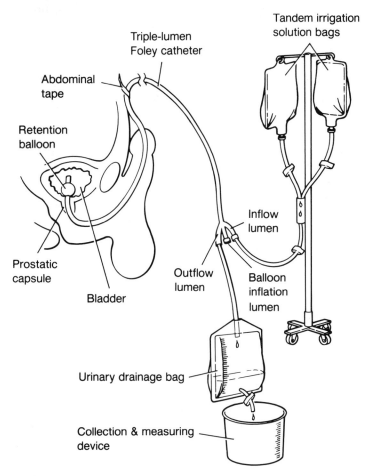

Fig. 29-2 Continuous bladder irrigation (Murphy drip).

8. Record amounts of irrigant and volume returned on intake and output record.	To determine the urinary output, subtract the volume of irrigant from the total volume returned.

RELATED NURSING CARE

NURSING ACTIONS	RATIONALE/AMPLIFICATION
1. Irrigate bladder manually using asepto or Toomey syringe to maintain patency of catheter if continuous irrigation does not control clotting and hemorrhage.	
a. Fill sterile container in irrigation set with sterile water.	
b. Clamp continuous irrigation infusion tubing.	
c. Put on sterile gloves.	
d. Draw 50 ml of sterile water into syringe.	
e. Disconnect tubing from inflow lumen and inject sterile water into bladder.	Do not contaminate the tubing and catheter connections.
f. Withdraw approximately 40 ml of fluid from bladder.	Leave a small amount of solution in the bladder to prevent the bladder wall from being sucked into the catheter, causing trauma.

g.   When catheter is patent, reconnect continuous irrigation tubing. Resume continuous irrigation.

Document catheter patency and resumption of continuous irrigation in the nurses' notes and notify the surgeon if bleeding is not controlled or if the catheter does not remain patent.

2.   If necessary, apply traction to bladder catheter to control bleeding by taping catheter to abdomen.

Apply traction cautiously and for short periods because of the potential for ischemia of bladder tissue.

3.   Keep accurate intake and output record.

Note the amounts of irrigant used on the intake and output record, including continuous and hand irrigation.

4.   To discontinue continuous irrigation, clamp solution port of triple-lumen catheter. Disconnect irrigation tubing. Drain catheter into regular urinary drainage bag.

Cover the port to protect it from contamination.

5.   Change incisional dressings as necessary using sterile technique.

If prostatectomy was performed using a surgical incision, incisional drains for urinary drainage will cause the dressing to become wet, causing client discomfort and a potential source of infection.

6.   Control postoperative pain with analgesics/passive exercises as necessary.

The client may experience back/leg pain because of the stretch on muscles that is caused by the use of the lithotomy position during surgery.

EVALUATION PHASE

ANTICIPATED OUTCOMES	NURSING ACTIONS
1. Prevention of complications of prostatectomy	
a. Hemorrhage	Monitor urinary output for blood postoperatively. Urine should be pink to light red during the immediate postoperative period. Hand irrigate the system using an asepto syringe if any of the following occur: clots, dark red urine, unusually viscous red urine, or client complaint of pressure. Apply traction as necessary for short periods. Evaluate hematocrit and hemoglobin results. Decreases result from postoperative bleeding and hemolysis caused by irrigating the bladder with hypotonic solutions.
b. Circulatory overload/electrolyte imbalance caused by use of hypotonic bladder irrigation	Monitor the client's vital signs and respiratory and cardiac systems for the following signs of circulatory overload: mental confusion, rales, shortness of breath, increased pulse rate, or elevated central venous pressures. Monitor for the following symptoms of electrolyte imbalances: hyperkalemia and dilutional hyponatremia.
c. Infection	Monitor for gram-negative septicemia/shock. Gram-negative bacteria implicated in preoperative urinary tract infections gain access to the bloodstream through prostatic veins that are exposed during surgery.

PRODUCT AVAILABILITY   URINARY IRRIGATION KITS

American McGaw
American Pharmaseal
Bard Inc.
Cutter Laboratories
Davol Inc.
Kendall Co.

Travenol Laboratories, Inc.
Welcon Inc.

URINARY IRRIGATION CATHETERS

Akron Catheter
Bard Inc.
Kendall Co.
Sherwood Medical Co.

IRRIGATING SOLUTIONS AND TUBING

Cutter Laboratories
Davol Inc.
Travenol Laboratories, Inc.

SELECTED REFERENCES
Lerner J, Karn Z: Manual of Urologic Nursing, pp 449–490. St. Louis, CV Mosby, 1982

VII

Integumentary techniques

30

Stoma and draining wound techniques

The client who has a stoma or draining wound can present challenges to nursing staff that can be overcome if proper supplies and appropriate techniques are used.

Before the development of odor-proof plastics and hypoallergenic adhesives, a stoma or draining wound was a handicap that made the client a social outcast. Often, the person had a distinctive odor, output leakage, and problems resulting from skin breakdown. As a result of improved products, the person with a stoma or chronic draining wound can lead a full and productive life. The nurse and client now have the advantage of a wide array of excellent products from which to choose. The quality of life for this group has also been enhanced by the growing nursing specialty of enterostomal therapy (ET). The ET nurse has been instrumental in improving client/family teaching and rehabilitation. The United Ostomy Association has many resources, including trained ostomy visitors who can provide immeasurable support and encouragement to the client and family (see list of resources for ostomy clients).

RESOURCES FOR OSTOMY CLIENTS

American Cancer Society, Inc.
National Headquarters
777 Third Avenue
New York, NY 10017
(212) 371-2900

International Association for Enterostomal Therapy
5000 Birch St., Suite 400
Newport Beach, CA 92660
(714) 476-0269

National Foundation for Ileitis and Colitis, Inc.
295 Madison Ave.   or   Western Region Office
New York, NY 10017   12012 Wilshire Blvd., #201
(212) 685-3440   Los Angeles, CA 90025
                                                          (213) 826-8811

United Ostomy Association
2001 W. Beverly Boulevard
Los Angeles, CA 90057
(213) 413-5510

Although the disease that resulted in the ostomy surgery may limit a client's activity, the ostomy itself need not be a handicap. Clients can be successful at all sorts of activities, such as sports, pregnancy, and all types of recreation and occupations. Occasionally, contact sports such as football are contraindicated, even though many persons with an ostomy have played without incident. The surgeon will advise the person according to individual circumstances.

In choosing the supplies and techniques to be used, thoroughly assess the client. History taking is an integral part of assessment. Pathophysiologic conditions as well as

411

psychosocial conditions play an important role in the adjustment and rehabilitation of the client. There are many diseases as well as birth defects and trauma that result in stomas and draining wounds. Improper site selection often results in additional surgery to achieve proper pouch adherence (Fig. 30–1).

Sterile technique is not usually necessary in stoma care or for most draining wounds. If sterile technique is indicated, carefully check each product's label for sterility, because most products in the ostomy line are considered to be clean rather than sterile.

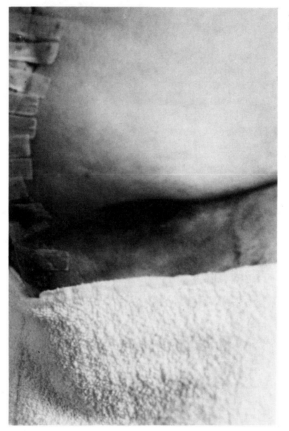

Fig. 30–1 Improper stoma site selection makes effective pouching impossible.

Recognize that even though pouching techniques for all types of procedures have similarities, the colostomy, ileostomy, urostomy, and draining wound must be dealt with as separate entities, each having unique differences.

COLOSTOMY

Depending on the portion of the bowel involved and the reason for surgery, there are several types of colostomies (Fig. 30–2). The colostomy may be in the ascending, transverse, sigmoid, or descending colon. It may be a loop, double-barrel, end, permanent, or temporary colostomy, depending on the circumstances and surgical procedure. The term *mucous fistula* is often used for the distal (nonfunctioning) stoma in a double-barrel colostomy.

There are a few important points to consider when working with the client who has a colostomy.

• All colostomies are not the same. Left-side and right-side colostomies are managed differently because of the characteristics of the fecal output.
• The left-side colostomy can often be controlled by the use of colostomy irrigation.
• Colostomy irrigation should be considered as only one method of care from which the client may choose.
• Right-side colostomies require a pouch at all times.

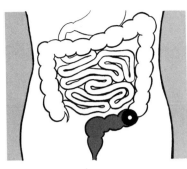

Sigmoid Colostomy

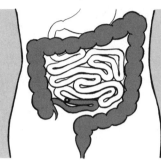

Descending Colostomy

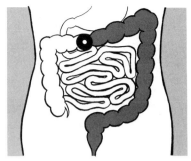

Transverse (Single B) Colostomy

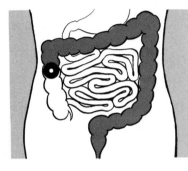

Ascending Colostomy

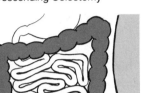

Ileostomy

Fig. 30-2 Location of various colostomies and an ileostomy. (After Types of Ostomies. Copyright © 1979. Hollister Incorporated. All rights reserved.)

- If a right-side colostomy must be irrigated to clean out for a procedure, use a lesser amount of irrigation water.

ILEOSTOMY

There are several conditions that result in ileostomy (see Fig. 30–2). The most common cause is inflammatory bowel disease (IBD). Other indications for ileostomy include familial polyposis, toxic megacolon, bowel necrosis, and birth defects.

UROSTOMY

The techniques used in urostomy stoma care are based on the same principles as the management of fecal stomas and draining wounds, with some differences unique to urostomy technique and supplies. The urostomy pouch selected should have an anti-reflux valve to decrease backflow into the pouch when the client is supine and an outlet-closure valve to allow connection to bedside drainage (Fig. 30–3). Because the

Fig. 30-3 Urostomy pouch may be connected to bedside drainage.

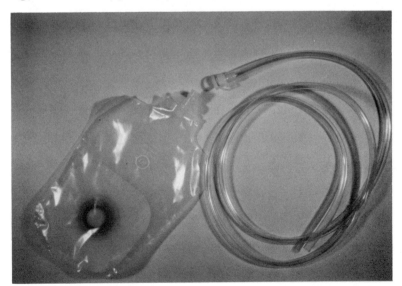

removed bladder was the first line of defense, the client with a urostomy must pay particular attention to signs of kidney infection. The stoma will not exhibit symptoms such as burning or painful urination as did the bladder. Keep in mind that mucus in the urine of a urostomy client is normal because the bowel segment used to construct the stoma is a mucus-secreting tissue.

Urine will flow from the urostomy at a rate in proportion to intake. If intravenous (IV) infusions are dripping at a rapid rate, urine output will be fairly constant, making it difficult to keep the client's skin dry while applying the pouch. The ideal time to change a urostomy pouch is when the client has had no intake (either IV or oral) for 2 hours to 8 hours. In the hospital setting, this is usually not practical. After discharge from the hospital, the best time for routine pouch change is right after the client awakens, before having anything to eat or drink. Use of a wick made of tissue or 4 × 4s will be helpful, although the wick must not be inserted into the stoma. Urine will be absorbed by the wick when it is held next to the stoma. This will keep urine from running onto the skin.

Stents are thin plastic tubes inserted during surgery that exit from each ureter through the conduit and stoma. Stents allow urine flow in spite of swelling at the ureteroileal anastomosis. They usually remain in place for 6 days to 10 days. It is not unusual for the stent to "wash out" into the pouch after swelling subsides. Although this is not usually cause for alarm, the surgeon should be notified.

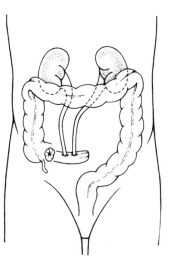

Fig. 30-4 Ileal conduit. (Brunner LS, Suddarth DS: Textbook of Medical–Surgical Nursing, 5th ed. Philadelphia, JB Lippincott, 1984)

The ileal conduit is a frequently used form of urinary diversion (Fig. 30-4). A segment of ileum is resected from the small bowel, leaving the blood supply from the mesentery intact. The bowel is reconnected and bowel function is unchanged. The proximal end of the bowel segment is sutured closed. The distal end is brought out, and a stoma is formed on the abdomen. The ureters are then implanted into the bowel segment, and urine passes from the kidneys, through the ureters, into the bowel segment (conduit), and from the stoma into the pouch.

General pouch application

Objectives
To provide an effective pouching system to contain output from an ostomy or draining wound

To preserve the integrity of the skin surrounding the stoma

To decrease the contamination of surrounding wounds by a draining wound

To keep the client odor free

ASSESSMENT PHASE

- What type of opening is present (*e.g.,* colostomy, ileostomy, urostomy [urinary diversion], draining wound [fistula, Penrose drain, gaping wound])? Wht modifications will be necessary for this client (Fig. 30–5)?
- Are there tubes, retention sutures, fat folds, skin valleys, or other obstacles to effective pouching (Fig. 30–6)?
- Does the client have a history of skin allergies that might necessitate patch testing of products to be used (Fig. 30–7)?
- Will the output be formed, liquid, or watery; high volume or low volume; mild or excoriating to the surrounding skin?

Fig. 30–5 Multiple and creative techniques may be required. (*A*) Salem-Sump tube draining intra-abdominal abscess. (*B*) Fecal fistula with Hollister Post-Op pouch. (*C*) Draining fistula with United Urostomy pouch, which can be conveniently connected to bedside drainage. (*D*) Small bowel fistula with Bongart Pediatric pouch to protect skin from excoriation.

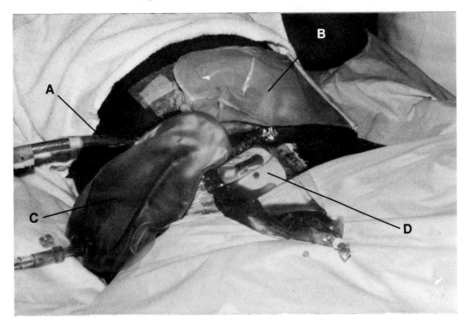

- Is it necessary to wear gloves to change the pouch? Routine use of gloves is unnecessary and conveys a negative attitude to the client. If a disease (such as hepatitis) is present, wear gloves.
- If the client has an ileostomy, consider the following:

  Is the nutritional level adequate for the wound to heal and for the client to gain strength?

  Has the client been receiving steroid therapy? A side-effect of steroid therapy is delayed healing.

  Does the client show signs of dehydration or electrolyte depletion because of ileostomy output and content?

  Are there any symptoms of folic acid or vitamin B_{12} malabsorption, especially if the terminal ileum has been resected?

  Does the client have enough bowel for the absorption of nutrients or is short-gut syndrome present?

- If the client has an urostomy, consider the following:

  Is there an abnormal amount of blood in the urine or is the urine pink tinged? Pink-tinged urine is expected 24 hours to 48 hours postoperatively.

  Is the hourly urine volume adequate for the intake?

  Are there stents in place to assist urine flow?

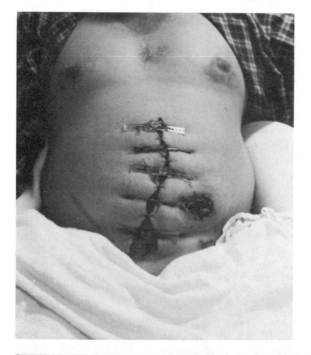

Fig. 30-6 Obstacles to effective pouch-ing.

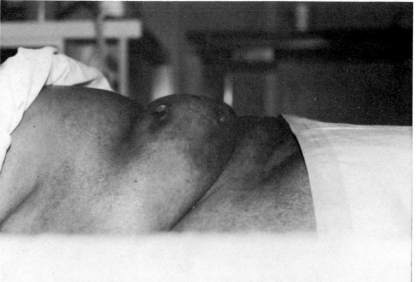

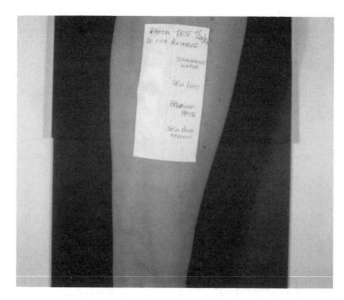

Fig. 30-7 Patch testing for product sensitivity.

PRECAUTIONS

- **Assess stoma color for adequate blood supply.**
- **The pouch and skin barrier opening must be slightly larger than the stoma to avoid pressure on the stoma.**
- **Nonverbal communication can convey negative attitudes to the client, making rehabilitation difficult.**
- **If the client has an ileostomy, strict adherence to a skin care regimen and a properly fitting appliance are mandatory to prevent rapid skin breakdown from digestive enzymes that are present in the output. Observe for symptoms of dehydration, sodium depletion, or blockage from a food bolus.**
- **If the client has a urostomy, do not take urine specimens from the pouch for any test.**

PLANNING PHASE

EQUIPMENT

Washcloth
Sterile 4 × 4s (if sterile technique is indicated)
Warmed sterile water or saline (if sterile technique is indicated)
Open-ended, drainable pouch*
Pouch clamp
Pectin-based skin barrier (if indicated; some brands of pouches include skin barrier)
Pectin-based paste (or karaya paste if pectin-based is not available)
2.5-cm (1-inch) microporus or waterproof tape
Scissors

CLIENT/FAMILY TEACHING

- Discuss the purpose of the proper pouching technique and supplies.
- Describe what will be felt and seen *before* the client and family observe the stoma or wound.
    The normal color of stoma tissue is red. It bleeds easily because of the rich blood supply.
    There will be sutures present.
    The stoma is swollen right after surgery but will become smaller after a few weeks.
    The stoma will always remain moist and slippery because it is normal for bowel tissue to secrete mucus.
    There will be discomfort where the skin has been excised, but the stoma will have no feeling, and even though it is red, it will not be tender.
- Encourage verbal communication of feelings, fears, and impressions, recognizing that negative statements and fears are a natural part of the path to acceptance. Once voiced, many fears begin to diminish.
- Encourage open communication and nonjudgmental attitudes from staff and family.
If the client has an ileostomy,
- Discuss the importance of compliance with steroid therapy (both maintenance and weaning).
- Explain the role of digestive enzymes in the output and the result of skin digestion (breakdown) if contact is allowed.
- Discuss the role of fluid and electrolyte balance. Explain the symptoms of dehydration, sodium depletion, and vitamin deficiencies.
- Inform the client that kidney stones are not uncommon because of chronic dehydration. Stress adequate fluid intake.
- Discuss dietary considerations to prevent food-bolus blockage. Foods that are difficult to digest (high-fiber foods) must be taken only in small amounts, chewed thoroughly, and accompanied by increased oral intake. These foods include mushrooms, nuts, coconut, peelings, foods with seeds (*e.g.,* tomatoes, strawberries, corn, popcorn, cabbage, Chinese food, and other similar foods.
- Inform the client that if a food-blous blockage occurs, an emergency situation exists and must be dealt with promptly. Relaxation techniques such as abdominal mas-

---

* If a brand with precut opening is being used, choose the side with an opening that is 3 mm to 6 mm (⅛ inch to ¼ inch) larger than the stoma.

sage, a warm bath, or the knee-chest position might allow the bolus to pass. If not, medical attention is mandatory, especially if vomiting or other signs of bowel obstruction are present.

- Stress prevention of skin breakdown, food-bolus blockage, dehydration, and sodium depletion. These are the most common problems in this group, yet they are ones that the client will ultimately control.

If the client has a urostomy,

- Stress the importance of preventing kidney infection by increasing oral intake of liquids and using proper pouch hygiene. The client must seek prompt medical attention if a kidney infection is suspected.

- Explain that the pouch contains urine that is inappropriate for *any* urine specimen. Routine urinalysis, samples for Clinitest and Acetest, and samples for culture and sensitivity can be collected only after the pouch has been removed and the area cleansed.

IMPLEMENTATION PHASE

NURSING ACTIONS	RATIONALE/AMPLIFICATION
1. Place client comfortably in lying or sitting position as condition allows. If abdominal perineal resection has been performed, do not sit client on toilet seat or inflatable ring — use pillow or foam pad.	Allow client to relax and watch the procedure when possible. Adequate visualization of the area to be pouched is important. Rings cause increased strain on the perineal suture line because of the spreading action of the buttocks when sitting.
2. Do not remove pouch presently in place until all supplies are at bedside and ready for use.	Because there is no spincter present, discharge or output cannot be controlled.
3. Open all packages. Remove paper or plastic protector from pouch.	
4. Gently remove pouch presently in place. Rather than pulling it away from client's skin, lift one corner and apply counterpressure to remove pouch (Fig. 30-8).	Counterpressure causes less discomfort/pain to the abdominal incision or stoma incision.

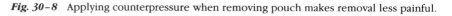

Fig. 30-8 Applying counterpressure when removing pouch makes removal less painful.

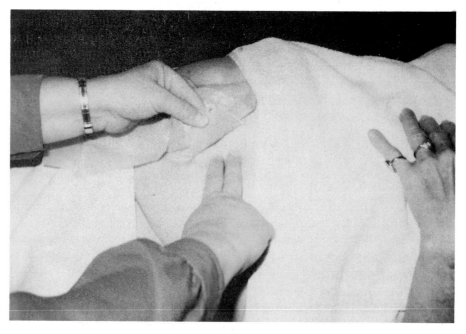

Fig. 30-9 Loop ostomy rod.

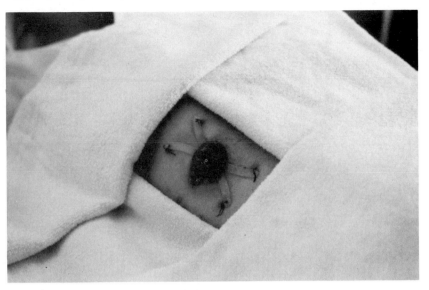

5. Remove present pouch and all products used as one unit, gently and with one motion. If client has undergone loop ostomy, locate rod and hold it in place while pouch is being removed (Fig. 30-9).

Unnecessary discomfort results if each product is removed one at a time. The loop rod is holding the bowel in place and must not be dislodged. (The rod is usually removed 7 days to 10 days postoperatively.)

6. Gently cleanse peristomal area and stoma with *warm* water and clean washcloth. If sterile technique is indicated, use 4 × 4 and *warmed* sterile water or saline. Remove all adhesive and pastes that remove easily.

Soap may be irritating to the skin.

If some of the products are not easy to remove completely, simply cleanse and leave the remainder in place rather than rubbing hard on the client's skin. Skin damage must be avoided to maintain a good seal.

7. If a pectin-based skin barrier is used, cut opening in barrier to fit shape of stoma or opening with approximately 2-mm (⅛-inch) clearance (Fig. 30-10).

The goal is to cover all of the skin adjacent to the stoma or opening to prevent skin breakdown caused by contact with the output. For an irregularly shaped stoma or

Fig. 30-10 Skin barrier cut to fit stoma.

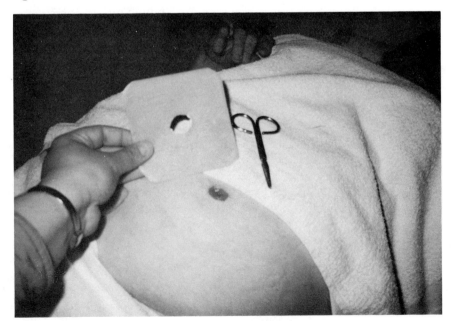

Fig. 30-11 Apply skin barrier over ring of paste.

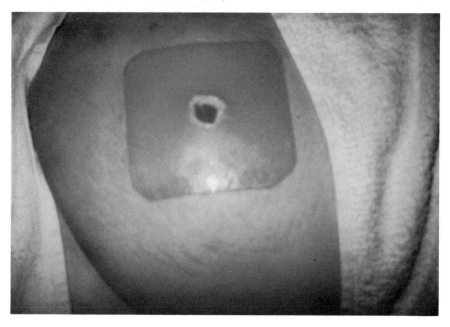

8. Apply paste in ringlike fashion around stoma or opening at junction where skin and stoma or opening meet. Do not spread paste on skin; leave it in ringlike form.

9. Remove release paper from skin side of skin barrier and apply to skin (Fig. 30-11).

10. Apply pouch with end pointing toward client's side if client is bedridden or toward client's feet if ambulatory (Fig. 30-12).

opening, first make a pattern and use it to obtain a better fit without the risk of wasting a skin barrier because of improper cutting.

When the skin barrier and pouch are applied, the paste acts as a filler that prevents output from seeping underneath the system.

Apply gentle pressure over the entire barrier to seal the barrier to the skin. Some brands of skin barriers have release paper on the pouch side of the barrier, which must be removed.

It is easier to empty the pouch into a bedpan or basin when it is pointed toward the side. If the client is able to sit to empty the pouch, it is more convenient if the pouch points downward.

Fig. 30-12 Pouch can be pointed at feet or toward side for convenience.

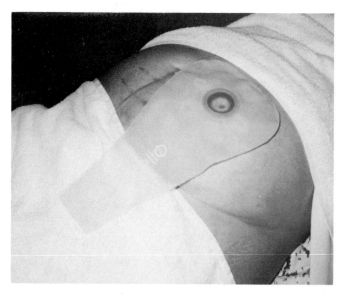
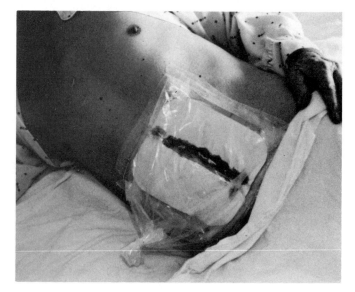

11. Apply pouch clamp according to package directions. Clamp will be used for several pouch changes and *must* be saved.

Each company manufactures clamps that are applied differently. If they are not applied properly, malfunction can occur.

12. Empty pouch of flatus and output as needed to prevent overexpansion.

Overexpansion will result in breaking of the seal and consequent leakage. To maintain the odor-proof quality of the pouch, always remove the clamp to empty the pouch rather than break the seal or use a pinprick to remove flatus.

13. If client has stoma, pour warm water into pouch opening to rinse inside of pouch if appropriate (Fig. 30–13).

Reflux of water into the stoma is unlikely and would not be harmful if it occurred. Reflux of water into a wound cavity could result in infection. If the client has a draining wound, do not rinse the pouch unless requested by the physician.

Fig. 30–13 Pouch can be rinsed without removal from body.

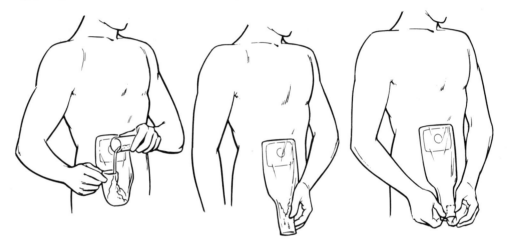

14. Remove odorous or soiled trash and linen from room after procedure is finished.

Odor control is extremely important to reduce client anxiety and fear.

15. Document the following on medical record:

    a. Stoma condition (*e.g.,* pink, red, pale, cyanotic, necrotic, moist)

The stoma is a mucous membrane with rich capillary blood supply. Report poor circulation to the stoma to the surgeon.

    b. Condition of peristomal skin (*e.g.,* clear, rash, irritated, excoriated)

    c. Description of output (*e.g.,* formed, liquid, or watery; color; odor; volume)

If output is liquid, record the amount on the intake and output record. Observe for signs of fluid and electrolyte imbalance.

    d. Client/family response and degree of involvement in objective terms

Care-givers must remember to be objective and non-judgmental in actions as well as in documentation.

RELATED NURSING CARE

NURSING ACTIONS	RATIONALE/AMPLIFICATION
1. Change pouch approximately every other day (during the first week after surgery, or immediately if leakage occurs. After first week, change pouch two times to three times per week.	Close observation of stoma color and the condition of peristomal skin is necessary in the early postoperative period. Change the pouch more frequently until the client is discharged so that adequate teaching can be given. After discharge, the pouch can be changed once or twice per week.

2. When client is free of IV infusions in upper extremities and of nasogastric tube, encourage client to begin doing increasing amounts of stoma care.

The client or a family member should be able to do stoma care by the time of discharge from the hospital.

3. Begin discharge planning early in hospitalization.

Assess the need for visiting nurses on discharge. Suggest a supplier of ostomy products for the client to use after discharge.

4. Teach stoma dilatation if ordered by physician.

Stoma dilatation is a controversial procedure. Stoma stenosis may cause symptoms of obstruction, and surgical revision may be necessary.

5. Do not use tincture of benzoin because of high incidence of skin irritation.

Tincture of benzoin causes stripping of the epidermis when the pouch is removed. Plasticized dressings made for skin preparation before pouching spare the epidermis and have a low incidence of skin irritation.

6. If allergic reactions to particular product occur, switch to different brand. This usually resolves problem.

7. Do not leave the pouch off to "air dry" irritated skin.

This usually makes skin irriation worse because of contact with output. Keeping the skin covered with an appliance that fits properly will allow healing because the skin is clean, dry, and protected from caustic output.

8. Do not use aspirin as deodorizer in pouch.

Aspirin can cause ulceration of the stoma. The pouch will remain odor proof if proper technique is used. Pouch deodorants that are safe and effective are available.

EVALUATION PHASE

ANTICIPATED OUTCOMES	NURSING ACTIONS
1. Prevention of odor and output leakage	Change leaking pouches immediately. Keep the pouch empty.
2. Prevention of skin breakdown	Evaluate for proper pouching techniques.
3. Prevention of contamination of surgical incisions by draining wounds	Evaluate for proper pouching techniques.

PRODUCT AVAILABILITY   FULL LINE OF OSTOMY PRODUCTS

Bard Home Health Division
P.O. Box 18
Berkeley Heights, NJ 07922

Coloplast, Inc.
6206 Benjamin Road
Tampa, FL 33614

ConvaTec, A Division of E.R. Squibb and Sons, Inc.
P.O. Box 4000
Princeton, NJ 08540

Dansac, Inc.
2920 Wolff St.
Racine, WI 53404

Hollister, Inc.
211 East Chicago Ave.
Chicago, IL 60611

Marlen Manufacturing and Development Co.
5150 Richmond Road
Bedford, OH 44146

Nu-Hope Laboratories, Inc.
2900 Rowena Ave.
Los Angeles, CA 90039

Vance Products, Inc.
Box 227
Spencer, IN 47460-0227

UNITED, Division of Howmedica, Inc.
P.O. Box 1970
Largo, FL 33540-0149

SELECTED REFERENCES

Broadwell DC, Jackson BS: Principles of Ostomy Care. St. Louis, CV Mosby, 1982

von Eschenbach AC, Rodriquez DB: Sexual Rehabilitation of the Urologic Cancer Patient. Boston, GK Hall Medical Publishers, 1981

Hill GL: Ileostomy: Surgery, Physiology and Management. New York, Grune & Stratton, 1976

Jeter KF: These Special Children. Palo Alto, CA, Bull Publishing Co., 1982

Shipes EA, Lehr ST: Sexual Counseling for Ostomates, Springfield, IL, Charles C. Thomas, 1980

31   *Thermal trauma techniques*

BACKGROUND

Thermal trauma encompasses injuries received from heat agents (flame, steam, electricity, caustic chemicals) or cold agents (frostbite, gases under pressure). Thermal trauma directly affects skin integrity and indirectly affects almost all other major body organ systems. Approximately 2 million persons suffer some form of thermal trauma each year in the United States. Of these, approximately 250,000 persons will require hospitalization, and approximately 12,000 persons will die from thermal trauma.

ASSESSMENT OF THERMAL INJURIES

In assessing the thermally injured person, obtain a history of the accident. This will provide information about the type of thermal agent, potential respiratory injury (caused by prolonged exposure to a smoky environment), and associated trauma (fractures, head and spine injuries, internal injuries).

CLASSIFICATION OF THERMAL INJURIES

Thermal injuries are classified according to the extent and depth of the injury. The extent of injury is based on the percentage of the total body surface area (TBSA) involved and is calculated by the Rule of Nines (Fig. 31–1) or by the Lund and Browder with Berkow formula chart (see example of chart on p. 425).

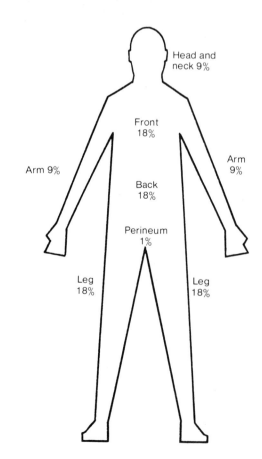

Head and neck 9%

Front 18%

Arm 9%

Arm 9%

Back 18%

Perineum 1%

Leg 18%

Leg 18%

Fig. 31–1   Rule of Nines for calculating total body surface area of thermal injury. (Brunner LS, Suddarth DS: Textbook of Medical–Surgical Nursing, 5th ed. Philadelphia, JB Lippincott, 1984)

The depth of injury is classified as superficial injury (first degree), partial-thickness injury (second degree), and full-thickness injury (third degree).

Superficial injury involves only the epidermis and is characterized by a dry, erythematous color that easily blanches on pressure. Pain is generally present because of irritated sensory nerve endings. Healing occurs in 10 days to 14 days, generally with little or no scarring.

Partial-thickness injury involves part of the dermis and is characterized by a moist, light pink to salmon color, blister formation (if epidermis is intact), and excruciating pain because of exposed nerve endings. Healing occurs within 14 days to 21 days, or longer if infection occurs, with variable amounts of scarring.

Full-thickness injury involves all of the dermis and may include injury to the

Lund and Browder with Berkow formula chart for assessing extent of burns.

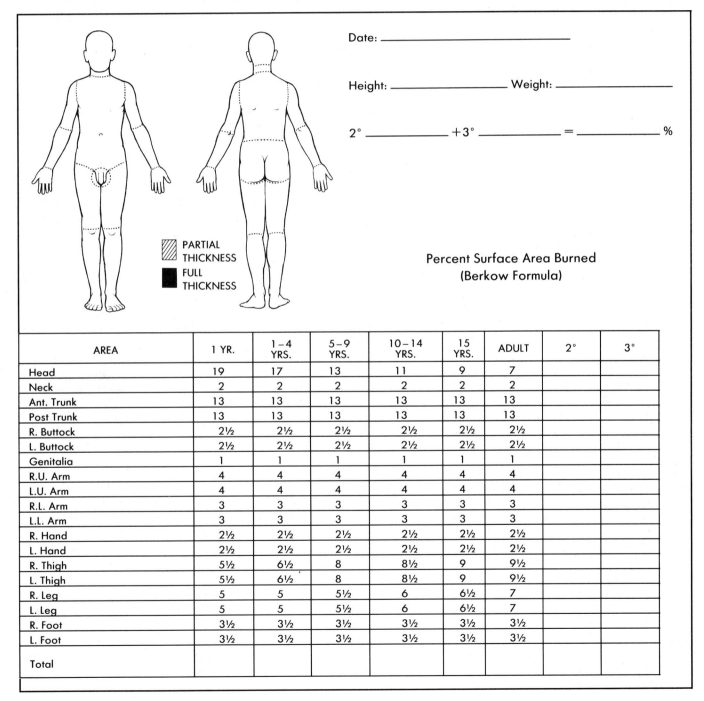

Date: _____

Height: _____ Weight: _____

2° _____ +3° _____ = _____ %

PARTIAL THICKNESS

FULL THICKNESS

Percent Surface Area Burned
(Berkow Formula)

AREA	1 YR.	1–4 YRS.	5–9 YRS.	10–14 YRS.	15 YRS.	ADULT	2°	3°
Head	19	17	13	11	9	7		
Neck	2	2	2	2	2	2		
Ant. Trunk	13	13	13	13	13	13		
Post Trunk	13	13	13	13	13	13		
R. Buttock	2½	2½	2½	2½	2½	2½		
L. Buttock	2½	2½	2½	2½	2½	2½		
Genitalia	1	1	1	1	1	1		
R.U. Arm	4	4	4	4	4	4		
L.U. Arm	4	4	4	4	4	4		
R.L. Arm	3	3	3	3	3	3		
L.L. Arm	3	3	3	3	3	3		
R. Hand	2½	2½	2½	2½	2½	2½		
L. Hand	2½	2½	2½	2½	2½	2½		
R. Thigh	5½	6½	8	8½	9	9½		
L. Thigh	5½	6½	8	8½	9	9½		
R. Leg	5	5	5½	6	6½	7		
L. Leg	5	5	5½	6	6½	7		
R. Foot	3½	3½	3½	3½	3½	3½		
L. Foot	3½	3½	3½	3½	3½	3½		
Total								

subcutaneous layer. The appearance of a full-thickness injury is dry, dull, leathery, and white, and black char deposits may be present. The full-thickness wound is anesthetic because sensory nerve endings are destroyed. Healing occurs only with surgical intervention (grafting) and often involves multiple surgical procedures.

TRIAGE FOR THERMAL INJURY

The American Burn Association classifies thermal injuries into the following three categories: minor, moderate, and major. Minor injury includes first-degree burns of less than 50% TBSA, second-degree burns of less than 15% TBSA, and third-degree burns of less than 2% TBSA. There is no associated trauma, preexisting diseases, or injuries to critical areas (*e.g.,* face, feet, hands, perineum). Minor injuries are easily treated on an outpatient basis.

Moderate injury includes first-degree burns of 50% to 75% TBSA, second-degree burns of 15% to 30% TBSA, and third-degree burns of 2% to 10% TBSA. There are no injuries to critical areas. Moderate injuries should be treated initially in a burn unit.

Major injury includes second-degree burns of more than 30% TBSA, third-degree burns of more than 10% TBSA, or burns that are complicated by extremes of age (<2 years and >45 years), respiratory injury, other associated major injury, preexisting diseases, or injuries to critical areas. Major injury receives optimal treatment in a burn center in which a multidisciplinary team approach to care is provided.

RESPIRATORY INJURY

Respiratory injury is classified into the following three categories: upper airway injury (nasopharynx–oropharynx to epiglottis), lower airway injury (below epiglottis), and carbon monoxide inhalation.

Upper airway injuries. Suspect upper airway injuries in persons with face and circumferential neck burns, singed nasal hairs, carbonaceous sputum, and dry, red oral mucosa. Laryngeal edema may cause mechanical airway obstruction and is characterized by increasing hoarseness and drooling of saliva. Early intubation is recommended to maintain airway patency (see Chap. 19, "Airway Management").

Lower airway injuries. Lower airway injuries, although they may result from inhalation of steam, more commonly occur as a result of inhalation of smoke. This results in a chemical pneumonitis of the tracheobronchial tree. Suspect injury to the lower airways in clients with carbonaceous sputum; wheezing cough; deteriorating arterial blood gases (ABGs), which reflect a worsening hypoxia; crackles (rales, rhonchi); and the presence of infiltrates, which may not be evident initially, on chest film.

Management of lower airway injury includes the administration of humidified oxygen, bronchodilators, and vigorous pulmonary toilet, which involves frequent tracheal suctioning or bronchoscopy to clear the debris from the bronchial tree (see Chap. 19, "Airway Management"). Steroids may also be used to decrease the inflammatory response. The complications of lower airway injury are pneumonia and adult respiratory distress syndrome (ARDS).

Carbon monoxide poisoning. Suspect carbon monoxide inhalation when the person has been exposed to a smoky environment for a prolonged period. Often, thermal skin injury is absent, but a significant amount of carbon monoxide, a by-product of combustion, may have been inhaled. Hypoxia results because carbon monoxide has an affinity for hemoglobin that is 20 times greater than that of oxygen. Significant carbon monoxide poisoning can be determined on the basis of the history of the accident; behavioral changes such as mental confusion, restlessness, or aggression; deteriorating blood oxygen levels; laboratory analysis for carboxyhemoglobin greater than 10%; and a cherry red skin color, which may not be visible because of black char deposits. The treatment involves early recognition and prompt administration of 100% oxygen.

EFFECTS OF THERMAL INJURY ON MAJOR BODY ORGAN SYSTEMS

In addition to cardiovascular changes caused by burn shock and respiratory complications caused by thermal injury to the respiratory tract, other major body organ systems are affected by thermal trauma. Assess the gastrointestinal (GI) system for paralytic ileus, hemorrhagic gastritis, and stress ulcer (Curling's ulcer). Evaluate the hematologic system for anemia. The client can lose as much as 15% of the circulating red blood cell mass because of exposure to direct heat (flame, scald, gases under pressure) at the time of injury. This can result in an anemia that is difficult to manage because the systemic bone marrow depression that results reduces the hematopoietic capabilities of the body. Additionally, the client with a major injury becomes immunosuppressed because of the overwhelming stress of the trauma, which results in bone marrow depression and consequent anemia and infection.

The metabolic demands of the client are greatly increased because of an increased secretion of catecholamines. The hypermetabolic state results in protein wasting and significant weight loss (20% or greater of preinjury weight). This gradually decreases as the wound is closed. Nutritional support is indicated in clients with a major thermal injury and is accomplished by enteral or parenteral routes (see Chap. 17, "Enteral Hyperalimentation," and Chap. 18, "Total Parenteral Nutrition").

FLUID RESUSCITATION OF BURN SHOCK

Burn shock is a major concern in persons who have sustained second- or third-degree burns of 20% TBSA or more. Immediately after thermal trauma, capillary permeability increases, resulting in a rapid loss of plasma into the burn wound. Additionally, there is an intravascular loss of sodium and water into normal muscle tissue that results in generalized edema formation. Burn shock is characterized by tachycardia, oliguria, paralytic ileus, and disorientation. Approximately 30% to 50% of the cardiac output (CO) can be decreased in the first hour after injury.

Fluid resuscitation of burn shock replaces body fluid volume during the acute phase of hypovolemia, until capillary integrity is restored approximately 24 hours after injury. Fluid resuscitation regimens are calculated to rapidly restore CO and include the crystalloid resuscitation formula (Baxter or Parkland formula), the Brooke formula, Moore's Burn Budget formula, Evans formula, and the hypertonic resuscitation formula (see Table 31-2).

WOUND MANAGEMENT

Wound-care objectives are directed toward early wound closure to decrease the possibility of wound sepsis. The thermal wound is initially cleansed and debrided. Wound coverings include topical antimicrobial therapy, biologic (physiologic) dressings, wet to dry soaks, and dry dressings. Hydrotherapy (once or twice daily) in conjunction with debridement of eschar (dead, burned skin) prepares the full-thickness wound for later grafting. Escharotomy may be required to release the tourniquetlike effect that eschar has on underlying tissues; that is, it results in arterial insufficiency.

INFECTION CONTROL

Infection is an ever-present problem in caring for clients with thermal trauma. The thermal wound generally does not become colonized with bacteria until 36 hours to 48 hours after the injury. Monitor the condition of the wound through burn-wound biopsies, which should be obtained three times per week. Burn-wound sepsis, which is defined as 10^5 organisms per gram of tissue, is promptly treated by systemic and subeschar antibiotic therapy. Prophylactic systemic antibiotic therapy, such as penicillin or cephalosporins, is initiated immediately after the injury to prevent colonization of the wound by gram-positive organisms.

Monitor environmental infection hazards to prevent cross-contamination between clients. Use reverse isolation techniques and meticulously clean the equipment and surroundings to decrease the risk of nosocomial infections.

Emergency burn care protocol

Objectives
To systematically assess and monitor the thermally injured client
To provide care in the immediate postburn period
To begin a fluid resuscitation protocol
To recognize the complications of thermal injury that are encountered in the immediate postburn period

ASSESSMENT PHASE

- Is the client experiencing airway, breathing, or circulation problems? Correct these problems immediately.
- Have baseline vital and neurologic signs been obtained? Baseline vital signs are important for evaluating fluid resuscitation in postinjury shock. Hypovolemia occurs rapidly. Changes in vital signs include tachycardia, tachypnea, and mental confusion. Blood pressure is generally normal, unless it is affected by associated injuries such as internal bleeding, and is not a reliable single indicator of post-thermal injury shock.
- Does the client have any associated injuries (*e.g.,* fractures, spinal cord trauma, internal bleeding)? Immobilize the spine before moving the client if spinal trauma is suspected.
- What are the circumstances surrounding the thermal injury? Determine the time of the accident, type of burning agent, environmental aspects (*e.g.,* enclosed space, explosions), associated falls, and loss of consciousness associated with the accident.
- What significant findings result from an evaluation of the past medical history? Is there a history of substance abuse, allergies, recent tetanus toxoid injection, or complicating chronic medical conditions, such as diabetes mellitus?
- What is the estimate of the percentage of TBSA burned? Use the Rule of Nines or the Lund and Browder with Berkow formula chart (see Fig. 31–1 and example of Lund and Browder chart). This is the first step in fluid resuscitation of thermal injury shock.
- Are arterial pulses present in the extremities? Evaluate and record the presence of pulses. Edema formation in the distal extremities can occlude arterial circulation.
- Are bowel sounds present? Gastric decompression may be required to avoid the risk of vomiting and aspiration.

PLANNING PHASE

EQUIPMENT

VASCULAR ACCESS EQUIPMENT

Sterile gloves
Vascular access tray
    Extra scalpel and blades
    Suture
Xylocaine 1%
Syringes—assorted sizes, including irrigating syringes
Ringer's lactate—12 liters
Angiocaths and intra-caths, 16 gauge and 18 gauge

URINARY DRAINAGE EQUIPMENT

Bladder catheterization tray
Urinary drainage bag with in-line urimeter

GASTROINTESTINAL DRAINAGE EQUIPMENT

Nasogastric (NG) tube
    Suction source
    Lubricant
    Tracheostomy tape (to secure tubes)
    Litmus paper
    Liquid antacid (as ordered)

ADVANCED CARDIAC LIFE SUPPORT (ACLS) EQUIPMENT

Endotracheal tube
    Topical anesthetic
    Laryngoscope
Suction catheters
Suction source
Tracheostomy tray (with tracheostomy tube assortment)
Humidified oxygen equipment

Cardiac monitor/defibrillator
ACLS drugs (see Chap. 3, "Mega Code [Advanced Cardiac Life Support])

WOUND CARE/POSITIONING SUPPLIES

Sterile sheets
Blankets, pillows—4 (sterilized or individually packaged from laundry)
Restraints
Sterile surgical gloves
Sterile surgical gowns
Masks, hair covers
Sterile 4 × 4s—10 or more packages
Sterile basins, large—2 or 3
Warmed sterile saline for irrigation or Hubbard tank
Iodophor or other cleansing agent
Topical antimicrobial cream
Kerlix
External radiant heat warmers
Bed scale

SUPPLIES FOR EYE INJURIES

Normal saline (intravenous) IV solution
IV tubing
Emesis basin
Fluorescein
Ophthalmic solutions (as ordered)

SUPPLIES FOR CHEMICAL BURNS

Shower facilities (trauma tank may be used)
Neutralizing agent (for chemical ingestion)
Petroleum-based antibiotic ointment (for hot tar or plastic burns)

CLIENT/FAMILY TEACHING

- Explain the immediate treatment protocols to the client and family to alleviate anxiety and to promote compliance with the treatment protocols. Client and family involvement with care will be essential to a successful resuscitation program.
- Support the family emotionally during the admission and immediate care processes. Use the chaplain, family pastor, and liaison nurse as available. Communicate frequently with the family about the condition of the injured client.
- Obtain information about the thermal injury and past medical history as necessary.

IMPLEMENTATION PHASE

NURSING ACTIONS	RATIONALE/AMPLIFICATION
1. Implement basic life support (BLS) and ACLS techniques as necessary (see Chap. 3, "Mega Code [Advanced Cardiac Life Support]").	Immediate life-threatening conditions supersede burn-wound care.
2. Implement emergency measures as necessary to prevent further injury.	Immobilize the spine in case of spinal injury; splint fractures.
3. Cut away clothing and remove jewelry if applicable.	
4. Cover client with blanket. Provide external heat source to maintain body temperature.	Loss of the skin's protective mechanism and the presence of shock predispose the client to hypothermia.
5. Obtain client's body weight.	Body weight provides a baseline for calculating fluid resuscitation.

6. Administer high-concentration, warm mist oxygen by face mask, unless intubation is required.

Intubation may be necessary in the presence of thermal injury to the upper or lower airways, or if burns of the face and neck are present.

7. Cannulate peripheral veins with large-bore (16- or 18-gauge) IV catheters. Suture lines in place to secure them.

Initially, burned areas are considered clean and may be used for IV cannulation. Colonization of the wound does not occur until 36 hours to 48 hours after the injury. Central venous cannulation is avoided initially. The decreased circulating blood volume makes central venous cannulation difficult. Central vessels may be required later for hyperalimentation.

8. Calculate requirements for postinjury fluid resuscitation (see following section on Fluid Resuscitation Protocol). Begin IV resuscitation.

Total requirements include reversing burn shock plus replacing blood lost from associated injuries.

9. Insert indwelling bladder catheter and attach to closed drainage system with in-line urimeter. Measure hourly urine output.

10. Obtain the following diagnostic studies for baseline profile: complete blood count (CBC), serology (Venereal Disease Research Laboratories [VDRL]), electrolytes, blood glucose, blood urea nitrogen (BUN), urinalysis, arterial blood gases (ABGS), chest film, electrocardiogram (ECG).

11. Insert NG tube and connect to low intermittent suction (see Chap. 13, "Gastrointestinal Intubation").

An NG tube prevents gastric dilatation and vomiting. If facial burns are present, secure the tube with wide tracheostomy tape positioned circumferentially above the ears. This allows for edema formation.

12. Administer narcotics (meperidine, morphine) in low-dose IV injections after fluid resuscitation is well established.

Titrate doses (meperidine in 10-mg increments; morphine in 2-mg increments) to provide optimum pain relief without vasodilatory effects, which may increase shock. Narcotics are given IV push because the shift of fluids into the interstitial spaces impairs peripheral circulation.

13. Cleanse wound in Hubbard tank or with warmed sterile saline and iodophor in sterile basins (see following sections on wound management techniques).

Wear sterile gloves, gowns, masks, and hair covering.

14. Apply topical antimicrobial cream as ordered.

15. Elevate thermally injured extremities.

Elevation of extremities prevents edema formation. Edema can occlude peripheral arterial circulation.

16. Administer tetanus toxoid 0.5 ml subcutaneously if client has not had booster in past 5 years.

If the client has never been immunized, give 250 units tetanus immune globulin in addition.

17. Implement special techniques for client with electric burns.

    a. Assess client's condition to determine entry and exit sites and path of current through body.

The client with electric burns may have minimal visible surface injury. Internal injury occurs to tissues along the axis of the current flow.

    b. Monitor continuous ECG tracing.

Dysrhythmias, particularly ventricular fibrillation, may occur as a result of electric current passing through the myocardium.

    c. Monitor urine for presence of hemochromogens.

The urine will be port-wine colored. Deep muscle damage occurs as a result of electric current passing through muscle masses, which results in a release of myoglobin

d. If hemochromogens are present in urine, proceed as follows:

from the damaged muscle cells. These pigments precipitate in the renal tubules and cause acute tubular necrosis.

(1) Administer additional fluid to flush kidneys (Ringer's lactate IV infusion) and to maintain urine output over 100 ml/hour.

(2) Give mannitol 12.5 g to 25 g IV infusion as ordered to generate osmotic diuresis.

Forced diuresis will not be indicated until hypovolemia is corrected.

(3) Administer sodium bicarbonate IV infusion as ordered to reverse accompanying acidosis caused by hemochromogen load and renal insufficiency.

Up to 400 mEq of sodium bicarbonate may be required in the first 4 hours after injury.

(4) Titrate sodium bicarbonate according to arterial *p*H determinations obtained on serial basis every 1 hour to 2 hours.

e. Evaluate client for long bone and vertebral fractures.

Electric injury often causes fractures, which result from extreme tetanic contractions that occur as the current passes through the body, or from a fall associated with the shock.

f. Assess body surface for multiple wounds, entry sites, one or more exit sites, arc injury, and flame or steam injuries.

g. Assess for peripheral pulses and elevate extremities.

Arterial insufficiency of the injured extremity due to extreme edema formation may require fasciotomy, which is an incision through all layers of the injured area, including the muscle fascia (Fig. 31–2) (see following section on Escharotomy Technique).

h. Apply topical antimicrobial cream as ordered.

Mafenide acetate (Sulfamylon) is commonly used to penetrate deep electric burn wounds.

18. Implement special techniques for chemical burns of skin or eye or those caused by ingestion.

Fig. 31–2 Fasciotomy to relieve arterial insufficiency of upper extremity following cold injury.

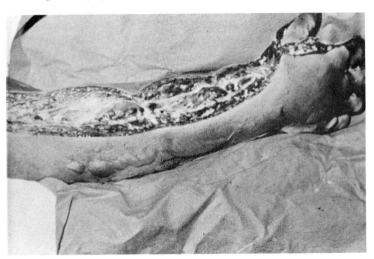

Chemical Injury to the Skin

a. Remove all clothing. Irrigate (shower) wound continuously for 30 minutes.

Copious amounts of water dilute and remove the chemical, which continues to damage tissue as long as it remains in contact with the skin. Alkaline chemicals continue to cause tissue destruction for up to 72 hours and require frequent showering (every 2 hours to 4 hours) for the first 24 hours to 72 hours.

b. Brush powdered chemicals from skin before irrigation.

c. Apply topical antimicrobial cream as ordered.

Chemical Injury to the Eye

a. Flush eye with copious amount of normal saline (1 liter in each eye).

Use normal saline IV infusion setup to facilitate eye irrigation.

b. After irrigation, stain cornea with fluorescein to identify injured area.

c. Apply ophthalmic solutions as ordered and patch eye if required.

Corticosteroids, antibiotics, and anesthetics may be ordered for ophthalmic instillation.

Ingestion of Chemicals

a. Do not induce emesis.

Emesis reintroduces the caustic agent to already injured tissues.

b. Administer appropriate neutralizing agent.

Consult the area poison-control center. Insertion of an NG tube for chemical removal is contraindicated because of the potential for emesis and the risk of perforation.

Injury with Hot Tar or Plastics

a. Cool burning agent with water.

Rapid cooling prevents further damage.

b. Liberally apply petroleum-based ointment (Neosporin, bacitracin) to debris.

Emulsification of the hardened tar or plastic will result, facilitating removal of the burning agent without causing further injury.

c. Apply topical antimicrobial cream, as ordered, after removal of debris.

RELATED NURSING CARE

NURSING ACTIONS	RATIONALE/AMPLIFICATION
1. Monitor gastric pH hourly. Withdraw specimen from NG tube and test with litmus paper. Administer antacid (Maalox, Amphojel, Riopan) as ordered. Clamp the tube 5 minutes to 15 minutes. Reconnect NG tube to low intermittent suction.	Administer antacids to maintain a gastric pH that is greater than 5. Hyperacidity is a result of physiological stress and may lead to a stress ulcer.
2. Administer histamine H_2 receptor antagonist (cimetidine [Tagamet] 300 mg IV piggyback infusion every 6 hours or ranitidine [Zantac] 50 mg IV piggyback infusion every 2 hours) as ordered.	Histamine H_2 antagonist therapy inhibits gastric acid secretion.

EVALUATION PHASE

ANTICIPATED OUTCOMES	NURSING ACTIONS
1. Early wound cover and prevention of nosocomial infection	Monitor sterile technique during debridement, tanking, and application of antimicrobial cream. Monitor the

2. Prevention of complications of thermal trauma, including airway occlusion, shock, arterial insufficiency, gastric dilation and vomiting, and stress ulcer

client's vital signs (including body temperature) and the condition of the wound for signs of infection.

Monitor the following on an hourly basis: output (NG, urine, blood loss), intake (by IV infusion and NG tube), sensorium (clouded sensorium in addition to decreased urinary output and tachycardia indicates inadequate fluid resuscitation), vital signs, peripheral pulses, voice quality (continual increasing hoarseness indicates tracheal edema), and gastric *p*H.

Fluid resuscitation protocol

Objectives
To prevent the development of burn shock (hypovolemia)
To correct the fluid-volume compositional defects of burn shock

ASSESSMENT PHASE

- Has the extent of the thermal injury been calculated using the Rule of Nines or the Lund and Browder with Berkow formula chart?
- Has the client been weighed?
- Have IV lines been inserted and secured?
- Has the time of injury been established? (This does *not* mean the time of arrival at the facility.)

PRECAUTIONS

- **The rapid infusion of large amounts of fluids may exacerbate cardiac and respiratory problems in clients with preexisting cardiopulmonary diseases. Monitor these clients closely for signs of heart failure.**
- **The development of arterial insufficiency may be hastened with rapid fluid administration, which requires escharotomy.**

PLANNING PHASE

EQUIPMENT

Ringer's lactate — 2 or more cases (crystalloid formula)
Ultrasound flowmeter (Doppler)
Clinitest and Acetest reagent tablets

CLIENT/FAMILY TEACHING

- Discuss the reason for IV fluid therapy.
- Explain that swelling will occur and may cause difficulty breathing (due to tracheal edema). If this occurs, endotracheal intubation may be necessary.
- Explain to the client that escharotomy may be necessary because of edema formation.
- Tell the client and family that the client's facial features may be swollen, causing eyelid and lip eversion.

IMPLEMENTATION PHASE

NURSING ACTIONS	RATIONALE/AMPLIFICATION

CRYSTALLOID RESUSCITATION REGIMEN

1. Calculate fluid requirements for first 24 hours using crystalloid resuscitation formula.

Because of the capillary leak (increased permeability) that causes the rapid movement of plasma protein and fluids into the burn wound, Ringer's lactate is the only fluid that is required in the first 24 hours. Ringer's lactate closely resembles the extracellular fluid and corrects the compositional defects found with fluid sequestration into the burn wound (Table 31–1).

Table 31–1
Composition of isotonic fluids for burn resuscitation

	Normal saline (mEq)	Lactated Ringer's (mEq)	Plasma/extracellular fluid (mEq)
Sodium	154	130	142
Chloride	154	109	103
Potassium		4	4
Calcium		3	5
Magnesium			3
Bicarbonate			27
Lactate		44*	

* Metabolized *in vivo* to bicarbonate.

4 ml Ringer's lactate × kg body weight × % TBSA burn

2. Infuse calculated amount of Ringer's lactate according to following schedule.

    a. One half of total amount is given in first 8 hours after burn injury.

    b. One quarter of total amount is given in second 8 hours after burn injury.

    c. One quarter of total amount is given in third 8 hours after burn injury.

3. Infuse aged plasma in fourth 8 hours after burn injury, using following formula:

0.35 ml to .5 ml plasma × kg weight × TBSA burn

4. Following resuscitation of burn shock (24 hours to 36 hours postburn), infuse dextrose 5% in water (D_5W) or dextrose 5% and 0.5 normal saline after plasma administration to replace insensible water loss (2 liters to 3 liters/day minimum).

An example of the crystalloid resuscitation formula is given below.

4 ml Ringer's lactate × 50 kg × 50% TBSA burn = 10,000 ml Ringer's lactate for the first 24 hours.

For example, if the total calculated amount of Ringer's lactate is 10,000 ml, in the first 8 hours 5000 ml (625 ml/hour) will be given. In the second 8 hours 2500 ml (313 ml/hour) will be given, and in the third 8 hours 2500 ml (313 ml/hour) will be given.

For example, if .5 ml plasma/kg/% TBSA burn will be given, the client weighs 50 kg, and TBSA of the burn is 50%, then 1250 ml total plasma volume will be given in the fourth 8-hour period. Eighteen hours to 24 hours after injury, capillary integrity is regained and infusion of plasma proteins will increase the circulating volume without further sequestration of fluid into the interstitial spaces.

See Table 31–2 for alternative fluid resuscitation formulas.

RELATED NURSING CARE

NURSING ACTIONS	RATIONALE/AMPLIFICATION
1. Measure and record intake and output hourly.	A reliable indicator for assessing adequate resuscitation is an adequate urinary output (50 ml to 70 ml/hour for adults; 1 ml to 2 ml/kg/hour for children). Increase the

Table 31–2
Burn resuscitation formulas (first 24 hours after burn)

Formula name	Formula
Crystalloid Resuscitation	4 ml Ringer's lactate × kg weight × % TBSA burn Infuse according to the following schedule: $\frac{1}{2}$ in the first 8 hours after burn $\frac{1}{4}$ in the second 8 hours after burn $\frac{1}{4}$ in the third 8 hours after burn
Brooke	
Electrolyte	1.5 ml Ringer's lactate × kg weight × % TBSA burn
Colloid	0.05 ml × kg weight × % TBSA burn
Water	2000 ml dextrose 5% in water (D_5W)
Modified Brooke	2 ml to 4 ml Ringer's lactate × kg weight × TBSA burn
Hypertonic Sodium	250 mEq Na/liter titrated to maintain urine output at 30 ml/hour
Evans	
Normal saline	1 ml × kg weight × % TBSA burn
Colloid	1 ml × kg weight × % TBSA burn
Water	2000 ml D_5W
Moore's Burn Budget	
Electrolyte	1000 ml to 4000 ml Ringer's lactate (titrated according to urine output) + 1200 ml 0.45 normal saline
Colloid	7.5% kg weight
Water	1500 ml to 5000 ml D_5W

2. Provide external heat source and cover burn wound.

rate of the IV infusion if the urine output is less than 30 ml/hour for 2 consecutive hours.

In the presence of a covered wound and external heat source, continued hypothermia indicates inadequate fluid resuscitation.

3. Monitor vital signs hourly during resuscitation phase.

Blood pressure is an unreliable indicator of resuscitation status because of compensatory vasoconstriction.

4. Monitor urine for presence of glucose and acetone every 4 hours.

Glycosuria commonly occurs after thermal trauma because of physiological stress and the release of glucocorticoids, which increases gluconeogenesis. Ketonuria may be present. It indicates metabolic acidosis, which accompanies burn shock and occurs as a result of decreased tissue perfusion, which leads to anaerobic metabolism and the production of ketone bodies. With adequate resuscitation, ketonuria should quickly resolve.

5. Elevate burned extremities. Monitor peripheral pulses and the sensory and motor function of peripheral muscles hourly. Use ultrasound flowmeter if you are unable to palpate pulses.

The absence of distal pulses indicates arterial occlusion caused by edema formation and the tourniquet effect of inelastic, burned skin. Arterial occlusion requires escharotomy to reestablish the circulation to the distal extremities (see following section on Escharotomy Technique).

EVALUATION PHASE

ANTICIPATED OUTCOMES	NURSING ACTIONS
1. Resuscitation/prevention of burn shock	Continually evaluate fluid resuscitation status by monitoring the following: urine output (50 ml to 70 ml/hour), normal core body temperature, absence of tachypnea (respiratory rate that is less than 20 breaths per

minute), absence of tachycardia (heart rate that is less than 120 beats per minute), and clear sensorium.

2. Prevention of complications of fluid resuscitation
   a. fluid overload

Clients with preexisting cardiopulmonary disease may not be able to tolerate the rapid infusion of Ringer's lactate and may show signs of cardiac failure or pulmonary edema. Auscultate breath sounds every 2 hours for crackles. Assess for neck vein distention. Monitor central venous pressure (CVP), pulmonary artery (PA) pressure, and pulmonary wedge pressure (PWP) if available (see Chap. 5, "Hemodynamic Pressure Monitoring").

Hydrotherapy

Objectives
To remove debris and topical creams from the burn wound
To aid in loosening eschar from the burn wound
To promote active range of motion

ASSESSMENT PHASE

- Are the client's vital signs stable? The client who is not hemodynamically stable cannot be tanked. If the client cannot be tanked, complete hydrotherapy with the client in bed using warmed normal saline and large sterile basins.
- Is the client's respiratory status stable? Do not tank the client who is in respiratory distress. Set up oxygen in the tank area and continuously administer oxygen and monitor oxygen delivery.
- Has the client received premedication? Administer meperidine 25 mg to 50 mg slow IV push or morphine sulfate 5 mg to 10 mg slow IV push (as ordered) 5 minutes to 10 minutes before hydrotherapy. If medication is given intramuscularly (IM), wait 30 minutes before beginning the procedure.

PRECAUTIONS

- **Hyponatremia may result from leaching of sodium from the burn wound during immersion in hypotonic solutions (*e.g.,* tap water).**
- **Prolonged exposure of open wounds results in hypothermia, increased metabolic rate, and increased oxygen demand.**
- **Clients who are hemodynamically unstable, who require paralyzing medications to facilitate ventilation, or who cannot maintain a core body temperature of 36.5°C should not be tanked.**

PLANNING PHASE

EQUIPMENT

Hydrotherapy tank
Mechanical lift
Plinth, end bars
Plastic liners for tank and plinth
In-line temperature gauge or thermometer
Water hose
Table salt
Transport stretcher
Radiant heat warmers—2
Iodophor scrub brushes or concentrate
Sterile 4 × 4s
Sterile gloves
Nonsterile gloves
Cap, mask, gown

> Sterile linens (sheets, blankets)
> Sterile scissors, forceps
> Bed scales
> Sterile plug for indwelling bladder catheter
> Sterile replacement catheter drainage system
> Adhesive plastic surgical drape (Steridrape) for covering surgical sites

CLIENT/FAMILY TEACHING

- Discuss the reasons for daily hydrotherapy.
- Describe the procedure to the client and family.
- Assure the client that premedication will be given to alleviate pain.
- Instruct the client on ways of increasing range of motion (ROM) when immersed in the warm solution. Reinforce the importance of active ROM to the maintenance of function.

IMPLEMENTATION PHASE

NURSING ACTIONS	RATIONALE/AMPLIFICATION
1. Prepare tank area before transporting client.	This shortens the period of time during which the client's wounds will be uncovered, decreasing the risk of hypothermia.
a. Scrub walls with detergent cleanser. Damp dust high and low places. Damp mop floor.	
b. Scrub tank with iodine-based or other detergent germicide.	
c. Scrub lift, plinth, bed scales, and transport stretcher with phenol-compound germicide.	
d. Line tank and cover plinth with plastic liners.	If plastic liners are not available for the tank, scrubbing with detergent germicide will suffice.
e. Pierce holes in plastic liner of plinth where agitation is desired.	The plinth used for the Hubbard tank incorporates air tubes connected to a compressor. Piercing the plastic liner will allow air bubbles to facilitate debridement.
f. Set up required oxygen.	
g. Prepare suctioning equipment.	
h. Warm environment with radiant heat warmers.	This decreases the risk of hypothermia.
i. Fill tank halfway with warm water 37.5°C (99.5°F).	
Add table salt (NaCl) to make balanced salt solution. Add iodophor concentrate to bath.	Add 681 g (1.5 pounds) NaCl to 20 gallons (76.8 liters) of water. Add 30 ml of iodophor concentrate per 20 gallons of water.
2. Prior to transporting client to tank area,	
a. Cover transport stretcher with sterile linen.	
b. Place plastic-covered plinth on top of stretcher.	
c. Put on cap, gown, and mask.	
d. Open sterile dressings for redressing after tanking. Use sterile field and cover with sterile drape.	Opening of the sterile dressings decreases the time during which the client is exposed to air.
e. Cover IV sites, chest tube insertion sites, and surgical incisions with adherent surgical drape (Steridrape).	

f. Position urinary drainage system to facilitate drainage, taking care to keep system out of tank.

g. Perform perineal care before placing client on table.

h. Put on nonsterile gloves. Remove soiled dressings, taking care not to contaminate wound.

i. Cover client with sterile blanket and transfer him to stretcher.

j. Transport client to tank room.

3. Place client in tank.

a. Attach end bars to plinth and attach lift securely.

Alternative method: Disconnect the catheter and plug it with a sterile catheter plug. Discard the drainage bag. Reconnect the catheter to a new drainage bag on completion of the tanking procedure.

Cleanse perineum with soap and water. Cleanse urinary meatus with iodophor solution if an indwelling bladder catheter is *in situ.*

Dispose of the dressings appropriately to decrease environmental contamination.

Fig. 31–3 Client in Hubbard tank.

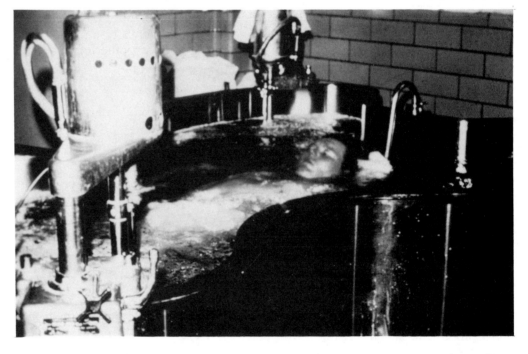

b. Lower client cautiously into warm water (Fig. 31–3).

c. Scrub wounds with iodophor sponges.

d. Connect air compressor tubing into plinth air tubes and lock into place around connections. Begin agitation.

e. Debride eschar during tanking (see following section on Debridement).

f. Reattach end bars to lift.

g. Raise client above water level. Gently tilt plinth to allow excess water to drain.

Alternative method: Lower the client into the unfilled tank and use the water hose for showering (Fig. 31–4). This technique decreases auto–cross-contamination from one infected body area to another. It also decreases the leaching of sodium, but is not conducive to softening eschar or facilitating ROM.

Set a time limit of 20 minutes for immersion to decrease sodium loss and hypothermia.

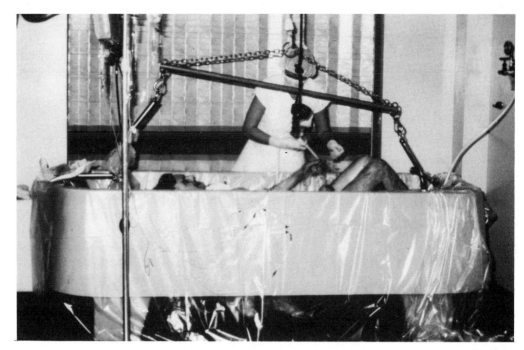

Fig. 31–4 Client in trauma tank. Note plastic liner in tank.

h. Raise plinth out of tank and place on bed scales.	Subtract the weight of the plinth from the total weight to obtain the client's weight.

4. Transport client to unit.

    a. Transfer client to stretcher.

    b. Cover client with sterile blanket before transporting him.

RELATED NURSING CARE

NURSING ACTIONS	RATIONALE/AMPLIFICATION
1. Drain tank. Discard plastic liners. Terminally, disinfect tank, floor, and other equipment.	
2. Shampoo client's hair at least twice weekly during tanking. If scalp is burned, cleanse daily.	

EVALUATION PHASE

ANTICIPATED OUTCOMES	NURSING ACTIONS
1. Removal of debris and topical creams; cleansing of burn wound	Monitor and document the appearance of the wound, client tolerance of the procedure, length of the procedure, cleansing agents used, and temperature of the bath.
2. Prevention of complications of hydrotherapy, including hypothermia and hyponatremia	Monitor and document the client's core body temperature. Evaluate electrolyte determinations and monitor the client for the following symptoms of hyponatremia: headache, apathy, confusion, nausea, vomiting, delirium, and coma.

Debridement

Objectives

To mechanically remove eschar from the thermal wound, thus hastening the healing process

To decrease bacterial proliferation beneath eschar

To prepare the granulating wound for definitive coverage (grafting)

ASSESSMENT PHASE

- Has premedication for pain been administered? Give IV push of medications 5 minutes before the procedure, and IM injections 30 minutes before the procedure.
- Has the wound been thoroughly cleansed? Debride the wound during or immediately after hydrotherapy (see previous section on Hydrotherapy).
- Has an external heat source been provided to warm the client during the procedure?
- Have dressing supplies been prepared in advance on a sterile field and covered with a sterile drape? Prepare dressings before the procedure to facilitate wound coverage quickly and to minimize exposure to air.

PRECAUTIONS

- **Excessive bleeding can occur during mechanical debridement. Digital pressure or the use of hemostatic agents are used to control bleeding.**
- **Hypothermia and excessive evaporation of water through the exposed wound can occur. Limit debridement to 15 minutes.**

PLANNING PHASE

EQUIPMENT

Sterile tray
Sterile Metzenbaum scissors—2
Sterile dissecting forceps—2
Sterile gloves
Cap, mask, gown
Hemostatic agent
    Microfibrillar collagen hemostat (Avitene)
    Oxidized cellulose (Oxycel)
    Absorbable gelatin sponge (Gelfoam)
    Thrombin
    Silver nitrate applicators or epinephrine-soaked (1:1000) sponges
Sterile 4 × 4s—6 or more packages
Sterile blankets—2
Sterile towels or drapes
Suture (chromic)
Electrocautery

CLIENT/FAMILY TEACHING

- Discuss the reason for mechanical debridement and explain the procedure fully to the client and family.
- Support the client psychologically throughout the procedure. Communicate progress continually throughout the procedure. Set reasonable time limits to avoid placing excessive stress on the client.
- Reassure the client that premedication for pain will be provided.

IMPLEMENTATION PHASE

NURSING ACTIONS	RATIONALE/AMPLIFICATION
1. Put on cap, gown, and mask. Wash your hands with antimicrobial soap.	
2. Open debridement tray on bedside table to provide sterile field. Open sterile supplies on sterile field.	

3. Drape area to be debrided with sterile towels or drapes. Expose only area to be debrided. Cover remaining areas with sterile blankets.

Unnecessary exposure results in hypothermia.

4. Use forceps to lift loose eschar. Trim away necrotic tissue with scissors (Fig. 31–5).

Debridement is the process of removing necrotic tissue from the wound at the interface of nonviable and viable tissue. Use a single edge of the forceps to facilitate loosening of the eschar from the underlying tissue.

Fig. 31–5 Debridement using instruments.

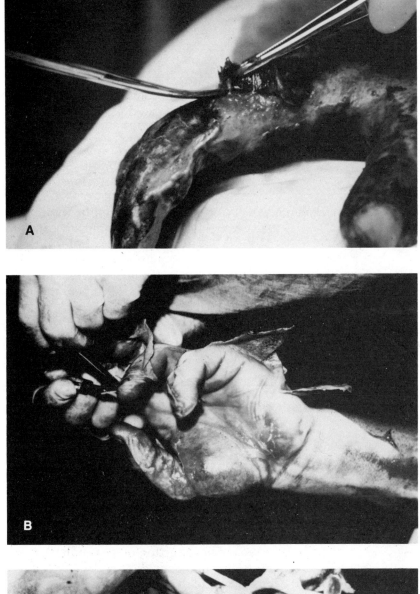

5. Inspect eschar for areas that may harbor accumulated purulent drainage.

Rub eschar gently with a gloved finger to identify areas of purulent accumulation. Debride the eschar over these areas and drain the exudate from these sites.

6. Control active bleeding.

Apply firm, constant, digital pressure to the bleeding area with a sterile 4 × 4 for 3 minutes to 5 minutes. Apply a hemostatic agent and continue digital pressure for an additional 5 minutes. Notify the physician of any continued bleeding, and prepare the suture and electrocautery.

7. Redress thermal wound on completion of procedure.

8. Dispose of contaminated supplies appropriately.

RELATED NURSING CARE

NURSING ACTIONS	RATIONALE/AMPLIFICATION
Monitor and record client's core body temperature before and after procedure.	Continue to provide an external head source as indicated.

EVALUATION PHASE

ANTICIPATED OUTCOMES	NURSING ACTIONS
1. Control of bacterial proliferation in wound	Document the location and appearance of the area debrided. Note any excessive bleeding and the measures used to control the bleeding. Note the location of any purulent areas that have been drained. Document the length of time of the procedure and the client's tolerance. Document the application of topical therapy.
2. Preparation of granulating wound for grafting	

PRODUCT AVAILABILITY   See following section on Escharotomy.

Topical antimicrobial therapy

Objectives
To control bacterial proliferation in the thermal wound
To prevent the conversion of partial-thickness wounds to full-thickness wounds through the infectious process
To prevent burn-wound sepsis

ASSESSMENT PHASE
- Has the thermal wound been thoroughly cleansed with the prescribed cleansing agents? See previous section on Hydrotherapy.
- Has the thermal wound been debrided?
- Has the appearance of the wound been documented?

PRECAUTIONS
- **Use strict aseptic technique when applying topical antimicrobial chemotherapeutic agents to avoid cross-contamination and nosocomial infections.**

PLANNING PHASE

EQUIPMENT
Cap, mask, gown
Sterile gloves
Topical agent

For light semiclosed dressings, include the following items:
　　Fine-mesh gauze
　　Sterile 4 × 4s
　　Sterile gauze rolls
　　Sterile drape (for sterile field)
For the open treatment method, include a bed cradle.

CLIENT/FAMILY TEACHING

- Discuss the rationale and the procedure for the application of topical antimicrobial cream.
- Describe the sensations that may be experienced. Sulfamylon causes pain or a burning sensation on application and removal. Betadine may sting when applied to partial-thickness wounds.

IMPLEMENTATION PHASE

NURSING ACTIONS	RATIONALE/AMPLIFICATION
1. Put on gown, cap, and mask. Wash your hands with antimicrobial soap.	
2. Prepare sterile field by opening sterile sheet on bedside table. Open sterile supplies on field. Open jars of topical cream and place in convenient location near client.	
3. Expose area to be treated. Put on sterile gloves.	
4. Apply topical agent to wound with gloved hand, using strict aseptic technique (Table 31–3).	To prevent contamination of the jar of cream, use one hand to transfer cream from the jar to the other hand, which is used to apply the cream to the wound. Be careful not to touch the wound or the other hand with the hand that you are using to obtain the cream (Fig. 31–6). Pay particular attention to the order of application in the client with positive wound biopsies. Apply the cream to the noninfected areas first, and then progress to the infected areas. Take precautions to prevent the transfer

Fig. 31–6 Technique for obtaining antimicrobial agent from jar without contaminating jar with hand used to apply cream to wound.

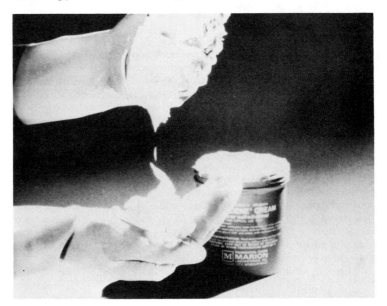

Fig. 31-7   Applying Silvadene to burn wound of lower extremity.

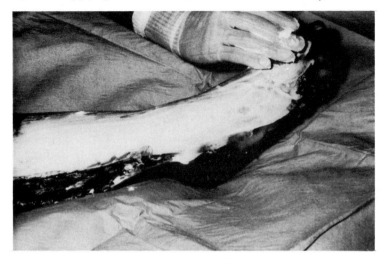

5. Leave cream-covered wound open to air using bed cradle to prevent adherence or cover it with layer of fine-mesh gauze and light gauze rolls.

6. Remove gloves. Dispose of contaminated supplies appropriately.

of microorganisms from one wound to another (Fig. 31-7).

Use fine-mesh gauze or 4 × 4s to prevent adjacent burned areas from touching.

Table 31-3
Topical antimicrobial agents

Agent	Application	Advantages	Disadvantages	Precautions
Silvadene (silver sulfadiazine 1%) Silvadene–Cerium (silver sulfadiazine and cerium) Silvadene–Furacin (silver sulfadiazine and nitrafurazone) alternating regimen	Apply 1 cm to 2 cm thick 2 times to 3 times daily after cleaning the wound.	Water soluble; effective against gram-positive and gram-negative organisms as well as yeast; pain-free application; easy removal; no systemic absorption	Development of resistant strains of organisms; fungal colonization of eschar may cause leukopenia; cerium nitrate may cause methemoglobinemia; nitrafurazone may cause renal failure	Use with caution in clients with hepatic or renal failure, in pregnant clients, or clients with hypersensitivity.
Sulfamylon (mafenide acetate)	Apply 3 mm thick every 12 hours after cleaning the wound.	Water soluble; effective against gram-positive and gram-negative organisms as well as some anaerobes; penetrates avascular necrotic tissue, providing deep antimicrobial coverage	Painful application and removal; may cause metabolic acidosis because of carbonic anhydrase inhibitor activity	Use with caution in pregnant clients and in clients with hypersensitivity to sulfonamides.
Betadine (povidone–iodine)	Apply ointment liberally to the wound 2 times to 3 times daily. Ointment will liquefy on reaching body temperature. Apply Helafoam by spraying the wound directly or by applying with the gloved hand. Spread to cover the wound 2 times to 3 times daily.	Water soluble; hardens eschar, facilitates excisional debridement; easily removed; causes translucence of the wound, allowing easy identification of the depth of injury	Decreases joint mobility; inhibits growth of bacteria *in vitro* if left on biopsy specimen; may cause elevation of triiodothyronine (T_3) and thyroxine (T_4) levels	Use with caution in clients with hypersensitivity to iodine.

RELATED NURSING CARE

NURSING ACTIONS	RATIONALE/AMPLIFICATION
Remove and reapply topical agent according to desired schedule.	Note signs of infection, including wound-margin cellulitis, excessive purulent exudate, and necrotic lesions, which indicate wound conversion from partial thickness to full thickness.

EVALUATION PHASE

ANTICIPATED OUTCOMES	NURSING ACTIONS
1. Prevention of bacterial proliferation of thermal wound	Document the appearance of the wound with each dressing change. Monitor for wound-margin cellulitis. Measure area of cellulitis in centimeters and record the measurement.
2. Prevention of burn-wound sepsis	Monitor and document signs and symptoms of burn-wound sepsis, including 10^5 bacteria per gram of tissue, marked wound-margin cellulitis, hypothermia or hyperthermia, disorientation, tachypnea, foul odor, change in wound color, decreased platelet count, increased or decreased white blood cell count, and glycosuria.
3. Prevention of complications of topical antimicrobial therapy	Monitor for side-effects of topical antimicrobial therapy. Side-effects of Silvadene include itching, rash, and burning. Monitor white blood cell count daily for potential leukopenia, a manifestation of allergic reaction. When Sulfamylon is used, monitor the client's respiratory rate, ABGs, and serum electrolyte levels for evidence of metabolic acidosis. Administer pain medication before the application and use of adjunct pain relief (*e.g.,* relaxation techniques). Remove Sulfamylon by gentle scraping with sterile tongue blades and gentle scrubbing during hydrotherapy. When Betadine is used, monitor the client's thyroid function; monitor the wound margin for evidence of iodine sensitivity (*e.g.,* rash, cellulitis).

PRODUCT AVAILABILITY

SILVER SULFADIAZENE

Marion Laboratories (Silvadene)

IODOPHOR OINTMENT

Purdue Frederick Co. (Betadine)

MAFENIDE ACETATE

Winthrop Laboratories (Sulfamylon)

CERIUM NITRATE

Marion Laboratories (Cerium)

Biologic dressings

Objectives
To protect against bacterial contamination of the wound
To provide a barrier against evaporative water losses through the open wound

To decrease protein losses in wound exudate

To decrease the pain of the thermal wound

To increase the ROM and to promote healing by protecting the underlying granulating tissue

To stimulate and prepare the granulation bed for autografting

ASSESSMENT PHASE

- Has the wound been thoroughly cleansed? See previous section on Hydrotherapy.
- Has the wound been thoroughly debrided? Adherence of the biologic dressing depends on a relatively clean granulating bed. See previous section on Debridement and following section on Wet to Dry Soaks.

PRECAUTIONS

- **The application of biologic dressings (primarily porcine grafts) to infected wounds or to wounds covered by eschar may cause acute febrile reactions, which require the removal of the dressing.**

PLANNING PHASE

EQUIPMENT

Biologic dressing rolls

    Porcine xenograft (heterograft)

    Allograft (homograft)

    Synthetic biologic dressing

    Autograft

Sterile drape

Sterile tray

    Suture scissors—2

    Dissecting forceps—2

    Sterile basin

Sterile normal saline—1 liter

Sterile 4 × 4s

Sterile cotton-tip applicators

Sterile gloves

Cap, mask, gown

Protective underpad

Scalpel blade (No. 11)

Optional items

    Antibiotic ointment-impregnated fine-mesh gauze rolls or antibiotic solution (for meshed graft)

    Sterile gauze roller bandage

    40-watt bulb heat lamp (for donor site care)

CLIENT/FAMILY TEACHING

- Discuss the purposes of biologic dressings with the client and family.
- Explain the procedure to the client.
- Tell the client that the dressings will decrease the pain in the wound and will make ROM easier.

IMPLEMENTATION PHASE

NURSING ACTIONS	RATIONALE/AMPLIFICATION
1. Place protective underpad beneath area to be grafted.	
2. Wash your hands with antimicrobial soap.	
3. Prepare sterile field by opening sterile tray on bedside table. Open sterile supplies on field.	
4. Open biologic dressing and 4 × 4s and place in sterile basin. Pour sterile normal saline into basin. Thaw frozen allograft and xenograft by placing in normal saline at room temperature for 30 minutes.	Normal saline prevents desiccation (drying) of the biologic material and removes the preservative agents.

5. Put on sterile gloves.

6. Place saline-soaked 4 × 4s over area to be covered.

Prevent wound drying by allowing saline-soaked 4 × 4s to remain over the wound until you are ready to apply the biologic dressing. Open only the amount of dressing needed. Once it is opened, label the dressing with the date and store the unused portion in a sterile container in the refrigerator for a maximum of 5 days.

7. Estimate length of biologic material needed. Cut this amount from roll; leave backing material intact.

8. Apply biologic material with dermal (shiny) side to wound (Fig. 31–8). Peel fine-mesh gauze or net backing from biologic dressing.

Fig. 31–8 Check biologic dressing for shiny or dermal side.

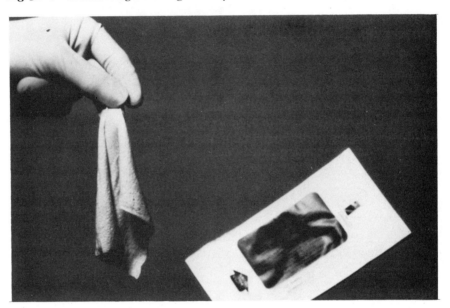

9. Smooth dressing with gloved fingers, flat end of the forceps, or cotton-tip applicators to remove wrinkles, air, or fluid pockets. Trim to fit wound margins.

10. Continue to apply in strips until area to be grafted is covered (Fig. 31–9).

Approximate the edges of the strips to prevent overlapping. Do not allow the strips to overlap with normal skin. Biologic dressings do not adhere to skin that is intact, but become dry and hardened.

11. Cover biologic dressing with strips of antibiotic ointment-impregnated fine-mesh gauze if appropriate.

Use fine-mesh gauze to decrease the bacterial contamination between the strips of the biologic dressing. Meshed biologic dressings are often used to obtain maximum coverage of the area. If meshed grafts are being used, apply fine-mesh gauze that has been soaked with antibiotic solution over the grafted areas. This provides antimicrobial coverage of the small open wound areas between the graft interstices.

12. Secure dressing with sterile gauze roller bandage or sterile net stretch bandage.

13. Apply splint if used.

Immobilization of the grafted area facilitates graft adherence. Splints are used primarily with autografts.

Fig. 31-9 Apply biologic dressing to wound in strips until entire wound is covered.

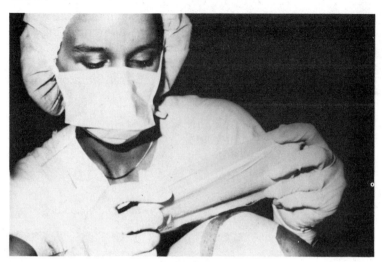

14. Elevate and position grafted area so that graft remains free of pressure.

15. Remove protective underpad. Change linen if it is soiled. Discard contaminated supplies appropriately.

RELATED NURSING CARE

NURSING ACTIONS	RATIONALE/AMPLIFICATION
1. Reapply antibiotic solution to gauze dressing every 4 hours to 6 hours to keep it moist.	This step is necessary only if meshed grafts are used.
2. Remove dressings down to top layer daily for inspection.	Clients with xenografts on partial-thickness wounds still receive daily hydrotherapy. Check the graft site at this time. Observe graft sites for signs of infection, including cellulitis, foul odor, or purulent drainage. Monitor the client's condition for temperature spikes.
3. Begin gentle ROM regimen as appropriate.	Regimen for ROM should begin on the fifth postgraft day for autografts, on the third postgraft day for allografts and xenografts (on full-thickness wounds), and on the first postgraft day for xenografts (on partial-thickness wounds).
4. Change allografts every 4 days to 5 days.	
5. Change xenografts every 3 days. Trim dried edges of porcine xenograft daily as healing of partial-thickness wound occurs.	Porcine xenograft is left in place on partial-thickness wounds until healing is completed, unless rejection or infection occurs. Porcine xenografts are changed every 72 hours on full-thickness wounds to prevent incorporation of porcine collagen into the wound.
6. Keep graft sites free of pressure and immobilize them until adherence occurs.	
7. If infection or rejection occurs, notify physician and prepare to remove graft, cleanse wound, and apply alternate topical agent.	
8. In first 48 hours after graft, remove exudate that has accumulated under grafted areas initially by rolling	Once the graft begins to adhere, rolling fluid may disrupt the adhering graft.

the graft with sterile cotton swabs. After procedure is completed, remove accumulated exudate by nicking graft with No. 11 scalpel blade and manually expressing fluid.

9. Provide donor site care.

The donor site is the area from which skin is harvested. It is essentially a partial-thickness injury. Donor sites are treated with a variety of methods, including fine-mesh gauze, porcine xenograft, and petroleum-based gauze.

   a. For the fine-mesh gauze–covered donor site, proceed as follows:

   (1) Expose donor site to air until area heals.

   (2) Position heat lamp 45 cm (18 inches) from site. Use lamp continuously until donor site is completely dry.

   b. For the porcine xenograft covered donor site, proceed as follows:

   (1) Expose donor site to air or use heat lamp until bleeding ceases and area is dry.

   (2) If covered with light gauze wrap, remove wrap after 24 hours by gently manipulating and moistening with saline as necessary.

   (3) Observe for accumulation of blood or fluid beneath xenograft.

   (4) Nick xenograft with No. 11 scalpel blade and express fluid as necessary.

   c. General care of donor sites is as follows:

   (1) Inspect daily for signs of infection, including foul odor, purulent drainage, marginal cellulitis, erythema, and fever.

   (2) Remove covering from infected donor site using saline to moisten adhered areas. Cleanse wound with iodophor and normal saline. Apply topical agent as ordered.

   (3) Wrap donor sites on lower extremities with elasticized bandages before ambulation.

Lower extremity burns and donor sites are covered with a distal-to-proximal wrap to prevent the pooling of blood and skin breakdown.

   (4) Keep donor sites dry and free of pressure.

Hydrotherapy will be interrupted for 7 days to 10 days while healing occurs.

10. Give bed baths to promote hygiene while hydrotherapy is interrupted.

Clients with xenografts on partial-thickness wounds continue to receive daily hydrotherapy.

EVALUATION PHASE

ANTICIPATED OUTCOMES	NURSING ACTIONS
1. Preparation of granulating wound bed for autografting	Evaluate the adherence of the biologic dressings. Adherence indicates that the granulating bed is ready for autografting.
2. Promotion of wound coverage and improved wound healing	Document the biologic dressing procedure, including the date and time of application, the area grafted, the appearance of the wound before the application of the

dressing, the type of biologic dressing applied, the type of dressing applied to secure the graft, the type of splint used, and the client's tolerance of the procedure. Monitor and document the appearance of the grafted area daily.

3. Prevention of wound infection

Monitor the client's vital signs every 4 hours. Monitor and report immediately any evidence of infection or rejection. For allografts and xenografts, fever, tachycardia, confusion, nausea, vomiting, and erythematous appearance of the wound indicate possible infection or rejection. For all types of grafts fever, marginal cellulitis, and purulent exudate indicate infection or rejection.

PRODUCT AVAILABILITY

PORCINE XENOGRAFT

Burn Treatment Skin Bank (available fresh, frozen, or lyophilized)
Genetic Laboratories Inc. (available fresh and frozen)

SYNTHETIC DRESSINGS

Parke–Davis and Co. (Epigard)
Abbott Laboratories (Hydron Barrier Dressing)
Derma-Lock Medical Corporation (Epi-Lock)
Woodroff Laboratories (Biobrane)

NET STRETCH BANDAGES

Surgifix Inc., (Surgifix)
Western Medical (BurnNet)

Wet to dry soaks

Objectives
To provide mechanical debridement of exudate and eschar from thermal wounds
To provide fine debridement of granulating wounds
To promote wound healing
To prepare the thermal wound for grafting

ASSESSMENT PHASE

- Has the wound been thoroughly cleansed with the prescribed cleansing agents? See previous section on Hydrotherapy.
- Has an external heat source, which is used to keep the client warm, been provided for the procedure?

PLANNING PHASE

APPLICATION

EQUIPMENT

Sterile basin (large)
Sterile coarse-mesh gauze (for exudate, eschar removal)
Sterile fine-mesh gauze (for fine debridement of granulation bed)
Sterile solution (normal saline, neomycin, bacitracin, as ordered)
Sterile gauze roll
Sterile gloves
Cap, mask, gown
Protective waterproof underpad
Solution warmer

REMOVAL

Weck blades
Nonsterile gloves
Sterile gloves

Cap, mask, gown
Sterile 4 × 4s
Sterile normal saline solution
Receptacle for contaminated dressings

CLIENT/FAMILY TEACHING   • Describe the procedure and explain the rationale for the procedure.
• Tell the client that medication will be given for pain before the dry dressings are removed.

IMPLEMENTATION PHASE

NURSING ACTIONS	RATIONALE/AMPLIFICATION
1. Put on gown, cap, and mask. Wash your hands with antimicrobial soap.	
2. Prepare sterile field by opening sterile package on bedside table. Open sterile supplies on sterile field. Place gauze into basin aseptically.	
3. Add specified solution to basin to soak gauze.	Warm the solution for client comfort, if heating is not contraindicated. Heat may destroy the antimicrobial properties of some solutions.
4. Place waterproof underpad beneath area to be treated.	
5. Put on sterile gloves. Apply saturated gauze to wound.	The gauze should be thoroughly wet but not dripping.
6. Secure gauze to wound by lightly wrapping with gauze roll.	Wrap from the distal end of the body part to the proximal end.
7. Remove gloves. Dispose of contaminated supplies appropriately.	
8. Remove wet linens from beneath client and place extra padding under moist dressings.	
9. Allow dressings to dry.	
10. Administer premedication for pain as ordered.	Analgesia is indicated before the removal of the dry dressing, which can be extremely painful. Wet to dry soaks are changed every 4 hours to 6 hours.
11. Put on gown, cap, and mask. Wash your hands with antimicrobial soap.	
12. Assemble equipment at client's bedside.	
13. Put on nonsterile gloves. Cut outer layer of gauze wrap away using Weck blade.	
14. Gently but firmly remove dry dressing, taking care not to touch wound with nonsterile gloves (Fig. 31–10).	Exudate and eschar that have adhered to the gauze will be automatically pulled away when the dressing is removed. Wetting the dressing for removal negates the purpose. If active, profuse bleeding occurs, moisten the dry, adhered dressing with normal saline to prevent further hemorrhage. Put on sterile gloves and control excess bleeding with digital pressure and sterile 4 × 4s.
15. Apply new wet soaks, if required, or other topical therapy.	
16. Remove gloves. Dispose of contaminated supplies appropriately.	Soiled dressings should be placed in doubled paper bags for incineration.

Fig. 31–10   Removal of dry dressing with adherent exudate.

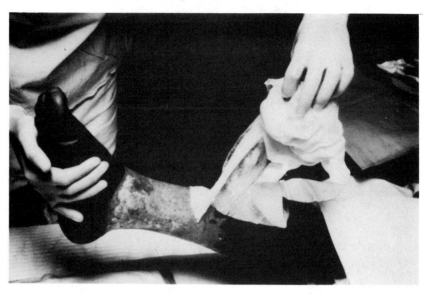

EVALUATION PHASE

ANTICIPATED OUTCOMES	NURSING ACTIONS
1. Removal of exudate and eschar from thermal wound	Document the color and appearance of the wound on application and removal of the dressings.
2. Preparation of clean granulation bed for grafting	Note any excessive bleeding on removal. Note the client's tolerance of the procedure.

Escharotomy technique

Objective

To reestablish circulation to distal extremities after arterial occlusion resulting from edema formation

ASSESSMENT PHASE

- Does the client have circumferential burns on the extremities or thorax? These patterns of thermal injury predispose the client to arterial occlusion and limit respiratory excursion.
- Are the arterial pulses on the extremity obliterated? Compare pulse assessments with baseline determinations on admission.
- Has the peripheral circulation ceased? This is determined by Doppler flow assessment (Fig. 31–11). (See Monitoring Blood Pressure and Peripheral Pulses using Doppler in Chap. 5.)
- Has the client reported deep, throbbing, aching pain of the distal extremities? This is a classic finding in arterial occlusion after thermal trauma.

PRECAUTIONS

- **The color and temperature of burned distal extremities are unreliable indicators of peripheral circulatory status.**

PLANNING PHASE

EQUIPMENT

Cutdown or minor-procedure tray
Sterile gloves
Syringes, 20 ml to 30 ml with 20- to 22-gauge needles
Sterile 4 × 4s — 10 or more packages
Topical hemostatic agent (See Product Availability at the end of this section.)

Fig. 31–11 Monitoring peripheral pulses using Doppler ultrasound.

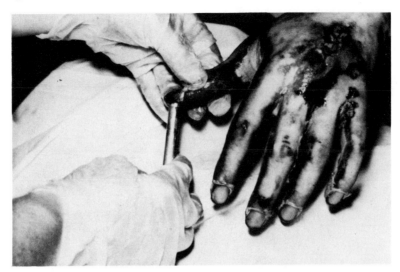

Electrocoagulation unit
Iodophor solution

CLIENT/FAMILY TEACHING
- Reinforce the physician's discussion of escharotomy with the client and family. Answer questions about the procedure.
- Reassure the client that the procedure should not be excessively painful, because it involves releasing burned rather than live tissue, and that a local anesthetic will be given as necessary.

IMPLEMENTATION PHASE

NURSING ACTIONS	RATIONALE/AMPLIFICATION
1. Prepare area to be incised with iodophor and sterile 4 × 4s. Wear sterile gloves.	Escharotomy consists of linear incisions along the circumferentially burned extremities or thorax. Incisions are made medially and laterally along the length of the burn wound, from the distal to the proximal joint (Fig. 31–12).
2. Open cutdown tray on bedside table to provide sterile field. Open sterile supplies on field.	
3. Assist physician with sterile gloves and help to draw up local anesthetic.	
4. Support client while planned incision is infiltrated with local anesthetic.	The local anesthetic is infiltrated into second-degree wounds. A third-degree wound is anesthetic because of the destruction of nerves. Local anesthetic is unnecessary.
5. Put on sterile gloves and help physician to control bleeding during procedure.	Hemostasis can be obtained by clamping the bleeding vessels with mosquito forceps, applying hemostatic agents, cauterizing small bleeders with silver nitrate applicators, ligating bleeders with sutures, or by electrocautery (Fig. 31–13).
6. After escharotomy, dress wound as ordered (see Wound Management Techniques.)	If the open method will be used, apply a light pressure wrap (using Kling) for 1 hour to assist with hemostasis. Remove the wrap and reapply topical antimicrobial cream as appropriate.

Fig. 31–12 (*A*) Escharotomy of medial aspect of lower extremity. (*B*) Escharotomies of thorax.

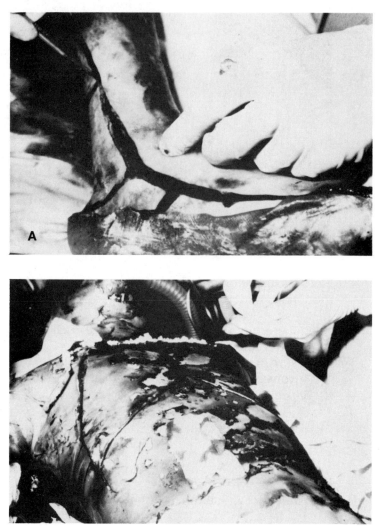

Fig. 31–13 Using clamps and microfibrillar collagen to obtain hemostasis.

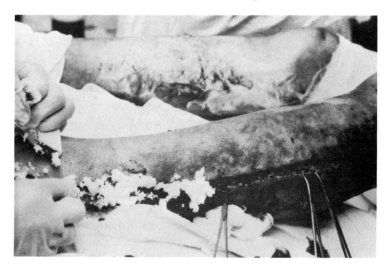

EVALUATION PHASE

ANTICIPATED OUTCOMES	NURSING ACTIONS
Increase in arterial circulation to distal extremities	Document the client's response to the procedure. Note and document the return of peripheral pulses. Evaluate the client's condition for relief of deep, aching pain of the extremity.

PRODUCT AVAILABILITY

HEMOSTATIC AGENTS

United States Pharmacopeia (Thrombin)
Parke–Davis (Thrombostat; available in 1,000-u, 5,000-u, 10,000-u, 20,000-u vials)
Armour Pharaceutical (Thrombinar; available in 1,000 u to 50,000 u vials)
Avicon Inc. — Microfibrillar collagen hemostat (Avitene; available in 1-g and 5-g jars)
Deseret (Oxycel)
Upjohn (Gelfoam)

Contracture prevention protocol

Objectives
To prevent the development of thermal-wound contractures
To maintain the functional position of the thermally injured area

ASSESSMENT PHASE

- Does the client have thermal injuries over joints? Wounds over joints predispose the client to the development of burn-wound contractures.
- Does the client have anterior neck burns? These predispose the client to flexion contracture of the neck.

PRECAUTIONS

- **Complete immobilization of the involved joints while maintaining the anatomic (functional) position may result in ankylosis (freezing) of the joint. Alternate the use of splints with ROM exercises and active use of the injured part.**
- **Clients will naturally assume a comfortable position, one which results in the least stretch of the wound. This causes flexion contractures.**

PLANNING PHASE

EQUIPMENT

NECK, HEAD, AND EARS

Small towel roll or short pediatric mattress placed on top of regular mattress
Foam doughnut

SHOULDERS

Shoulder boards, overbed tables, or abduction splints

ELBOWS

Extension splints

HANDS

Volar positioning splints
4×4s
Gauze roller bandages — 2

TRUNK

Towel or sheet roll

HIPS

Trochanter rolls

KNEES

Extension splints

ANKLES AND FEET

Footboard or dorsiflexion splints
Foam heel protectors

CLIENT/FAMILY TEACHING

- Discuss the importance and purpose of splinting and positioning. Elicit the cooperation of the client and family in the rehabilitation program.
- Assure the client that pain medication will be given to decrease discomfort as needed.
- Encourage the client to perform as many activities of daily living (ADL) as possible to maintain function. Explain that the splints will be applied at intervals and are worn during periods when the client is asleep.

IMPLEMENTATION PHASE

NURSING ACTIONS	RATIONALE/AMPLIFICATION
1. Place client in supine position, which maximizes wound stretch and maintains functional position.	
a. For burns of neck, head, and ears,	
(1) Extend neck by using small towel roll or short mattress on top of regular mattress.	Do not place a pillow under the client's head. Use a towel roll if the client has respiratory or spinal problems.
(2) Place foam doughnut under client's head to prevent pressure on external ears.	Burned ears are susceptible to costochondritis, which may be encouraged with pressure.
b. For burns of shoulders, abduct shoulders to 90° to 110° using shoulder boards, overbed tables, or abduction splints (Fig. 31–14).	
c. For burns of elbows, position anterior elbow burns fully extended with palms facing upward.	Splint the elbow with an extension splint if ordered. Prevent flexion of the elbow by frequently encouraging

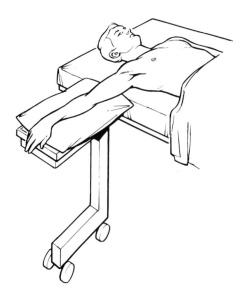

Fig. 31–14 Abduction of shoulder on overbed table.

d. For burns of hands, splint with volar positioning splint, or position client's hand holding gauze roller bandage, and wrap with roller bandage.

Pad the splint with gauze to prevent pressure on the burn wound. Wrap the digits individually to prevent "webbing" of the adjacent burn surfaces. Encourage the client to alternately flex and extend the metacarpal and interphalangeal joints. Encourage thumb to finger opposition ROM.

the client to keep his elbows extended. Monitor the client's condition for the development of ulnar palsy in the noncompliant client. This is caused by flexion and compression of the posterior elbow.

e. For burns of the trunk, position torso in proper alignment. Place sheet or towel roll lengthwise along spine.

This prevents internal rotation of the shoulders.

f. For burns of hips, abduct thighs approximately 15°.

Prevent external rotation of the thighs by using trochanter rolls.

g. For burns of knees, apply extension splints or position with knees extended with patellae facing upward.

External rotation of the thighs and flexion of the knees (frog-leg postion) places pressure on the lateral fibula head and can result in peroneal nerve palsy.

h. For burns of the ankles and feet, position feet in dorsiflexion (90°) by using footboard or dorsiflexion splints. Apply foam heel protectors.

This prevents plantar flexion, which may result in the shortening of the Achilles tendon.

2. Position client prone, giving attention to following:

a. Shoulders. Abduct shoulders and position arms above the head (keeping the elbows extended).

Alternate periods of positioning and avoid prolonged supine positioning to prevent brachial nerve palsy.

b. Feet. Allow feet to dorsiflex 90° over edge of mattress.

RELATED NURSING CARE

NURSING ACTIONS	RATIONALE/AMPLIFICATION
1. Encourage client to comply with exercise and positioning program.	
2. Encourage client to perform active ROM exercises and assist with passive ROM every 4 hours to 6 hours while client is awake.	Do not exercise joints that have exposed bone or tendon until surgical coverage is obtained. Dry tendons are brittle and can be damaged if they are exercised. Keep exposed tendons moist until they are covered.
3. Apply splints at nap times and at bedtime.	Flexion and stiffening tends to occur most often during sleep.
4. Change client's position frequently and alternate periods of ambulation and sitting.	

EVALUATION PHASE

ANTICIPATED OUTCOME	NURSING ACTIONS
Maintenance of function of thermally injured areas of body	Evaluate and document contracture prevention protocol. Evaluate the function of the involved joints.

PRODUCT AVAILABILITY

SPLINTS

Fred Sammons Inc. (Orthoplast preformed splints)
Roylan Medical Products (Polyform/Ezeform preformed splints)

Infection control protocol

Objectives
To monitor and control bacterial proliferation in the burn wound
To prevent colonization of the wound by β-hemolytic streptococci
To prevent septicemia caused by nosocomial infection

ASSESSMENT PHASE

- What are the client's baseline vital signs? Hyperthermia and tachycardia generally occur initially with local infections. Hypothermia may occur with sepsis.
- Is there any evidence of wound infection? Cellulitis, necrotic lesions, foul odor, and purulent exudate are indicators of wound infection.
- What is the pattern of serial white blood cell counts? Leukopenia may be a side-effect of certain medications (*e.g.,* silver sulfadiazine). Leukocytosis generally occurs with local infection; leukopenia may occur with overwhelming sepsis.
- What is the client's clinical status? Systemic manifestations of sepsis include hypotension, tachycardia, tachypnea, paralytic ileus, altered sensorium, thrombocytopenia, hyperglycemia, glycosuria, metabolic acidosis, and hypoxia.

PRECAUTIONS

- **Systematic invasion of the burn wound by bacteria occurs through the lymphatic system, not through the bloodstream. Blood cultures may continue to be negative even when a fatal infection is present.**

PLANNING PHASE

SUBESCHAR CLYSIS

EQUIPMENT

Solution administration sets (volutrols) — 5 or more
Antibiotic (as ordered; amount will depend on sensitivity reports)
0.45% normal saline or 0.9% normal saline IV infusion
22-gauge needles — 20 or more
Saline solution
Iodophor sponges
Sterile 4 $\times$ 4s
Sterile gloves
Cap, mask, gown
Rubber bands
IV stand

BURN-WOUND BIOPSY

Scalpel
No. 11 blade
Sterile dissecting forceps
Sterile specimen container
Iodophor solution
Sterile 4 $\times$ 4s
Nonsterile gloves
Hemostatic agent

SYSTEMIC ANTIBIOTIC THERAPY

Antibiotic (as ordered)
Iodophor solution

ENVIRONMENTAL INFECTION CONTROL

Reverse isolation supplies
Gowns
Caps, masks
Nonsterile gloves
Antiseptic hand wash

CLIENT/FAMILY TEACHING
- Discuss the procedure and the reasons for subeschar clysis, wound biopsies, and IV antibiotics.
- Explain the reason for reverse isolation to the client and family. Demonstrate to family members the procedures for putting on a gown and proper use of the cap, mask, and gloves. Encourage the family to comply with isolation procedures and inform them of the danger of exposing the client to family members with upper respiratory infections and flulike viruses.

IMPLEMENTATION PHASE

NURSING ACTIONS	RATIONALE/AMPLIFICATION

WOUND INFECTION CONTROL PRECAUTIONS

1. Wash your hands with antimicrobial soap before all procedures.

Frequent, proper handwashing reduces the risk of cross-contamination.

2. Put on cap, mask, and gown for all contact with client. Use sterile gloves for all procedures involving direct contact with wound. Use nonsterile gloves for procedures involving indirect contact.

3. Use strict aseptic technique when applying dressings, taking care not to contaminate jar of antimicrobial cream. Take precautions to prevent cross-contamination from one body area to another.

4. Provide meticulous oral and perineal care daily.

Meticulous oral and perineal care decreases the risk of wound contamination from normal body flora.

5. Trim or shave hair from burned areas; shave facial hair of male client with facial burns daily.

Trim or shave hair to decrease the possibility of contamination by organisms residing around hair follicles.

6. Administer subeschar antibiotic clysis when ordered.

Subeschar clysis deposits antibiotics directly into the subeschar space. It is indicated for burn-wound sepsis or control of bacterial proliferation, and it aids in separating the eschar from the burn wound.

   a. Premedicate client with pain medication.

   b. Prepare solution as ordered (carrier fluid and antibiotic).

Usually, the maximum daily dosage of antibiotic is ordered.

   c. Divide total amount of solution into 100-ml aliquots (portions). Fill the volutrols aseptically.

If the amount of carrier solution ordered is 500 ml, fill five volutrols with 100 ml each.

   d. Suspend volutrols from IV stand, using rubber bands as hangers.

   e. Prime volutrol tubings and cap each with 22-gauge needle.

   f. Put on sterile gloves. Cleanse topical agent from area to be treated using sterile saline-soaked 4 × 4s. Wipe needle insertion sites with iodophor sponges.

   g. Insert 22-gauge needles at 45-degree angles into the eschar at 15-cm intervals (Fig. 31–15).

   h. Infuse 25 ml of solution into each area. Change needles and rotate sites until entire amount of solution has been delivered.

This amount of solution covers an area in the subeschar space that is approximately 8-cm square.

   i. Reapply topical agent when clysis is concluded.

Fig. 31–15 Subeschar clysis setup.

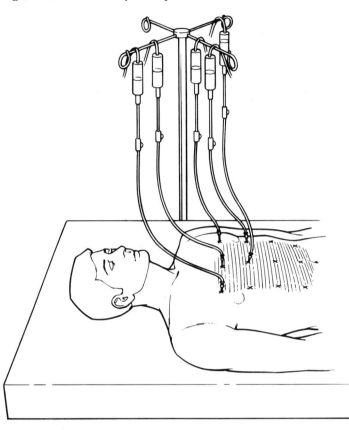

j. Dispose of all contaminated equipment appropriately.

k. Document area infused, type and amount of fluid and antibiotic, appearance of eschar, and client tolerance of procedure.

Note the infusion on the intake and output record also.

7. Obtain burn-wound biopsies three times per week from representative areas of burn wound.

Biopsies provide information about the type and amount of invading organisms (bacteria, fungi, yeast), and about the efficacy of topical antimicrobial therapy, subeschar antibiotic clysis, and systemic antibiotic therapy.

a. Open all supplies at bedside.

b. Put on sterile gloves. Remove topical agents with saline-soaked 4 × 4s.

c. Cleanse area to be excised with iodophor solution. Rinse residual iodophor from wound with saline-soaked 4 × 4s.

d. Using scalpel, make two parallel incisions that are 1 cm to 2 cm long and 0.5 cm apart.

Full-thickness samples of eschar are excised and sent to the laboratory for quantitative and qualitative analysis.

e. Using forceps, lift specimen and excise it from subcutaneous tissue. Include minute portion of unburned tissue. Place specimen in sterile container and transport to laboratory (Fig. 31–16).

The specimen will generally weigh between 20 mg and 50 mg. Qualitative analysis and identification of the organisms will be completed in 24 hours; sensitivity reports are ready in 48 hours.

f. Control excess bleeding from site with digital pressure or hemostatic agent. Dispose of contaminated supplies appropriately.

Fig. 31–16 Obtaining burn-wound biopsy.

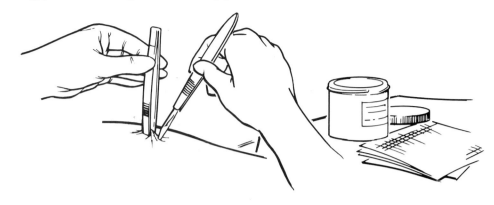

g. Document time and site of biopsy excision, amount of bleeding, hemostasis, and client tolerance of procedure.

SYSTEMIC ANTIBIOTIC THERAPY

1. Provide meticulous pulmonary toilet every 2 hours to 4 hours. Instruct client to turn, cough, and breathe deeply at least every 2 hours. Administer intermittent positive pressure breathing (IPPB) as ordered (see Chap. 19, "Airway Management"). Administer bronchodilators as ordered.

The risk of pneumonia is increased in the client with respiratory injury, tube feedings, artificial airways, or central nervous system (CNS) depression caused by analgesics.

2. Cleanse urinary meatus with iodophor solution every 6 hours if indwelling urinary catheter is in place.

Cleanse the urinary meatus to decrease the risk of a urinary tract infection.

3. Inspect burned ears daily for signs of costochondritis, such as redness, foul odor, protrusion from head, necrotic appearance, and intense pain.

The ears can be a source of systemic sepsis. Report signs of costochrondritis to the physician.

4. Inspect IV sites daily for signs of phlebitis, such as redness, swelling, pain, and localized warmth.

IV sites can be a source of systemic sepsis. Insert a new IV line and discontinue the present IV line.

5. Obtain following cultures as indicated: sputum, urine, wound, IV sites, and IV catheter tips.

6. Administer antibiotics as required.

Antibiotics are ordered on the basis of sensitivity reports.

7. Monitor renal function studies for clients receiving aminoglycosides.

Renal toxicity is a side-effect of aminoglycosides.

8. Support vital systems as indicated during acute septic shock period.

ENVIRONMENTAL INFECTION CONTROL

1. Place client on reverse isolations.

A private room is most conducive to decreasing cross-contamination. Use of laminar-flow isolation units have been found to decrease exogenous organisms.

a. Wear cap that completely covers hair, mask over nose and mouth, and gown for each contact with client.

b. Monitor compliance with isolation procedure for all persons who come into contact with client.

c. Keep handwashing supplies near client's room.

2. Monitor daily environmental cleaning. Damp dust high and low places in client's room. Damp mop floors. Dispose of trash properly and dispose of uneaten food. Store bedside snacks in closed containers. Keep cut flowers and potted plants outside room.

Do not permit open outside windows. If window screens are unavailable, keep the client's door closed continuously.

EVALUATION PHASE

ANTICIPATED OUTCOMES	NURSING ACTIONS
1. Prevention of nosocomial infections	Monitor and document the appearance of the wound with each dressing. Monitor the client's vital signs every 4 hours. Evaluate white blood cell count and platelets daily. Evaluate the color and appearance of IV sites, sputum, and urine daily for signs of infection. Monitor daily chest films. Monitor culture and sensitivity reports.
2. Prevention of burn-wound sepsis	Monitor isolation and aseptic techniques.
3. Control of bacterial colonization	Evaluate wound-dressing techniques to prevent the contamination of burn wounds from one site to another. Different organisms may be cultured from different sites on the same client.

SELECTED REFERENCES

Baxter CR, Curreri PW, Marvin JA: The control of burn wound sepsis by the use of quantitative bacterial studies and subeschar clysis with antibiotics. Surg Clin North Am 53(6):1509–1518, December 1973

Dowling M: Developing a Nursing Care Plan. In Wagner M (ed): Care of the Burn-Injured Patient: A Multidisciplinary Involvement, Littleton, MA, PSG Publishing Co., Inc., 1981

Johnson C, Cain V: Burn care: The rehabilitation guide. Am J Nurs 85(1):48–50, January 1985

Kenner C: Burn injury. In Kenner C, Grizetta C, and Dossey B: Critical Care Nursing: Body–Mind–Spirit, 2nd ed. Boston, Little, Brown, 1985

Kenner C: Patients with Thermal Injuries. In Beyers M, Dudas S (eds): The Clinical Practice of Medical Surgical Nursing, 2nd ed. Boston, Little, Brown, 1984

Robertson KE, Cross P, Terry J: Burn care: The crucial first days. Am J Nurs 85(1):29–45, January 1985

32

Positioning/immobility techniques

PRESSURE SORE MANAGEMENT

BACKGROUND

There are many terms and treatments used in the prevention and care of pressure sores. The term *decubitus* is defined as "the act of lying down." The terms *decubitus ulcer* and *bedsore* both give the impression that these lesions are acquired from lying in bed. Although this frequently occurs, there are many other ways that pressure causes skin breakdown due to cellular necrosis. It is not unusual to see lesions caused by sitting, an improperly fitting prosthesis, or undue pressure from a cast.

A bedsore or decubitus ulcer can easily be misunderstood by clients and families. When the term pressure sore is used, it is more likely to convey the meaning and understanding that pressure (from any source) causes problems and should be avoided.

Each pressure sore should be classified as stage I, II, III, or IV, and then a systematic approach to treatment should be initiated. In many institutions there are no set rules for identifying, assessing, and managing the at-risk client. There may be a vague term such as "decubitus care" on the Kardex. Often the result is that the client is subjected to a variety of treatment methods.

Although methods such as heat lamps, povidone–iodine (Betadine), sugar, egg whites, and so forth do eventually work in many cases, the trend is to promote a moist, physiologically compatible environment within the wound. There are several studies that show that use of transparent dressings, hydroactive dressings, absorption dressings, and other similar products promote wound healing better than do the drying methods that are traditionally used. When necrotic tissue is present, these products often eliminate the need for surgical debridement. There are also enzymatic debridement ointments that can be used.

A moist environment in the wound prevents eschar formation and tissue desiccation, allowing a more rapid epithelial migration. There is also less trauma to the newly formed granulation tissue during routine care of the pressure sore. If one stops to consider that it is abnormal for any tissue below the epidermis to be dry, it makes sense that a moist environment would enhance wound healing. Epithelialization occurs more slowly in the presence of local tissue dehydration and when physical, chemical or bacteriologic wound complications are present.

Pressure sores can take months and even years to heal. Not only are time and money important issues, but pressure sores may even cause the death of the client. The threat of septicemia, nutritional imbalances, and energy expenditure can be significant in the client who has a pressure sore of any severity. Early and frequent assessment, the use of prevention protocols with every at-risk client, and early intervention when a pressure sore does occur will enhance successful treatment.

Pressure sore prevention protocol

Objectives
To determine which clients are at risk of developing pressure sores
To initiate the prevention protocol when appropriate

ASSESSMENT PHASE

- What is the client's nutritional level? Is enteral or parenteral hyperalimentation indicated? Adequate nutrition promotes healing.
- What is the client's level of mobility? Spontaneous movement aids blood flow to dependent parts. Are there mobility restrictions (*e.g.,* protheses)?
- Is the client incontinent of feces or urine?
- Is the client alert? Are the client and family willing to take an active role in care?
- Does the client exhibit additional health-care needs? Multiple problems (*e.g.,* diabetes, pulmonary infections) increase risk factors.
- Is the client thin or obese? Either condition causes increased pressure over bony prominences (Fig. 32–1).

Fig. 32–1 Assess all bony prominences.

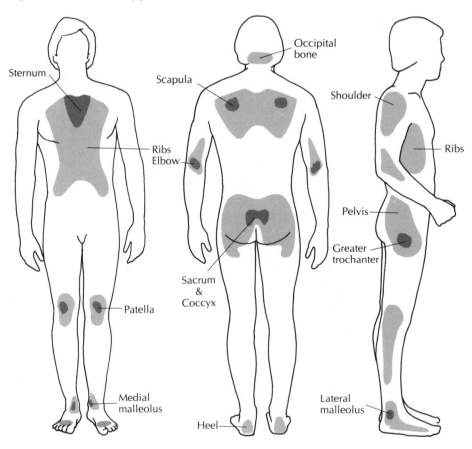

PRECAUTIONS

- **Reevaluate the client if the client's general condition deteriorates.**
- **If enteral feedings are started, monitor for diarrhea.**

PLANNING PHASE

EQUIPMENT

Pressure sore assessment form (See example of pressure sore evaluation form.)

CLIENT/FAMILY TEACHING

- Discuss the principles of how pressure causes a lack of blood flow to an area, resulting in cellular necrosis.

Pressure sore assessment form. (© Dynamic Dimensions in Health Care, Columbia, MD. Reprinted with permission)

PRESSURE SORE EVALUATION
Profiling the Patient "At Risk"
(on admission, weekly and p.r.n.)

ASSESSMENT Identify any patient at risk to develop pressure sores by assessing the six clinical condition parameters and assigning a score. Patients with a score of 8 or above should be considered at risk to develop pressure sores. Initiate prevention protocol.

Clinical Condition Parameters	Score
General Physical Condition (health problem)	
Good (minor)	0
Fair (major but stable)	1
Poor (chronic/serious-not stable)	2
Level of Consciousness (to commands)	
Alert (responds readily)	0
Lethargic (slow to respond)	1
Semi-comatose (responds only to verbal or painful stimuli)	2
Comatose (no response to stimuli)	3
Activity	
Ambulant without assistance	0
Ambulant with assistance	2
Chairfast	4
Bedfast	6
Mobility (extremities)	
Full active range	0
Restricted movement (moves with limited assistance)	2
Moves only with assistance	4
Immobile	6
Incontinence (bowel and/or bladder)	
None	0
Occasional (less than 2 per 24 hrs.)	2
Usually (more than 2 per 24 hrs.)	4
Total (no control)	6
Nutrition (for age and size)	
Good (eats/drinks adequately - 50% or more of meal)	0
Fair (eats/drinks inadequately - 50% or less)	1
Poor (unable/refuses to eat/drink - less than 50%)	2
Total:	

DOCUMENTATION Circle location of ulcer on figure at left. Number ulcer as and when seen. Record ulcer as and when seen.

Stage I   Reddened area
II   Blister, skin break
Stage III   Skin break exposing subcutaneous tissue
IV   Skin break exposing muscle and bone

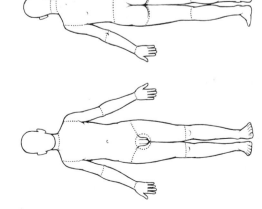

DATE				
Location				
Stage (I, II, III, or IV)				
Appearance*				
Size (cm.)				
Drainage**				
Odor**				
Inflammation				
Undermining				
Comments				

*p = pink/red   s = slough   e = eschar   **s = serosanguineous   p = purulent   0 = none   ***0 = none   m = mild   f = foul

- Discuss the purpose of initial and ongoing assessment during the course of the illness or debilitation.
- Stress that assessment should continue after discharge for the client who is at risk. Teach the client and family how to assess for pressure areas.
- Inform the client or a family member of the purpose and importance of each clinical-condition parameter.
- Encourage active participation and return demonstration of assessment for pressure sores by the client or a family member.
- Stress basic skin care, adequate nutrition, fluid and electrolyte balance, and exercise.

IMPLEMENTATION PHASE

NURSING ACTIONS	RATIONALE/AMPLIFICATION
1. Thoroughly review medical record for information concerning health needs and history of client.	Admission diagnosis, height, weight, diet, general state of health, and symptoms are important background information.
2. Assess client's general physical condition.	The number of health problems increases the client's risk factors.
3. Determine level of consciousness and degree of alertness.	Determine at what level the client will be able to follow directions and participate in care.
4. Assess degree of activity client will have.	Encourage the maximum amount of activity possible according to the client's condition. Use pressure relief devices when indicated.
5. Assess mobility of extremities. Encourage frequent range of motion (ROM) at least every 2 hours to 4 hours.	A physical therapy consult may be beneficial.
6. Assess bowel and bladder continence. Maintain clean, dry skin. Use skin care products to maintain skin integrity.	Control diarrhea if present. Consider a bowel training program, or an indwelling or external bladder catheter when indicated.
7. Assess nutritional level. Begin supplemental nutrition when appropriate.	Consider a dietitian consult. Monitor the client's weight and nutritional intake. Observe for signs of nutrition depletion (*e.g.,* diarrhea, wound output, poor appetite). Check laboratory values such as hemoglobin, hematocrit, and serum protein. Observe for negative nitrogen balance.
8. Assess all bony prominences.	
9. If pressure sore or reddened area that does not return to normal color in approximately 5 minutes is found, initiate the treatment protocol described in following section on Pressure Sore Treatment Protocol.	Early implementation of treatment increases the effectiveness of care and decreases the severity of damage.

RELATED NURSING CARE

NURSING ACTIONS	RATIONALE/AMPLIFICATION
1. If bowel or bladder incontinence is found, administer perianal care after each episode.	Avoid perianal skin breakdown.
2. Maintain soft, supple skin over entire body.	Avoid the overuse of soap. Use moisturizing products in the bath and provide back care during at least every shift.
3. Although most pressure sores occur over bony prominences, observe for less obvious locations of pressure sores.	Nasogastric tubes that are taped too tightly, armboards, side rails, and tubing can cause pressure sores in a short period.

EVALUATION PHASE

ANTICIPATED OUTCOMES	NURSING ACTIONS
1. Early detection of at-risk client and implementation of prevention protocol	Assess the client's condition on admission, weekly, and prn.
2. Increase in client and family awareness of their responsibility in prevention of pressure sores	Ensure ongoing education and reinforcement by nursing staff.

Pressure sore treatment protocol

Objective
To provide an effective, consistent, and systematic approach to the management and treatment of pressure sores

Fig. 32–2 Assessing wound for undermining. (*A*) Extent of wound can be determined with a cotton swab and marked with a magic marker. (*B*) Measure and record diameter of pressure sore.

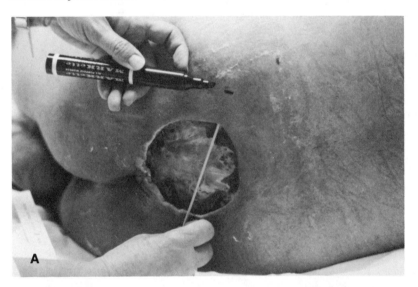

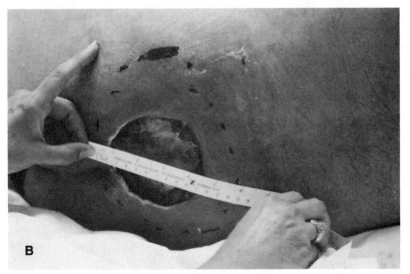

ASSESSMENT PHASE
- Does the client have adequate nutritional support? Enteral or parenteral hyperalimentation may be necessary.
- Is the client able to follow directions and to understand the reasons for breakdown and consequent treatment?
- Is the client incontinent of urine or feces?
- Are there multiple health-care needs that complicate treatment? Diabetes, pulmonary problems, casts, and traction increase risk factors.
- Is eschar, slough, or undermining present (Fig. 32–2)?
- Is a pressure relief device indicated? An alternating pressure air mattress, a water bed, air-fluidized therapy, or kinetic therapy is often indicated (see following sections on Air-Fluidized Therapy and Kinetic Therapy.)

PRECAUTIONS
- **Cellular necrosis can begin in the at-risk client in less than 1 hour.**
- **All pressure sores are contaminated, but few are actually infected. Although sterile technique is usually not indicated, adherence to clean technique is mandatory to prevent further introduction of contaminants into the wound.**
- **Occlusive dressings are contraindicated when clinical infection exists.**
- **Wounds secrete an exudate that is frequently mistaken for pus.**
- **The eschar covering is often mistaken for a scab and is incorrectly thought to protect the wound. *Pressure sores cannot be staged if eschar is present.***
- **An eggcrate mattress should be considered a comfort item only, because it is not adequate for pressure relief.**

PLANNING PHASE

EQUIPMENT

Wound dressing
Pressure sore flow sheet (See example of pressure sore flow sheet.)
Pressure relief device (if appropriate)

CLIENT/FAMILY TEACHING
- Explain the role of nutrition in wound healing.
- Discuss the importance of good skin care over the entire body. Encourage frequent use of moisturizing lotions to maintain soft, supple skin.
- Stress the avoidance of irritants such as soaps, chemicals, perspiration, fecal and/or urinary incontinence.
- Promote active and passive exercise and discuss the role of exercise in prevention and treatment of pressure sores.

IMPLEMENTATION PHASE

NURSING ACTIONS	RATIONALE/AMPLIFICATION
1. Assess pressure sore and determine if it is stage I, II, III, or IV.	Consult other health-team members (*e.g.,* enterostomal therapist or dietitian).
2. Document objective findings on pressure sore flow sheet (see sample pressure sore flow sheet).	Ensure accurate and consistent use of flow sheet. Reevaluate treatment as pressure sore changes.
3. Thoroughly cleanse wound.	If pink granulation base is present, use physiological solution such as saline or water to minimize damage to the new tissue.
	If necrotic debris is present in the wound, cleanse with antiseptic solution (hydrogen peroxide, povidine–iodine). Then rinse thoroughly with normal saline or water. Use antiseptic sparingly on healthy tissue not protected by dermis to prevent damage to migrating epithelial cells.

Pressure sore flow sheet. (© Dynamic Dimensions in Health Care, Columbia, MD. Reprinted with permission)

Instructions: Write in schedule of care beneath each title. Use product names where applicable. Date column daily. Initial each shift indicating that patient was evaluated and care was provided according to schedule.

Patient Name _____

Date							
Pressure Relief							
Skin Care							
Patient Movement							
Nutritional Care							
Patient Teaching							
Cleansing							
Treatment							
Covering							

4. Debride wound if necessary to remove necrotic tissue, eschar, or slough. Sharp debridement (scalpel, scissors) followed by enzymatic therapy is most effective method. Enzymatic agents include casein (Travase), and fibrinolysin and deoxyribonuclease (Elase).

5. Choose type of wound products suited to stage and degree of drainage.

Necrotic tissue promotes bacterial growth and causes an unpleasant odor. Whirlpool therapy is beneficial. Before using enzymatic agents, rinse the wound of antiseptic. Follow product instructions. Discontinue use of enzymatic agents when pink granulation base is present.

Follow all package directions and precautions.

a. *Absorption dressings* are used for wounds with excessive drainage (usually stages III and IV). Change at least daily.

An absorption dressing helps to clean, deodorize, and maintain moisture in the wound and to absorb excess wound fluid.

b. *Hydroactive dressings* should be changed every 5 days to 7 days or if gel leaks around edges (usually stages I, II, and III).

The hydroactive dressing interacts with the wound fluid to form a gel that maintains a moist environment and protects the wound.

c. *Nontransparent occlusive dressings* should be changed every 5 days to 7 days or if fluid leaks around edges (usually stages I, II, and III).

A nontransparent dressing maintains a moist environment and protects the wound.

d. *Semipermeable transparent adhesive film* should be changed every 5 days to 7 days or if leakage occurs (usually stages I and II).

Fluid that collects under the film can be aspirated to reduce leakage around the edges.

6. Monitor progress of treatment.

If improvement is not noted, try another method that provides a moist environment for the wound yet keeps the environment outside the wound clean and dry.

7. Obtain culture and sensitivity of fresh wound drainage if client exhibits symptoms of infection. (Do not mistake normal wound fluid for pus.)

Cleanse the wound thoroughly and rinse well with normal saline or water. Compress the edges of the wound to obtain fresh drainage. Send drain to laboratory immediately.

RELATED NURSING CARE

NURSING ACTIONS	RATIONALE/AMPLIFICATION
1. Observe for additional pressure sores.	Clients frequently develop more than one pressure sore.
2. Ensure accurate and consistent use of flow sheet.	Use of the flow sheet enables effective monitoring of wound progress and concise, objective documentation that is easily accessible.

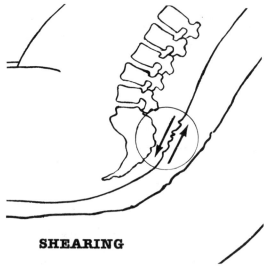

Fig. 32–3 Shearing occurs when client is pulled upward in bed over sheet.

SHEARING

3. Avoid shearing action when changing client's position and when pulling client up in bed (Fig. 32–3).

Encourage the client to use the overhead bar with a trapeze bar when appropriate. The use of a draw sheet is helpful. Avoid wrinkles in the bed linen.

EVALUATION PHASE

ANTICIPATED OUTCOMES	NURSING ACTIONS
1. Decrease in severity of tissue damage	Begin the treatment protocol immediately.
2. Improvement in wound healing	Use techniques that provide a moist environment inside the wound yet keep the client clean and dry and with soft, supple skin.
3. Early identification of at-risk client and monitoring of risk factors	Reevaluate and assess the client's condition on an ongoing basis using the flow sheet.
4. Instruction of client or family member in principles of pressure sore prevention and treatment	

PRODUCT AVAILABILITY

DRESSINGS

American Pharmaseal (HydraGran absorbent dressing)
Bard Home Health Division (Bard absorption dressing)
ConvaTec, A Division of E.R. Squibb and Sons, Inc. (DuoDerm hydroactive dressing, Stomahesive skin barrier)
Hollister, Inc., (Thin Film transparent dressing, Hollihesive skin barrier)
United, Division of Howmedica, Inc. (Uniflex transparent dressing and skin care kit)

FLOW SHEETS

Dynamic Dimensions in Health Care, Columbia, MD

ENZYMATIC AGENTS

Flint Pharmaceutical Company (Travase)
Parke–Davis Pharmaceutical Company (Elase)

SELECTED REFERENCES

Alterescu V: Debriding Enzymes. Journal of Enterostomal Therapy II(3):122–124, May/June 1984

Broadwell DC, Jackson BS: Principles of Ostomy Care. St. Louis, CV Mosby, 1982

Coodley E et al: Management of decubitus ulcers. Compr Ther 9(7):61–66, 1983

Cooper DM et al: Guide to Wound Care. Libertyville, IL, Hollister Inc., 1983

Fowler E: Pressure sores: A deadly nuisance. J Gerontol Nurs 8:(12):680–685, December 1982

Fowler E and Goupil DL: Comparison of the wet-to-dry dressing and a copolymer starch in the management of debrided pressure sore. Journal of Enterostomal Therapy, 11(1):22–25, January/February 1984

Spence WR, Bates I: New Absorption Dressing for Secreting Ulcers. Dallas, Texas Medical Association, Forum of Original Research, BHHD 127, 1981

PRESSURE CONTROL DEVICES

BACKGROUND

EFFECTS OF IMMOBILITY

Persons experiencing decreased mobility are predisposed to complications involving multiple body systems, including the skin and the pulmonary, cardiovascular, gastrointestinal, musculoskeletal, genitourinary, and psychological systems.

Tissue ischemia can develop within 20 minutes of continuous pressure; skin breakdown can occur within 1 hour to 2 hours. Atelectasis quickly develops because of the pooling of secretions in the lungs. Deep vein thrombosis due to venous stasis can result in pulmonary embolism. Decreased peristalsis causes problems with constipation. Muscle atrophy results from nonuse of muscles, and osteoporosis occurs with demineralization of the bone. Resorption of bone elevates serum calcium levels, which predispose the immobilized client to renal calculi. In addition, urinary stasis results in urinary tract infections. Prolonged immobility can also result in mental depression.

<table>
<tr><td>CURRENT PRESSURE
CONTROL DEVICES</td><td>Several methods are used to slow the onset of complications of immobility, including the use of foam-rubber mattresses, eggcrate mattresses, air or water mattresses, flotation pads, intermittent inflation mattresses, pillows, and rigorous turning schedules. CircOlectric beds and Stryker frames are used to prevent problems that are caused by immobility in clients with spinal injuries.*</td></tr>
</table>

CURRENT PRESSURE CONTROL DEVICES

Several methods are used to slow the onset of complications of immobility, including the use of foam-rubber mattresses, eggcrate mattresses, air or water mattresses, flotation pads, intermittent inflation mattresses, pillows, and rigorous turning schedules. CircOlectric beds and Stryker frames are used to prevent problems that are caused by immobility in clients with spinal injuries.*

ADVANCEMENTS IN PRESSURE CONTROL DEVICES

Recent advancements have been made in the delivery of nursing care to the immobilized client, including air-fluidized support therapy and kinetic therapy.

Air-fluidized support therapy. Air-fluidized support therapy (Clinitron, KINAIR) is useful in the treatment of clients receiving intensive therapy. The Clinitron support system is composed of a tank that is filled with 1500 to 2000 pounds of soda lime glass beads (microspheres). An air compressor draws ambient air into the system through a 5-micron filter and is then heated or cooled as desired. Air passes through a porous diffuser and rises through a 30-cm (12-inch) layer of microspheres, setting them in dry, fluidized motion. The system exerts 11 mm Hg of pressure or less, which is below capillary closure pressure, thus enabling continuous blood flow to all recumbent areas. The KINAIR provides controlled air suspension therapy through support of the body, which lies on cushions inflated with air. This system allows for low contact pressure on the skin and underlying tissues.

Other purported benefits of air-fluidized therapy include elimination of shear and friction forces, elimination of maceration, reduction or elimination of the need for narcotics or sedatives, and thermal control. Disadvantages include increased evaporative water losses, increased potential for pulmonary congestion, and the potential for microsphere leakage, which can result in pulmonary and corneal irritation because of the presence of foreign bodies.

Kinetic therapy. Activity has been found to be important to well-being and health. It has been determined that the average, healthy person moves or changes position during sleep approximately every 11 minutes. This has been defined as essential activity and is called the minimum physiologic mobility requirement (MPMR). Kinetic therapy provides a continuous side-to-side motion with a range of 124° every 3.5 minutes. This schedule meets the client's MPMR, thus decreasing the problems associated with immobility.

Air-fluidized therapy

Objectives
To prevent skin breakdown
To provide a clean air environment and to promote healing of skin lesions (burns, decubiti)
To increase the client's comfort
To provide stable support for orthopaedic alignment

ASSESSMENT PHASE

• Is the client at risk of developing pressure sores?
• Does the client have a condition that will benefit from air-fluidized therapy? Clients who have pressure sores, burns, fractures, multiple trauma, or who are comatose will be managed more easily on air-fluidized therapy.

PLANNING PHASE

EQUIPMENT

Air-fluidized bed
Foam wedge
Regular bed linen
Manufacturer's instruction manual

* Refer to King E, Wieck L, Dyer M: *Illustrated Manual of Nursing Techniques,* 3rd ed. Philadelphia, JB Lippincott, 1986, for techniques used with the CircOlectric bed and Stryker frame.

CLIENT/FAMILY TEACHING
- Explain the reason for placing the client on air-fluidized therapy and the expected benefits.
- Discuss the sensations that the client will experience. These include a gentle floating sensation with warmed air circulating through the filter sheet and linen, and a soft humming sound caused by the air compressor.

IMPLEMENTATION PHASE

NURSING ACTIONS	RATIONALE/AMPLIFICATION
1. Prepare Clinitron therapy unit. Turn on unit to fluidize it. Set temperature control at comfortable setting (between 32°C and 34.5°C).	Obtain the manufacturer's instruction manual. Prepare the unit before placing it in the client's room, because it takes 12 hours or more to reach the desired temperature range (27.7°C to 39.9°C). An alternative air-fluidized support system in KINAIR (Kinetic Concepts). Refer to the manufacturer's instruction manual for proper use.
2. Place client on air-fluidized therapy unit (Fig. 32–4).	

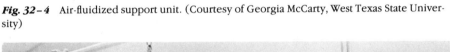

Fig. 32–4 Air-fluidized support unit. (Courtesy of Georgia McCarty, West Texas State University)

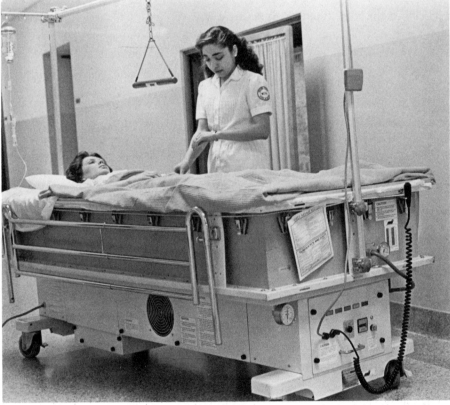

a. Place regular flat bed sheet on top of filter sheet.	Do not secure the sheet to avoid interfering with the flotation effect. Do not use plastic linen savers to avoid interfering with the circulation of clean, warm air.
b. Defluidize unit before transferring client in or out of unit.	This prevents possible damage to the diffuser board, which is contained within the tank.
c. Fluidize unit.	

3. Position client using bed sheet.

    a. Pull filter sheet loose from beneath client.

    b. Turn client by taking hold of hospital sheet at client's hip and shoulder.

    c. Pull client to side of unit.

    d. Turn client by pulling sheet upward and over.

    e. Defluidize unit to maintain position for procedural ease (*e.g.,* to give back care or intramuscular (IM) injection).

    f. Refluidize unit on completion of procedure.

    g. To leave client in side-lying position, cross top leg over bottom leg and use pillow to support top leg.

    h. Place client in semi-Fowler's position by using following method:

        (1) Place wedge in accessible position.

        (2) Pull client to head of unit using under sheet.

        (3) Hold under sheet at client's shoulders bilaterally and pull client up into sitting position, while simultaneously defluidizing unit.

        (4) Position wedge to provide back support. Make certain that wedge is resting on filter sheet, not on bed sheet.

        (5) Refluidize unit.

4. Position client for special procedures using following method:

    a. Place client in desired position.

    b. Defluidize unit while simultaneously pushing down into microsphere beads and creating well space in desired area. Continue pushing down into beads for 3 seconds to 5 seconds until unit hardens.

    c. Place client in Trendelenberg's position using following method:

        (1) Grasp sheet at level of client's hips bilaterally and pull up while simultaneously pushing down on pillow beneath client's head and shoulders. Defluidize unit while continuing to push down for 3 seconds to 5 seconds.

        (2) Remove pillow from beneath client's head. Place wedge under legs to obtain maximum elevation and support of legs.

Do not position the client when the unit is defluidized. This negates the purpose of the therapy.

This aids in the ease of moving the client and allows the sheets to move with the client, eliminating shear and friction forces.

You can turn the client toward or away from you.

The microspheres will conform to the client's body shape and will hold the client in the desired position. The unit automatically refluidizes after 30 minutes.

Use of a foam wedge provides four levels of elevation (13°, 20°, 30°, and 67°).

Depending on the client's condition, the client can assist using a trapeze bar.

The foam wedge remains in position more securely when it is placed directly on the filter sheet. To reposition the client, remove the wedge and repeat the maneuvers used to prevent shear and friction forces, which might be encountered if the client is pulled up on the wedge.

Special procedures include dressing changes or urinary bladder catheterizations.

d. Place client in position to perform cardiopulmonary resuscitation (CPR) using following method:

    (1) Hyperextend head by placing one hand on client's forehead and pushing downward while lifting back of neck and simultaneously defluidizing unit.

    (2) Begin CPR.

Unplug the unit to prevent automatic refluidizing in 30 minutes. A cardiac board is unnecessary. The first chest compression will compact the beads into a firm surface.

5. Transfer client to stretcher using following method:

a. Move client to side of unit.

b. Lift client using bed sheet while simultaneously defluidizing unit.

c. Ease client onto unit, which is now solid.

d. Move stretcher alongside unit and transfer client using bed sheet.

RELATED NURSING CARE

NURSING ACTIONS	RATIONALE/AMPLIFICATION
1. Protect unit from damage. Do not allow oils or petroleum- or silver-based products to absorb through filter sheet into tank.	Pad the filter sheet with absorbent material when damaging compounds are being used.
2. Do not allow client to smoke while unit is fluidized.	This protects the filter sheet from ashes.
3. Avoid pinning or clamping items to filter sheet.	
4. If leak develops, defluidize unit and wipe loose beads with damp towel. Damp mop floor immediately. Temporarily repair any leaks with adhesive tape. Notify maintenance representative.	Beads are very slippery and may cause a fall if they are left on the floor.
5. Encourage ROM exercises while client is receiving air-fluidized therapy.	Contractures of the extremities can develop when the client is in a comfortable position.
6. Monitor intake and output while air-fluidized therapy is being given.	Dehydration may occur because of increased evaporative water loss resulting from the continuous circulation of warm, dry air through the unit.
7. Perform pulmonary toilet as necessary (see Chap. 19, "Airway Management").	Aggressive pulmonary toilet is indicated for the client with pulmonary congestion.
8. Defluidize unit for firm support during chest physiotherapy.	

EVALUATION PHASE

ANTICIPATED OUTCOMES	NURSING ACTIONS
1. Prevention/resolution of skin breakdown	Monitor the integrity of the client's skin.
2. Promotion of comfort	Monitor vital signs, complaints of pain, and the need for narcotics and sedatives.

3. Control of temperature

Monitor the client's body temperature, and control the temperature of the unit. For control of hypothermia or hyperthermia, allow 1 hour for each .5°C to 1°C change in the bed temperature.

PRODUCT AVAILABILITY

CLINITRON THERAPY UNIT

Support Systems International

KINAIR

Kinetic Concepts

Kinetic therapy

Objectives

To stabilize fractures, particularly cervical fractures

To prevent skin breakdown through coninuous change of pressure distribution

To provide continuous postural drainage

To prevent thrombus formation while preventing venous stasis

To prevent the development of postural hypotension through the continuous physiologic effect on the vasculature

To reduce muscle wasting and resorption of bone

To reduce urinary stasis

ASSESSMENT PHASE

• Does the client have a condition that would benefit from kinetic therapy? Clients with spinal cord injury, head injury, and multiple trauma will benefit from kinetic therapy.

• Will the client need to be immobilized because of injuries? Stabilization of injuries while decreasing the severity of, or preventing the complications of, immobility is achieved with kinetic therapy.

• Is the client immobilized because of illness? Acute, progressively debilitating neurologic disorders such as Guillain–Barré syndrome and multiple sclerosis will benefit from kinetic therapy.

PRECAUTIONS

• **Clients with true claustrophobia may experience an acute exacerbation of claustrophobia while receiving kinetic therapy.**

• **Comatose clients who are easily agitated will become more agitated while receiving kinetic therapy because of the additional stimulation.**

• **Kinetic therapy can worsen severe diarrhea because kinetic therapy stimulates peristalsis.**

• **Adjust the angle of rotation to avoid weight bearing on the affected side for clients experiencing acute pain during rotation onto the injured side.**

PLANNING PHASE

EQUIPMENT

Kinetic treatment table

Foam supporter

Manufacturer's instruction manual

CLIENT/FAMILY TEACHING

• Explain the purpose of kinetic therapy and the anticipated benefits to the client.

• Describe the sensations that the client will experience. The client may feel a gentle, rocking, side-to-side motion as the table rotates approximately 62° from side to side. The client may also experience a sliding sensation. Tell the client and family of the safety aspects to reassure them that the client will not fall.

• Explain to the client that the kinetic therapy will be continuous, with the exception of special procedures (*e.g.,* feeding, bathing, chest physiotherapy).

IMPLEMENTATION PHASE

NURSING ACTIONS	RATIONALE/AMPLIFICATION

1. Prepare kinetic treatment table for client. Figure 32–5 illustrates positioning of client with clamps and pads in place.

Fig. 32–5 Kinetic treatment table in lateral rotation position.

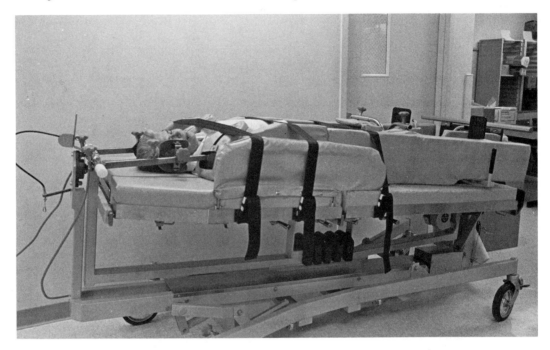

a. Lock table in horizontal position.

b. Lock wheels. Move all side supports to extreme lateral position, and then remove them from table.

Keep side supports separated to facilitate replacement.

c. Remove knee packs and abductor packs. Slide foot and knee assemblies to foot of table.

d. Loosen shoulder clamp assembly and swing it upright to vertical position. Retighten.

e. Cover cervical, thoracic, and rectal pads with disposable absorbent underpads.

2. Transfer client gently and smoothly to kinetic treatment table.

Be careful to maintain correct body alignment during transfer. Avoid skin injury when transferring across metal posts.

3. Position client on kinetic treatment table.

a. Center client on surface of table by aligning pubis, umbilicus, and nose with center post.

The client must be centrally positioned for proper balance.

b. Replace thoracic side supports with client's arms abducted to 90°.

Be careful to avoid placing the thoracic supports too snugly against the axilla to prevent brachial nerve palsy.

c. Adjust client's longitudinal position to allow 2.5 cm (1 inch) of space between axilla and side support.

d. Move thoracic side support medially to snugly support client's chest and lock cam arms securely.

e. Adjust knee assembly to position that is 3 cm to 5 cm above client's knees; lock cam handle into place.

f. Place foam leg support under each leg without allowing heels to touch foam surface.

Proper positioning of the foam leg support avoids pressure on the heels, preventing skin breakdown.

g. Place foot supports in foot assembly and adjust so that foot is supported in anatomic position. Lock foot assembly by closing cam handle.

The foot support is necessary to prevent foot drop, but should be left in place no longer than 2 hours at a time to prevent pressure sores on the soles of the feet.

h. Install abductor packs.

i. Place leg side supports and move them medially to fit snugly against client's hips.

j. Install knee packs; adjust them to rest 3 cm to 5 cm above client's knees.

k. Lower head and shoulder assembly into position and move medially to rest against client's head. Adjust shoulder pack to rest 3 cm to 5 cm above client's shoulders. Adjust head pack to prevent pressure on client's ears. Tighten head and shoulder assembly securely.

l. Place foam arm support under each arm, allowing hand to rest in anatomic position on rounded edge of support.

The foam arm support places the hand in the functional position and protects the ulnar nerve at the elbow from excessive pressure.

Fig. 32-6 Check pressure points before beginning rotation.

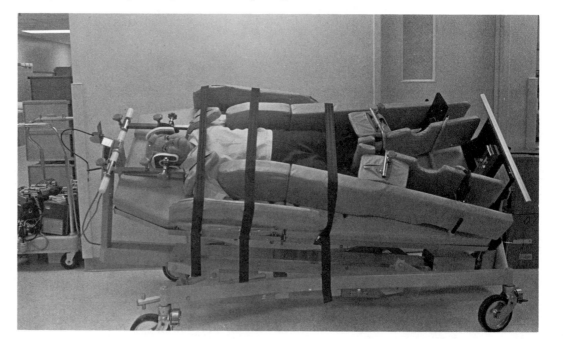

m. Install arm side supports.

n. Secure safety straps across client.

o. Place drainage tubes through appropriate holes.

Tubing for urinary bladder drainage and chest drainage can be positioned through the appropriate holes in the treatment table by lowering the appropriate hatch in the table.

p. Balance table.

Refer to the manufacturer's instruction manual.

q. Check pressure points with table in 62-degree position bilaterally (Fig. 32–6).

A space of 1.25 cm of the uppermost aspect of the body should be present to ensure complete pressure relief during rotation.

4. Start rotations.

Warn the client before beginning or stopping the rotation.

a. Plug table into the electric source.

b. Hold footboard firmly and pull out locking pin.

c. Push connecting arm cam handle into locking position, then rotate table slowly until connecting assembly locks into place.

This begins automatic rotation.

RELATED NURSING CARE

NURSING ACTIONS	RATIONALE/AMPLIFICATION
1. Bathe client daily with warm water and mild soap. Cleanse all surfaces of kinetic treatment table during bath with warm water and mild soap.	Rinse both the client and the treatment table thoroughly to remove soap residue and prevent contact dermatitis. Dry thoroughly. With the table in the extreme lateral position, drop the appropriate hatches to cleanse the posterior aspects of the client.
2. Assess client's skin every shift for areas of redness or blister formation.	Redness or blisters indicate incorrect position adjustment or wrinkled linen beneath the client.
3. Monitor healing of abrasions or pressure sores daily.	
4. Control hyperthermia with built-in fan on treatment table, in addition to sponging client with tepid water.	Monitor client's temperature every 4 hours. Leave the fan on unless the client is hypothermic and cannot maintain normal body temperature.
5. Monitor drainage systems (*e.g.,* bladder catheter) and note that proper clearance between table frame and drainage systems is present.	
6. Provide full ROM to all joints twice daily to prevent ankylosis of joints.	

EVALUATION PHASE

ANTICIPATED OUTCOMES	NURSING ACTIONS
1. Stabilization of fractures	Monitor the client's alignment and the table adjustments daily.
2. Prevention of complications of immobility	
a. Pressure sores	Monitor the skin condition daily. Check pressure points daily with the table in extreme lateral positions. Alternate the use of footboards every 2 hours.

b. Pulmonary congestion

Assess the respiratory system every shift. Perform pulmonary toilet as necessary, and provide chest physiotherapy as necessary. The table can be manually positioned to facilitate postural drainage.

c. Venous stasis

Monitor peripheral edema and peripheral pulses during each shift.

d. Constipation

Assess bowel sounds during each shift. Initiate bowel program for the client with spinal cord injury.

e. Urinary tract infection

Observe and note urine color and presence of sediment during each shift. Maintain the acidity of the urine to decrease the risk of urinary tract infection and urinary calculi by giving the client acidifying agents (*e.g.,* cranberry juice).

PRODUCT AVAILABILITY

KINETIC TREATMENT TABLE

Kinetic Concepts (Roto Rest kinetic treatment table)

SELECTED REFERENCES

Adelstein W, Watson P: Cervical spine injuries. J Neurosurg Nurs 15(2):65–71, April 1983

Milazzo V, Resh C: Kinetic nursing: A new approach to the problems. J Neurosurg Nurs 14(3):120–124, June 1982

Parish LC, Witkowski JA: Clinitron therapy and the decubitus ulcer: Preliminary dermatologic studies. Dermatology 19(9):517–518, November 1980

Sanchez DG, Bussey B, Tetorak M: How air fluidized beds revolutionize skin care. RN, June 1983, pp 46–48.

Scheulen JJ, Munster AM: Clinitron air fluidized support: An adjunct to burn care. Journal of Burn Care and Rehabilitation, July–August 1983, pp 271–275

VIII

Miscellaneous techniques

33

Safety techniques

Electric safety protocol

BACKGROUND

The critical care nurse, the biomedical technician, and the hospital that is purchasing equipment each have a responsibility in ensuring the electric safety of all who use electric equipment in the critical care unit. All hospitals should have stringent guidelines for purchasing and monitoring electric equipment. Regular function checks should be performed by a biomedical technician who is qualified to judge the equipment's effectiveness and safety. A record of safety checks should be visible on the equipment. The nurse must be informed of considerations and risks involved in working with electric equipment.

Refer to the manufacturer's instruction manual when using equipment for the first time to be aware of potential safety hazards. Report malfunctioning or broken equipment to the biomedical department, no matter how minute the problem is. An intact ground wire serves to carry escaping current away from the client. Consider each frayed cord or broken ground wire a potential killer.

MICROSHOCK

Clients with implanted transvenous devices such as pacemakers or indwelling cardiac, pulmonary artery, or arterial lines are referred to as electrically sensitive, because the skin barrier has been bypassed. These clients are at risk of being subjected to microshocks. A microshock is a low-voltage electric shock, generated from various grounding defects. These small currents of .1 ma or less are imperceptible to touch, yet if they are carried directly into the heart by a line filled with an electric conductor such as saline, they can induce ventricular fibrillation and cause death.

There are several easily identifiable sources of microshock in the critical care unit. Two-pronged plugs lacking a ground wire facilitate a direct pathway from the outlet to the client's heart if the right conditions exist (Fig. 33–1). A broken ground wire presents the same hazard as a lack of a ground wire. Staff members can be excellent conductors of electricity if they touch faulty equipment, the client, the client's bed, or each other at the same time (Fig. 33–2).

An indwelling pacemaker requires an electric impulse of 10 ma to cause contraction of myocardial muscle, yet an electric current of only .1 ma can induce ventricular fibrillation. The difference in the response of the myocardium to these stimuli results because of the type of current involved and because the pacemaker impulse is a controlled synchronous electric impulse that is emitted only one at a time. The electric current that can travel to the heart from grounding defects is an AC current, a common household current that is emitted in 60 cycles/second. The rapid, uncontrolled impulses of AC current are most likely to cause myocardial muscle to fibrillate. A 60-cycle pattern on the oscilloscope indicates a current leakage that could lead to microshock (see Fig. 1–11*B*).

Objective
To prevent injury to clients and personnel from electric equipment

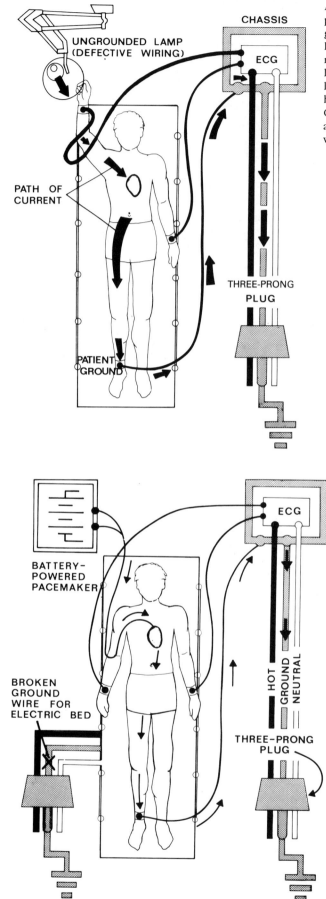

Fig. 33-1 Electrical hazard caused by providing alternative pathway for grounding current. As defectively wired lamp is touched, electricity that has accumulated in metal frame takes alternative low-resistance pathway and a potentially lethal current passes through patient's heart to ground lead. (After Directions in Cardiovascular Medicine. 7. The Heart and Electrical Hazards, p 22. Sommerville, NJ, Hoechst Pharmaceutical, 1973)

Fig. 33-2 An electrical hazard in the CCU. The nurse can complete circuit by simultaneously touching metal portion of electrical bed (which is leaking current) and external ends of patient's pacemaker catheter. Current flows from electrical bed to ECG ground through low-resistance pathway (pacemaker electrode) through patient's heart. (After Directions in Cardiovascular Medicine. 7. The Heart and Electrical Hazards, p 22. Sommerville, NJ, Hoechst Pharmaceutical, 1973)

ASSESSMENT PHASE
- Does any of the equipment have loose connections, frayed wires, or broken ground wires?
- Is the client in a nonelectric bed? Electric beds in the critical care area are an additional hazard.
- Is the client electrically sensitive because of indwelling lines or leads?
- Is wet linen present? This is an excellent conductor of electricity.
- Is water, blood, or fluid present on the floor?

PRECAUTIONS
- **If tingling, smoke, or sparks are noted when using equipment, remove the equipment from service.**

PLANNING PHASE

CLIENT/FAMILY TEACHING
- Instruct the client and family that there should be no equipment brought in from outside the hospital, because these are often improperly grounded and are sources of current leakage. Also, they often use two-pronged plugs.
- Instruct the client and family that smoking is not allowed if oxygen equipment is present. (No smoking is usually a policy in critical care units.)

IMPLEMENTATION PHASE

NURSING ACTIONS	RATIONALE/AMPLIFICATION
1. Use safety techniques described below during defibrillation.	
a. Make sure that conductive gel is *not* on paddle handles or smeared across client's chest.	The gel might function as a circuit for the discharge of current from the machine, causing the current to arc from paddle to paddle across the client's chest or to the hands of the nurse holding the paddles.
b. Avoid contact with bed, client, or electrode surface of paddles when defibrillating.	
c. Be certain that care-giver who is performing defibrillation is not standing in any blood, urine or saline.	All of these fluids are ionizable and can provide a path for electric current.
d. If Ambu bag is being used, stop ventilating client, shut off oxygen, and move away from bed during defibrillation.	A spark from the defibrillator could cause an explosion and fire in an oxygen-rich atmosphere.
e. Call ''all clear'' before discharging defibrillator.	Other personnel at the bedside should avoid contact with the bed or client to prevent accidental shock.
f. Use conductive gel or pad and apply enough force to ensure good skin contact during defibrillation.	A conductive agent and firm skin contact are essential to prevent arc or contact burns caused by improperly placed paddles.
g. Do not place paddles over electrocardiogram (ECG) monitoring electrodes.	This could divert the current and cause severe burns.
h. Test defibrillators daily for proper discharging.	
(1) Follow manufacturer's instructions for proper technique.	
(2) Never discharge current into air or by holding paddles together.	This may cause arcing or damage to the paddles or internal circuitry of the defibrillator.
2. Safety techniques for temporary transvenous pacemaker are as follows:	
a. Place client in nonelectric bed and use no electric appliances.	The catheter and electrodes of a transvenous pacemaker are excellent conductors of electricity, and a small amount of leakage of current from other electric appli-

b. Cover front panel of pacemaker with clear plastic cover or wrap.

c. Cover all catheter connections and external wires with rubber glove.

d. Wear rubber gloves when adjusting pacemaker settings or connections.

3. Safety techniques for indwelling cardiac, pulmonary artery, or arterial lines are as follows:

a. Check all cords and plugs for grounding defects.

b. Do not use metal stopcocks in lines.

4. To ensure electric safety with supplemental oxygen make sure that television is always at least 10 feet from and above bed of client receiving oxygen therapy.

5. Safety techniques for cardiac monitors are as follows:

a. Check for clean tracing on oscilloscope.

b. Do not place wet items such as wet towels, beverages, or solutions on top of monitors or other electric equipment.

6. Use general precautions described below to ensure electric safety.

a. Do not touch client and electric device at same time.

b. Touch bed rails before touching client with intravascular lines or pacemaker.

c. Ground all metal beds.

d. Do not use any equipment that has not been approved for use in hospital and that does not have visible inspection tag.

e. Do not remove plug from outlet by pulling on cord.

f. Do not use two-pronged extension cords or plugs in hospital. These bypass ground wire.

g. Use three-pronged extension cords only if absolutely necessary. Request biomedical department to extend length of cord so that this will not be necessary.

ances could be lethal because of the possibility of microshock.

This will prevent accidental changing of the pacemaker settings and act as an insulator from an electric conductor.

Rubber acts as an insulator.

Electric hazards begin at the transducers of these lines. Although the plastic tubing and catheters act as insulators, the column of fluid (especially saline) is an excellent conductor. The transducer site where current leakage is likely to enter.

If the metal stopcock comes in contact with a metal object that is not properly grounded, microshock can occur.

Oxygen is highly volatile, and television receivers have high voltage circuits in which arcing is common.

If 60-cycle interference occurs, make sure that all electrode pads have adequate conductive gel and good skin contact, all cables are intact with no loose wires, and all plugs are three-pronged and properly grounded. Evaluate for possible current leakage from a nearby machine. Water is a good conductor of electricity.

Stray current can flow through the care-giver and the client to ground.

This dissipates any static electricity.

Metal is a good conductor of electricity.

This fractures wires in the cord and causes shorting of the device.

If a three-pronged extension cord is used, tape the cord to the floor to prevent falls and damage to the plug.

h. Do not use "cheater" connectors that permit three-pronged plug to be used in two-pronged outlet.

This bypasses the ground.

i. Return any piece of equipment that has been dropped, even if it appears to be intact, to biomedical department for servicing.

EVALUATION PHASE

ANTICIPATED OUTCOME	NURSING ACTIONS
Prevention of electric shock to clients or personnel	Monitor the electric safety and inspection program. Evaluate nursing techniques for correct electric safety measures. Use manufacturer's instruction manuals. Provide in-service programs related to electric safety.

SELECTED REFERENCES
Buchsbaum WH, Goldsmith B: Electrical Safety in the Hospital. Oradell, NJ, Medical Economics Company, 1975

Hoenig SA, Scott DH: Medical Instrumentation and Electrical Safety: The View from the Nursing Station. New York, John Wiley, 1977

Miscellaneous infection control techniques (contact isolation, strict isolation, drainage/secretion precautions)

Objectives
To prevent the spread of multiresistant bacteria that have been judged to be of epidemiologic importance (contact isolation)
To prevent nosocomial infections that are spread through contact with infectious drainage or secretions (drainage/secretion precautions)
To prevent the transmission of highly contagious or virulent infections that are spread by direct contact or airborne methods (strict isolation)

ASSESSMENT PHASE

- Is a private room required? A private room is not necessary to implement drainage/secretion precautions.
- Is the client cooperative? Does the client practice good hygiene?
- Is the client incontinent? Does the client have an indwelling urinary device?
- Have multiresistant bacteria been cultured from the client (*e.g.,* resistant strains of *Pseudomonas, Serratia,* or *Klebsiella*)?
- What category of isolation/precautions is required? (See the lists of diseases requiring isolation or precautions.)

PLANNING PHASE

EQUIPMENT

Isolation cart
Isolation sign
    Contact isolation—orange
    Strict isolation—yellow
    Drainage/secretion precautions—green
Gowns
Gloves
Masks (not required for drainage/secretion precautions)

CLIENT/FAMILY TEACHING

- Inform the client and family of the precautions required and the reasons behind them.
- Assure the client that nursing care will not be compromised. Emphasize that it is the infectious agent that is being isolated—not the client.

Diseases or conditions requiring contact isolation*

Acute respiratory infections in infants and young children, including croup, colds, bronchitis, and bronchiolitis caused by respiratory syncytial virus, adenovirus, coronavirus, influenza viruses, parainfluenza viruses, and rhinovirus

Conjunctivitis, gonococcal, in newborns

Diphtheria, cutaneous

Endometritis, group A *Streptococcus*

Furunculosis, staphylococcal, in newborns

Herpes simplex, disseminated, severe primary or neonatal

Impetigo

Influenza, in infants and young children

Multiply-resistant bacteria, infection, or colonization (any site) with any of the following:

1. Gram-negative bacilli resistant to all aminoglycosides that are tested. (In general, such organisms should be resistant to gentamicin, tobramycin, and amikacin for these special precautions to be indicated.)
2. *Staphylococcus aureus* resistant to methicillin (or nafcillin or oxacillin if they are used instead of methicillin for testing)
3. *Pneumococcus* resistant to penicillin
4. *Haemophilus influenzae* resistant to ampicillin (beta-lactamase positive) and chloramphenicol
5. Other resistant bacteria may be included in this isolation category if they are judged by the infection control team to be of special clinical and epidemiologic significance.

Pediculosis

Pharyngitis, infectious, infants and young children

Pneumonia, viral, in infants and young children

Pneumonia, *Staphylococcus aureus* or group A *Streptococcus*

Rabies

Rubella, congenital and other

Scabies

Scalded skin syndrome (Ritter's disease)

Skin, wound, or burn infection, major (draining and not covered by a dressing or dressing does not adequately contain the purulent material), including those infected with *Staphylococcus aureus* or group A *Streptococcus*

Vaccinia (generalized and progressive eczema vaccinatum)

* A private room is indicated for contact isolation; in general, however, patients infected with the same organism may share a room. During outbreaks, infants and young children with the same respiratory clinical syndrome may share a room.

Diseases requiring drainage/secretion precautions*

Infectious diseases included in this category are those that result in production of purulent material, drainage, or secretions, unless the disease is included in another isolation category that requires more rigorous precautions. (If you have questions about a specific disease, see the listing of infectious diseases in Guideline for Isolation Precautions in Hospitals, Table A, Disease-Specific Isolation Precautions.)

The following infections are examples of those included in this category provided they are *not* a) caused by multiply-resistant microorganisms, b) major (draining and not covered by a dressing or dressing does not adequately contain the drainage) skin, wound, or burn infections, including those caused by *Staphylococcus aureus* or group A *Streptococcus,* or c) gonococcal eye infections in newborns. See Contact Isolation if the infection is one of these three.

Abscess, minor or limited

Burn infection, minor or limited

Conjunctivitis

Decubitus ulcer, infected, minor or limited

Skin infection, minor or limited

Wound infection, minor or limited

* A private room is usually indicated for drainage/secretion precautions.

Diseases requiring strict isolation*

Diphtheria, pharyngeal
Lassa fever and other viral hemorrhagic
  fevers, such as Marburg virus disease†

Plague, pneumonic
Smallpox†
Varicella (chickenpox)
Zoster, localized in immunocompromised
  patient, or disseminated

* A private room is indicated for strict isolation; in general, however, patients infected with the same organism may share a room (CDC Guidelines).
† A private room with special ventilation is indicated.

IMPLEMENTATION PHASE

NURSING ACTIONS	RATIONALE/AMPLIFICATION
1. Place Centers for Disease Control (CDC) isolation/precautions card on client's door.	If drainage/secretion precautions are being implemented and a private room is not available, place the sign in a conspicuous place beside the client's bed.
2. Label outside of client's record "Isolation/precautions" or place duplicate copy of CDC sign on front of chart.	Labeling alerts personnel to specific precautions.
3. Label all interdepartmental communication (*e.g.,* laboratory or x-ray film requests) "Isolation/precautions.	Labeling alerts other departments to the specific precautions required.
4. Follow specifications on front of CDC card (see lists of isolation/precautions protocols).	

EVALUATION PHASE

ANTICIPATED OUTCOME	NURSING ACTION
Prevention of cross-infection with multiresistant bacteria or transmissible diseases	Monitor compliance with the CDC requirements for the particular category of isolation.

Contact isolation

VISITORS—REPORT TO NURSES' STATION BEFORE ENTERING ROOM

1. Masks are indicated for those who come close to patient.
2. Gowns are indicated if soiling is likely.
3. Gloves are indicated for touching infective material.
4. HANDS MUST BE WASHED AFTER TOUCHING THE PATIENT OR POTEN-TIALLY CONTAMINATED ARTICLES AND BEFORE TAKING CARE OF ANOTHER PATIENT.
5. Articles contaminated with infective material should be discarded or bagged and labeled before being sent for decontamination and reprocessing.

Strict isolation

VISITORS—REPORT TO NURSES' STATION BEFORE ENTERING ROOM

1. Masks are indicated for all persons entering room.
2. Gowns are indicated for all persons entering room.
3. Gloves are indicated for all persons entering room.
4. HANDS MUST BE WSHED AFTER TOUCH-ING THE PATIENT OR POTENTIALLY CONTAMINATED ARTICLES AND BEFORE TAKING CARE OF ANOTHER PATIENT.
5. Articles contaminated with infective material should be discarded or bagged and labeled before being sent for decontamination and reprocessing.

Drainage/secretion precautions

VISITORS—REPORT TO NURSES' STATION BEFORE ENTERING ROOM

1. Masks are not indicated.
2. Gowns are indicated if soiling is likely.
3. Gloves are indicated for touching infective material.
4. HANDS MUST BE WASHED AFTER TOUCHING THE PATIENT OR POTENTIALLY CONTAMINATED ARTICLES AND BEFORE TAKING CARE OF ANOTHER PATIENT.
5. Articles contaminated with infective material should be discarded or bagged and labeled before being sent for decontamination and reprocessing.

SELECTED REFERENCES

Garner JS, Simmons BP: CDC guidelines for the prevention and control of nosocomial infections: Guidelines for isolation precautions in hospitals. Am Infect Control 12(2):103–166, April 1984

34

Bedside blood glucose monitoring

BACKGROUND

The rapid assessment of blood glucose is often important in clients in critical care units. The technique may be used to determine blood glucose in a comatose person admitted to the emergency room or to titrate an insulin drip.

In fasting clients, venous, capillary, or arterial blood glucose concentrations are essentially identical. The concentrations are higher in capillary blood after ingestion of glucose. The use of reagent strips to test blood glucose should not replace laboratory determinations, but should be used to guide therapy until these tests are available. Blood is obtained by a fingerstick and is placed on a reagent strip. The strip may be read against a color chart or placed in a glucose meter for interpretation. Because equipment and reagent strips from each manufacturer are different, it is important to use the correct color chart and glucose meter.

Home blood glucose monitoring (HBGM) is used by selected diabetics at home as a substitute for, or supplement to, urine testing. It is particularly useful for clients who have an altered renal threshold for glucose, when urine testing would not provide accurate results, and for clients using an insulin pump.

Blood glucose determination

Objective
To obtain rapid assessment of blood glucose

ASSESSMENT PHASE

• Is bedside assessment of blood glucose appropriate for this client (*e.g.,* diabetic coma with insulin drip, coma of unknown origin)?

PRECAUTIONS

• **Timing and rinsing techniques must be precise to avoid inaccurate results.**

PLANNING PHASE

EQUIPMENT

Reagent test strips
Cotton balls
Paper towel (if applicable)
Wash bottle (if applicable)
Stopwatch
Color chart or glucose meter and calibration equipment

CLIENT/FAMILY TEACHING

• If the client's condition permits, explain the reason for monitoring blood glucose
• Tell the client that a fingerstick will be required to obtain a blood sample.
• If the client will be discharged using HBGM, begin teaching the technique to the family or client. If the client's condition permits, a family member may begin performing the test under supervision.

IMPLEMENTATION PHASE

NURSING ACTIONS	RATIONALE/AMPLIFICATION
1. Warm up and calibrate glucose meter (if used).	Follow the manufacturer's instructions. Warm-up and calibration are not required by Glucoscan.
2. Remove reagent strip from bottle and immediately replace cap and tighten.	Note the date on the bottle when opening a new bottle of reagent strips. Discard bottles after 4 months. Do not store in bright light (*e.g.,* window sill).
3. Compare unreacted reagent area of strip with zero block on color chart.	If the reagent area is discolored, discard the strip and use another one.
4. Clean puncture area thoroughly.	See Fingerstick in following section.
5. After performing puncture, allow drop of blood to form and wipe it away with clean, dry cotton ball.	
6. Allow second drop of blood to form.	Avoid excessive manipulation of the puncture site to obtain blood. Perform a second fingerstick if the blood is not free flowing.
7. Apply large drop of blood sufficient to cover entire reagent area of strip.	Keep the surface level to avoid spilling the drop of blood. Always use a large drop of blood. If a small drop is spread over the entire reagent area to give a thin film, color development will be paler than with a large drop, and lower results will be obtained. Also, using a thin layer causes a tendency to overwash the strip, which results in low readings.
8. Immediately begin timing for 60 seconds (Dextrostix or Chemstrip bG).	Follow the specific instructions for the product in use.
9. Prepare reagent strip for comparison with color chart or interpretation with glucose meter.	Follow the specific instructions for the product in use.
Dextrostix	
a. Immediately wash reagent area for 2 seconds with sharp, constant stream of water using wash bottle.	Direct the stream of water across the entire reagent area. It is not necessary to remove every trace of blood from around the edges of the strip. Rinsing under the tap results in overwashing and false low results.
b. Immediately compare with color chart on package.	The range should be from 0 to 250 mg/dl. Do not compare strips from one bottle with the color chart on another.
c. Blot on clean paper towel and insert into prepared Dextrometer.	The result is displayed on a digital readout. The range should be from 0 to 399 mg/dl.
Chemstrip bG	
a. Wipe blood from reagent strip with cotton ball.	
b. Time for additional 60 seconds.	
c. Compare with color chart on package.	The range should be from 20 mg to 800 mg/dl.
10. Interpolate results that fall between two color blocks on color chart.	
11. Record results on diabetic flow sheet.	

RELATED NURSING CARE

NURSING ACTIONS	RATIONALE/AMPLIFICATION
Correlate results of bedside determinations of blood glucose with client's clinical condition and blood glucose tests performed in laboratory.	If the results do not reflect the client's clinical condition, obtain a stat blood glucose.

EVALUATION PHASE

ANTICIPATED OUTCOMES	NURSING ACTIONS
Accurate assessment of blood glucose	Follow specific product instructions to avoid inaccurate results. Monitor for hypoglycemia or hyperglycemia. Normal fasting specimens will show color development that is greater than the 45 mg/dl color block. After a high-carbohydrate meal or measured challenge, normal results are generally below 130 mg/dl after 2 hours. Monitor serial bedside glucose determinations and titrate therapy as ordered.

PRODUCT AVAILABILITY

GLUCOSE METERS

(Biodynamics Stat Tek meter
Lifescan Glucoscan System
Ames Dextrometer Reflectance Colorimeter

REAGENT TEST STRIPS

Ames Dextrostix
Biodynamics Chemstrip bG

SELECTED REFERENCES

Plasse NJ: Monitoring blood glucose at home: A comparison of three products. Am J Nurs 81(11):2028–2029, November 1981

Stevens AD: Monitoring blood glucose at home: Who should do it. Am J Nurs 81(11):2026–2027, November 1981

Fingerstick

BACKGROUND

Two methods are available for obtaining capillary blood for blood glucose determinations. A spring-loaded device called an Autolet can be used, or blood can be obtained manually by performing a fingerstick with a lancet. The Autolet is ideal for clients on HBGM, but it is also effective for use by staff for obtaining frequent blood samples.

Objective
To produce regular capillary blood samples to monitor blood glucose

ASSESSMENT PHASE

• Does the client require bedside monitoring of the blood glucose, or would laboratory determinations be more appropriate? Bedside monitoring will be helpful in titrating an insulin drip or for obtaining an estimate of the blood glucose in the comatose client.
• Will the client be discharged on HBGM? Early client/family teaching will be necessary.

PRECAUTIONS

• **Use a new lancet for each fingerstick to prevent the risk of infection.**
• **Use soap and water to prepare the skin rather than alcohol if samples are to be taken over an extended period. Punctures made through wet alcohol**

can increase peripheral neuropathies, and alcohol tends to toughen the skin.

PLANNING PHASE

EQUIPMENT

Autolet
Platforms
Autolet lancets
Fingerstick lancets (if Autolet is not used)
Alcohol swabs or soap and water
Cotton swabs
Sterile vaseline (optional)

CLIENT/FAMILY TEACHING

• Explain to the client and family the reasons for frequent fingersticks to obtain blood.
• Begin predischarge teaching if the client is to be discharged on HBGM.
• Supervise the client in performing fingersticks when his condition allows.

IMPLEMENTATION PHASE

NURSING ACTIONS	RATIONALE/AMPLIFICATION

AUTOLET

1. Take platform runner from box and twist off platform and insert into slot ensuring that recessed side of platform is facing downwards (Fig. 34–1 *a* and *b*).

Two platforms are available, allowing different depths of penetration. The yellow or standard puncture platform allows tissue penetration to a maximum depth of 2.4 mm (Fig. 34–1, *inset*). The orange or superpuncture platform allows deeper penetration to a maximum depth of 3 mm. Use the orange platform if sufficient blood flow cannot be obtained with the yellow platform.

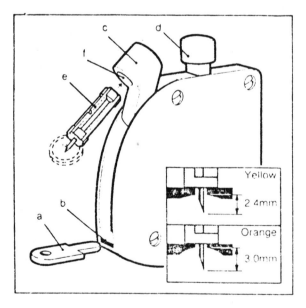

Fig. 34–1 Autolet components. (Courtesy Ames Division, Miles Laboratories, Inc., Elkhart, IN)

2. Pull arm back toward activating button until it clicks into position (Fig. 34–1 *c* and *d*).

3. Insert lancet into sprung socket in arm and push firmly into position. Take up any slackness in seating by rotating lancet by approximately one quarter turn (Fig. 34–1 *e* and *f*).

Use a new lancet for each operation in which the Autolet is used by one client only. Use a new lancet and platform to prevent cross-infection for multiple users.

4. Remove plastic disk from end of lancet by twisting it off and exposing needle.

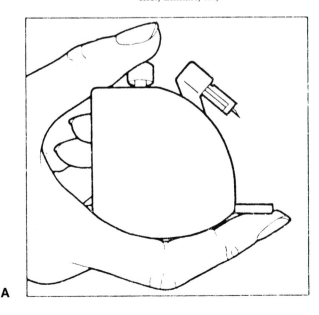

Fig. 34–2 Puncture sites for obtaining capillary blood. (Courtesy Ames Division, Miles Laboratories, Inc., Elkhart, IN)

5. Select puncture site (Fig. 34–2).

6. Clean and dry puncture site with warm water and soap or clean with alcohol swab.

7. Ensure good blood supply to site by gentle manipulation.

8. Apply thin layer of sterile vaseline to site (optional).

9. Place recessed surface of platform against site so that tissue protrudes into hole in center of platform.

10. Apply slight pressure to activating button (see Fig. 34–1*d*), allowing lancet to puncture skin and retract clearly (Fig. 34–3).

The earlobe is used exclusively in some countries on the grounds that it is less painful than the fingers.

Warm water promotes peripheral dilation and easier blood flow.

Sterile vaseline enhances blood-drop formation and facilitates collection.

Fig. 34–3 Self-use of Autolet. (*A*) Applying pressure to activating button. (*B*) Alternatively, pressure can be applied to activating button by pressing on hard surface. (Courtesy Ames Division, Miles Laboratories, Inc., Elkhart, IN)

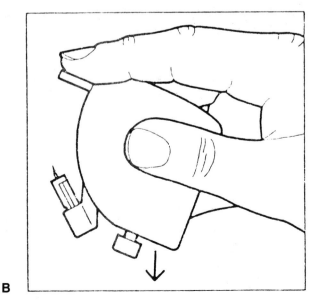

A   B

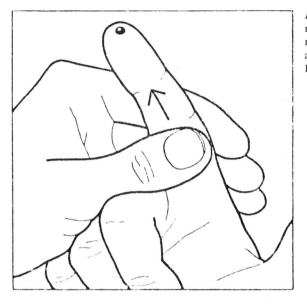

Fig. 34–4 Blood flow is increased by manipulating tissue toward puncture site. Direct manipulation at puncture site should be avoided. (Courtesy Ames Division, Miles Laboratories, Inc., Elkhart, IN)

11. Wait few seconds to allow blood to begin to flow by opening up small puncture.

Facilitate blood flow by manipulating the surrounding tissue toward the puncture site (Fig. 34–4). Do not squeeze directly at the puncture site because this may cause contamination of the sample with tissue fluid.

12. Wipe away first drop of blood with cotton ball and collect second drop.

Use the second drop to prevent contamination of the sample.

13. Apply drop to reagent strip and begin capillary glucose determination.

14. Clean and swab site to close wound. Hold pressure with cotton ball if necessary.

MANUAL FINGERSTICK

 1. Select puncture site (see Fig. 34–2).

 2. Prepare client's skin with alcohol swab or soap and water.

 3. Peel protective wrapper from lancet, keeping sharp point sterile.

 4. Support puncture site with one hand and instruct client that a stick will be felt.

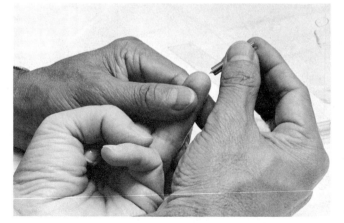

Fig. 34–5 Apply gentle pressure to distal joint of finger to ensure adequate blood supply to fingertip. Lancet guard prevents lancet from being inserted too deeply.

5. Holding lancet in opposite hand, quickly stick puncture site to depth of approximately 3 mm (Fig. 34-5).

6. Wait few seconds to allow blood to begin to flow.

Encourage blood flow by gentle manipulation of the surrounding tissue (*e.g.,* firm but gentle massage at the base of the fingers and thumb or stroking movements on the thumb in the direction of the puncture site). Do not squeeze directly at the puncture site because this may cause the sample to be contaminated with tissue fluid.

One large drop will be needed to perform the test.

7. Wipe first drop with cotton swab and collect second drop for glucose determination.

8. Apply large drop of blood sufficient to cover entire reagent area of test strip.

9. Perform capillary blood glucose test.

10. Stop blood flow by holding pressure over wound with cotton ball.

11. Clean puncture site with alcohol or soap and water.

RELATED NURSING CARE

NURSING ACTIONS	RATIONALE/AMPLIFICATION
Rotate puncture sites to maintain skin integrity.	

EVALUATION PHASE

ANTICIPATED OUTCOME	NURSING ACTIONS
1. Production of capillary blood sample with minimal trauma to client	
2. Prevention of infection	Monitor puncture sites for signs of infection, such as redness, swelling, or pain. Use a new platform and lancet for multiple use of Autolets.

PRODUCT AVAILABILITY Ames Division, Miles Laboratories Inc. (Autolet)

SELECTED REFERENCES Stevens AD: Monitoring blood glucose at home: Who should do it. Am J Nurs 81(11):2026–2027, November 1981

35 *Organ harvesting*

BACKGROUND

Organ transplantations have, in recent years, gained national attention among health-care professionals and health-care consumers, specifically because of the number of successful transplants. Frequently, however, this attention is focused on the lack of available donor organs that are needed by persons who are awaiting transplantation. Factors that contribute to the success of transplantations are early recognition of potential donors, prompt initiation of an effective referral and retrieval system, and advances made in surgical and medical therapeutics.

CURRENT STATUS OF ORGAN TRANSPLANTATIONS

More than 6900 renal transplants are performed yearly; of these, approximately 75% involve cadaver organ donations. Currently, the number of persons receiving hemodialysis is increasing by more than 6000 per year. The increase in the number of renal transplants is only 400 per year, and an estimated 12,000 persons who are dependent on hemodialysis are awaiting transplants. The success rate for renal transplants 1 year after transplantation varies from 55% to 95% among transplantation centers.

Cardiac disease is the leading cause of death in the United States; over 792,000 persons die yearly. Approximately 350 cardiac transplants are performed each year; of these, 7% are cardiopulmonary transplants. Without cardiac transplants, life expectancy for persons with end-stage cardiac disease is 1 month to 3 months. With cardiac transplants, cardiac-graft survival statistics currently approximate survival statistics for renal transplants, with some transplantation centers reporting an 80% survival rate 1 year after transplant (see Chap. 12, "Heart Transplantation").

As with end-stage cardiac disease, the only alternative to transplantation in end-stage liver disease is death. With increasing public awareness, a fourfold increase in the number of donor livers has enabled approximately 500 liver transplants to be performed per year. Liver-graft survival 1 year after transplantation is approximately 70%. The primary population that has benefited most from advances made in liver transplantations comprises children who suffer from congenital biliary anomalies.

Pancreatic transplants, first performed in 1966, have not achieved the success rates of other solid organ transplants, mainly because of infection and rejection of the graft. With the advent of improved immunosuppressive therapy, current investigative methodologies for pancreatic transplantation include composite organ grafts (whole pancreas, spleen, and duodenal segment) or segmental transplants with occlusion of the pancreatic duct. There is, at present, inconclusive data about which method has the most success.

Another group awaiting donor organ transplants are the 20,000 persons who need corneal transplants. An estimated 30,000 persons who are potential organ donors die yearly. Of these, only approximately 15% donate organs. Recent legislation (Public Law 98-507) has been passed to strengthen coordination of referrals, promote public awareness, and examine medicolegal and ethical issues. In addition, a ban on the buying and selling of donor organs is a feature of the current legislation. Some states (*e.g.,* Oregon and New York), in an effort to increase public awareness, have passed legislation requiring hospital officials to ask families of patients who die whether they wish to donote the deceased person's organs for transplant purposes.

REFERRAL AND RETRIEVAL

Currently, two referral and retrieval communication systems developed by the North American Transplant Coordinators Organization (NATCO) are in use. The first is a national telephone network (1-800-24-DONOR) that directs health-care professionals to the nearest organ retrieval center 24 hours per day, 7 days per week. The second is 24-ALERT, a network made up of recorded, updated telephone communications that provide listings of needed extrarenal organ donors. Access to 24-ALERT is available through any of the 18 participating transplantation centers. The service operates 24 hours per day, giving details of donor requirements, including organs needed, blood type, age, geographic recovery area, and 24-hour referral number.

CRITERIA FOR BRAIN DEATH

Organ donors must be pronounced brain dead, yet must have intact cardiopulmonary functioning (which may be artificially maintained) to minimize ischemia of donor organs. Brain death is defined as the irreversible cessation of function of brain structures, including the cerebrum, cerebellum, and main stem to spinal segment C1. Donor exceptions to the continuous need for perfusion and oxygenation are corneal, skin, and bone donors, all of which can be harvested after brain death and the cessation of cardiopulmonary functioning.

The following criteria serve as guidelines in determining brain death:

Deep coma with irreversible etiology in the absence of induced hypothermia or pharmacologically induced central nervous system depression

Absence of spontaneous movements

Absence of response to deep painful stimuli, including no decerebrate or decorticate posturing

Apnea with the absence of spontaneous respiration in 3 minutes without respiratory support, in the presence of a normal $PaCO_2$ level, and in the absence of pharmacologically induced respiratory-muscle paralysis

Absence of cranial nerve reflexes, including fixed and dilated pupils, and absence of corneal, oculocephalic, oculovestibular, and gag and swallowing reflexes

Electrocerebral silence as documented by an electroencephalogram (EEG) tracing recorded for no less than 30 minutes, in part at full gain

Cessation of cerebral circulation as documented by cerebral flow studies, which should be performed if there is a possibility of pharmacologic effect or uncertainty regarding the nature of the pathology of the intracranial lesion

Spinal reflexes, which may be present in the event of complete brain death, are of no diagnostic value in determining brain death.

General protocol for organ harvesting

Objectives

To provide early recognition of potential organ donors

To initiate prompt, effective referral and retrieval systems in persons with irreversible cessation of cerebral function

ASSESSMENT PHASE

- Has the donor been pronounced brain dead by the attending physician? Documentation of the date and time of death is made in the donor's chart.
- Is the donor normotensive and maintained on adequate life supports? Perfusion and oxygenation of vital organs must be maintained to prevent ischemia.
- Does the family have a support system available to aid them in making the decision to donate organs and to cope with the loved one's death? Notify the hospital chaplain, the family's pastor, the psychiatric liaison nurse, the transplant coordinator nurse, or other family members to provide support as needed.
- Has written consent for organ donation been obtained from the next of kin? In the case of multiple organ donations, list each organ to be donated on the consent form.

- Has a written consent for operation been obtained from the next of kin? Combining these written consents may or may not be acceptable. Consult hospital policy. Written consents may not be obtained until the donor is pronounced dead.
- Has verbal consent been obtained from the county coroner or medical examiner's office? Consent must be given before the surgical removal of organs and is documented in the donor's chart. Include the official's name and the time that permission was granted.
- Has the organ recovery center been notified? The recovery center will provide consultation on specific problems related to the maintenance and retrieval of the organs.
- Have temporary operating room privileges been granted by the hospital administration representative for the visiting retrieval-team surgeons?
- Have transportation arrangements been made for the retrieval team both to and from the airport and hospital?

IMPLEMENTATION PHASE

NURSING ACTIONS	RATIONALE/AMPLIFICATION

PREOPERATIVE PHASE

1. Maintain donor's organ viability by restoration and maintenance of organ perfusion and oxygenation.

Satisfactory cardiopulmonary status is imperative to ensure organ viability.

2. Restore and maintain blood pressure to 100 mm Hg systolic or greater.

Organ perfusion is adequate with a systolic blood pressure of 100 mm Hg.

3. If blood pressure is less than 100 mm Hg, infuse Ringer's lactate or normal saline 5 ml/kg over 10 minutes; repeat as needed until blood pressure is greater than or equal to 100 mm Hg and central venous pressure (CVP) is 10 cm to 20 cm water pressure (cm H_2O).

4. Maintain blood pressure at or above 100 mm Hg, infusing 1 milliliter Ringer's lactate per ml urine output, plus 50 ml/hour for adults to account for insensible loss.

For children (<33 kg [75 lbs]), infuse the amount of hourly urine output plus 20 ml/hour to account for insensible loss.)

5. Infuse volume expanders as ordered (*i.e.,* dextran, Plasmanate, hetastarch, albumin).

Volume expanders aid in restoring circulatory dynamics through osmotic volume expansion.

6. For sustained hypotension (blood pressure <100 mm Hg), administer low-dosage dopamine (<10 mcg/kg/minute) and titrate to restore and maintain blood pressure at or above 100 mm Hg.

Low-dose administration of dopamine increases heart stroke volume and perfusion pressure, without causing vasoconstriction of the renal arteries.

7. Maintain adequate urinary output of 50 ml to 70 ml/hour.

Adequate urinary output is a reliable sign of organ perfusion.

8. For sustained low urinary output (<50 ml/hour) in presence of satisfactory rehydration, administer intravenous (IV) infusion of furosemide 100 mg or mannitol 12.5 g.

Diuretics stimulate diuresis through excretion of water, sodium, potassium, and chloride.

9. If urinary output is greater than 250 ml/hour, infuse 0.45 normal saline plus 15 mEq potassium chloride (KCL) per liter at rate to replace urine output plus 50 ml/hour.

After diuresis, the infusion of adequate amounts of IV solution plus electrolytes prevents hypovolemia and electrolyte imbalances. Measure the urine output each hour and add 50 ml to determine the amount to be infused for the following hour.

10. Monitor serum electrolytes every 4 hours.

This identifies electrolyte imbalances.

11. If serum potassium is less than 3.5 mEq, administer 10 mEq KCl/100 ml solution in IV piggyback infusion over 1 hour to 2 hours.

This identifies electrolyte imbalances. Administration of a bolus of potassium over a controlled period aids in the correction of hypokalemia. Administer the potassium solution using an IV pump to control the rate.

12. If urinary output is consistently greater than 200 ml/hour and has low specific gravity (1.000 to 1.005), administer Pitressin 50 units/500 ml IV infusion at 50 ml/hour. Titrate infusion to maintain urinary output of 100 ml to 200 ml/hour.

Diabetes insipidus may occur with brain death. Administration of an antidiuretic hormone (Pitressin) will control urinary output and prevent electrolyte imbalances and dehydration.

13. Maintain adequate oxygenation and normal acid–base balance. Normal ranges follow:

These allow for sufficient exchange of O_2 and CO_2 in the alveoli.

    a. 70 mm Hg to 100 mm Hg PaO_2

This ensures adequate O_2 availability for the tissues.

    b. O_2 saturation greater than or equal to 95%.

    c. pH within normal limits (7.35 to 7.45) Obtain arterial blood gases (ABGs) every 4 hours as needed.

This evaluates acid–base balance.

14. Monitor ventilator settings and regulate as needed to maintain oxygenation and acid–base balance.

Ventilator settings will vary depending on body size and ABG values. Guidelines for determining ventilator settings are

    a. Tidal volume of 10 ml to 20 ml/kg

    b. F_1O_2 of 40% to 100% as needed

    c. Respiration rate of 10 breaths to 20 breaths per minute

    d. Positive end expiratory pressure (PEEP) of 5 cm H_2O to 15 cm H_2O.

15. Auscultate breath sounds bilaterally every 4 hours and document presence and quality. Also document presence of adventitious sounds.

The presence of breath sounds bilaterally denotes ventilation bilaterally. Adventitious sounds may indicate pulmonary pathology or infection.

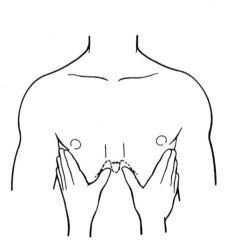

Fig. 35–1 Technique for assessing chest wall excursion. Place thumbs together over lower anterior chest during inspiration cycle of ventilator. Record number of centimeters between thumbs.

16. Assess and document chest wall excursion every 8 hours and as required (Fig. 35–1).

Asymmetrical chest wall excursion with a decrease in breath sounds unilaterally may indicate pneumothorax or misplacement of the endotracheal tube.

17. Obtain and assess chest film every 24 hours or as needed.

The chest film is useful in determining tube placement and the development of pneumonia, pneumothorax, or congestive heart failure.

18. Suction endotracheal tube and oropharynx every 2 hours and as necessary.

The removal of secretions is necessary for adequate diffusion of gases across the alveolar membrane, to prevent the multiplication of bacteria in pooled secretions and to prevent atelectasis.

19. Reposition client every 2 hours.

Frequent changes in position assist in preventing atelectasis and pooled secretions.

20. Administer broad-spectrum antibiotics as ordered.

Prophylactic administration of antibiotics guards against infection, specifically pneumonia, which would result in the rejection of the cadaver as a donor.

21. Assess for peripheral cyanosis (*i.e.,* circumoral, nailbeds) continuously.

Cyanosis is a late sign of hypoxia and requires immediate and aggressive action to prevent or decrease ischemia of vital organs.

22. Type and crossmatch 4 units to 6 units of packed red blood cells and keep on standby for operative procedure.

During multiple organ donation, blood loss is replaced to maintain the circulating blood volume and the perfusion of donor organs.

INTRAOPERATIVE PHASE

1. Prepare operating room for standard laparotomy with addition of following equipment:

Cadaver organ harvesting is performed using strict surgical asepsis.

  a. Vascular instruments and vascular suture

  b. Red-top blood tubes

Donor blood samples will be supplied to the retrieval team for use in tissue-matching procedures.

  c. Temperature probe, rectal or esophageal

  d. 50-ml syringes with 16- or 18-gauge needles —2

2. Prepare sterile area for organ maintenance.

This provides a separate area for the maintenance and preservation of donor organs.

  a. Large back table

  b. Table with sterile waterproof drape

  c. Sterile lap basin set, opened on waterproof drape

  d. Mosquito clamps—4 (2 straight, 2 curved)

  e. Vascular forceps—2 pairs

  f. Large hemostat

  g. Allis forcep

  h. Babcock forcep

  i. Metzenbaum scissors—small (blunt tip)

  j. Ringer's lactate—4 liters chilled (not frozen)

  k. Extra IV poles

  l. Bucket of unsterile ice

Equipment supplied by the retrieval team includes

  a. *In situ* flush tubing

  b. Cannulas/catheters

  c. Collin's or Euro–Collins' solution

Intracellular solution is used for flushing of all donor organs.

  d. Sterile plastic bags

  e. Ice chest for organ transport or organ perfusion machine

3. Prepare following medications for administration as ordered.

    a. Phentolamine mesylate (Regitine) 10 mg to 20 mg IV push

    b. Mannitol 12.5 g to 25 g IV infusion or furosemide 20 mg to 100 mg IV push

    c. Heparin 10,000 units to 20,000 units IV push (300 U/kg body weight)

    d. Methylprednisolone sodium succinate 250 mg to 1 g IV push

4. Document time that organ flushing commences.

5. Rapidly perfuse donor organs with 1 liter to 4 liters chilled Ringer's lactate (4°C) with added dextrose (30 ml/liter) and heparin (5000 U/liter).

6. Infuse intracellular-type solution (Collins' or Euro–Collins') as ordered (Fig. 35–2).

7. After removal of donor organs from cadaver, quickly cool external surface of organs by placing organs in splash basin filled with iced Ringer's lactate or chilled Collins' solution.

The medications will be given in rapid succession, therefore, prepare them in advance.

Phentolamine mesylate provides maximum vessel dilation before the cessation of donor organ circulation.

Mannitol or furosemide promotes active diuresis.

Heparin prevents coagulation of donor organ vessels.

Methylprednisolone reduces the possibility of rejection.

The surgeon will cool and perfuse donor organs by an *in situ* flush technique using cannula placement for the en bloc cadaver organ perfusion.

The surgeon will notify you about when to commence the perfusion of the donor organs. Rapid cooling to 25°C to 30°C core body temperature lowers metabolism and decreases ischemia. The appearance of the cooled organs should be pale.

Document the time that donor organs are placed into the splash basins.

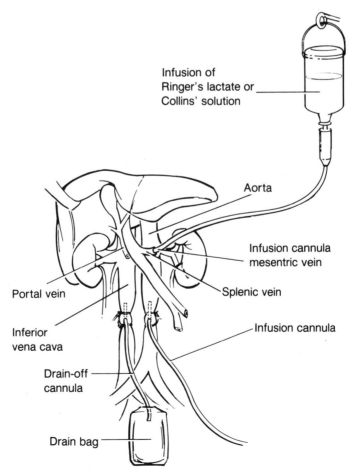

Fig. 35–2 *In situ* flush cannulation sites for multiple cadaveric organ retrieval.

Infusion of Ringer's lactate or Collins' solution

Aorta

Infusion cannula mesentric vein

Portal vein

Splenic vein

Inferior vena cava

Infusion cannula

Drain-off cannula

Drain bag

8. Package organs for transportation (refer to specific organ donor protocol in following sections for preferred packaging).

Proper packaging will aid in organ viability.

POSTOPERATIVE PHASE

1. Discontinue life-support systems when ordered by physician.

After the removal of the donor organs from the cadaver, artificial cardiopulmonary support is no longer necessary.

2. If cadaver is coroner's case, leave all IV catheters and tubes in place.

3. Administer postmortem care according to hospital policy.

4. Transport body to morgue.

EVALUATION PHASE

ANTICIPATED OUTCOMES	NURSING ACTIONS
Successful organ retrieval and maintenance	Upon completion of organ harvesting, the retrieval surgeon will document the condition of the organs removed and the evidence of any pathology.

Renal donor protocol

ASSESSMENT PHASE

- See Assessment Phase under General Protocol for Organ Harvesting in previous section
- Does the cadaver donor meet the following criteria for acceptability?
  Aged 2 years to 50 years
  No history of renal disease, diabetes mellitus, hypertension, or cancer (exceptions may be made for skin, lip, or central nervous system tumors)
  No bacteremia or diseases of viral or unknown causes
  Normotensive donor (BP $\geq$ 100 mm Hg systolic) with satisfactory urinary output (50 ml to 70 ml/hour)

IMPLEMENTATION PHASE

NURSING ACTIONS	RATIONALE/AMPLIFICATION

PREOPERATIVE PHASE

1. Obtain following diagnostic studies within 24 hours before procurement:

Diagnostic studies identify potential pathology that may exclude the use of the cadaver as an organ donor. Urine tests and creatinine levels should be within normal limits.

    a. Blood chemistry studies every 4 hours

    b. Serum creatinine and blood urea nitrogen (BUN)

    c. Urinalysis

    d. Urine cultures

Cultures, urinalysis, complete blood count (CBC), hepatitis-associated antigen (HAA), and serology identify the presence of infectious processes.

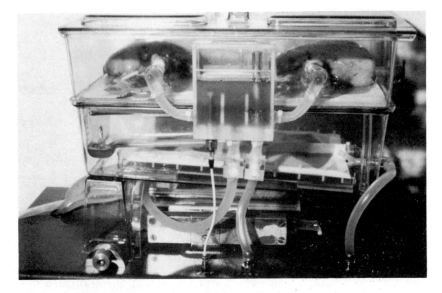

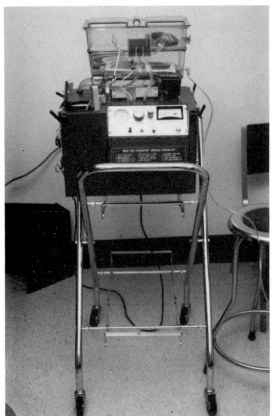

Fig. 35-3 Cold perfusion of kidneys. (Courtesy Southwest Organ Bank, Dallas, TX)

e. Blood cultures obtained from two separate sites

f. Chest film

g. ABO typing

h. HAA and serology

i. CBC every 12 hours   CBC assesses hydration status and O_2 carrying capacity.

j. ABGs every 4 hours and prn (when required)   ABGs assess respiratory status and acid–base balance.

2. See previous section on General Protocol for Organ Harvesting for guidelines on cadaver donor maintenance.

INTRAOPERATIVE PHASE

1. See previous section on General Protocol for Organ Harvesting for intraoperative actions, including *in situ* flushing.

2. Package kidneys for maintenance and preservation according to preferred technique.

    a. Continuous cold storage by ice immersion at 0°C. Package kidneys separately in sterile plastic bags that contain Collins' or Euro–Collins' solution. Then pack in ice in styrofoam or polyesterene ice chest.

    b. Continuous cold perfusion at 5°C to 10°C with iso-osmolar or hyperosmolar intracellular solutions (Collins' or Euro–Collins') (Fig. 35–3).

    c. Continuous cold storage by ice immersion at 0°C plus adjunct support of tissue respiration through persufflation of kidney by oxygen.

Current methods of kidney preservation allow 72 hours between procurement and transplantation.

Continuous cold storage reduces metabolism to minimal cell function and results in a renal core temperature of 0°C. This is the most commonly used storage technique.

The use of an organ perfusion machine provides reduced metabolism and the removal of end products.

Continuous bubbling of oxygen through the kidney by the renal vessels improves preservation and initial function of the revascularized kidney. The technique requires a portable oxygen tank, flowmeter, and oxygen-delivery tubing.

POSTOPERATIVE PHASE

See previous section on General Protocol for Organ Harvesting.

EVALUATION PHASE

ANTICIPATED OUTCOMES	NURSING ACTIONS
Successful retrieval and preservation of viable kidneys for transplantation	

Liver donor protocol

ASSESSMENT PHASE

- See Assessment Phase under General Protocol for Organ Harvesting in previous section.
- Does the cadaver donor meet the following criteria for acceptability?
  - Aged 2 months to 50 years
  - Donor liver size compatible with recipient's hepatic cavity
  - Donor ABO-type compatible with recipient ABO types. ABO-mismatched livers are used in emergency situations.
  - Normotensive donor (BP ≥ 100 mm Hg systolic)
  - Acceptable donor liver function as determined by the following laboratory values within normal limits: liver enzymes; bilirubin, total and direct; albumin; prothrombin; fibrinogen; urobilinogen, and ammonia
  - No history of acute infectious processes or malignancies (except for primary brain tumor)

IMPLEMENTATION PHASE

NURSING ACTIONS	RATIONALE/AMPLIFICATION

PREOPERATIVE PHASE

1. Obtain following diagnostic studies within last 24 hours before procurement:

These diagnostic studies assess donor liver function and identify potential pathology that may exclude the use of the cadaver as an organ donor. Liver function tests should be within normal limits. CBC, urinalysis, cultures, HAA, and serology identify the presence of infectious processes.

    a. CBC every 12 hours

    b. Prothrombin time, partial thromboplastin time

    c. Serum glutamic-oxaloacetic transaminase (SGOT), serum glutamic-pyruvic transaminase (SGPT)

    d. Alkaline phosphatase, lactate dehydrogenase (LDH)

    e. Ammonia, urobilinogen

    f. Total and direct bilirubin

    g. Serum albumin

    h. ABO typing

    i. ABGs every 4 hours and as required

    j. HAA and serololgy

    k. Urinalysis

    l. Blood cultures obtained from two separate sites

2. See previous section on General Protocol for Organ Harvesting for guidelines on cadaver donor maintenance.

INTRAOPERATIVE PHASE

1. See previous section on General Protocol for Organ Harvesting for intraoperative actions, including *in situ* flushing.

Current methods of liver preservation allow a 6- to 10-hour lapse between donor procurement and recipient transplantation.

2. Prepare liver for maintenance and preservation by double-bagging in sterile plastic bags containing cold Collins' solution and pack in ice in styrofoam or polyesterene ice chest.

The technique of cold solution flush infusion and hypothermic storage is preferred over methods using continuous cold perfusion because endothelial cell disruption occurs after 8 hours of perfusion. The cause of cell disruption is due to uneven distribution of the perfusate.

POSTOPERATIVE PHASE

See previous section on General Protocol for Organ Harvesting.

EVALUATION PHASE

ANTICIPATED OUTCOME	NURSING ACTIONS
Successful retrieval and preservation of viable liver for transplantation	

Pancreas donor protocol

ASSESSMENT PHASE
- See Assessment Phase in previous section on General Protocol for Organ Harvesting.
- Does the donor meet the following criteria for acceptability?
  Aged 3 months to 55 years
  Donor ABO type is compatible with recipient ABO type
  Normotensive donor (blood pressure ≥ 100 mm Hg systolic)
  No history of diabetes mellitus, pancreatitis, malignant neoplasms (except primary brain tumor), hypertension, infection, transmissible diseases, or abdominal injuries or surgery that may have damaged the pancreas
- Does the donor meet the criteria for research purposes? Any donor pancreas will be accepted for research.

IMPLEMENTATION PHASE

NURSING ACTIONS	RATIONALE/AMPLIFICATION

PREOPERATIVE PHASE

1. Obtain following diagnostic studies within 24 hours before procurement:

These diagnostic studies assess donor pancreatic function and identify pathology that may exclude the use of the cadaver as an organ donor. Pancreatic function should be within normal limits. CBC, HAA, serology, cultures, and urinalysis identify the presence of infectious processes.

  a. Serum glucose

  b. Serum amylase

  c. BUN

  d. CBC every 12 hours

  e. ABO typing

  f. ABGs every 4 hours and prn

  g. HAA and serology

  h. Urinalysis

  i. Blood cultures obtained from two separate sites

2. See previous section on General Protocol for Organ Harvesting for guidelines on cadaver donor maintenance.

INTRAOPERATIVE PHASE

1. See previous section on General Protocol for Organ Harvesting for intraoperative actions, including *in situ* flushing.

2. Package pancreas for maintenance and preservation by placing composite graft in cold bath of Collins' solution.

The pancreas, spleen, and duodenum are removed jointly as a composite organ graft. Preservation times are limited to 2 hours to 3 hours before revascularization by transplantation.

POSTOPERATIVE PHASE

See previous section on General Protocol for Organ Harvesting.

EVALUATION PHASE

ANTICIPATED OUTCOMES	NURSING ACTIONS
1. Successful retrieval and preservation of viable pancreas or pancreatic tissues for transplantation	
2. Procurement of donor pancreas for purposes of research	

Corneal, skin, and bone donor protocol

ASSESSMENT PHASE

• Does the cadaver donor meet the following criteria for acceptability?
  Any age is acceptable.
  No history of corneal disease, communicable diseases (*e.g.,* hepatitis, syphilis), leukemia, malignant neoplasms, tuberculosis, or systemic infections
  Written consent obtained from next of kin

IMPLEMENTATION PHASE

NURSING ACTIONS	RATIONALE/AMPLIFICATION
CORNEAL DONOR	
1. Keep eyes of comatose donor closed and instill 2 drops normal saline every 2 hours.	This prevents drying and ulceration of the corneal tissues.
2. After death, close eyes and apply ice packs.	Application of cold will prevent pooling of fluids. Elevating the head of the bed is recommended for decreasing the potential fluid pooling.
3. Transport body to morgue and place in refrigerated vault as soon as possible after death.	Refrigeration slows metabolism, keeping the corneal tissue viable. The results of transplantation are improved when harvesting occurs within 6 hours postmortem.
4. Enucleation and removal of cornea is performed in morgue, usually by eye bank personnel.	After removal, the corneas are put into a sterile metal container and transported in an ice chest. Examination and preservation of the corneas will be done at an eye bank. Cultures will be obtained; corneas are irrigated with antibiotic solutions and then preserved using the tissue culture method. Refrigeration at 4°C is maintained.
SKIN DONOR	
1. Transport body to morgue.	Removal of the skin can be accomplished up to 18 hours postmortem because of the skin's low metabolic rate.
2. Scrub torso and legs with antiseptic solution (*e.g.,* iodophor, Hibiclens) and rinse. Shave area to be harvested.	Preparation of the area to be harvested will reduce the bacterial count of the tissue. Harvesting of the skin generally involves removal of the skin circumferentially from the torso and legs.
3. Split-thickness skin is removed by dermatome, usually by a skin bank technician.	
4. After removal of skin, place harvested skin in cool normal saline solution.	Saline solution maintains viability because it prevents drying. On arrival at the skin bank, the skin is placed in a cryopreservative medium (which may also contain an

antibiotic to decrease bacterial growth). The tissue is then rolled in fine-mesh gauze and packaged. Packaged skin is stored in liquid nitrogen at 196°C. Long-term preservation is achieved by this method.

BONE DONOR

1. Transport body to morgue.

Bone harvesting can be accomplished up to 16 hours postmortem.

2. Bone harvesting is performed by bone bank technicians.

The most commonly harvested bones are the iliac crest, femur, tibia, fibula, ribs, and joints. Preservation is accomplished by viable or nonviable methods.

a. The bone may be frozen after culturing and placed into a sterile container. Cryoprotectant may be used. The packaging process includes trimming the bone to the desired shape and size. Viable, frozen bone can be maintained up to 12 months.

b. The bone may be cleaned and dried and processed by ethylene oxide sterilization. The nonviable bone can be maintained up to 12 months, with resterilization at 6 months.

EVALUATION PHASE

ANTICIPATED OUTCOMES	NURSING ACTIONS
Successful retrieval and preservation of usable corneal, skin, and bone tissues for transplantation	

SELECTED REFERENCES

AORN Recommended Practices Subcommittee. Recommended practices: Storing, preserving, and maintaining skin, bone, cartilage, and blood vessel tissue. AORN, September 1984, pp 392–396

Cunningham SM: When a transplant team comes to your operating room. AORN, Januray 1984, pp 50–54

Rosenthal JT, Shaw BW, Hardesty RL, Griffith BP et al: Principles of multiple organ procurement from cadaver donors. Ann Surg, November 1983, pp 617–621

Skelley L: Organ donation process. Focus on Critical Care, August 1983, pp 44–46

Southwest Organ Bank. Cadaver Organ Recovery Manual, Dallas, Southwest Organ Bank, September 1984

INDEX

Numbers followed by an *f* indicate a figure; *t* following a page number indicates tabular material.